Property of:
Roger D. Freeman, M.D.
Neuropsychiatry Clinic, BCCH
rfreeman@cw.bc.ca

Gates and Rowan's
Nonepileptic Seizures
Third Edition

Gates and Rowan's
Nonepileptic Seizures

Third Edition

Edited by
Steven C. Schachter
W. Curt LaFrance, Jr.

CAMBRIDGE UNIVERSITY PRESS

CAMBRIDGE UNIVERSITY PRESS
Cambridge, New York, Melbourne, Madrid, Cape Town,
Singapore, São Paulo, Delhi

Cambridge University Press
The Edinburgh Building, Cambridge CB2 8RU, UK

Published in the United States of America by
Cambridge University Press, New York

www.cambridge.org
Information on this title: www.cambridge.org/9780521517638

First edition (1993) and second edition (2000) Published by Butterworth
Heinemann, © A. James Rowan and John Gates
Third edition Published by Cambridge University Press, © S. C. Schachter
and W. C. LaFrance, Jr. 2010

This publication is in copyright. Subject to statutory exception
and to the provisions of relevant collective licensing agreements,
no reproduction of any part may take place without the written
permission of Cambridge University Press.

This edition published 2010

Printed in the United Kingdom at the University Press, Cambridge

*A catalog record for this publication is available from the
British Library*

Library of Congress Cataloging in Publication data
Gates and Rowan's nonepileptic seizures. – 3rd ed. / edited by Steven C.
Schachter, W. Curt LaFrance Jr.
    p. ; cm.
Rev. ed. of: Non-epileptic seizures / edited by John R. Gates, A. James Rowan.
2nd ed. c2000.
Includes bibliographical references and index.
ISBN 978-0-521-51763-8 (hardback)
1. Convulsions.   2. Convulsions – Psychological aspects.
I. Gates, John R.   II. Schachter, Steven C.   III. LaFrance, W. Curt.
IV. Non-epileptic seizures.   V. Title: Nonepileptic seizures.
[DNLM: 1. Seizures – diagnosis.   2. Diagnosis, Differential.
3. Neurobehavioral Manifestations.   4. Seizures – physiopathology.
5. Seizures – therapy. WL 340 G259 2010]
RC394.C77N66   2010
616.8′45 – dc22   2009032957

ISBN 978-0-521-51763-8 Hardback

Cambridge University Press has no responsibility for the
persistence or accuracy of URLs for external or third-party
internet websites referred to in this publication, and does
not guarantee that any content on such websites is, or will
remain, accurate or appropriate.

All material contained within the DVD is protected by copyright and other
intellectual property laws. The customer acquires only the right to use the
DVD and does not acquire any other rights, express or implied, unless these
are stated explicitly in a separate licence.

To the extent permitted by applicable law, Cambridge University Press is not
liable for direct damages or loss of any kind resulting from the use of this
product or from errors or faults contained in it, and in every case Cambridge
University Press's liability shall be limited to the amount actually paid by the
customer for the product.

Every effort has been made in preparing this publication to
provide accurate and up-to-date information which is in accord with
accepted standards and practice at the time of publication. Although case
histories are drawn from actual cases, every effort has been made to disguise
the identities of the individuals involved. Nevertheless, the authors, editors,
and publishers can make no warranties that the information contained
herein is totally free from error, not least because clinical standards are
constantly changing through research and regulation. The authors, editors,
and publishers therefore disclaim all liability for direct or consequential
damages resulting from the use of material contained in this publication.
Readers are strongly advised to pay careful attention to information provided
by the manufacturer of any drugs or equipment that they plan to use.

Contents

List of contributors   *page* vii
Preface   xi
Dedications   xiii
Remembrances   xvii

Section 1: Recognition, diagnosis, and impact of nonepileptic seizures

1. **Epidemiology and classification of psychogenic nonepileptic seizures**   3
   Nathan M. Griffith and Jerzy P. Szaflarski

2. **Psychogenic nonepileptic seizures: historical overview**   17
   Michael Trimble

3. **The burden of psychogenic nonepileptic seizures (PNES) in context: PNES and medically unexplained symptoms**   27
   James C. Hamilton, Roy C. Martin, Jon Stone, and Courtney B. Worley

4. **Clinical features and the role of video-EEG monitoring**   38
   Selim R. Benbadis and W. Curt LaFrance, Jr.

5. **Comorbidity of epileptic and psychogenic nonepileptic seizures: diagnostic considerations**   51
   Peter Widdess-Walsh, Siddhartha Nadkarni, and Orrin Devinsky

6. **Nonepileptic paroxysmal neurological and cardiac events**   62
   Fergus J. Rugg-Gunn and Josemir W. Sander

7. **Parasomnias: epileptic/nonepileptic parasomnia interface**   77
   Roderick Duncan and Aline Russell

8. **The use of hypnosis and linguistic analysis to discriminate between patients with psychogenic nonepileptic seizures and patients with epilepsy**   82
   John J. Barry and Markus Reuber

9. **Diagnostic issues in children**   91
   Tobias Loddenkemper and Elaine Wyllie

10. **Diagnostic issues in the elderly**   110
    Christoph Kellinghaus and Gabriel Möddel

Section 2: Nonepileptic seizures: culture, cognition, and personality clusters

11. **Cultural aspects of psychogenic nonepileptic seizures**   121
    Alfonso Martínez-Taboas, Roberto Lewis-Fernández, Vedat Sar, and Arun Lata Agarwal

12. **Psychogenic nonepileptic seizures: why women?**   131
    Bettina Schmitz

13. **Use of neuropsychological and personality testing to identify adults with psychogenic nonepileptic seizures**   136
    Carl B. Dodrill

14. **Cognitive complaints and their relationship to neuropsychological function in adults with psychogenic nonepileptic seizures**   142
    George P. Prigatano and Kristin A. Kirlin

15. **Health Related Quality of Life: utility and limitation in patients with psychogenic nonepileptic seizures**   149
    Gemma Mercer, Roy C. Martin, and Markus Reuber

16 **Legal medicine considerations related to nonepileptic seizures** 157
Roy G. Beran, John A. Devereux, and W. Curt LaFrance, Jr.

Section 3: Psychiatric and neuropsychological considerations in children and adolescents with psychogenic nonepileptic seizures

17 **Psychiatric features and management of children with psychogenic nonepileptic seizures** 163
Rochelle Caplan and Sigita Plioplys

18 **Neuropsychological and psychological aspects of children presenting with psychogenic nonepileptic seizures** 179
Ann Hempel, Julia Doss, and Elizabeth Adams

19 **Adolescents' and parents' perceptions of psychogenic nonepileptic seizures** 187
Manjeet S. Bhatia and Ravi Gupta

20 **Munchausen syndrome** 190
Ghislaine Savard, Frederick Andermann, and Renée Fugère

Section 4: Psychiatric considerations in adults with psychogenic nonepileptic seizures

21 **Classification of nonepileptic seizures** 199
W. Curt LaFrance, Jr. and Mark Zimmerman

22 **Posttraumatic stress disorder, abuse, and trauma: relationships to psychogenic nonepileptic seizures** 213
Elizabeth S. Bowman

23 **Comorbidities in psychogenic nonepileptic seizures: depressive, anxiety, and personality disorders** 225
Adriana Fiszman and Andres M. Kanner

Section 5: Treatment considerations for psychogenic nonepileptic seizures

24 **Historical approaches to treatments for psychogenic nonepileptic seizures** 237
W. Curt LaFrance, Jr. and Steven C. Schachter

25 **Managing psychogenic nonepileptic seizures in patients with epilepsy** 247
Roderick Duncan and Meritxell Oto

26 **Models of care: the roles of nurses and social workers in the diagnosis and management of patients with psychogenic nonepileptic seizures** 253
Noreen C. Thompson and Patricia A. Gibson

27 **Who should treat psychogenic nonepileptic seizures?** 260
Andres M. Kanner

28 **Designing treatment plans based on etiology of psychogenic nonepileptic seizures** 266
W. Curt LaFrance, Jr. and Helge Bjørnæs

29 **Cognitive behavioral treatments** 281
Laura H. Goldstein, W. Curt LaFrance, Jr., Craig Chigwedere, John D. C. Mellers, and Trudie Chalder

30 **Group psychotherapy treatment for psychogenic nonepileptic seizures** 289
Kim D. Bullock

31 **Hypnosis in the treatment of psychogenic nonepileptic seizures** 297
Franny C. Moene and Jarl Kuyk

32 **Pharmacological treatments for psychogenic nonepileptic seizures** 307
W. Curt LaFrance, Jr. and Dietrich Blumer

33 **Family therapy for patients diagnosed with psychogenic nonepileptic seizures** 317
Richard C. Archambault and Christine E. Ryan

Appendix 327
Index 336

Contributors

Elizabeth Adams, PhD
Minnesota Epilepsy Group, P.A., St. Paul, MN, USA

Arun Lata Agarwal, MD
Assistant Professor, Department of Psychiatry, Maulana Azad Medical College and G.B. Pant Hospital, New Delhi, India

Frederick Andermann, OC, MD, FRCP(C)
Professor of Neurology and Pediatrics, Montreal Neurological Hospital and Institute, McGill University, Montreal, Canada

Richard C. Archambault, EdD
Clinical Assistant Professor, Department of Psychiatry and Human Behavior, Brown School Medical, Providence, RI, USA

Miya Asato, MD
Children's Hospital Pittsburgh, Pittsburgh, PA, USA

John J. Barry, MD
Professor of Psychiatry and Behavioral Sciences, Stanford University Medical Center, Stanford, CA, USA

Selim R. Benbadis, MD
Professor, Department of Neurology, Director, Comprehensive Epilepsy Program, University of South Florida & Tampa General Hospital, Tampa, FL, USA

Roy G. Beran, MB BS, FRACGP, FRACP, Grand Dip (Further Ed), Grad Dip (Text Ed), MD, FAKPHM, BLegS, FACLM, FRCP, FACBS, MHL, Accredited Sleep Physician, PFFLM(Hons)
Liverpool Hospital, Sydney, New South Wales, Australia

Manjeet S. Bhatia, MD
Professor and Head, Department of Psychiatry, University College of Medical Sciences and Guru Teg Bahadur Hospital, Dilshad Garden, Delhi, India

Helge Bjørnæs, PhD
The National Centre for Epilepsy Sandvika and Department of Neuropsychiatry and Psychosomatic Medicine, Division of Neuroscience, Oslo University Hospital, Oslo, Norway

Dietrich Blumer, MD
Professor of Psychiatry and Head of Neuropsychiatry, University of Tennessee, Memphis School of Medicine, Memphis, TN, USA

Elizabeth S. Bowman, MD
Consulting Psychiatrist, Indiana University Adult Epilepsy Clinic and Adjunct Professor of Neurology, Indiana University School of Medicine, Indianapolis, IN, USA

Kim D. Bullock, MD
Clinical Assistant Professor, Department of Psychiatry and Behavioral Sciences, Stanford University, Stanford, CA, USA

Rochelle Caplan, MD
Professor, Semel Institute for Neuroscience and Human Behavior, University of California, Los Angeles, CA, USA

Trudie Chalder, PhD, MSc
Professor of Cognitive Behavioural Psychotherapy, Institute of Psychiatry, King's College London, London, UK

Craig Chigwedere, BSc, MA, MSc
Cognitive Behavioural Psychotherapist/Clinical Lecturer in CBT, St Patrick's Hospital and Trinity College, Dublin, Republic of Ireland

John A. Devereux, BA, LLB, DPhil
Professor of Common Law, T.C. Beirne School of Law, University of Queensland, St. Lucia, Qld, Australia

List of contributors

Orrin Devinsky, MD
Professor of Neurology, Neurosurgery, and Psychiatry, Director, NYU Comprehensive Epilepsy Center and Director, Institute of Neurology and Neurosurgery at Saint Barnabas, NYU School of Medicine, New York, NY, USA

Carl B. Dodrill, PhD
Regional Epilepsy Center, Departments of Neurology and Neurological Surgery, University of Washington School of Medicine, Seattle, WA, USA

Julia Doss, PsyD
Minnesota Epilepsy Group, P.A., St. Paul, MN, USA

Roderick Duncan, MD, PhD, FRCP
Consultant Neurologist, Institute of Neurological Sciences, Southern General Hospital, Glasgow, UK

Adriana Fiszman, MD
Investigator and Attending Psychiatrist, Laboratory of Stress-Related Disorders, Institute of Psychiatry of the Federal University of Rio de Janeiro, Rio de Janeiro, Brazil

Renée Fugère, MD, FRCPC
Medical Director, National Mental Health Unit for Women (federal jurisdiction) and Assistant Professor, Department of Psychiatry, University of Montreal, Montreal, Canada

Patricia A. Gibson, MSSW
Associate Professor, Department of Neurology, Wake Forest University School of Medicine, Winston-Salem, NC, USA

Laura H. Goldstein, BSc, MPhil, PhD
Professor of Clinical Neuropsychology, Institute of Psychiatry, King's College London, London, UK

Nathan M. Griffith, PhD
Research Postdoctoral Fellow in Neuropsychology, UCLA Semel Institute for Neuroscience and Human Behavior, Los Angeles, CA, USA

Ravi Gupta
Assistant Professor, Department of Psychiatry, National Institute of Medical Sciences, Shoba Nagar, Delhi Road, Jaipur, Rajasthan, India

James C. Hamilton, PhD
Associate Professor of Psychology, Clinical Affiliate Associate Professor of Internal Medicine, University of Alabama, Tuscaloosa, AL, USA

Ann Hempel, PhD
Minnesota Epilepsy Group, P.A., and Adjunct Assistant Professor, Department of Neurology, University of Minnesota Medical School, Minneapolis, MN, USA

Andres M. Kanner, MD
Professor of Neurological Sciences and Psychiatry, Rush Medical College, Director, Laboratory of EEG and Video-EEG-Telemetry, and Associate Director, Section of Epilepsy and Rush Epilepsy Center, Rush University Medical Center, Chicago, IL, USA

Christoph Kellinghaus, MD
Staff Physician, Department of Neurology, Klinikum Osnabrück, Osnabrück, Germany

Kristin A. Kirlin, PhD
Section of Clinical Neuropsychology, Barrow Neurological Institute, St. Joseph's Hospital and Medical Center, Phoenix, AZ, USA

Jarl Kuyk, PhD
Department of Psychology, Epilepsy Institute of the Netherlands Foundation (SEIN), Heemstede, The Netherlands.

W. Curt LaFrance, Jr., MD, MPH
Director of Neuropsychiatry and Behavioral Neurology, Rhode Island Hospital, and Assistant Professor of Psychiatry and Neurology (Research), Brown Medical School, Providence, RI, USA

Roberto Lewis-Fernández, MD
Associate Professor, Department of Psychiatry, Columbia College of Physicians and Surgeons, and Director, NYS Center of Excellence for Cultural Competence and Hispanic Treatment Program, New York State Psychiatric Institute, New York, NY, USA

Tobias Loddenkemper, MD
Assistant Professor of Neurology, Harvard Medical School, Division of Epilepsy and Clinical Neurophysiology, Children's Hospital, Boston, MA, USA

List of contributors

Roy C. Martin, PhD
Associate Professor of Neurology, University of Alabama at Birmingham, AL, USA

Alfonso Martínez-Taboas, PhD
Associate Professor, Carlos Albizu University, Puerto Rico

Gemma Mercer, ClinPsyD, CPsychol
Clinical Neuropsychologist, Department of Clinical Neuropsychology, Salford Royal Hospital, Salford, Manchester, UK

John D. C. Mellers, MBBS, MRCPsych
Consultant Psychiatrist, Maudsley Hospital, London, UK

Gabriel Möddel, MD
Department of Neurology, University Clinics of Münster, Münster, Germany

Franny C. Moene, PhD
Clinical Psychologist/Psychotherapist, De Grote Rivieren, Organization for Mental Health, Dordrecht, The Netherlands

Siddhartha Nadkarni, MD
Assistant Professor of Neurology and Psychiatry, NYU School of Medicine, New York, NY, USA

Meritxell Oto, MRCPsych
Research Fellow, Regional Epilepsy Service, Institute of Neurology, Southern General Hospital, Glasgow, UK

Sigita Plioplys, MD
Children's Memorial Hospital, Chicago, IL, USA

George P. Prigatano, PhD
Newsome Chair of Clinical Neuropsychology, Barrow Neurological Institute, St. Joseph's Hospital and Medical Center, Phoenix, AZ, USA

Markus Reuber, MD, PhD, FRCP
Senior Clinical Lecturer in Neurology, University of Sheffield, Sheffield, UK

Anastasia Sullwold Ristau, PhD
Licensed Psychologist of Pediatric Psychology Services with the Integrative Medicine and Pain Programs of the Children's Hospitals and Clinics of Minnesota, Minneapolis, MN, USA

Fergus J. Rugg-Gunn, MBBS, MRCP, PhD
Consultant Neurologist, The National Hospital for Neurology and Neurosurgery, London, UK

Aline Russell, FRCP
Consultant Clinical Neurophysiologist, Department of Neurology Institute of Neurological Sciences, Southern General Hospital, Glasgow, UK

Christine E. Ryan, PhD
Director, Family Research Program, Assistant Director, Mood Disorders Program, Rhode Island Hospital, and Assistant Professor, Department of Psychiatry & Human Behavior, Brown Medical School, Providence, RI, USA

Jay Salpekar, MD
Children's National Medical Center, Washington, DC, USA

Josemir W. Sander MD, PhD, FRCP
Professor of Neurology, Honorary Consultant Neurologist, University College London, Institute of Neurology, London, UK

Vedat Sar, MD
Professor of Psychiatry, Director, Clinical Psychotherapy Unit and Dissociative Disorders Program, Department of Psychiatry, Istanbul University, Istanbul Faculty of Medicine, Istanbul, Turkey

Ghislaine Savard, MD, FRCP
Neuropsychiatrist, Associate Professor, Department of Neurology, Montreal Neurological Hospital and McGill University, Montreal, Canada

Steven C. Schachter, MD, FAAN
Professor of Neurology, Harvard Medical School, Chief Academic Officer and Director of NeuroTechnology, CIMIT and Department of Neurology, Beth Israel Deaconess Medical Center, Boston, MA, USA

Bettina Schmitz
Department of Neurology, Vivantes Humboldt Klinikum Berlin, Charité, Humboldt University, Berlin, Germany

Jon Stone, MB, ChB, FRCP, PhD
Consultant Neurologist and Honorary Senior Lecturer, Department of Clinical Neurosciences, Western General Hospital, Edinburgh, UK

List of contributors

Jerzy P. Szaflarski, MD, PhD, FAAN
Associate Professor, Departments of Neurology, Neuroscience and Psychiatry, Cincinnati Epilepsy Center, University of Cincinnati Academic Health Center, Cincinnati, OH, USA

Noreen C. Thompson, RN, MSN, PMHCNS-BC
Psychiatric Consultation Liaison Nurse, University of Kansas Hospital and Assistant Clinical Professor, University of Kansas School of Nursing, Kansas City, KS, USA

Michael Trimble, MD, FRCP, FRCPsych
Professor of Behavioural Neurology, Institute of Neurology, London, UK

Robert T. Wechsler, MD, PhD
Medical Director, Idaho Comprehensive Epilepsy Center, Boise, ID, USA

Peter Widdess-Walsh, MA, MB, MRCPI
Assistant Professor of Neurology (Research), NYU School of Medicine, Institute of Neurology and Neurosurgery at Saint Barnabas, Livingston, NJ, USA

Courtney B. Worley, MPH
Clinical Health Psychology, The University of Alabama, Tuscaloosa, AL, USA

Elaine Wyllie, MD
Professor of Pediatrics and Director, Center for Pediatric Neurology, Cleveland Clinic, Cleveland, OH, USA

Mark Zimmerman, MD
Director of Outpatient Psychiatry, Rhode Island Hospital and Associate Professor of Psychiatry, Brown Medical School, Providence, RI, USA

Preface

The first edition of *Non-Epileptic Seizures* was published in 1993 and edited by Drs. A. James Rowan and John R. Gates. Based on a 1990 symposium called "The Dilemma of Non-Epileptic (Pseudoepileptic) Seizures," this instant classic synthesized the available knowledge and hypotheses regarding all facets of nonepileptic seizures into four sections: neurological, psychiatric and neuropsychological aspects, and fundamentals of treatment. The second edition was published in 2000 and reflected the continued outgrowth of the 1993 symposium as well as a second conference – "Non-Epileptic Seizures: A Consensus Conference on Diagnosis and Treatment" – held in Bethesda in 1996.

A third conference, the 2005 Psychogenic Nonepileptic Seizures (PNES) Treatment Workshop, sponsored by the National Institute of Neurological Disorders and Stroke (NINDS), the National Institute of Mental Health (NIMH), and the American Epilepsy Society and chaired by W. Curt LaFrance, Jr., brought together experts from around the world, representing many disciplines. The enthusiasm emanating from that landmark meeting reverberated widely amongst professionals interested in the evaluation and treatment of persons with PNES. Sadly, the field soon afterwards lost its pioneers: John Gates on September 28, 2005 and Jim Rowan on August 27, 2006.

Recognizing the increasingly rapid developments since the second edition, the importance of *Non-Epileptic Seizures* as the embodiment of the field, and the singular contributions of Drs. Gates and Rowan, we endeavored to organize a new edition and to forever link the names of Gates and Rowan with this topic by their inclusion in the book title. It is therefore most fitting that this edition includes dedications from Rita Meyer Gates and Rita Rowan, with our gratitude, as well as personal remembrances of Drs. Gates and Rowan.

Historically, neurology and psychiatry were practiced as a unitary model, addressing patients with neurological and psychogenic disorders with equal attention. Unfortunately, as neurologic and psychiatric practices became dichotomized in the twentieth century, the topic of PNES fell between the borderlands of neurology and psychiatry.

Bridging neurology and psychiatry again, the primary aim of this edition is to educate physicians, psychologists, clinicians, allied health providers and researchers about the diagnosis and treatment of children and adults with nonepileptic seizures. Building on the groundwork laid in the first two editions, the editors and authors of this third edition provide a multidisciplinary approach to the neuropsychiatric disorder of psychogenic nonepileptic seizures. The authors are the foremost experts in their respective fields and provide an update on the current knowledge of nonepileptic seizures from the neurologic, neuropsychological, psychological, psychiatric, and social perspectives. The structure of the book sections allows an in depth appraisal of diagnostic semiology, clinical characteristics, issues in children, comorbidities, and, finally, a significant expansion of treatment for PNES. The addition of the DVD provides video samples of different seizure types and vignettes to aid clinicians with the differential diagnosis and treatment of nonepileptic seizures.

It is our hope that *Gates and Rowan's Nonepileptic Seizures*, 3rd edn. will honor the memories and legacies of its founding editors, and serve to reflect as well as influence the continued development of the field, informing clinicians and inspiring researchers to improve the care of persons with nonepileptic seizures today and in the future.

Steven C. Schachter and W. Curt LaFrance, Jr.

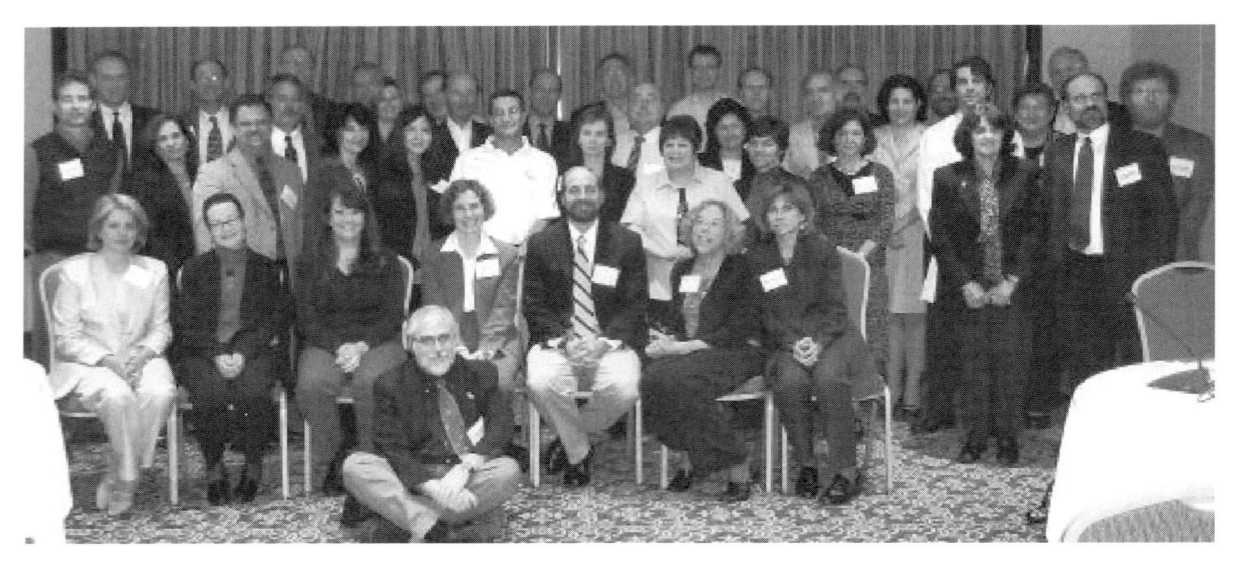

Participants, 2005 Psychogenic Nonepileptic Seizures Treatment Workshop, sponsored by National Institute of Neurological Disorders and Stroke, National Institute of Mental Health, and American Epilepsy Society.

Sitting: (left to right) Sigita Plioplys, Rochelle Caplan, Brenda Burch, Andy Kanner (floor), Joan Austin, Curt LaFrance, Margaret Jacobs, Debra Babcock
Row 2: Roy Martin, Claudia Moy, Roberto Lewis-Fernández, Daphne Simeon, Valerie Voon, Selim Benbadis, Elaine Wyllie, Donna Andrews, Patty Shafer, Linda Street, Phyllis Gilbert, Michael First
Row 3: Ken Alper, Mark Hallett, Mark Rusch, Lynn Rundhaugen, Michael Trimble, David Spiegel, John Gates, Laura Goldstein, Gabor Keitner, Cynthia Harden, Charles Zaroff, Helena Kraemer, Chris Sackellares
Row 4: Gregory Mahr, Peter Gilbert, Randall Stewart, Greer Murphy, Richard Brown, Jonathan Halford, Paul Desan, Steve Schachter, John Barry

Not pictured: John Campo, Orrin Devinsky, Frank Gilliam, Dalma Kalogjera-Sackellares, John Mellers, and Markus Reuber contributed significantly prior to the workshop but were unable to attend.

Dedication for Dr. A. James Rowan

On the Friday afternoon before his last admission to the hospital, Jim Rowan presided over his weekly pediatric epilepsy conference. He insisted on it. He dressed himself carefully though every small movement cost more energy than he had to spare – but this was his favorite conference of the week.

More effort and energy was expended getting him into a taxicab and then up to the EEG laboratory where the conference was held. It was well attended. Jim was clearly fatigued, yet, the moment he was given the first case the "old" Dr. Rowan was again in charge – no fatigue, no effort, just joy in his competence and knowledge, and yes, his love of it. He sat before the computer screen reading EEGs, and without any evident struggle, expounded as usual on case after case. It was a dazzling performance.

Epilepsy, understanding it, treating it, and teaching about it was the work to which Jim gave his life. That afternoon he gave his last share of energy to it. He would not have had it any other way. The pediatric conference, concerning epilepsy at the beginning of life, his geriatric research, concerning epilepsy at the end of life, and this work on nonepileptic seizures suggests the range of his interests and the depth of his dedication. It is fitting that the new edition continues to advance this very important work.

Rita Rowan

Dedication for Dr. John R. Gates

John was an intentional man who woke each morning with an explicit commitment to proffer his best in every circumstance, to everyone; who went to sleep each night weighing the day's successes and challenges, probing the "what and how" for an inspiration that might give rise to the next opportunity. What he took as a matter of course – expertise, indefatigable energy, imagination, and hustle – others found remarkable, and he devoted himself to patient care, research, writing, teaching, and organizational, volunteer, and committee work.

John was fascinated by the workings of the brain, and he believed that neurology, rather than psychiatry, held more potential for effective intervention. For this reason, as a young intern he chose to specialize in epilepsy so that he could make a difference. His wish and ambition to make that decisive difference in individual lives and in the field of epilepsy came to permeate his work, which in turn became his life. John's interests and efforts included advancing surgical techniques to improve surgical outcomes, pharmaceutical and device research, mentoring a broad range of students, physicians, and adjunct individuals, and membership in local, regional, and national organizations advancing quality assurance, professional practice, fiscal strength, and community resources.

His 25 years of work in the field of psychogenic nonepileptic seizures (PNES) were of a special order; he was determined to mitigate the primary and secondary causes of distress within this special population. The origin of his passion, the impetus that fueled his concern and commitment, was his mother's PNES. And it was his resolve to make a difference, coupled with his compassion and enthusiastic optimism, which compelled him in his work with PNES.

Based on John's vision of model collaboration, he organized and convened the initial interdisciplinary PNES consensus conferences in 1990 and 1993. These conferences were the milestones that set the stage for years of joint effort among epileptologists, psychiatrists, and neuropsychologists to ensure the best diagnostic and treatment parameters for PNES. This early work defined and continues to influence the multifactorial, multicultural, and multidisciplinary emphases in the treatments for these patients. He would have been particularly pleased that this new volume was edited by an epileptologist and a neuropsychiatrist.

John was unabashed in his esteem and admiration for his colleagues, his respect and regard for his patients, and his love for his family and friends. He was often generous, exuberant, and forgiving to a fault. His conviction of the inherent value and goodness of people gave meaning to his life and heartened those around him.

He set great store by his Jersey street-fighter roots, which he credited for his "backbone." He had the ability to stand his ground, often alone, under terrific pressures. Never one to uphold the status quo, he made 'thinking outside the box' his mantra long before it was part of popular culture. John was always keen to work out an impossible situation. But then a brain tumor appeared at the age of 53. This was a terrific blow. Though his commitment to his treatment was 100+%, there would be no recovery. He would not live long enough to appreciate the testimonials, honors, and awards that were bestowed to pay tribute to him; he would not be cognizant of the expressions of respect, appreciation, and love he had engendered during his life.

John would applaud publication of this third edition and then press for continuation of the work. With John, whether flying his plane, guiding boy scouts, fishing in the cold of a Minnesota winter, advocating for his special needs son, writing poetry, or absorbed in his work, it was always upwards and onwards.

May his life and dedication to patients with PNES continue to be an inspiration.

Rita Meyer Gates

In remembrance of Dr. A. James Rowan

Steven C. Schachter

Dear Jim,

You were one of my closest friends, and I miss you terribly. Your advice and genuine kindness and concern brought me through difficult times. Your fatherly pride in anything I accomplished made me try even harder to please you. You shouldered many burdens with grace, and shared a few of your own along the way, but you always kept your focus on the task at hand and on the well-being of others.

Everything important to you about the field of epilepsy became important to us, whether through your impassioned lectures, your impromptu conversations, or your writings. Your wisdom and perspectives will be passed on from us to those who follow. You had that penetrating way of looking at people in the audience, your glasses half down your nose. You wouldn't release your gaze until you were sure they understood the importance of what you were saying. Who can forget the essence of successful aging after seeing your that picture of Kin and Gin Narita, the Japanese twin sisters, joyously celebrating their 100th birthday?

The Veterans Affairs Cooperative Study was your baby. I served on the Data Safety Monitoring Board, which conducted periodic checkups during the study's gestation. I can still picture you pacing back and forth outside the door while the committee met, like an expectant parent. And I can also see you glowing when presenting the results of this landmark study.

You never knew it, but you were the inspiration behind the Epilepsy Foundation's Seniors and Seizures Initiative, and the Board of Directors wanted you to know the Foundation authorized half a million dollars for research in the area of epilepsy in the elderly, which should make you very proud.

We shared many wonderful times together, personal and professional. Sue and I will never forget when you and Rita flew our family to New York to have Christmas dinner with you.

Whenever I recommend one of your books to one of our fellows, I say "That book was written by a good friend of mine, Jim Rowan." And now, with a few of your favorite words and phrases, I add "He was a terrific physician, and a wonderful human being, as a matter of fact."

Farewell, Jim. Your memory will always remain with us. God rest your soul.

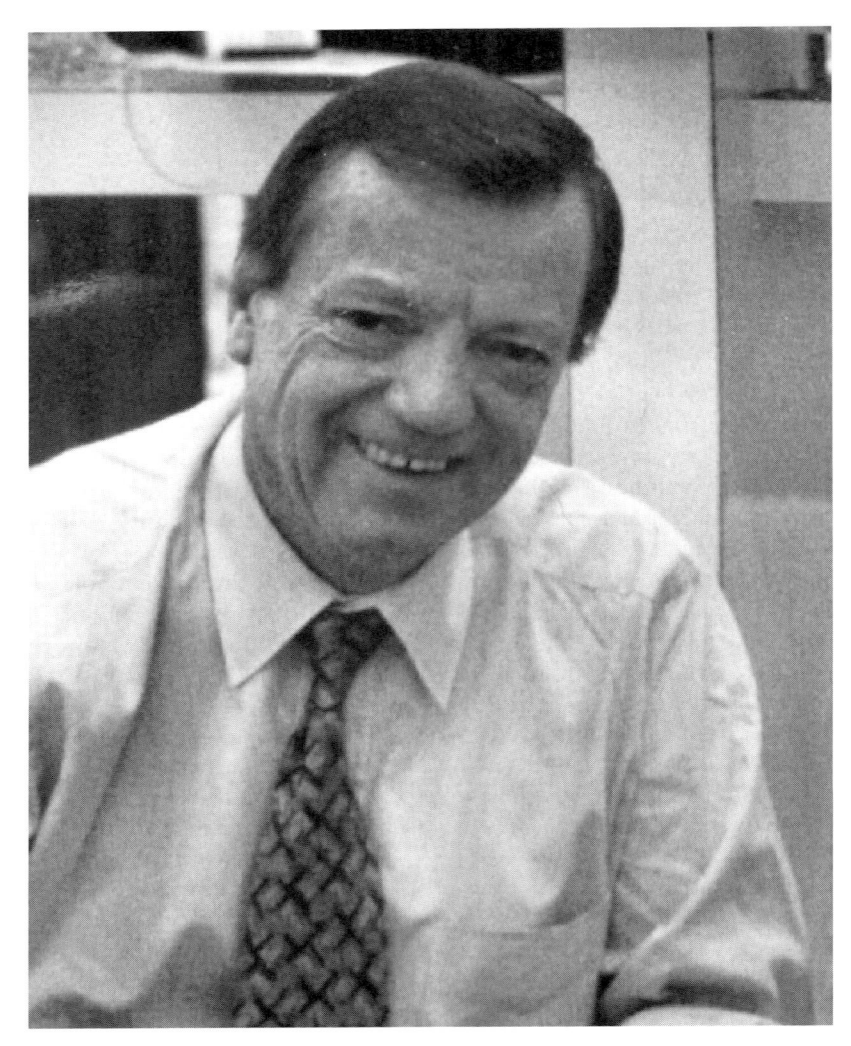

Dr. A. James Rowan

In remembrance of Dr. John R. Gates

Steven C. Schachter

John R. Gates, MD died September 28, 2005, at age 54 from a brain tumor. A moving memorial service was attended by over one thousand people, and centered around readings, poetry, and music – all artistic favorites of John's. He was survived by his beloved sweetheart and wife of 15 years, Rita; children, Jason, Rachel, and Stuart; and an extended family. Friends, family, patients, and colleagues around the world remember a wonderful man who made numerous and substantial contributions to the field of epilepsy and the practice of neurology. With contributions from many of those who were closest to John, I offer this appreciation.

A champion fighter from an early age

Born in the inner city of Trenton, New Jersey, John emerged from humble surroundings to graduate Magna Cum Laude from Harvard University. He was brought up by his grandparents. After both his grandparents passed away when he was 15 years old, a teacher who recognized his brilliance helped him get a scholarship for disadvantaged youth. He went on to attend elite schools in Massachusetts and England, where he excelled academically. I believe it was because of this unique background that he was able to challenge the establishment with confidence. Indeed, from his childhood until his untimely death, John "never gave up the fight." He was "an enthusiastic paladin for the wars against epilepsies, and more."

Standout trainee

At the University of Minnesota Medical School, John perfected his ability to question, challenge, and shake up the status quo. John was a 4th year medical student, rotating through neurology. At that time, Dr. A. B. Baker was the chairman of the Neurology Department, and a very demanding teacher and world class scholar with tremendous clinical experiences in neurology. It is very unusual to hear a neurology resident arguing with Dr. Baker, not to mention a 4th year medical student. But John did. He once said to Dr. Baker during a teaching round, "Dr. A. B. Baker, I don't think so. . . . " We all held our breath, and didn't know what to expect. I believe even Dr. Baker was caught by surprise as well. I can't recall the detail of the conversation then, but I remember he was able to present his view in a calm and logical manner, though I don't think he was able to win the case. His unique way of dealing with authority left me with an indelible impression.

His fellow residents and teachers witnessed the growth and development of a stellar and compassionate clinician who sought the truth, sometimes in unconventional ways. I happened to be the very first chief resident he had to work with. In the beginning, it was truly a disaster; he almost constantly argued with me in the diagnosis and clinical management of cases. Sometimes in front of the whole crew in the sign-out rounds in the evening, he would challenge me for saying something not well founded. The results of these numerous arguments were that we both went to the library to look for references to back up what we said, and then Xeroxed articles for each other to prove our points. By the end of his three-month rotation at the Minneapolis VA Hospital, we both had piles of references from each other, and that is how we learned "evidence-based medicine" in the 1970s.

One of my most poignant memories is when John was chief resident. I was the attending. The case was that of a young woman with subarachnoid hemorrhage. John's team had been pared to a minimum over the holidays by scheduled vacations, and John was filling many roles – including single-handedly managing all aspects of critically ill patients, including the young woman. He invested everything of himself in an effort to stave off what was inevitable. He also became exhausted. Late on Christmas Eve we took a break in my office to discuss plans for the night. John told me that the young woman had just deteriorated, and he did not know what he was going to tell her family. He put his head down and cried. I think I did too. Although he projected unflappable bravado, his complete personal investment in his patients and their families was also his gift and his emotional Achilles' heel.

There is the apocryphal tale of the burr hole drilled by John in an emergency room for suspected extracerebral hemorrhage. It was dry, but a legend was born of the most swash-buckling of all neurology residents, ever. He always knew more than his fellow residents and usually more than his attendings. Even when he did not, he thought he did. He was at once the most inspiring of trainees and the most challenging, and always a force to be reckoned with.

Passion for patients and their doctors

John co-founded the Minnesota Epilepsy Group in St. Paul, a practice that grew into a world-renowned, comprehensive epilepsy center noted for clinical and research excellence, and widely emulated. A clinical professor of neurology at the University of Minnesota, John was "passionate in his commitment to patient care," tried "his hardest to be the best doctor" for his patients, and believed "the treatment of epilepsy had no boundaries" and that "people with epilepsy deserved first rate care."

Over the years, John recruited and attracted "technically superior and enormously caring staff – all of whom were a reflection of John's core values, and who will carry on his legacy through their work." John's coworkers were "dedicated to him and held him in such high esteem. Nurses, psychologists, neurologists, support staff – at every place he worked – would spontaneously talk about John and his dedication to patients. They truly held him in a special spot in their hearts for years and that is something one rarely sees."

His "strong advocacy for compassionate treatment of people with nonepileptic seizures" was widely recognized and appreciated. "Far too often, these patients are dismissed and treated as second class citizens by epileptologists. John hated that attitude."

His influence on patient care and the epilepsy movement spread out from St. Paul to around the world. "John was one of those special people, and there are very few, who made a critical difference at all levels in the epilepsy movement – patient care, research, public policy, and volunteerism." He was a "powerful and effective voice in the world of epilepsy, one who spoke for the needs of clinicians who are truly devoted to the care of their patients."

Prodigious scholarship, impactful teaching, and a zest for work

John authored hundreds of publications and perhaps is best known for his writings and edited books on psychogenic nonepileptic seizures, efficacious use of antiepileptic drugs (AEDs), and the surgical management of epilepsy.

Everyone who knew John was impressed by his energy and commitment to "whatever the task, old or new." He "always had a smile on his face, and a zest and enthusiasm for his work," which was "marked by breadth, honest service, and courage."

Several months before he died, John participated in a National Institutes of Health (NIH)-sponsored workshop on nonepileptic seizures (NES). While he thought of himself as "one of the 'old dogs' in the pack," he was regarded as the brightest luminary in this field by the many accomplished international, interdisciplinary workshop participants. "In typical John fashion, he broke the ice very early on, with a few bold comments about the differences between neurology and psychiatry. Once the smoke settled, it proved to be a perfect entrée, loosening up everyone for an intense and invaluable discussion on NES treatment research."

He excelled at lecturing and was a "masterful teacher" who "never stood on formalities and shared his knowledge and experience with young neurologists and foreign doctors". His enthusiasm for teaching continued even after his constitutional energy was nearly depleted. "John couldn't "turn it off" even when critically ill. To the end, John was lecturing and educating even when he needed help walking up to the podium."

Leadership and dedication to American Epilepsy Society (AES) and International League Against Epilepsy (ILAE)

John was president of numerous organizations, including the Minnesota Epilepsy Group, the American Academy of Neurology Congress of Neurosocieties, the Association of Neurologists of Minnesota, and the Ramsey County Medical Society. He served on the ILAE Commission for Neurosurgery and participated in projects of the Subcommission for Pediatric Epilepsy Surgery. He chaired the Practice Committee of the American Epilepsy Society and served on a number of other AES committees and task forces, as well as the AES Board of Directors while courageously battling his cancer. "John's voice on the AES board always reflected his passion and commitment to the needs and best interests of individuals with epilepsy."

As his wife Rita remarked in accepting the AES J. Kiffin Penry Award for Excellence in Epilepsy Care on John's behalf,

John loved this society. If John were here, he would turn the tables, and, looking out at you, would make it about you. He would thank you for being such great colleagues. He would talk about how much each of you contributed; how he so appreciated your hard work; how key people working together make something come alive; how grateful he was that you shared his passion for this work, work that makes such a difference for so many; and how much fun it was to "play with you in this sandbox."

A warm and friendly guy who occasionally tilted at windmills

Each of us who knew John remembers something special about him, whether serious or humorous, profound or simple. He was the kind of guy who would wake up one morning with an idea and then a few hours, days, weeks, or months later, it would become a reality. He was a grass roots organizer who gave untold time and energy to innumerable epilepsy-related projects, including summer camp for kids, assisted living for young adults, funding for the less well-off for affordable medications, and "inventing" local, regional, and national training and mentoring programs. Above all else, "he was a warm and friendly guy who made many people, especially his patients, feel special."

When I think of John, his email address always pops into my mind: gaterair@aol.com. It was so appropriate. He seemed to swoop into a room as if he was a plane landing or, under some circumstances, as a dive bomber when he wanted to destroy opposition to some point he held dearly. Gaterair@aol.com also conveys to me the sense of soaring, which also captures his personality to me. He was always a presence in any meeting, no matter how large the group. He never just went through the motions of showing up. He was always in the mix of any discussion speaking out about the issues near and dear to him; his patients, the profession of epileptology, and the economics of running a practice.

I remember his ability to cut through or circumvent nonsense and get to the heart of any matter quickly, and directly, without causing antagonism, which is a great skill. Even when he was very sick, we appreciated his ability to do this.

The two things I will most remember about John are his jokes, mostly aimed at hospital and HMO administrators; and his unfailing willingness to serve as counselor, friend, or mentor. His passion for completing projects (the ultimate goal of which was always to help patients) was matched only by his kindness and collegiality.

A trademark of John that I appreciated was his ability to connect with whomever he was speaking to. His deep voice conveyed a deportment of seriousness, which however was countered by his wide smile and straight look into your eyes that made you feel welcomed to his attention.

John was an interesting combination of great brilliance, professional dedication, impeccable ethics and still a lovable nature.

He was deep, funny, irreverent, lovable and infuriating, all in one day. He was the brightest bulb in every group and knew it. He had vast energy, and his personal and professional agendas were always way more ambitious than most mortals would or should take on. He had enormous ego strength and self-confidence. If he thought an unproven or unconventional approach made sense for his patient, he forged directly ahead, full speed, against all resistance.

He was intense and very perceptive. He knew what he wanted and went after it with all his energy, and usually got what he wanted. I admired him for his intelligence, intense energy, drive, and his unique capacity to think on a grand scale. He was not afraid to be unconventional.

I didn't always agree with him, but I sure appreciated his passion. I also appreciated that he did not mind if you disagreed with him and I recognized that he sometimes went over the top just to spark some movement. Just like when he flew his plane, he always wanted to be moving towards some goal and he hated getting bogged down on technicalities.

As you know, he was a pilot. He flew into Seattle for one of the meetings. Apparently there are others named Gates in the Seattle area, and with John's last name, he told me with great amusement that he was treated very well indeed at the airport.

His kind face, warm smile, and ability to inspire confidence in less endowed friends were the sparks that spread the epilepsy gospel into a wheat field in the middle of the country.

I remember his saying that the first thing he told people moving to Minneapolis was to get a new Sears Diehard battery, no matter how old their current car battery was. Sort of a "Don't fool yourself" approach.

I regarded him as a minor renegade with a sense of humor. John was a real gentleman who occasionally liked to tilt at windmills.

Farewell

John will be missed enormously. Many of us can still hear him say "Hi guy, how are you doing!" As one close colleague said, "He was special to me. I am not exactly sure why. Maybe it is some form of love." One of his many grateful patients said, "You were the best doctor. I had such faith in you and I know God will be with you always."

Farewell, John. Your memory and inspiration live on, and we are all better for having known you.

Legacies

Several funds have been established in memory of John Gates: the Minnesota Medical Foundation, Dr. John R. Gates Memorial Award in Neurology, 200 Oak St. SE, Suite 300, Minneapolis, MN 55455-2030; Epilepsy Foundation of Minnesota, John R. Gates MD Project Fund, 1600 University Ave. W., Suite 205, St. Paul, MN 55104; and Minnesota ABC, Dr. John R. Gates Scholarship Fund, 8761 Preserve Blvd, Eden Prairie, MN 55344, attn: Gardner Gay.

Acknowledgments: Remembrances of John were generously submitted by the Minnesota Epilepsy Group, members of the American Epilepsy Society and its Board of Directors, David Anderson, Joan Austin, Greg Barkley, Elinor Ben-Menachem, Martin Brodie, Helen Cross, Richard Gilmartin, Mark Granner, Bruce Hermann, John Hughes, Barry Johnson, W. Curt LaFrance, Chi-Wan Lai, Ken Laxer, Ron Lesser, Gary Mathern, Dick Mattson, Rita Meyer, Georgia Montouris, Venkat Ramani, Jim Rowan, Elson So, Mike Sperling, Mark Spitz, and Bill Theodore.

Adapted from Schachter S.C. John Gates: An Appreciation. *Epilepsy Behav* 2006;**9**:545–8. With permission from Elsevier.

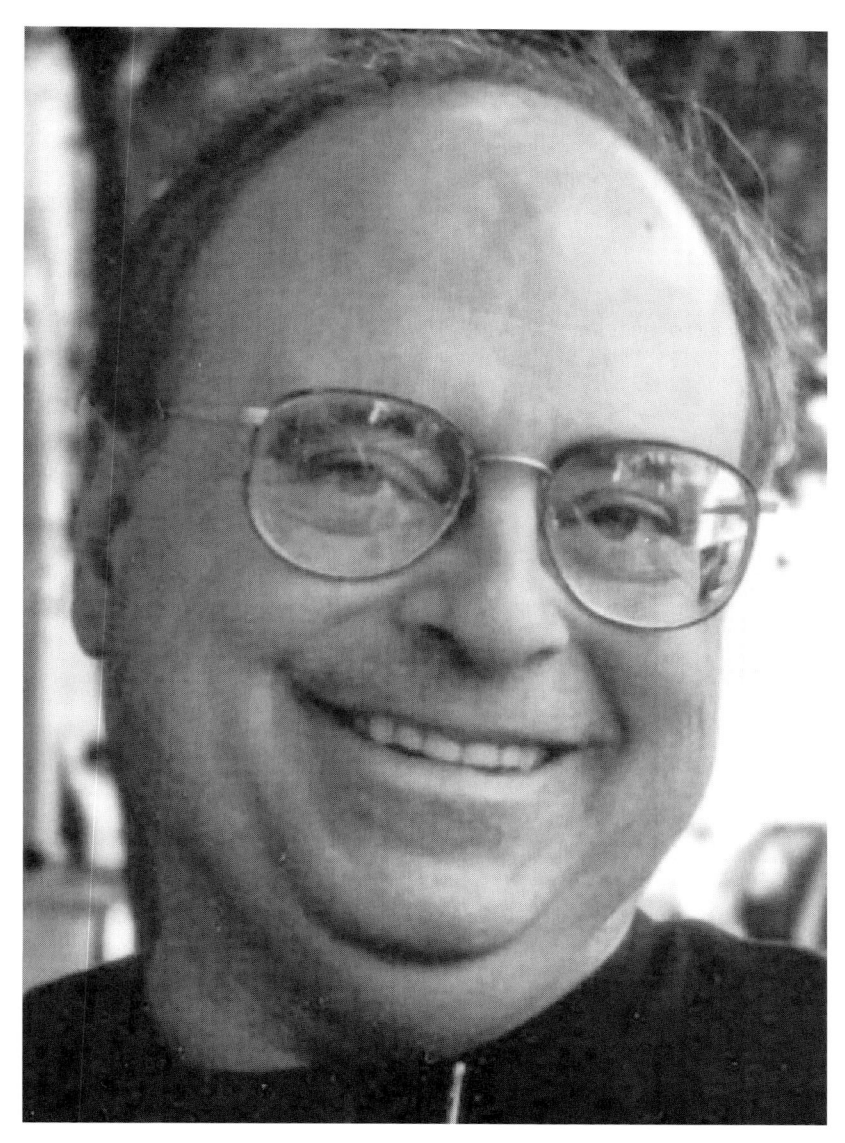

Dr. John R. Gates

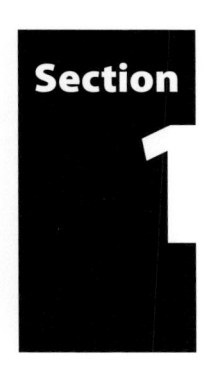

Section 1 Recognition, diagnosis, and impact of nonepileptic seizures

Section 1 Chapter 1

Recognition, diagnosis, and impact of nonepileptic seizures

Epidemiology and classification of psychogenic nonepileptic seizures

Nathan M. Griffith and Jerzy P. Szaflarski

Psychogenic nonepileptic seizures (PNES) are events that resemble epileptic seizures (ES) but without epileptiform activity and with psychological underpinnings [1]. Clinicians have been fairly able to reliably distinguish PNES from ES based on clinical characteristics of the disease [2], but a definitive distinction between ES and PNES was not possible until an improved diagnostic tool – prolonged video-EEG (VEEG) monitoring – became available. Video-EEG allowed the correct diagnosis of PNES in a considerable percentage of patients with poorly controlled seizures. The diagnosis of PNES, referred to as hystero-epilepsy in the past (see Chapter 2), however, has existed for millennia.

A survey of British neurologists in the late 1980s revealed that preferred nomenclature for unexplained neurological symptoms included "functional," "psychogenic," and "hysteria" [3]. Scull cites 15 synonyms for PNES, including, among others, "pseudoseizures" (suggesting that there is something spurious or false about the events), "hystero-epilepsy" (indicating that the uterus is the origin of the nonepileptic events), "hysterical pseudoseizures," "pseudoepileptic seizures," and "psychogenic seizures" [4]; more recently terms such as PNES, "nonepileptic attack disorder," and "stress seizures" have also been used. The emergence of new, less pejorative labels such as PNES indicates an increasing understanding and acknowledgment that the events are very real to the patient, witnesses, and physicians, but these events have different and variable pathophysiology or etiology as compared to ES. The term *psychogenic* nonepileptic seizures emphasizes the distinction between psychogenic and *physiological* nonepileptic seizures (or events) as seen in patients with migraine or other neurological conditions, sleep disorders or cardiac events (see Chapters 6 and 7). Consistent with the first two editions of this book and with research on terminology, the term psychogenic nonepileptic seizures is currently the most appropriate term for this condition, moving beyond the pejorative connotation that "pseudoseizure" carries; this term will be used throughout the rest of this chapter and book, where appropriate.

Epidemiology of PNES

The diagnosis of PNES is based on a history consistent with conversion disorder and confirmation of the diagnosis on VEEG. Monitoring reveals the lack of epileptiform EEG changes during clinical events associated with alteration of consciousness or motor, sensory, and/or autonomic phenomena; normal alpha rhythm (or no change in background rhythm) with or without the alteration of consciousness; and nonstereotypic nature of the events. Typically, no sustained response to antiepileptic drugs (AEDs) is found. A history consistent with PNES is also used in making the diagnosis [5, 6]. Some patients who have possible or confirmed diagnosis of ES are considered to carry a dual diagnosis of PNES/ES.

Until recently, no population-based studies of PNES had been performed, and most estimates of incidence and prevalence of PNES were based on VEEG reports from tertiary care epilepsy centers. By default, the incidence and prevalence reported from such estimates were heavily dependent on referral patterns to the epilepsy centers and vigilance of the clinicians evaluating the patients in the outpatient clinics who later referred them for VEEG monitoring. Further, these estimates were likely to underreport PNES because patients with PNES may not always be evaluated by epilepsy specialists since the nature of their events may be variable and include symptoms suggestive of pain syndromes, sleep disorders, movement

---

Gates and Rowan's Nonepileptic Seizures, 3rd edn. ed. Steven C. Schachter and W. Curt LaFrance, Jr. Published by Cambridge University Press. © S. Schachter and W. C. LaFrance, Jr. 2010.

disorders or multiple sclerosis, and stroke-like events (see Chapter 4). Further, the average delay in making the diagnosis of PNES is approximately 7 to 8 years [1, 5, 7]. Video-EEG is usually performed in patients who experience frequent or medication-resistant events that raise the suspicion of the clinician as possibly nonepileptic; patients with infrequent or controlled events, even when suspicious for PNES in description, do not usually undergo VEEG monitoring because of the high cost and low yield of such studies. Frequently, patients with poorly controlled seizures are referred to epilepsy centers for possible surgical evaluation or other interventions and are diagnosed with PNES only after the full evaluation including the VEEG is completed. Further, many patients undergo multiple VEEG evaluations as they may be searching for confirmation of a diagnosis or they may be referred to various centers for second opinions by physicians who are either unaware of the previous evaluations or diagnoses, or who are dubious of the diagnosis of PNES [8]. Therefore, epidemiological studies of PNES are difficult to generalize and, by definition, can include only patients who underwent VEEG. Therefore, estimations based on the results of VEEG likely lead to underestimates of the true incidence and prevalence of PNES, as referring patients for VEEG monitoring depends on availability of the testing, vigilance of the referring and evaluating physicians and frequency of the events.

Incidence of PNES

Incidence is broadly defined as the number of new cases of a disease occurring per unit of time in a specific population. Only two true epidemiological studies of incidence of PNES were performed to date. The first study was performed in Iceland in the mid 1990s. In this country with a very stable population, all patients with new-onset seizures were considered for VEEG, which was performed in the only available laboratory [9]. The authors of this study identified 14 patients ages 16 to 54 with definite PNES; the majority of these patients (78.6%) were women. The incidence of PNES was calculated as 1.4 per year per 100 000. The highest incidence of PNES was noted in the 15 to 24 years age group (3.4/100 000 person–years), with no patients above the age of 55 diagnosed with PNES. The incidence of PNES was highest in female patients 15 to 24 years of age (5.9/100 000 person–years). The authors estimated that patients with PNES constitute about 5% of all patients with new-onset seizures. For comparison, the authors estimated the incidence of epilepsy in the Icelandic population over 15 years old to be 35/100 000 person–years.

The second study was performed in Hamilton County, Ohio [5]. The authors found the mean incidence of PNES to be about 3.03/100 000 person–years, which is about 2 times higher than the incidence reported by Sigurdardottir and Olafsson [9]. The highest incidence in the Szaflarski *et al.* study was in the 25 to 44 years age group (4.38/100 000 person–years) [5]. The gender ratio of 73% women was similar to the Iceland study and to previous reports [10]. This incidence of PNES was compared to the population incidence of epilepsy in Rochester, Minnesota of 44/100 000 person–years [11]. Interestingly, the incidence of PNES in this study was twice that of the incidence of PNES in the Icelandic population, while the overall incidence of epilepsy in the US study was also higher when compared to that reported from Iceland. The similarities between the two studies indicate that the proportion of patients with newly diagnosed PNES may be fairly similar when compared to the overall incidence of epilepsy. In addition, the results indicate a fairly similar approach to the evaluation of patients with new-onset seizures/spells between the two studies. There also may be similar awareness and vigilance of the physicians regarding the possibility of a diagnosis other than epilepsy in patients with new-onset seizures. Finally, the study by Szaflarski *et al.* also found increasing incidence of PNES over the study period, indicating higher awareness of clinicians and familiarity with the diagnosis of PNES and of possibly improved access to VEEG in the US, assuming that the actual incidence was stable over time.

Prevalence

Prevalence is defined as the number of active cases of a disease per unit of population at risk. Obviously, it is difficult to estimate the prevalence of disease when diagnosis is based on VEEG, which is costly, time consuming, and sometimes difficult to obtain, as compared to clinical criteria. Nevertheless, there are many reports that indicate the prevalence of PNES to be between 10% and 20% in children and 10% and 58% in adults who are referred to epilepsy centers, with the most frequently quoted numbers between 20% and 30% [12]. A recent study proposed an estimate of the prevalence of PNES based on a calculation using known prevalence of epilepsy of 0.5% to 1%, a proportion of intractable epilepsy among epilepsy patients of 20% to 30% (with 20% to 50% of these patients referred to epilepsy centers), and assumed 10% to 20% of patients referred to epilepsy centers would be diagnosed with PNES [13]. Using the available data, the estimated prevalence of PNES was between 1/50 000 and 1/3000 or 2 to 33 per 100 000. Therefore, PNES is not a rare disorder and its economic impact related to medication and treatment expenses is estimated to be high, probably similar to the economic impact of epilepsy (see Chapter 3). Correct diagnosis and appropriate patient education may lead to a better understanding of the disease by patients and physicians and, therefore, may lower the economic impact by 69% to 97% [14].

Prevalence of comorbid epilepsy and PNES

The reported prevalence of comorbid epilepsy in patients diagnosed with PNES varies considerably and was reported to be as low as 9% and as high as 63% [5, 15], with the higher number reported in one of the first studies reporting the results of VEEG in patients with medication-resistant epilepsy. In this study a total of only eight patients with PNES were identified (five had comorbid epilepsy). In an epidemiological study of PNES incidence, Sigurdardottir and Olafsson reported that 50% of patients diagnosed with PNES had comorbid epilepsy [9]. This number appears to be very high as other recent studies reported much lower incidence/risk of epilepsy in patients with PNES. In the second incidence study reported above, only 16/177 (9%) patients were diagnosed with comorbid PNES and epilepsy [5], which is much more in line with a later estimate from a study that found coexistence of epilepsy in about 9.4% of patients with PNES [16]. Therefore, it appears that about 10% of patients with PNES have comorbid epilepsy. Most importantly, in patients with well characterized epilepsy and abnormal EEG showing epileptiform discharges, PNES are still possible and should be considered if the patient is not responding to standard treatments.

To summarize, the diagnosis of PNES is not uncommon, with about 5% to 10% of patients with spells/seizures having nonepileptic events. Clinicians should be vigilant in monitoring the description of events and particularly aware of unusual phenomena that may be atypical in ES but suggestive of PNES. Unusual characteristics of seizures or lack of medication response should prompt VEEG evaluation as a means of clarifying the diagnosis and designing an optimal treatment plan.

Clinical classification schemes of PNES

Since the introduction of VEEG, epileptologists have had increased diagnostic capability, especially as regards the differentiation of ES from nonepileptic seizures, which has led to many of the advances in the understanding and treatment of nonepileptic seizures [17]. Studies have identified heterogeneity in the psychological background and profile of patients with nonepileptic seizures. However, commonalities are found in many patients with nonepileptic seizures, including a history of trauma or abuse, psychiatric comorbidities, and family or social dysfunction. Studies have identified and proposed differentiation of discrete subtypes of nonepileptic seizures [18, 19]. For example, in his introduction to the second edition of this book, Gates divided nonepileptic events into a dichotomy – physiologic and psychogenic [20]. The ability to classify patients within subtypes of nonepileptic seizures is important because there is evidence that subtypes are clinically relevant in terms of predicting outcome [19], informing nosology [18, 19], and, perhaps most importantly, potentially directing treatment [21, 22].

Studies of subtypes of nonepileptic seizures have utilized a wide range of methodologies and criteria. The following broad categories of subtypes that do not conform to existing psychiatric taxonomy will be reviewed: (a) classifications based on clinical semiology, (b) classifications based on personality testing, (c) classifications based on both semiology and personality testing, and (d) classifications based on suspected psychological mechanism/etiology. In this section, we survey the literature on classifications as an introduction to further discussions in subsequent chapters.

Classifications based on semiology

Characterizing seizure-like events by their semiology has a long history that can be traced back to initial theorizing by Charcot and Janet about "hysterical" reactions [23]. The earliest classifications of PNES resulting from descriptive accounts of semiology were dichotomous. These classifications of PNES were borne out of conceptualizations of PNES as expressions of basic human needs or drives. For example, Kretschmer, following the ideas of Freud, characterized spells as either hypermotor or atonic [24]. As summarized by Blumer and Adamolekun, Kretschmer postulated that PNES appear "...in the form either of a motility storm consisting of regression in a state of terror with hyperkinesis, trembling, and convulsing, or of sham death with stupor, immobilization, or a hypnoid state" [25; p. 498]. Similarly, Szondi described a polarity of paroxysmal drives oriented around the locus of perceived source of danger. Szondi postulated that PNES represented either a "protective drive," with the epileptiform reaction as a response to perceived internal danger, or a hysteriform reaction in response to perceived danger in the external world [25].

This basic classification of PNES as either hypermotor or atonic has survived within differing terminology ("catatonic" vs. "thrashing," "convulsive" vs. "nonconvulsive") and underlies modern classification schemes of PNES [19].

Some early attempts to classify subtypes of PNES by semiology followed this theorized dichotomy fairly closely. For example, Meierkord *et al.* categorized spells as attacks of collapse and attacks with prominent motor activity [10]. Interestingly, several authors have reported that two-thirds of patients with PNES have the hypermotor type and the remaining one-third of patients has the atonic type of spells [10, 26]. Other classifications of PNES included both motor and affective components of PNES. For example, Wilkus and Dodrill categorized PNES as mostly motor/limited affect and limited motor/prominent affect groups [27].

Other semiology-based classifications of PNES introduced finer, but differing distinctions between types of spells. In an early study of semiology, PNES were characterized into four major patterns associated with the events: bilateral motor, unilateral motor, multiple behavior phenomena, or impaired responsiveness with no observable behavior [28]. In contrast, Henry and Drury, in a study of whether stereotyped behavior during PNES represents learned behavior, characterized events as convulsive, hypotonic ("sudden falls, or leaning limply/leans onto a bed or other nearby support"), automatistic ("simple or complex movements that are symmetric or nonconvulsive"), or hypokinetic ("motionless or nearly motionless staring with unchanging posture") [29]. In a study of whether closed eyes during spells indicated psychogenic etiology in the context of seizure provocation, Flugel *et al.* used video and EEG to classify patients into the following three semiology-based groups: strong movements particularly of the extremities (similar to a generalized tonic-clonic seizure [GTCS]), spells with mild, less pronounced motor activity, and almost motionless unresponsiveness [30]. In contrast, Gumnit and Gates mention the importance of differentiating PNES that resemble complex partial seizures (CPS) from those that resemble GTCS [31]. In a review of cases described in other studies, van Merode *et al.* categorized PNES as resembling GTCS, resembling CPS, or resembling a combination of both categories [32]. In one of the first studies to use cluster analysis (a specific statistical technique allowing for identification of "symptom clusters"), Groppel *et al.* classified patients with PNES via VEEG into three semiology-based clusters: psychogenic motor seizures, psychogenic minor motor or trembling seizures, and psychogenic atonic seizures [33].

Reuber *et al.* in an outcome study involving long-term follow-up classified patients with PNES into the following groups: positive motor, negative motor, and purely sensory [22]. However, a subset of recent studies has excluded PNES characterized exclusively by sensory phenomena from their classification schemes due to the limited sensitivity of scalp electrodes for detection of simple partial seizures [18, 34]. This problem renders the differentiation of ES and PNES, in the case of sensory or subjective PNES, extremely difficult, thus compromising the designation of these events as PNES versus ES.

More recent studies have further expanded the number and complexity of delineations between types of PNES in order to better understand the natural history and pathogenesis of PNES. For example, Selwa *et al.* introduced a classification of PNES into six types: catatonic, thrashing, automatisms, tremor, intermittent, and subjective. This study was unique in that it focused on the utility of subtype with regard to outcomes, such as remission of seizures and discontinuation of AEDs [19]. Although there are six subtypes in the proposed Selwa *et al.* classification, their study focused on comparisons between catatonic and thrashing, the two most conceptually opposite categories. Recently, Griffith *et al.* modified the Selwa scheme to a four subtype scheme, consisting of catatonic, major motor, minor motor, and subjective [18]. The Griffith *et al.* classification is more parsimonious and resulted in better interrater reliability than the Selwa *et al.* scheme [18, 19].

In summary, recent attempts to classify PNES by semiology have expanded upon earlier dichotomous distinctions between, for example, "atonic" and "hypermotor" events, by identifying three to four distinct subtypes of PNES, with the most useful of these schemes demonstrating good interrater reliability; these new classifications schemes have been reported to be related to outcome (see Section 5).

Classifications based on personality testing

Some investigators have used psychological testing, especially personality testing, to identify subtypes of patients with intractable seizure disorders. The most commonly used measure of personality and psychopathology in both ES and PNES populations is the Minnesota Multiphasic Personality Inventory (MMPI) [35, 36]. Other personality measures have also been used in these populations [26, 35]. For example, in a sample of presurgical patients with intractable seizure disorders, a subset of whom (about 20 of 90) were likely to have PNES or both PNES and ES, King et al. identified three groups based on personality profiles (in order of greatest frequency): minimal psychological complaints, generalized clinical elevations (high psychological complaints), and intermediate elevations with a tendency to emphasize somatic complaints or depression [37].

Several authors have emphasized the heterogeneity of personality profiles among patients with PNES [35, 37, 38]. For example, studies have found that a majority of patients with PNES have personality abnormalities on psychometric tests [26, 39], but there is not a single characteristic personality profile that can be attributed to these patients [40]. Barrash et al. analyzed MMPI profiles of patients with PNES and identified seven discrete personality clusters: histrionic, depressed, nonaffective serious psychopathology, disinhibited, decompensated, somatisizers, and asymptomatic [41]. In another study involving personality testing with the MMPI, Gumnit and Gates analyzed interviews, MMPI, and projective testing results among patients with PNES. They found five underlying etiology-based subtypes based on suspected etiology or function of PNES: (a) psychological distress-emotional conflict, (b) inappropriate coping mechanisms, (c) misinterpretation of normal physiological stimuli, (d) psychotic behavior, and (e) an epileptic aura or seizure followed by PNES. They also reported that these subtypes were useful for selecting patients for appropriate treatments [31].

Of note, the model employed by the Diagnostic and Statistical Manual of Mental Disorders (DSM) has been criticized by some authors [26, 42, 43]. For example, Reuber et al. favored a dimensional system that would consider personality disorders as extremes on a continuum of common personality traits. These authors also noted considerable symptomatic and behavioral overlap and poor interrater reliability between DSM personality disorders [26]. In addition, Reuber et al. and other investigators have criticized use of the MMPI for categorizing personality subtypes, especially among inpatient groups.

The same authors stated that the MMPI is difficult to interpret because it simultaneously measures both personality characteristics and psychopathological syndromes, such as hypochondriasis and conversion [26]. In contrast to studies utilizing the MMPI, Reuber et al. used the Dimensional Assessment of Personality Pathology-Basic Questionnaire (DAPP-BQ [44]) to measure personality in patients with PNES as compared to patients with ES and healthy subjects. They found three distinct "typical pathological personality profiles" via cluster analysis (in order of size): similar to borderline personality disorder, overly controlled personality, and similar to avoidant personality disorder.

There has been increasing attention in behavioral medicine paid to the importance of measuring "normal" personality traits. Cragar et al. emphasized the relationships of normal personality traits to health status, health outcomes, and behavior patterns [21]. Moreover, normal personality traits, such as optimism and pessimism, have been found to be relevant to investigations of both etiology and outcome in both medical and psychological disorders [45, 46]. Cragar et al. studied normal personality traits in patients with PNES by means of personality dimensions derived from the five factor model as measured by the Revised NEO Personality Inventory (NEO-PI-R) [47]. Using cluster analysis of both MMPI and NEO-PI-R results, Cragar et al. found three personality clusters in patients with PNES: depressed neurotics, somatic defenders, and activated neurotics [21].

It is therefore clear that classification of PNES by personality testing has underscored the heterogeneity of personality profiles in patients with PNES. Although some earlier work focused on pathological personality profiles, a more recently employed approach has been to investigate personality traits/dimensions/clusters, which may inform etiology and outcomes.

Classifications based on both semiology and personality testing

A few studies have combined personality, psychological testing and semiology in identifying subtypes of PNES. In perhaps the best example of this approach, Wilkus and Dodrill classified patients with PNES into the following groups: (1) mostly motor and limited/none affectual and (2) limited motor/prominently affectual. These two PNES subgroups had different composite MMPI profiles; moreover, 76% of patients in the study could be classified into one of these two groups [27].

By simultaneously considering/classifying both behavioral and affectual aspects of the presentation of PNES, the classification of PNES by both semiology and personality testing may represent an important evolution in the classification of PNES.

Classifications based on etiology/suspected psychological mechanism

Some investigators have classified patients with PNES via behavioral and interpersonal factors believed to contribute to the development of PNES – in other words, by etiology or suspected psychological mechanism. On a patient-by-patient basis, PNES may have a single-factor or multifactorial etiology; that is to say, in a given patient, PNES are believed to manifest from one or more of several distinct causal pathways [48, 49]. Ford identified several factors that may individually or jointly contribute to the etiology of somatoform disorders, including: (a) secondary gain, (b) behavioral manifestations of ineffective communication/inability to adequately identify and express strong emotion, and (c) disturbed family systems [50].

Studies of patients with PNES have produced similar findings related to etiological factors (i.e., interpersonal, communication, and/or family problems). For example, Lesser summarized the etiological factors of PNES described in the literature as follows: (a) interpersonal, (b) intrinsic emotional problems or internalized conflicts (e.g., somatization, dissociation, posttraumatic stress), (c) psychosis, (d) personality disorder, and (e) cognitive difficulties or history of head trauma [49]. Similarly, Alsaadi and Marquez classified PNES by suspected psychological causal pathway, while emphasizing that all PNES function as a coping mechanism [48]. They classified the etiology of PNES as follows: (1) caused by misinterpretation of physical symptoms, (2) the result of psychopathological processes (e.g., somatization, dissociation), (3) response to acute stress (in patients with absence of psychopathology), and (4) reinforced behavior pattern in cognitively impaired patients.

On the other hand, some authors have conformed more closely to psychodynamic theory in classifying patients with PNES by etiology. For example, one group of authors described four "psychodynamic pathways" to PNES: (a) history of childhood physical or sexual abuse, (b) recent sexual assault, (c) multiple life stresses that overwhelm coping abilities, and (d) panic attacks mistaken for PNES [51, 52]. These authors noted that for all of these categories, the manifestation of PNES was often triggered by recent trauma. Other studies conformed more closely to formal psychological diagnostic categories and processes. For example, one study identified six categories, or "symptom patterns," of patients with PNES, based in part on the most effective psychotherapeutic interventions used with each group [53]. Rusch *et al.*'s findings were reformulated by LaFrance and Devinsky as the following: (1) anxious, (2) abused (subclassified into 2a – abused [borderline personality disorder] and 2b – afraid [as in posttraumatic stress disorder]), (3) somatic, (4) dysthymic/depressed, and (5) mentally retarded [54].

Classification of PNES by suspected etiology brings into focus common risk factors, such as recent trauma, and the multifactorial nature of the development and maintenance of PNES. Examining elements that may explain the differential effectiveness of psychotherapeutic interventions with subgroups of patients with PNES may inform our understanding of nosology.

Neurological events mimicking PNES

There is no single diagnostic test that allows certain differentiation of PNES, ES, physiological nonepileptic events, or other types of psychiatric diagnoses. Even VEEG, the gold standard in distinguishing between PNES and epilepsy, is not always correct as it may be difficult to distinguish, for example, between bizarre ictal behaviors associated with frontal lobe/supplementary motor seizures and PNES [55, 56]. Certainly, VEEG, in association with other tests and clinical observation(s), is a valuable tool in differentiating PNES from other neurological or non-neurological conditions. But before such testing is scheduled, as with all patients presenting for initial evaluation or follow-up, a detailed general history is essential for correct diagnosis. A focused, symptom-oriented approach alone may lead to incorrect diagnosis. Description of the events obtained from the patient may be very sketchy or plainly inaccurate. Therefore, a detailed description of the event(s) from witnesses may be of significant value. Information about duration of the events may be the first clue to the correct diagnosis as PNES are usually prolonged, lasting sometimes more than 30 minutes [29]. Further, seizure precipitants and the presence or absence of certain phenomena, such as prolonged waxing and waning course of the events, screaming, hearing but not being able to respond, ictal eye closure or crying, asynchronous or asymmetric extremity movements, pelvic thrusting, etc. may be helpful in coming to the right diagnosis. Further, the presence of EEG abnormalities including epileptiform discharges is not necessarily indicative of epilepsy [57] (see Chapter 4).

The differential diagnosis of PNES also includes physiological nonepileptic events. These are usually paroxysmal events with physiological explanation. These etiologies include syncope, nonepileptic myoclonus, dysautonomia, and various sleep disorders (parasomnias), including sleepwalking, confusional arousals, and REM sleep behavior disorders. This list also includes other neurological phenomena, including transient ischemic phenomena and migraine, and non-neurological phenomena such as organic hallucinations and psychosis-related, e.g., to medication or substance toxicity.

Syncope, especially convulsive syncope, is likely the most frequent physiological phenomenon that is confused with PNES. Overall, convulsive syncope is a relatively common event. In one study of unselected blood donors, convulsive syncope occurred in 0.03%. The donors frequently experienced convulsive tonic extensor spasm(s); other epileptic phenomena simulating epileptic seizure occurred less frequently. Up to 11.9% of these events were associated with convulsive phenomena. Further, the authors did not find any significant differences between the "early" and the "delayed" responses [58]. In another VEEG study, 10 of 22 syncopal episodes precipitated by cardiac arrhythmias were associated with regular or irregular tonic movements. Although generalized EEG changes were observed in some patients (usually generalized slowing), no ictal or interictal epileptiform discharges were noted [59]. Therefore, in patients with syncope or when the description of events is not clear, a detailed cardiac evaluation, including either 24-hour Holter monitoring or even up to 30 days of cardiac event monitoring, should be considered. Figure 1.1 depicts the EEG and EKG of a patient who experienced vasovagal syncope in response to hyperventilation. Generalized EEG changes are noted in response to CNS hypoperfusion.

Transient ischemic events that may mimic epilepsy include not only transient ischemic attack (TIA) but also migrainous phenomena. As these events are fairly frequent, and migrainous sensory phenomena that are not associated with headache may be sometimes difficult to distinguish from simple partial sensory seizures, clinicians need to utilize detailed clinical history to reach the diagnosis. With the incidence of TIAs approximating 83/100 000 person–years [60] and the incidence of migraine averaging in males between 6.6/1000 and 10.1/1000 person–years and in females between 14.1/1000 and 18.9/1000 person–years [61], there is a high chance that neurologists will encounter several patients per year that have somewhat unusual presentations of the respective disease that will require differentiation from ES or PNES.

Physiological events that require differentiation from PNES and ES are further described in Chapters 6 and 7. It is very important for the practicing clinician not to assume that patients with unusual events have PNES without proper evaluation, as there are many other clinical entities that mimic ES and PNES that need to be excluded based on thorough clinical history and supplementary testing.

Classification of PNES via existing psychiatric schemes

Consensus on a descriptive nosology of PNES has been elusive. A well-accepted descriptive nosology fosters meaningful classification, facilitates differential diagnosis, and may aid in the understanding of the etiology of a disorder, thereby leading to the development of treatments. However, despite repeated and ongoing attempts to classify PNES as psychiatric phenomena, the classification of PNES within existing psychiatric taxonomies continues to be controversial [62–64]. The classification of PNES is difficult because patients with PNES do not fall into a single, distinct psychopathological category. In fact, researchers have suggested that PNES is not a unitary disorder, but instead may have multiple etiologies and manifestations [40]. Moreover, the etiology of PNES is

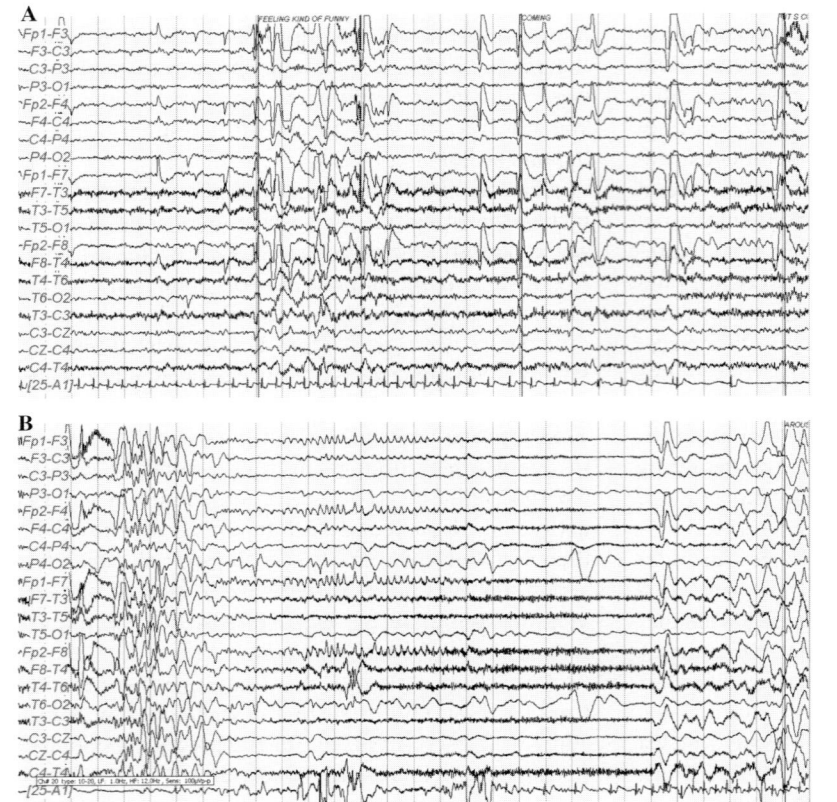

Figure 1.1. EEG/EKG tracing of a patient with history of events of loss of consciousness associated with myoclonic jerks (grey vertical lines represent 1 second markers; each panel represents 30 seconds of recording). While the patient undergoes video-EEG monitoring he is asked to hyperventilate. Panel A shows clear tachycardia ([25-A1] channel) and gradual prolongation of the QRS with pause lasting approximately 20 seconds (extends to panel B). Generalized slowing of the background EEG is noted with a burst of generalized theta/delta activity without epileptiform discharges in the first part of panel B followed by suppression of the EEG activity and then gradual recovery (not shown).

multifaceted and includes the interaction of predisposing, precipitating, and perpetuating factors [65, 66].

Sources of confusion underlying classification of PNES

A review of the literature reveals several interrelated sources of confusion that complicate the diagnosis and classification of PNES. The reality of the diagnostic process in clinical practice is that PNES are often diagnosed based on the nature of presenting symptoms and the *exclusion* of nonpsychogenic etiologies, rather than the identification of relevant psychological factors with histories consistent with conversion or dissociative disorders and documentation of non-neuroanatomical findings on examination. The result is that PNES often are diagnosed negatively ("not ES") as opposed to positively ("is PNES"). This contributes to uncertainty as to the diagnostic features that comprise PNES. Moreover, the classification of PNES is hampered by several unresolved philosophical and semantic dilemmas concerning the nature and underlying causes of PNES. These include: (a) whether somatization or dissociation is the primary underlying etiology of PNES, (b) a descriptive vs. etiological approach to psychiatric classification, and (c) whether PNES should be conceptualized and classified as a symptom of a psychiatric disorder or as a separate disease entity.

Somatization vs. dissociation as the primary underlying etiology of PNES

Disagreement as to whether PNES should be characterized as primarily a somatoform or dissociative disorder complicates the classification of PNES [50, 62, 67]. Several reviews have examined the differential role and impact of dissociation and somatization in PNES [40, 63]. The results of these studies have been mixed. One study of a sample including patients with ES, PNES, and mixed disorder (ES + PNES) found that patients with PNES had a higher level of dissociation than the other groups [68]. Another study reported more dissociative experiences among patients with newly developed PNES than newly developed ES [69]. Indeed, the comorbidity of dissociative disorders among patients with PNES has been reported to be as high as 91% [52]. Several studies have concluded that patients with PNES have high rates of psychiatric disorders such as those found in traumatized groups and closely resemble patients with dissociative disorders [70, 71]. Another study found that a "depersonalization/derealization" subscale that resulted from factor analysis of the Dissociative Experiences Scale (DES) differentiated patients with PNES from patients with CPS [72]. However, in a study of somatization, dissociation, and general psychopathology in patients with ES vs. PNES, measures of somatization, but not dissociation, were associated with seizure outcome and severity [64]. Several other studies have found that PNES are best characterized as a manifestation of somatization [73–75]. Moreover, dissociation and somatization may not be entirely separable [52, 62]. For example, dissociation and somatization were positively correlated in a recent study of patients with PNES [74]. Another study postulated that PNES may be "a specific form of dissociation which involves a conversion-like trigger in its manifestation" [76; p. 154].

This conflict between somatization or dissociation as the primary underlying etiology of PNES is best exemplified by a noticeable schism in the classification of PNES under the world's two leading psychiatric classification systems: the DSM [42] and the International Classification of Diseases (ICD) [77]. The DSM-IV-TR classifies PNES under somatization; in contrast, the ICD-10 classifies PNES under dissociation. Although at least one study expressly endorses the ICD approach to the classification of PNES [63], the classification of PNES is most often discussed in terms of classification via the DSM.

Descriptive vs. etiological approach to psychiatric classification

The uncertainty related to whether somatization or dissociation should be considered the primary underlying etiology of PNES has been influenced by a change in the orientation of the DSM to psychiatric classification. In particular, a shift in recent editions of the DSM away from considerations of etiology and towards a more "descriptive" approach to classification has impacted the classification of PNES by conflating somatization and dissociation. The descriptive approach involves grouping disorders based on similarities of manifestation/symptomatology and overlap of occurrence. The Somatoform Disorder category was introduced in DSM-III to emphasize the importance of excluding medical (e.g., neurological) etiologies of symptoms believed to have a psychological origin in the differential diagnosis of these disorders. These disorders, which had been categorized under the conversion (cf. dissociation) subtype of Hysterical Neurosis in DSM-II [78], were reclassified in DSM-III [79] as Conversion Disorder, a subcategory of Somatoform Disorder. According to the DSM, the differentiation of somatoform and dissociative disorders introduced in DSM-III is more a practical than a conceptual division. However, despite descriptive use of the terms "conversion" and "dissociation" in DSM, these terms are generally interpreted by mental health professionals as indicating both a group of psychiatric syndromes *and* the psychological processes by which those syndromes are brought about [62]. Moreover, the contents of the criteria for Conversion Disorder in DSM-IV (i.e., conflicts, stressors, psychological factors) indicate implicit endorsement of this assumption [62].

Thus, PNES straddle the diagnostic line between somatization and dissociative disorders in DSM. "Nonepileptic seizures" are not included as diagnostic entities or classification criteria in DSM-IV. However, DSM-IV does refer to "seizures," both in the description of a subtype of Conversion Disorder ("with seizures or convulsions") and in a list of "pseudoneurological" symptoms that indicate Somatization Disorder. Of note, dissociative symptoms also are listed as a pseudoneurological symptom that indicates Somatization Disorder in DSM-IV. Thus, as summarized by Martin and Gates and others, DSM-IV is guilty of a logical inconsistency by including dissociative symptoms as a criterion for a somatoform disorder [80].

Frequent comorbidities of PNES

A descriptive approach to classification often includes a consideration of frequent comorbidities in the definition/description of a disorder. There is consensus that patients with PNES have an increased risk of comorbid psychiatric disorders [43]. Several authors have summarized the frequency of psychiatric comorbidities in patients with PNES. A wide range of DSM-IV disorders are reported as comorbid, the most common being somatoform disorders, dissociative disorders, affective disorders, and anxiety disorders, especially posttraumatic stress disorder (PTSD) [40,

43, 52, 81]. It should be noted, however, that methodological weaknesses have been identified in studies of psychiatric morbidity in patients with PNES, including that these studies are often undertaken in patients with intractable seizures in specialized epilepsy centers, they utilize poorly defined or less-than-optimal methods of psychiatric diagnosis, and there is inconsistent differentiation of current and lifetime psychiatric diagnosis [40].

Other studies have reported the frequency of comorbidity of personality disorders in patients with PNES [82]. Studies have reported that a majority of patients with PNES have personality abnormalities on psychometric tests, with up to 86% of patients with PNES reported to have comorbid personality disorders [26, 39]. There is no characteristic disordered personality profile that predominates among patients with PNES. However, the predominant DSM personality disorder cluster among patients with PNES is cluster B, which consists of Borderline, Histrionic, Narcissistic, and Antisocial personality disorder, and is characterized by hostility, impulsivity, and instability of relationships, self-image, and emotions. There is evidence to suggest that Borderline personality disorder is the most common personality disorder among patients with PNES [82].

In the literature on psychiatric classification of PNES, comorbidities of PNES seem to have indirectly informed the understanding of the etiology of PNES. An example of this is the association between PTSD, a frequent comorbidity of PNES, and the assertion that dissociation, rather than somatization, is the basic underlying etiology of PNES [63, 76]. In addition, some statements made in the PNES literature have perpetuated confusion as to the direction of causation between comorbidities and PNES (e.g., "the most common psychiatric disorder *resulting in* PNES is…" [83; p. 498]). Other statements have called into question whether PNES subsumes, or is subsumed by, psychiatric diagnostic categories (e.g., "The PNES group *includes a number of DSM-IV diagnostic categories*" [84; p. 28]).

Proposed dissociative subtype of PNES

Some authors have proposed recognition of a dissociative subtype of PNES [71, 85]. In fact, Brewin *et al.* proposed that PNES may be a dissociative variant of PTSD [86]. Many authors have reported similarities between patients with PNES and PTSD related to dissociative symptomatology and a history of trauma/abuse [51, 52, 71]. Moreover, patients with PNES are more likely to report a history of trauma than patients with ES [68, 70] or other groups of patients with "functional" symptoms [66].

Conceptualization of PNES as symptom vs. disease

Most current approaches to classification of PNES within existing psychiatric classification schemes conceptualize PNES as either a symptom of a psychiatric disease or as a distinct disease entity. Some authors consider PNES to be an *atypical* symptom or manifestation of an existing disorder [54, 87]. On the other hand, some authors suggest that PNES represent a qualitatively distinct category of symptom, such as "medically unexplained symptoms (MUS)," that are often part of a more chronic, complex disorder, such as somatoform or dissociative disorder [62]. In terms of conceptualizing PNES as a symptom, many studies provide a list of diagnostic categories into which PNES may be classified or report proportions of patients with PNES that meet diagnostic criteria for various DSM disorders [81]. Authors who conceptualize PNES as a distinct disease entity are likely to advocate adapting existing classification schemes [62, 80].

In summary, classification of PNES based on psychiatric phenomena that either precipitate or lead to PNES may be helpful in understanding the etiology of PNES and selecting treatment. Designing such classification is challenging, as semiology and etiology of PNES vary; moreover, there is no single psychiatric condition to which PNES can be reliably/uniquely attributed. Despite these issues, however, the majority of patients with PNES fall in the existing categories of conversion or dissociative disorders.

Suggestions for changing the classification of PNES in DSM

Several authors have suggested changing DSM-IV in order to foster more detailed, accurate, and logically consistent classification of PNES. For example, Martin and Gates proposed amending DSM-IV via a detailed, DSM-compatible nosology and classification of "seizure-like events" [80]. This model is discussed and updated in Chapter 21. The original scheme suggested by Martin and Gates, which includes a decision tree for differential diagnosis, classifies all "seizure-like events" into the following categories: ES, symptomatic seizures (i.e., nonepileptic seizures of physiological origin), and PNES. In contrast, a recent, comprehensive review of the issue by Brown *et al.* suggested that the authors of the upcoming DSM-V move "pseudoneurological" (i.e., conversion) symptoms from the Somatoform to the Dissociative Disorders [62]. Their reasoning for this proposed shift was that pseudoneurological and dissociative symptoms may result from the same psychological process, and may be best regarded as different symptoms of the same underlying syndrome. Others have suggested that it would be better to make finer distinctions between and within somatoform and dissociative categories than to lump different presentations together into a single "functional" syndrome [88].

Summary

Psychogenic nonepileptic seizures have been recognized for millennia, but not until recently have diagnostic tools, such as VEEG allowed clinicians a greater degree of certainty in confirming the diagnosis. Patients with PNES are frequently encountered by clinicians – it is important for epileptologists to be aware of this diagnosis and to be willing to provide appropriate diagnostic evaluation and subsequent treatment disposition. With a history of trauma or abuse, the majority of patients with PNES are classified under the Conversion Disorder diagnosis. Further research is needed to determine if diagnostic schemes subdividing PNES based on clinical characteristics or results of personality testing, risk factors, or psychiatric diagnoses may be helpful in identifying subsets of patients who may respond to certain therapeutic interventions. Moreover, subdividing patients with PNES into reliable, commonly recognized subgroups may allow additional insight into the etiology of this challenging clinical entity, beyond what is already established.

References

1. Szaflarski JP, Hughes C, Szaflarski M, *et al.* Quality of life in psychogenic nonepileptic seizures. *Epilepsia* 2003;**44**(2):236–42.
2. King DW, Gallagher BB, Murvin AJ, *et al.* Pseudoseizures: diagnostic evaluation. *Neurology* 1982;**32**(1):18–23.
3. Mace CJ, Trimble MR. 'Hysteria', 'functional' or 'psychogenic'? A survey of British neurologists' preferences. *J R Soc Med* 1991;**84**(8):471–5.
4. Scull DA. Pseudoseizures or non-epileptic seizures (NES); 15 synonyms. *J Neurol Neurosurg Psychiatry* 1997;**62**(2):200.
5. Szaflarski JP, Ficker DM, Cahill WT, Privitera MD. Four-year incidence of psychogenic nonepileptic seizures in adults in Hamilton County, OH. *Neurology* 2000;**55**(10):1561–3.
6. Vanderzant CW, Giordani B, Berent S, Dreifuss FE, Sackellares JC. Personality of patients with pseudoseizures. *Neurology* 1986;**36**(5):664–8.
7. Reuber M, Fernandez G, Bauer J, Helmstaedter C, Elger CE. Diagnostic delay in psychogenic nonepileptic seizures. *Neurology* 2002;**58**(3):493–5.
8. Harden CL, Burgut FT, Kanner AM. The diagnostic significance of video-EEG monitoring findings on pseudoseizure patients differs between neurologists and psychiatrists. *Epilepsia* 2003;**44**(3):453–6.
9. Sigurdardottir KR, Olafsson E. Incidence of psychogenic seizures in adults: a population-based study in Iceland. *Epilepsia* 1998;**39**(7):749–52.
10. Meierkord H, Will B, Fish D, Shorvon S. The clinical features and prognosis of pseudoseizures diagnosed using video-EEG telemetry. *Neurology* 1991;**41**(10):1643–6.
11. Hauser WA, Annegers JF, Kurland LT. Incidence of epilepsy and unprovoked seizures in Rochester, Minnesota: 1935–1984. *Epilepsia* 1993;**34**(3):453–68.
12. Sirven JI, Glosser DS. Psychogenic nonepileptic seizures: theoretic and clinical considerations. *Neuropsychiatry Neuropsychol Behav Neurol* 1998;**11**(4):225–35.
13. Benbadis SR, Hauser AW. An estimate of the prevalence of psychogenic non-epileptic seizures. *Seizure* 2000;**9**(4):280–1.
14. Martin RC, Gilliam FG, Kilgore M, Faught E, Kuzniecky R. Improved health care resource utilization following video-EEG-confirmed diagnosis of nonepileptic psychogenic seizures. *Seizure* 1998;**7**(5):385–90.
15. Sutula TP, Sackellares JC, Miller JQ, Dreifuss FE. Intensive monitoring in refractory epilepsy. *Neurology* 1981;**31**(3):243–7.
16. Benbadis SR, Agrawal V, Tatum IV, WO. How many patients with psychogenic nonepileptic seizures also have epilepsy? *Neurology* 2001;**57**(5):915–17.

17. LaFrance Jr WC. Psychogenic nonepileptic seizures. *Curr Opin Neurol* 2008;**21**(2):195–201.
18. Griffith NM, Szaflarski JP, Schefft BK, et al. Relationship between semiology of psychogenic nonepileptic seizures and Minnesota Multiphasic Personality Inventory profile. *Epilepsy Behav* 2007; **11**(1):105–11.
19. Selwa LM, Geyer J, Nikakhtar N, *et al.* Nonepileptic seizure outcome varies by type of spell and duration of illness. *Epilepsia* 2000;**41**(10):1330–4.
20. Gates J. Epidemiology and classification of non-epileptic seizures. In: Gates JR, Rowan AJ, eds. *Non-Epileptic Seizures*, 2nd edn. Boston, MA: Butterworth-Heinemann. 2000; 3–15.
21. Cragar DE, Berry DT, Schmitt FA, Fakhoury TA. Cluster analysis of normal personality traits in patients with psychogenic nonepileptic seizures. *Epilepsy Behav* 2005;**6**(4):593–600.
22. Reuber M, Pukrop R, Bauer J, *et al.* Outcome in psychogenic nonepileptic seizures: 1 to 10-year follow-up in 164 patients. *Ann Neurol* 2003;**53**(3): 305–11.
23. Trimble MR. Pseudoseizures. *Neurol Clin* 1986;**4**(3): 531–48.
24. Kretschmer E. *Hysteria*. New York: Nervous and Mental Disease Publ. Co., 1926.
25. Blumer D, Adamolekun B. Treatment of patients with coexisting epileptic and nonepileptic seizures. *Epilepsy Behav* 2006;**9**(3):498–502.
26. Reuber M, Pukrop R, Bauer J, Derfuss R, Elger CE. Multidimensional assessment of personality in patients with psychogenic nonepileptic seizures. *J Neurol Neurosurg Psychiatry* 2004;**75**(5):743–8.
27. Wilkus RJ, Dodrill CB. Factors affecting the outcome of MMPI and neuropsychological assessments of psychogenic and epileptic seizure patients. *Epilepsia* 1989;**30**(3):339–47.
28. Gulick TA, Spinks IP, King DW. Pseudoseizures: ictal phenomena. *Neurology* 1982;**32**(1):24–30.
29. Henry TR, Drury I. Ictal behaviors during nonepileptic seizures differ in patients with temporal lobe interictal epileptiform EEG activity and patients without interictal epileptiform EEG abnormalities. *Epilepsia* 1998;**39**(2):175–82.
30. Flugel D, Bauer J, Kaseborn U, Burr W, Elger C. Closed eyes during a seizure indicate psychogenic etiology: a study with suggestive seizure provocation. *J Epilepsy* 1996;**9**:165–9.
31. Gumnit RJ, Gates JR. Psychogenic seizures. *Epilepsia* 1986;**27** Suppl 2:S124–9.
32. van Merode T, de Krom MC, Knottnerus JA. Gender-related differences in non-epileptic attacks: a study of patients' cases in the literature. *Seizure* 1997;**6**(4): 311–6.
33. Groppel G, Kapitany T, Baumgartner C. Cluster analysis of clinical seizure semiology of psychogenic nonepileptic seizures. *Epilepsia* 2000;**41**(5):610–4.
34. Dworetzky BA, Strahonja-Packard A, Shanahan CW, *et al.* Characteristics of male veterans with psychogenic nonepileptic seizures. *Epilepsia* 2005;**46**(9):1418–22.
35. Cragar D, Berry D, Fakhoury T, Cibula J, Schmitt F. A review of diagnostic techniques in the differential diagnosis of epileptic and nonepileptic seizures. *Neuropsychol Rev* 2002;**12**(1):31–64.
36. Dodrill C, Wilkus R, Batzel L. The MMPI as a diagnostic tool in nonpileptic seizures. In: Rowan AJ, Gates JR, eds. *Non-Epileptic Seizures*. Boston, MA: Butterworth-Heinemann. 1993; 211–19.
37. King TZ, Fennell EB, Bauer R, *et al.* MMPI-2 profiles of patients with intractable epilepsy. *Arch Clin Neuropsychol* 2002;**17**(6):583–93.
38. Kalogjera-Sackellares D, Sackellares JC. Personality profiles of patients with pseudoseizures. *Seizure* 1997;**6**(1):1–7.
39. Kuyk J, Swinkels WA, Spinhoven P. Psychopathologies in patients with nonepileptic seizures with and without comorbid epilepsy: how different are they? *Epilepsy Behav* 2003;**4**(1):13–8.
40. Reuber M, Howlett S, Kemp S. Psychologic treatment of patients with psychogenic nonepileptic seizures. *Expert Rev Neurother* 2005;**5**(6):737–52.
41. Barrash J, Gates J, Heck D, Benial T, eds. MMPI subtypes among patients with nonepileptic events. Annual Meeting of the American Epilepsy Society; 1989. Boston, MA; New York: Raven Press, Ltd.
42. American Psychiatric Association. *Diagnostic and Statistical Manual of Mental Disorders*, 4th edn., Text Revision (DSM-IV-TR). Washington, DC: American Psychiatric Association, 2000.
43. Reuber M. Psychogenic nonepileptic seizures: answers and questions. *Epilepsy Behav* 2008;**12**(4): 622–35.
44. Livesley WJ, Jackson DN, Schroeder ML. Factorial structure of traits delineating personality disorders in clinical and general population samples. *J Abnorm Psychol* 1992;**101**(3):432–40.
45. Chang E, ed. *Optimism & Pessimism: Implications for Theory, Research, and Practice*. Washington, DC: American Psychological Association, 2002.
46. Gillham J, ed. *The Science of Optimism and Hope: Research Essays in Honor of Martin E. P. Seligman*. Philadelphia: Templeton Foundation Press, 2000.
47. Costa P, McCrae R. *NEO-PI-R Professional Manual*. Odessa, FL: Psychological Assessment Resources, Inc., 1992.

48. Alsaadi TM, Marquez AV. Psychogenic nonepileptic seizures. *Am Fam Physician* 2005;**72**(5):849–56.
49. Lesser RP. Treatment and outcome of psychogenic nonepileptic seizures. *Epilepsy Curr* 2003;**3**(6): 198–200.
50. Ford C. Somatization and nonepileptic seizures. In: Rowan AJ, Gates JR, eds. *Non-Epileptic Seizures.* Boston, MA: Butterworth-Heinemann. 1993; 153–64.
51. Bowman ES. Etiology and clinical course of pseudoseizures. Relationship to trauma, depression, and dissociation. *Psychosomatics* 1993;**34**(4):333–42.
52. Bowman ES, Markand ON. Psychodynamics and psychiatric diagnoses of pseudoseizure subjects. *Am J Psychiatry* 1996;**153**(1):57–63.
53. Rusch MD, Morris GL, Allen L, Lathrop L. Psychological treatment of nonepileptic events. *Epilepsy Behav* 2001;**2**(3):277–83.
54. LaFrance WC, Jr, Devinsky O. Treatment of nonepileptic seizures. *Epilepsy Behav* 2002; **3**(5 Suppl):19–23.
55. Kanner AM, Morris HH, Luders H, et al. Supplementary motor seizures mimicking pseudoseizures: some clinical differences. *Neurology* 1990;**40**(9):1404–7.
56. Saygi S, Katz A, Marks DA, Spencer SS. Frontal lobe partial seizures and psychogenic seizures: comparison of clinical and ictal characteristics. *Neurology* 1992;**42**(7):1274–7.
57. Zivin L, Marsan CA. Incidence and prognostic significance of "epileptiform" activity in the EEG of non-epileptic subjects. *Brain* 1968;**91**(4):751–78.
58. Lin JT, Ziegler DK, Lai CW, Bayer W. Convulsive syncope in blood donors. *Ann Neurol* 1982;**11**(5): 525–8.
59. Aminoff MJ, Scheinman MM, Griffin JC, Herre JM. Electrocerebral accompaniments of syncope associated with malignant ventricular arrhythmias. *Ann Intern Med* 1988;**108**(6):791–6.
60. Kleindorfer D, Panagos P, Pancioli A, et al. Incidence and short-term prognosis of transient ischemic attack in a population-based study. *Stroke* 2005;**36**(4):720–3.
61. Stewart WF, Linet MS, Celentano DD, Van Natta M, Ziegler D. Age- and sex-specific incidence rates of migraine with and without visual aura. *Am J Epidemiol* 1991;**134**(10):1111–20.
62. Brown RJ, Cardena E, Nijenhuis E, Sar V, Van Der Hart O. Should conversion disorder be reclassified as a dissociative disorder in DSM V? *Psychosomatics* 2007;**48**(5):369–78.
63. Brown RJ, Trimble MR. Dissociative psychopathology, non-epileptic seizures, and neurology. *J Neurol Neurosurg Psychiatry* 2000;**69**(3):285–9.
64. Reuber M, House AO. Treating patients with psychogenic non-epileptic seizures. *Curr Opin Neurol* 2002;**15**(2):207–11.
65. Reuber M, Elger CE. Psychogenic nonepileptic seizures: review and update. *Epilepsy Behav* 2003;**4**(3):205–16.
66. Reuber M, Howlett S, Khan A, Grunewald RA. Non-epileptic seizures and other functional neurological symptoms: predisposing, precipitating, and perpetuating factors. *Psychosomatics* 2007;**48**(3): 230–8.
67. Torem M. Non-epileptic seizures as a dissocative disorder. In: Rowan AJ, Gates JR, eds. *Non-Epileptic Seizures.* Boston, MA: Butterworth-Heinemann. 1993; 173–9.
68. Prueter C, Schultz-Venrath U, Rimpau W. Dissociative and associated psychopathological symptoms in patients with epilepsy, pseudoseizures, and both seizure forms. *Epilepsia* 2002;**43**(2):188–92.
69. van Merode T, Twellaar M, Kotsopoulos IA, et al. Psychological characteristics of patients with newly developed psychogenic seizures. *J Neurol Neurosurg Psychiatry* 2004;**75**(8):1175–7.
70. Fleisher W, Staley D, Krawetz P, et al. Comparative study of trauma-related phenomena in subjects with pseudoseizures and subjects with epilepsy. *Am J Psychiatry* 2002;**159**(4):660–3.
71. Kuyk J, Van Dyck R, Spinhoven P. The case for a dissociative interpretation of pseudoepileptic seizures. *J Nerv Ment Dis* 1996;**184**(8):468–74.
72. Alper K, Devinsky O, Perrine K, et al. Dissociation in epilepsy and conversion nonepileptic seizures. *Epilepsia* 1997;**38**(9):991–7.
73. Alper K, Devinsky O, Perrine K, Vazquez B, Luciano D. Psychiatric classification of nonconversion nonepileptic seizures. *Arch Neurol* 1995;**52**(2): 199–201.
74. Reuber M, House AO, Pukrop R, Bauer J, Elger CE. Somatization, dissociation and general psychopathology in patients with psychogenic non-epileptic seizures. *Epilepsy Res* 2003;**57**(2–3): 159–67.
75. Tojek TM, Lumley M, Barkley G, Mahr G, Thomas A. Stress and other psychosocial characteristics of patients with psychogenic nonepileptic seizures. *Psychosomatics* 2000;**41**:221–6.
76. Harden CL. Pseudoseizures and dissociative disorders: a common mechanism involving traumatic experiences. *Seizure* 1997;**6**(2):151–5.
77. WHO. World Health Organization. *The ICD-10 Classification of Mental and Behavioural Disorders: Clinical Descriptions and Diagnostic Guidelines.*

Geneva, Switzerland: World Health Organization, 1992.

78. American Psychiatric Association. *Diagnostic and Statistical Manual of Mental Disorders*, 2nd edn. (DSM II). Washington, DC: American Psychiatric Association, 1968.

79. American Psychiatric Association. *Diagnostic and Statistical Manual of Mental Disorders*, 3rd edn. (DSM III). Washington, DC: American Psychiatric Association, 1980.

80. Martin R, Gates J. Nosology, classification, and differential diagnosis of nonepileptic seizures: an alternative proposal. In: Gates JR, Rowan AJ, eds. *Non-Epileptic Seizures*, 2nd edn. Boston, MA: Butterworth-Heinemann. 2000; 253–67.

81. Bowman ES. Nonepileptic seizures: psychiatric framework, treatment, and outcome. *Neurology* 1999;**53**(5 Suppl 2):S84–8.

82. Lacey C, Cook M, Salzberg M. The neurologist, psychogenic nonepileptic seizures, and borderline personality disorder. *Epilepsy Behav* 2007;**11**(4):492–8.

83. Chabolla DR, Krahn LE, So EL, Rummans TA. Psychogenic nonepileptic seizures. *Mayo Clin Proc* 1996;**71**(5):493–500.

84. Gates JR. Nonepileptic seizures: classification, coexistence with epilepsy, diagnosis, therapeutic approaches, and consensus. *Epilepsy Behav* 2002;**3**(1):28–33.

85. Fiszman A, Alves-Leon SV, Nunes RG, D'Andrea I, Figueira I. Traumatic events and posttraumatic stress disorder in patients with psychogenic nonepileptic seizures: a critical review. *Epilepsy Behav* 2004;**5**(6):818–25.

86. Brewin CR, Andrews B, Rose S, Kirk M. Acute stress disorder and posttraumatic stress disorder in victims of violent crime. *Am J Psychiatry* 1999;**156**(3):360–6.

87. LaFrance WC, Jr, Barry JJ. Update on treatments of psychological nonepileptic seizures. *Epilepsy Behav* 2005;**7**(3):364–74.

88. Wessely S, White PD. There is only one functional somatic syndrome. *Br J Psychiatry* 2004;**185**:95–6.

Section 1 Chapter 2

Recognition, diagnosis, and impact of nonepileptic seizures

Psychogenic nonepileptic seizures: historical overview

Michael Trimble

Hysteria, as the condition is fondly called, is as old as the earliest medical texts from Egyptian and Greek cultures. Originally this referred to a concept of the origin of symptoms, found exclusively in women, due to the wandering womb, which, being frustrated by lack of proper use, leaves its anatomical position and travels around the body causing pressure in anomalous places, and hence symptoms. Although there has been an academic debate about what the Egyptians and subsequently the Greeks actually were referring to when they discussed the wandering womb, the early history reflects on three important points: symptoms such as are seen today were seen over 2000 years ago, across at least two different cultures, and that the postulated mechanism was gender related.

Examples of the reported symptoms include the classical globus hystericus, caused by pressure from the wandering uterus on the throat, and paralyses, but central to the evolving history of the subject was convulsions.

Middle Ages

The Middle Ages, with its neo-Platonic papal stranglehold on developing scientific thought, and thus on the medical sciences, conflated the manifestations that we would now view as hysteria with those of witchcraft. The *Malleus Maleficarum* was used since the late 1400s as a text on identification of signs of witchcraft, including the presence of seizures [1]. Witchcraft became a statutory crime in 1541 in Europe, a date which heralded two hundred years of witch-hunting and persecution. The detection of witches became paramount, and stigmata were identified. In particular, "witches-patches" – areas of sensory anesthesia were recorded, but the muscular contortions and convulsions of the afflicted were well noted.

Edward Jorden (1569–1632), a physician of London and Bath, wrote a treatise in 1603 called "A brief discourse of a disease called the suffocation of the mother" [2] (alluding to comments from ancient Greece, by Aretaeus [3]), essentially to counteract the prevailing mood which was to attribute such symptoms to possession by some supernatural power. His view was that the so-thought stigmata of hysteria were in fact signs of mental illness, thus reclaiming, for the first time since Hippocrates, the essentially medical, somatic nature of the phenomena.

His book was occasioned by a trial in 1602, in which a charwoman, Elizabeth Jackson, was accused of bewitching the 14-year-old Mary Glover. The latter had convulsions, episodes of loss of speech, periodic blindness, paralysis and loss of sensation of the left side of the body, aggressivity, and personality changes. Jorden recognized the polymorphous nature of the symptoms, its link to the female sex, and the importance of "perturbations of the mind" in the cause of the disorder.

Outbreaks of mass hysteria, in which groups of people manifested mainly motor abnormalities, were well described in the Middle Ages, and culminated in the grand chorea epidemics of Europe. Outbursts of St. Vitus' dance, Tarantism, *convulsionnaires* and the like referred to groups of people, from half a dozen to several hundred, who would display exaggerated movements, dance, and convulse until they dropped exhausted. Many episodes were noted in relation to natural disasters, for example after the spread of the great plague, but other outbreaks came in closely knit social groups, often united by some strong religious belief. These phenomena emphasized the imitative nature of many hysterical afflictions, and the powerful role of social and cultural pressure, and contagion in their pathogenesis.

Gates and Rowan's Nonepileptic Seizures, 3rd edn. ed. Steven C. Schachter and W. Curt LaFrance, Jr. Published by Cambridge University Press. © S. Schachter and W. C. LaFrance, Jr. 2010.

Willis and the beginnings of neurology

Concepts of etiology thus slowly moved from the supernatural to the natural. The uterus remained popular, but several other shifts of emphasis occurred. The uterine theories slowly gave way to two interpenetrating themes, namely that the main organ involved in hysteria was the brain, and that somehow emotions were highly relevant. The English neurologist Thomas Willis (1621–75) was one of the first to espouse the central importance of the brain. He reflected that "this passion comes not from the vapours rising into the head from the uterus or spleen, nor from a rapid flow of blood into the pulmonary vessels, but has its origin in the brain itself" [4, p. 87]. He was led to this conclusion, not only following postmortem examinations and by his clinical observations of the disorder in prepubertal and senile women, but by the irreconcilable fact that he observed hysteria in men! For Willis the condition was primarily convulsive: "the distemper named from the womb is chiefly and primarily convulsive, and chiefly depends on the brain and nervous stock being affected." Hysterical fits were caused by "spirits inhabiting the brain, now being prepared for explosions" [5]. Since in further studies Willis came to the conclusion that it was the animal spirits in the middle part of the brain that were disturbed in epilepsy, he must have thought that both epileptic and non-epileptic convulsions have a similar iatrochemical basis.

The emphasis on the emotions was taken up by several writers, including Willis and Thomas Sydenham (1624–89). The later opined that of all chronic medical conditions, next to infections, hysteria in his practice was the commonest, afflicting one-sixth of patients. Not only did Sydenham suggest the chronic nature of the condition, but he hinted at personality contributions. Patients were prone to irritability and anger outbursts, they were capricious, and labile in their moods and affections. He firmly placed the origins of hysteria in the mind, referring to "over-ordinate commotions of the mind," with a "faulty disposition of the animal spirits" [6, p. 85].

Associations with what we may now refer to as depression were noted in Burton's *Anatomy of Melancholy* [7], and the concept that the mind could influence the body, a precursor of twentieth-century psychosomatic concepts, became well accepted. The Scottish physician Sir Robert Whytt (1714–66), discoverer of reflex activity in the nervous system, and one who recognized that the mind could cause actions not appreciated by consciousness, discussed the newly invented term "nervous disorders," namely those "which, on account of an unusual delicacy, or unnatural state of the nerves, are produced by causes, which, in people of a sound constitution, would either have no such effects, or at least in a much less degree" [8, p. 102]. In a passage which antedated the later importance given to psychologically traumatic events, he opined: "Thus doleful or moving stories, horrible or unexpected sights, great grief, anger, terror and other passions, frequently occasion the most sudden and violent nervous symptoms…" [8, p. 206].

Eighteenth and nineteenth centuries

The close links between hysteria and epilepsy continued throughout the eighteenth and nineteenth centuries. Boerhaave (1668–1738) felt that hysteria could degenerate into epilepsy, and Cheyne, in his book *The English Malady or a Treatise of Nervous Diseases of all Kinds as Spleen, Vapours, Lowness of Spirits, Hypochondriacal and Hysterical Distempers, etc.* [9], noted few differences between epilepsy and hysteria, saying that the former "differs very little or not at all, or at most in a few circumstances only, from Hypochondriacal and Hysteric Fits: which last when violent, terminate always in these Epileptik Fits, as they, on the other hand, when they become weak, dwindle into the Hysterik Kind" [9].

Themes of either sexual frustration or sexual excess in hysteria, while tending to wane in the eighteenth century, and inherent in such names as the *hysteria libidinosa* (Boissier de Sauvages 1706–67), or *furor uterinus* continued to resurface. Thomas Laycock (1812–76), teacher of Hughlings Jackson (1835–1911), wrote about the reciprocal relationships between the body and mind, developing a biologically orientated scientific psychology. He believed that in hysteria the nervous system was implicated, that it was seen in the majority of cases in females of childbearing ages, and therefore the generative organs were involved in the pathogenesis. The condition often came on following grief, terror, fear, or disappointment in love; these emotional events exciting deranged actions in the generative system and thence the hysterical phenomena [10].

Laycock's investigations took him to speculate into the nature of the mind, and on the role of consciousness in these phenomena. Following on from Whytt's studies of reflex activity, and Marshall Hall's

(1790–1857) demonstration in animals of the spinal reflex arc, Laycock suggested that the cerebrum (cranial ganglia) was also a reflex center like the spinal ganglia, and he developed his law of the unconscious functional activity of the brain. This was several decades before the Freudian elaboration.

The general practitioner, later ophthalmologist, Robert Brudenell Carter (1828–1918), divided hysteria into two main forms, simple, which manifest essentially as hysterical seizures, and complicated. The latter, foreboding the later Briquet's form, "generally involves much moral and intellectual, as well as physical derangement, and when it is fully established, the primary convulsion, the *fons et origo mali* is sometimes suffered to fall into obeyance…being arrested by the urgency of new maladies" [11, pp. 28–9]. He implicated sexual emotions as causative, and shifted the whole debate away from pathology of the sexual organs to inhibited sexual passions. This was, according to Veith [12], the first theory of repression. Emotions led to physical disorders by somatic discharge, affects provoking the wide range of motor and sensory states seen in the condition. Interestingly, Carter also observed the factitious nature of the illness in many patients, some using leaches in the mouth to produce bleeding, or bandages to cause limb swellings and the like. Although since the time of Sydenham, the chameleon-like nature of hysteria was recognized, and its simulative nature alluded to, this seems one of the first texts to raise the question of patient motives and actions more directly.

Thus, summarizing the history of hysteria to the mid-nineteenth century, several statements can be made. The condition hysteria had been recognized for centuries, and had been the source of much speculation regarding etiology and pathogenesis. Certainly, it is not clear how many patients falling under this diagnosis given by earlier physicians were in reality not suffering from now recognized neurological disorders, and many diagnostic and nosological confusions existed. However, trends and general statements can be noted. Causation shifted away from the uterus to the brain, and then to the mind. Psychosomatic concepts were readily accepted, emotions, but especially sexual emotions, discharging through the somatic apparatus provoked the polymorphous, often bizarre symptomatology recognized as hysteria. The potential chronicity of the condition was recognized, as was its occurrence in males. Certain types of people, that is certain personality types, seemed more susceptible, and external exciting causes such as accidents could be relevant. Convulsions were often specifically discussed as an emblem.

Further developments: the French school

The mid- to late-nineteenth century saw a further blending of hysteria with epilepsy with the introduction by the French physicians of the term "hystero-epilepsy." This implied an association of the two disorders, and while most accepted that there were *accés-distincts*, where a clear differential diagnosis between an epileptic attack and a hysterical seizure was possible, others claimed the existence of *accés-distincts – complexes* in which both epileptic and hysterical symptoms were combined, so as to make a distinction between these two impossible. At the same time, the concept of epilepsy became expanded, to include a wide range of clinical phenomena. Todd (1809–60) used the term "epileptiform" to describe seizures in which consciousness was not impaired, and in which unilateral convulsive movements were noted, which may "pass into the true epileptic fit" [13]. The German neuropsychiatrist Griesinger (1817–68), who introduced the term psychomotor, referred to "epileptoid" conditions, and Hughlings Jackson discussed at length the associated phenomena of epilepsy. For him there were many epilepsies as opposed to one discrete disease, and the borderland covered "all conditions in which there is a transient impairment of voluntary motor power, sensation or consciousness," which included not only an episode of migraine but also a sneeze [14].

As the nineteenth century progressed, there was an explosion of interest in hysteria, but the main writings came not from England, but from France. Not only did the sexual theme become revived, but also the concept of posttraumatic hysteria crystallized. Some of the early-nineteenth-century French physicians, such as Pinel (1745–1826), Louyer-Villermay (1776–1837), and Landouzy (1845–1917) reverted to uterine theories, challenging the concept of male hysteria. However, cerebral origins of hysteria found increasing support through Georget (1795–1828) and Pierre Briquet (1796–1881). The latter was chief physician to the Paris *Charité*, and he readily admitted that he undertook to study hysteria as a matter of duty, on account of the frequency of cases that he reluctantly had to examine. His book *Traité Clinique et Thérapeutique de l'Hystérie*

Section 1: Recognition, diagnosis, and impact

[15] reported on the results of personal examinations of nearly 450 patients, and stands as the nineteenth-century landmark in hysteria studies, having a considerable influence on Charcot and his school.

Briquet firmly rejected uterine theories, and described a series of cases in males. He outlined the multifarious symptoms, including the spasms, anesthesias, convulsions, paralyses, and contractures, which by then had become familiar in descriptions of patients diagnosed with hysteria. In one table he refers to the length of time that the symptoms lasted. Of 418 patients, 179 had the condition for between six months and four years, 81 between five and ten years, and of the rest, lasting a longer time, in 59 patients the condition lasted longer than 20 years, in 5 patients for 55 years. These patients were polysymptomatic, "des troubles permanents qui portent sur presque tous les organes" [15, p. 519]. Thus, these descriptions were clearly forerunners of the later christened Briquet's hysteria.

As to pathogenesis, he was clear that it was a condition of that portion of the brain which received sensations and affective impressions, and he described hysteria as a nervousness (neurosis) of the encephalon. However, he recognized many interacting factors. These included heredity and emotional predisposition; impressionability and emotional lability were also characteristic. He cited several antecedents, including the excitement of accidents and physical abuse. Incidentally, Briquet was critical of the term hysteria, but felt it should be continued to be used because it had been in use so long and everyone understood its meaning.

The hysteria mantle then fell to Charcot (1825–93), the doyen of mid- to late-nineteenth-century French neurology, and his school of successors, many of whom also wrote on the subject of hysteria. Working at the Salpêtrière, where he became chief of neurology, he observed in detail the clinical phenomenology of cases of hysteria. It was his view that hysteria should be treated as any other neurological condition, and by sufficient and detailed observations it should be possible to define its cause and course, the former being sought in the brain. Hysteria major (*la grande hystérie*) was hysteria with convulsions. He documented the physical stigmata of hysteria in considerable detail. These included anesthetic patches, often involving the whole of one side of the body, contraction of the visual fields, and, interestingly, ovarian tenderness, a reversion to the genital region. Hysteria in his view was rarely monosymptomatic, and often chronic.

It is known that Charcot's later theories moved towards a more psychological approach. This was partly due to his work with hypnotism, but also because of his observations of traumatic hysteria. He tended away from the use of the term hysteria, and preferred the expression "neurosis." By hypnotizing patients, he was able to demonstrate that symptoms of hysteria could be produced, or resolved, but importantly, that in posttraumatic cases, the identical symptoms to the posttraumatic symptoms could be reproduced. He therefore did not accept any fundamental difference between hysteria of traumatic and nontraumatic origin.

For Charcot and his school, it remained the nervous system which was abnormal, and his invocation of hereditary factors was related to the predominant place of degenerative theories in nineteenth-century neurology. Not all people would succumb to hysteria, or could be hypnotized, only those with certain nervous constitutions, which reflected hereditary and sometimes moral degeneration. Although it is often contended that Charcot never moved away from his neurological approach to understanding the symptoms of hysteria, his ideas are clearly a herald to some of the later developed Freudian theories. They are also a reaffirmation of the importance placed on suggestion in the evolving symptomatology.

With regards to hysterical convulsions, Briquet felt that hysteria with mixed attacks was in reality a particular form of hysteria, namely very intense hysteria, and the prognosis was that of this condition, and not that of epilepsy. Charcot distinguished epilepsy from hysteria, and noted in particular alterations of temperature that were different following repeated attacks in the two disorders. As an alternative to hystero-epilepsy, he used the term "hysteria major" to describe hysteria that presented with convulsive patterns. By careful clinical observation, the Salpêtrière school outlined several stages of the convulsive attacks, called respectively the prodromal stage, the epileptoid stage, the period of clownism, the period of emotional attitudes, and the period of delirium. In the third stage, the characteristic "*arc de cercle*" was seen, in which the trunk is raised, and the body rests on the feet and occiput only (Figure 2.1).

By defining the other stigmata of hysteria, Charcot heightened the differential diagnosis between different forms of attacks. In particular,

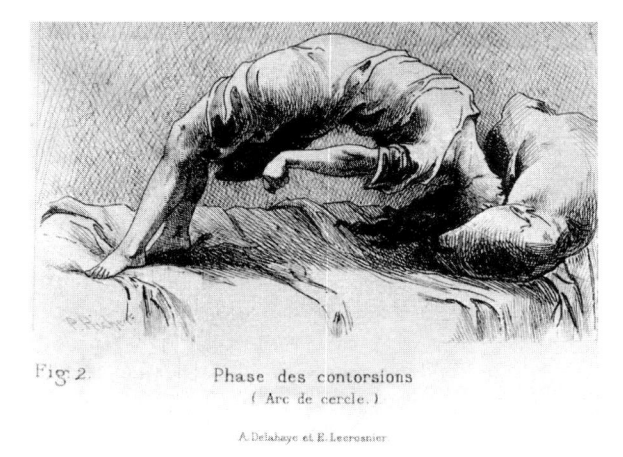

Figure 2.1. Arc de cercle.

an accompanying nonanatomical anesthesia was important for the diagnosis of hysteria: "its well established existence is, therefore, a valuable indication, one which will often reveal the real nature of many symptoms, which would otherwise remain doubtful" [16].

Another important investigator from the French school was Pierre Janet (1859–1947). His theories became overridden by Freudian ideologies, but in recent times, with a renewal of interest in the phenomenon of dissociation, a revival of Janet's views has occurred. He initially studied philosophy, but started experimenting with hypnosis at Le Havre, and then studied medicine in Paris, spending time at the Salpêtrière where he examined Charcot's patients. Charcot encouraged him to study experimental psychology, and patients with hysteria and neurasthenia became his main interest. By careful analysis of the patients' symptoms and the content of their mental states, he developed a scheme that related to subconscious mental ideas, which themselves were related to traumatic events, and which could become replaced by symptoms. The mechanism was through a narrowing of the patients' consciousness, related to a weakening of psychological synthesis. Subconscious fixed ideas could be clarified through hypnosis (or by examining dreams), and their exposure provided a therapeutic avenue (Janet always claimed that psychoanalysis was an extension of his ideas, and that he discovered the method of cathartic cure).

Janet also emphasized the importance of patients' predispositions, an elaboration of the degeneracy ideas, as these abnormal tendencies were not only preponderant in hysteria, but were related to fundamental properties of the brain. He developed further the concept of symptoms being dependent on ideas, noting that suggestibility is important, but there also existed "a number of mental states anterior to suggestibility" [17, p. 227]. Suggestion, in which there is "complete and automatic development of an idea," takes place "outside the will and personal perception of the subject" [17, p. 251]. These were, for him, subconscious acts. In the same way that ideas can become associated, so they can be dissociated, and dissociated ideas can have their own independent existence. There is a dissociation of mental unity, and "at the moment of suggestion there is a shock, an emotion which destroys the feeble personal synthesis of the subject. The suggested idea remains isolated, more or less completely separated from the other ideas; it can then develop and suppress all else, or even foreign thoughts…a tendency to suggestion and subconscious acts is the sign of mental disease, but it is above all, the sign of hysteria" [17, pp. 275–6]. These fixed ideas grow, and install themselves in the mind, in a phrase of Charcot's, quoted by Janet, "like parasites." The links with the later developed Freudian idea of repression is clear. For Janet, convulsive episodes were a variety of somnambulism beginning as somnambulisms, particularly related to events which excited the affect. He discussed association of ideas in which perceptions and remembrances would bring on the seizure as they were linked in the patient's mind [17]. He discussed "associations of ideas" in which "the dreaded perception and the remembrances which bring on the fit" are linked in the patient's mind [17]. The actual pattern of the seizure was thus an ensemble of emotional expressions, such as anger but also eroticism.

Freud and his followers

The story of how the Viennese neurologist Sigmund Freud (1856–1939) went to Paris for five months in 1885/6 to study with Charcot is well known. Although he still busied himself with neuropathology, he swiftly fell under Charcot's spell, and his interest in psychology crystallized. He returned to Vienna, and presented to the local society of physicians a case of traumatic hysteria in a male that he had seen with Charcot. This was not well received. Although hysteria in males was by that time accepted, to equate male hysteria with traumatic neurosis was unacceptable. Freud then felt obliged to present a case of his own, which he did a month later. The reception of this presentation was also lukewarm. Notwithstanding this rejection, as Freud saw it, from the medical establishment, he then pursued his interest in hypnosis with Joseph Breuer (1842–1925). The story, which led on to the development of psychoanalysis and his psychological elaborations of the structure of the human psyche, is well known. Hysterical symptoms related to traumatic ideas, absent from consciousness, could be uncovered by the analytic method. The unconscious mind, riven with conflicts, converted energies into physical symptoms, the latter resolving the psychic tension. To quote in full:

Our experiences have shown us, however, that the most various symptoms, which are ostensibly spontaneous and, as one might say, idiopathic products of hysteria, are just as strictly related to the precipitating trauma as the phenomena to which we have just alluded and which exhibit the connection quite clearly. The symptoms which we have been able to trace back to precipitating factors of this sort include neuralgias and anesthesias of various kinds, many of which had persisted for years, contractures and paralyses, hysterical attacks and epileptoid convulsions, which every observer regards as true epilepsy, petit mal and disorders in the nature of tic, chronic vomiting and anorexia, carried to the pitch of rejection of all nourishment, various forms of disturbance of vision, constantly recurring visual hallucinations, etc. The disproportion between the many years duration of the hysterical symptom and the single occurrence which provoked it is what we are accustomed invariably to find in traumatic neuroses. Quite frequently it is some event in childhood that sets up a more or less severe symptom which persists during the years that follow [18, 1893, p. 88].

Often the connection between the trauma and the symptom was a symbolic one. While initially Freud attributed the childhood event to some actual sexual seduction, he later turned to a fantasized trauma, leading him on to his theories of the developmental phases of the human mind, with its tripartite division into id, ego and superego, and the concepts of libidinal fixation and the Oedipus complex. One consequence of all of this was to reaffirm a common link between the pathogenesis of hysteria and traumatic hysteria. The memory of the trauma remains buried, but still working pathogenetically, hence the famous remark, "hysterics suffer mainly from reminiscences" [18, p. 91]. It was epigenetic; that is, postnatal and developmental factors, rather than any degenerative diathesis of the brain, were the keys to understanding these patients.

Mechanisms invoked included pathological association, dissociation, suppression – later to become repression, and primary gain, through which unconscious conflicts are resolved by symptom formation. The latter were causal, as opposed to secondary gains, which were seen as maintaining the symptoms, bringing relief from some disagreeable social situation or relationship. Conversion, a term not used originally by Freud, but which was used in an original way by him, thus referred to the psychologically converted physical symptoms. By now, neurosis had become a psychoneurosis, and hysteria was a paradigm.

Freud regarded the motor phenomena of hysterical attacks as appropriate to the affect that accompanied the memory of some past trauma and which was of importance in bringing about the hysteria. However, there clearly were relationships between epileptic and hysterical convulsions, which he explained as follows:

In infants, apart from the respiratory action of screaming, affects only produce and find expression in uncoordinated contractions of the muscles of the primitive kind – in arching the body and kicking about. As development proceeds the muscular passes more and more under the control of the power of co-ordination and the will, but the opisthotonus, which represents the maximum of motor effort of the total somatic musculature, and the clonic movements of the kicking and thrashing about persist throughout life as a form of reaction for the maximal excitation of the brain – for the purely physical excitation in epileptic attacks, as well as for the discharge of maximal affects in the shape of more or less epileptoid convulsions (viz. the purely motor part of hysterical attacks) [19].

A similar association between epilepsy and hysteria was observed and explained by other psychoanalytically inclined physicians. Pierce-Clarke [20] attempted to present a psychobiological theory of epilepsy, which used later Freudian ideas in attempting to explain certain types of epilepsy. He pointed out that in many cases of epilepsy no pathological disorder could be demonstrated, and from his own studies of patients with epilepsy he was able to discern certain patterns of developmental traits prior to the onset of epilepsy. He suggested that the fit itself served as an unconscious gratification for the libido. Thus in both epilepsy and the neuroses, infantile motives and the inadequate development of the individual's affects and instincts led to the development of symptoms.

Jelliffe and White in their 1929 textbook also considered this relationship by discussing energy and its flow within the nervous system [21]. This could be blocked at any level – psychic, sensory motor, and physicochemical – and in the classic epileptic attack all levels were involved. However, different "levels" could also be involved in other varieties of attacks. "The hysterical convulsion offers an example of a high level convulsive type of reaction…next lower in the scale of levels are the psycho-asthenic convulsions of Oppenheim (compulsion neurosis type), which are expressions of a more severe grade of neurosis…then come the very interesting affect epilepsies…distinctly epileptoid types of reaction conditioned by purely psychological situations." The epileptic seizure itself was considered as "a flight into unconsciousness," when occurring at times of stress. The fit was "…therefore a break in the life demand for adaptation or attempt at escape from an intolerable stimulus whether from within (toxin, tumour), or from without (live situation) (pages 101–102)."

Freud further discussed the mechanisms with regards to epilepsy and psychologically induced seizures with his study of Dostoevsky [22], linking his epilepsy to the Oedipus complex, suggesting its content as a punishment for fantasist parricide, and noting how the seizure satisfied guilt through masochism. Fenichel [23] reflected on the narcissistic regression of epilepsy, the energy tension in the brain being an expression of sadistic impulses. Stekel [24] described the epileptic seizure as an escape from an unbearable situation, the traumatic events that form the point of crystallization often residing in childhood events.

The twentieth century

Such ideas lived on well into the twentieth century, and became imbricated with the concept of the epileptic personality, which originally was seen as a psychoanalytic concept as opposed to a personality change linked with a chronic pathological disorder, as it is viewed at the present time. Another theme running through these writings is the concept of the seizure being precipitated by stress, hence the use of such terms as "affect epilepsy" [25]. It is now well recognized that stress cannot only be a precipitator of an epileptic seizure, but also is closely linked with nonepileptic seizures psychogenic (PNES). Stress can also alter the EEG. Unfortunately the whole concept of stress is rather nebulous, but as the twentieth century proceeded, the discovery of central nervous system circuits for arousal and emotion, such as the reticular formation and the limbic system, led to neurobiological speculations not only with regards to the causes of epilepsy, but to PNES. The value of the EEG in making a diagnosis of epilepsy only really came to prominence with the introduction of prolonged monitoring, particularly video-EEG monitoring. It is now recognized that abnormal EEG patterns, in the interictal phase of attacks, are quite unhelpful at making a diagnosis of epilepsy, and are misleading when irregularities, particularly in temporal structures, are used to fortify a diagnosis of temporal lobe epilepsy when the clinical evidence is wanting.

The idea that hysteria disappeared from medical eyes with the death of Charcot is totally dispelled by the profusion of cases of classical hysteria noted in soldiers who broke down during the First World War. Further, these clinical syndromes rather negated the developing Freudian theories that all neuroses were at the heart related to sexual traumas.

The clinical pictures of the war neuroses were varied, but typical. There were acute and chronic forms, but somatic symptoms were predominant. Convulsions, paralyses, contractures, anesthesias, tics, choreas, loss of sight or hearing, stammering, neurasthenias – essentially the full house of symptoms seen over the centuries allied to the diagnosis of hysteria – were recorded.

The end of the First World War did not see the end of the problem. First, many chronic cases remained, and they not only required ongoing care, but also pensions. A school of thought developed that many such people would have adapted poorly to civilian life in any case, even if they had not been in the war, and the possibility of a pension perpetuated the problem.

Other wars followed. Classical patterns of hysterical breakdown were seen in the Second World War, and then in the wars in Korea, Vietnam and the Falklands. By the time of the Second World War, shell shock, as a physical concept, had been officially abandoned, and the recognition of the psychological nature of the condition led to the widespread introduction of psychological interventions. These treatments may have been more effective than earlier ones, but in addition to psychological interventions, psychiatrists such as William Sargant and Eliot Slater introduced new physical therapies for hysteria for soldiers returning from the front, including prolonged sedation and barbiturate-induced abreaction. John Huston's 1946 documentary film, commissioned by the US Army Signal Corps, "Let There Be Light," vividly captures the conditions and treatments described above in returning WWII veterans with "psychoneuroses." [Editor's note: a scene from the movie showing a barbiturate-induced abreaction is included with permission in the DVD accompanying this edition.]

New hysteria studies

The "new hysteria studies" refer to the socio-historical studies of hysteria that have been published mainly in the last twenty or so years. The inspiration for these studies has little to do with medicine, and has been driven by feminist interpretations of the literature. Essentially hysteria is viewed as a diagnosis made by men (doctors) about women (patients), and is in essence a social construct of the historical timeframe of medical theories. Diagnosis is seen as a method of social control, doctors as agents of the status quo.

Psychiatry has come in for particular criticism, with diagnosis based largely on subjectively based symptomology, and insistence on madness as a medical rather than a social construct. The substantial and influential contribution of Elaine Showalter, in *The Female Malady: Women, Madness and the English Culture, 1830–1980* [26], gave pride of place to hysteria as the quintessential female disorder. Feminist reformers were seen as psychologically ill, while the hysterical personality, portrayed in such characters as Blanche Dubois (from Tennessee Williams' *A Streetcar Named Desire*) to Scarlet O'Hara (Mitchell's *Gone with the Wind*), was seen as the epitome of feminine characterization, the *femme fatal* with succubic exuberance which demands suppression.

Another interpretation, adopted for example by Edward Shorter [27], is that hysteria is a recognizable psychiatric disorder, the symptoms of which vary over different social epochs. In a mistaken analysis of the clinical situation he suggests that the Victorian faints, swoons, and convulsions are now rare, and that various psychosomatic disorders have come to take their place. He documents several case histories of the Victorian couch invalids, confined to their beds, often for years, including well-known examples such as Elizabeth Barrett Browning. He concluded that these pictures disappeared from the literature after 1900, based in his view on the culmination of several factors. These included the unconscious selection of symptoms by patients, which was susceptible to various social and cultural pressures, assisted by a shifting medical paradigm, in which doctors influenced patients' behaviors.

In fact, although elegant and well argued, these texts are based on mistaken facts, and fail to acknowledge the continued existence of hysteria in the twentieth century, not only in countless hundreds of thousands of men who came to medical attention in the various war settings, but also in the continued existence of classical hysterical presentations over the decades. The nineteenth-century polysymptomatic Victorian invalid is simply a variant of today's Briquet's hysteria, the somatization disorder of Diagnostic and Statistical Manual of Mental Disorders Fourth Edition (Text Revision) (DSM IV-TR) [28]. In fact, far from disappearing after 1900, the numbers of cases of hysteria rose phenomenally in the twentieth century, and in the last 20 years, the swoons and convulsions have once again become an important part of neurological practice, historically referred to as pseudoseizures, or as psychogenic nonepileptic seizures, as has been adopted since the first edition of this textbook [29].

Conclusions

The history of hysteria is long and distinguished, and it is closely woven within the texture of epilepsy. Patients with medically unexplained syndromes have been recognized in many different cultures for over 2000 years, and the term hysteria has been used successfully to describe such patients. As early as the seventeenth century, the contribution of the emotions to the development of symptoms was discussed, and the pertinent role of trauma and accidents was an early observation.

The contributions of the personality were commented on, and notably adjectives such as capricious, labile, emotionally unstable, and suggestible were descriptors. The role of unconscious forces, and of physical abuse, was also discussed, well before the contributions of Freud, but the latter's more extensive consideration of sexual trauma for a time came to dominate ideas. However, the phantasized nature of the trauma and the role of epigenetic intra-psychic forces had to give way to some extent to alternative theories from the extensive observations of shell shock and later war-related syndromes. Further, in a civilian setting, the role of extrinsic motivations, especially compensation, became central to these discussions, especially medico-legal debates, as the cost of compensation began to rise.

The debates and arguments of Victorian physicians and surgeons over whether a patient's symptoms were "organic" or not echo down to us today, shielding and revealing a lack of knowledge about these fascinating medical syndromes. The introduction of new investigatory techniques in the latter part of the twentieth century, particularly video-EEG monitoring, has led to the recognition that many patients with epilepsy are misdiagnosed, and the misdiagnosis relates in part to a reliance on the EEG rather than on careful clinical descriptions and history-taking when the patient is seen. Since the time of Charcot or before, attempts have been made to separate epileptic from nonepileptic seizures. A commonality of findings, with regards, for example, to impaired performance on neuropsychological tests, an overrepresentation of left-handers, a history of minor head injuries, and the recognized combination of epileptic and nonepileptic seizures in 10% to 30% of patients who have PNES, continues to emphasize the psychobiology of PNES, and the long historical tradition of a link between these disorders. Hysteria, over two millennia, has not simply arisen from the ashes of the past – the fires have been burning brightly all along.

References

1. Institoris H, Sprenger J, Sommers H. *Malleus Maleficarum*. London: Pushkin, 1948.
2. Jorden E. *A Disease Called the Suffocation of Mother*. London: John Windet, 1603.
3. Aretaeus. On hysterical suffocation. In: *The Extant Works of Aretaeus, the Cappadocian*. London: Sydenham Society. 1856; 285–7.
4. Dewhurst K. *Thomas Willis' Oxford Lectures*. Oxford: Sanford Publications, 1980.
5. Willis T. *An Essay of the Pathology of the Brain and Nervous Stock in which Convulsive disease are treated*. Trans. Pordage S. Dring. London: Leigh and Harper, 1684.
6. Sydenham T. *The Works of Thomas Sydenham*. London: Sydenham Society, 1850.
7. Burton R. *The Anatomy of Melancholy*. Oxford, 1621.
8. Whyte R. *Observations on the Nature, Causes and Cure of Those Disorders Which Have Been Called Nervous, Hypochondriac, or Hysteric, to Which are Prefixed Some Remarks on the Sympathy of the Nerves*. Edinburgh: Becket and Du Hodt, 1751.
9. Cheyne G. *The English Malady; or a Treatise of Nervous Diseases of All Kinds, as Spleen, Vapours, Lowness of Spirits, Hypochondriacal and Hysterical Distempers etc*. London: Strahan and Leake, 1733.
10. Laycock T. *An Essay on Hysteria*. Philadelphia: Barrington and Haswell, 1840.
11. Carter RB. *On the Pathology and Treatment of Hysteria*. London: Churchill, 1853.
12. Veith I. *Hysteria. The History of a Disease*. Chicago: University of Chicago Press, 1965.
13. Todd RB. *Clinical Lectures on Paralysis, Certain Diseases of the Brain and other Affections of the Nervous System*. London, 1856.
14. Hughlings Jackson J. In: Taylor J, ed. *Selected Writings of John Hughlings Jackson*. London: Staples Press, 1958.
15. Briquet P. *Traité Clinique et Thérapeutique de l'Hystérie*. Paris: J-B Baillière et fils, 1859.
16. Charcot JM. *Lectures on the Diseases of the Nervous System*. Trans. Sigerson G. New Sydenham Society. London 1877.
17. Janet P. *The Mental State of Hystericals*. Trans CR Corson. New York: GP Putnam's Sons, 1901.
18. Breuer J, Freud S. (1893–1895). *Studies on Hysteria*. Standard Edition, 2. London: Hogarth Press, 1955.
19. Breuer J, Freud S. (1893–1895). *Studies on Hysteria*. Standard Edition, 2. London: Hogarth Press, 1955.
20. Pierce-Clarke L. A psychological interpretation of essential epilepsy. *Brain*, 1929;**43**:38–49.
21. Jellife SE, White WA. *Diseases of the Nervous System*. London: HK Lewis, 1929.
22. Freud S. *Dostoevsky and Parracide*. Realist 1. 1929.
23. Fenichel O. *Hysterie und Zwangsneurosen*. Wien, 1931.
24. Stekel W. *Der epileptische Symptom-Complex. Nervoese Angstzustaend*. Wien, 1924.
25. Bratz H, Leubuscher H. Die Affekt-epilepsie. Eine klinische, von der echten Epilepsie abtrennbare Gruppe. *Dt med Wschr* 1907;**33**:592–3.
26. Showalter E. *The Female Malady: Women, Madness and the English Culture, 1830–1980*. New York: Pantheon, 1985.
27. Shorter E. *From Paralysis to Fatigue: A History of Psychosomatic Illness in the Modern Era*. New York: Free Press, 1992.
28. American Psychiatric Association. *Diagnostic and Statistical Manual of Mental Disorders*, 4th edn., Text Revision (DSM-IV-TR). Washington, DC: American Psychiatric Association, 2000.
29. Rowan AJ, Gates JR, eds. *Non-Epileptic Seizures*, 1st edn. Stoneham, MA: Butterworth-Heinemann, 1993.

Recommended reading

Charcot J-M. *Clinical Lectures on Diseases of the Nervous System*, Vol. 3. Trans T Savill. London: New Sydenham Society, 1889.

Charcot J-M, Marie P. Hysteria. In: *D Hake Tuke, Dictionary of Psychological Medicine*. London: Churchill, 1892.

Ellenberger HF. *The Discovery of the Unconscious*. New York: Basic Books, 1970.

Griesinger W. *Mental Pathology and Therapeutics*. Trans C Lockhart Robertson and J Rutherford. London: New Sydenham Society, 1862.

Hecker JFC. *The Epidemics of the Middle Ages*. Trans BG Babbington. London: The Sydenham Society, 1844.

Hunter R, MacAlpine I. *Three Hundred Years of Psychiatry*. Oxford: Oxford University Press, 1963.

Janet P. *The Major Symptoms of Hysteria*. London: Macmillan Company, 1907.

Merskey H. *The Analysis of Hysteria*, 2nd edn. London: Gaskell, 1995.

Micale MS, *Approaching Hysteria*. New Jersey: Princeton University Press, 1995.

Micale MS, Lerner P. *Traumatic Pasts*. Cambridge: Cambridge University Press, 2001.

Owen AGR. *Hysteria, Hypnosis and Healing. The Work of J-M Charcot*. London: Dennis Dobson, 1972.

Pierce-Clarke L. A psychological interpretation of essential epilepsy. *Brain* 1929;**43**:38–49.

Reynolds JR. Remarks on paralysis and other disorders of motion and sensation, dependant on an idea. *Br Med J* 1869;ii:483–5.

Ross TA. *Lectures on War Neuroses*. London: Edward Arnold and Co., 1941.

Sackellares JC, Kalogjera-Sackellares D. Psychobiology of psychogenic pseudoseizures. In: Trimble MR and Schmitz B, eds. *The Neuropsychiatry of Epilepsy*. Cambridge: Cambridge University Press. 2004; 210–26.

Shephard B. *A War of Nerves*. London: Johnathan Cape, 2000.

Stone M. Shellshock and the psychologists. In: Bynum WF, Porter R, Shepherd M, eds. *The Anatomy of Madness*, Vol. 2. London: Tavistock Publications. 1985; 242–71.

Temkin O. *The Falling Sickness*. Baltimore: Johns Hopkins University Press, 1951.

Trimble MR. *Post-Traumatic Neurosis*. Chichester: J Wiley and Sons, 1981.

Section 1 Chapter 3

Recognition, diagnosis, and impact of nonepileptic seizures

The burden of psychogenic nonepileptic seizures (PNES) in context: PNES and medically unexplained symptoms

James C. Hamilton, Roy C. Martin, Jon Stone, and Courtney B. Worley

This chapter provides information on the costs and burdens associated with psychogenic nonepileptic seizures (PNES). Usually discussions of this sort are framed against the specific backdrop of epileptology, i.e., the proportion of patients with epileptic seizures (ES) who also have PNES, and the costs of treating PNES compared with those of treating ES.

However, we wish to broaden the view of PNES for the purposes of this chapter by placing them in the larger contexts of medically unexplained signs and symptoms in neurology and in general medicine. The premise of this approach is that it is worth considering the possibility that PNES reflect a specific expression of the more general problem of medically unexplained physical signs and symptoms that appears to pervade almost every division of clinical medicine. In taking this approach we hope to stimulate a cross-fertilization of ideas between the study of PNES and the burgeoning study of medically unexplained symptoms (MUS).

The landscape of medically unexplained symptoms

The connection of PNES to the larger category of MUS begins with the diagnosis of conversion disorder [1]. The majority of patients with PNES are assigned this diagnosis [2]. Conversion disorders, in turn, belong to the broader Diagnostic and Statistical Manual of Mental Disorders, Fourth Edition (DSM-IV) category of somatoform disorders. The somatoform disorders, particularly somatization disorder, pain disorder, hypochondriasis, and undifferentiated somatoform disorder, share in common with conversion disorder the presence of medical complaints for which no adequate physical explanation can be found. By definition these medical complaints are either so persistent, numerous, or disabling that they cause significant subjective distress or functional impairment. Well-controlled epidemiological studies of the somatoform disorders have been limited to somatization disorder and hypochondriasis [3]. However, studies of primary care settings suggest that approximately 15% of patients meet either DSM-IV or The International Classification of Diseases, Tenth Edition (ICD-10) criteria for a somatoform disorder [4, 5]. Several researchers in this field have defined and studied clinically significant variants that do not reach DSM or ICD criteria for a somatoform disorder, and which are much more common (e.g., abridged somatization disorder [6], multisomatoform disorder [7]). The prevalence of these specific conditions among primary care patients has been estimated to range between 2% and 22% [6, 8].

Also lying outside the somatoform disorder category are medical syndromes that are characterized by subjective medical complaints that have no clear medical explanation [9, 10]. These functional somatic syndromes include chronic fatigue syndrome, irritable bowel syndrome, myalgic encephalomyelitis, fibromyalgia, multiple chemical sensitivities, and Gulf War syndrome. Chronic fatigue syndrome and fibromyalgia have received the most research attention. Population studies suggest a point-prevalence rate of 0.2% to 3%, with higher rates among primary care patients [11]. Although research on all of these syndromes has produced some suggestive evidence of pathophysiological mechanisms, a set of definitive biological markers that distinguish patients from well persons and psychiatric patients has not yet emerged. On the other hand, there is substantial and consistent evidence that these syndromes show a high degree of overlap with one another, and similarly high levels of psychiatric comorbidity [2, 12].

Two other related phenomena, namely, factitious disorder and malingering, bear mentioning. Factitious disorder is diagnosed in patients whose signs and symptoms have been proved to be intentionally exaggerated, feigned, simulated, or self-induced. The presumed motive for medical deception in these cases is the satisfaction of a psychological need [1]. Factitious disorder cases may constitute as much as 1% of all medical inpatient admissions [13, 14]. Cases of intentional medical deception are considered malingering when the motives for medical deception are primarily instrumental, such as avoiding military service, securing disability status, or procuring addicting prescription medicines. In practice, the line between internal and external motives is unclear and arbitrary, and in many cases multiple motives may contribute to sick role enactment (see Chapters 16 and 20).

The burden of medically unexplained symptoms

Research reports from the US and Europe confirm the high medical costs associated with unexplained medical problems [15, 16]. Barsky and colleagues found that primary care patients with apparent high levels of unexplained medical complaints had higher costs for primary care, specialty visits, emergency visits, outpatient procedures, and hospital admissions compared to patients without MUS [17]. They estimate that annual healthcare costs in the US associated with MUS may exceed $200 billion. Fink studied a group of patients with frequent hospitalizations and compared those with and without evidence of MUS. He found that admissions related to unexplained medical symptoms were associated with rates of surgical and medical treatment comparable to the admissions for well-defined illness [18]. The patients with MUS also had poorer treatment outcomes. In a separate paper, Fink reported that 56 patients found to be "persistent somatizers" accounted for 3% of all medical hospital admissions in the entire nation of Denmark over the 8-year study period [19]. Cohen *et al.* undertook a study to test a clinical impression that women diagnosed with what was historically referred to as "hysteria" undergo an excessive number of surgical procedures. The patients with hysteria had about three times as many operations as did the healthy control patients and twice as many as did the medically ill control patients [20].

One might intuitively imagine that self-reported illness with no defined medical cause would be less disabling and costly than those with a clear medical basis. However, studies that compare patients with functional disorders to those with a related, but well-defined, medical disorder consistently show that patients with MUS have comparable, and sometimes greater, disability and healthcare costs. For example, patients with irritable bowel syndrome show levels of distress and disability comparable to those of patients with inflammatory bowel diseases, like Crohn's disease [21–23]. Similarly, patients with fibromyalgia show comparable levels of impairment to patients with rheumatoid arthritis [24, 25]. Not surprisingly then, patients with PNES had similar disability rates (approximately 40%) to those with epilepsy [26].

Studies that use symptoms or medical visits as their units of analysis probably overestimate the burden of MUS by including complaints that turn out to be benign and self-limiting. The symptoms remain unexplained because they go away on their own, obviating the need to explain them. In other cases, these studies of medical records might capture MUS for which medical attention was appropriately sought, such as symptoms suggesting heart attack or stroke. However, the studies that use patients as their level of analysis and carefully identify persons with chronic or multiple MUS more accurately capture the scope of the problem. The bottom line is that 10% to 15% of patients in primary care settings present with significant physical suffering and disability that cannot be linked to a specific disease or injury. These patients received many surgical and medical investigations and treatments that may do them little good while exposing them to potential iatrogenic harm, which may compound their suffering and disability.

Medically unexplained symptoms in neurology

Medically unexplained symptoms are also common in neurology practice. Studies in the UK [12, 27], The Netherlands [28], and Denmark [29] have found that around one-third of newly seen neurology outpatients have symptoms rated by their neurologist as only "somewhat explained" or "not at all explained" by measurable disease. Looking at the narrower group of patients with "conversion symptoms," Perkin, a neurologist in London, made this diagnosis in 3.8% of 7836 consecutive new neurology outpatients [30]. Schiffer found an identical proportion in a US outpatient sample [31]. Studies suggest that between one-third and one-half of patients with conversion symptoms have PNES [32]; suggesting that perhaps 1% to 2% of all neurology outpatients may carry this diagnosis. The frequency of conversion symptoms in neurology inpatients has typically been reported in the range 5% to 9% [31, 33–35]. In one UK study, PNES accounted for 63% of these admissions [28].

Patients with MUS in neurology clinics, including patients with PNES, therefore represent a huge public health problem, about which there has been little publicity or large-scale research [32, 36]. Studies conducted in neurological clinics in Scotland found that, compared to patients with medically explained neurological symptoms, patients with medically unexplained neurological symptoms:

1. Are predicted by higher numbers of physical symptoms at presentation [27]
2. Have similar self-reported levels of disability [27]
3. Have higher rates of distress [27]
4. Are found to be "more difficult to help" by neurologists [37].

Other unexplained symptoms in patients with PNES

Studies examining the frequency of other somatic symptoms in patients with PNES highlight the fact that PNES is usually not an isolated symptom in an individual patient. Several authors have highlighted the frequency of pain disorders in patients with PNES. Ettinger *et al.* [38] found that 77% of 56 patients with PNES had moderate to severe pain in one or more areas of their body. Headache and neck and back pain were most common. Interestingly, patients with a pain syndrome were more likely to have a poor outcome for their PNES. Similarly, Benbadis found that a history of chronic pain or fibromyalgia had a 75% positive predictive value for identifying PNES in patients undergoing diagnostic video-EEG (VEEG) monitoring [39].

Additional studies have examined other conversion symptoms in patients with PNES. Lempert *et al.* reported additional conversion symptoms in 60% of their 50 subjects (30% stance and gait; 22% sensory; 16% paresis; 16% pain; 10% visual symptoms; 6% bladder dysfunction; 4% contracture; 2% globus) [40].

Bowman reported even higher proportions in her series (e.g., 49% weakness) [41]. Meierkord reported 21% of 110 patients with PNES had another conversion symptom [42]. Another study found 50% of children with PNES had another conversion symptom [43]. Conversely, 23% of patients with motor conversion symptoms also had PNES [44]. However, these studies probably overestimate the frequency of other conversion symptoms because of sampling bias. Series from tertiary centers or series of patients undergoing VEEG monitoring are likely to reflect more patients with severe or chronic PNES, who in turn are more likely to score higher on measures of somatization [45]. However, even in a series closer to primary care, patients with PNES still had a median of one other neurological symptom (including pain and fatigue) [46].

Burden of PNES

Although we now know more about the frequency of PNES in neurological practice [47], the costs associated with PNES, both direct and indirect, are not well studied. Estimating from our best comparison population, patients with ES [48, 49], the costs associated with PNES are suspected to be considerable given that both groups have comparable assessment paths to eventual diagnosis (i.e., clinic visits, emergency room visits, neuroimaging) and that PNES can frequently be refractory even after definitive diagnosis [46]. The complications that arise from attempting to calculate these costs are highlighted by Begley and Beghi [49] in their review of the economic costs associated with epilepsy (e.g., mapping disease progression and accounting for the costs associated with comorbid conditions, such as stroke, depression, other medically explained symptoms). Such issues are also germane to cost estimations in PNES, and the PNES literature lacks these types of high-caliber formal cost-of-illness investigations.

The establishment of economic costs associated with PNES is important because these patients represent a substantial proportion of patients seen for seizure disorders by neurologists and primary care physicians (see Chapter 1). Sophisticated cost analyses of epilepsy, based on both incidence and prevalence estimates, have demonstrated multi-billion dollar costs associated with intractable ES [49, 50]. It has been estimated that persons with intractable ES have lifetime direct costs over one million dollars, along with indirect cost estimates of over seven million

Table 3.1 Time to diagnosis for patients with PNES

Author	Year	Country	Sample	Time to diagnosis
Martin et al. [52]	1998	US	20 PNES	6.8 years (range 6 months to 33 years)
De Timary et al. [67]	2002	Belgium	50 PNES 53 PNES + ES	8.7 years (SD = 1.3) 16.5 years (SD = 1.4)
Reuber et al. [57]	2003	Germany	164 total 98 PNES, 66 PNES + ES	8.3 years (SD = 10.3)
Oto et al. [54]	2005	UK	160 PNES	7 years
D'Alessio et al. [68]	2006	Argentina	24 PNES	8.8 years
Arain et al. [69]	2007	US	48 PNES	9 years (range 1 – 52 years)
Binder & Salinsky [53]	2007	US	Not cited (review paper)	1994 patient series – 4 years 2004 patient series – 2 years
Bodde et al. [61]	2007	Netherlands	22 PNES	7.2 years
Finlayson et al. [55]	2007	Canada	50 PNES	<1 year (26%) 1–3 years (26%) 3–5 years (8%) 5–10 years (12%) 10+ years (26%)
O'Sullivan et al. [70]	2007	Ireland	20 PNES 18 PNES + ES	1.7 years (SD = 1.9) 3.8 years (SD = 3.8)
Duncan & Oto [71]	2008	Scotland – UK	25 PNES + learning disability 263 PNES	10.7 years 6.9 years
Kuyk et al. [72]	2008	Netherlands	22 PNES	6.7 years (median 4.5 years)

PNES, psychogenic nonepileptic seizures; ES, epileptic seizures; SD, standard deviation.

dollars [50]. Although no studies to date have explicitly examined the comparative economic costs of epilepsy and PNES, a few studies have presented data in a form that provides clues to these costs. For example, patients with PNES commonly exhibit high-frequency seizures that are resistant to treatment [51] and often require intensive and potentially expensive procedures (i.e., emergency room admissions). Patients with PNES often receive antiepileptic drugs (AEDs) for protracted periods of time prior to and even after definitive diagnosis [48]. The following sections highlight some of the direct cost and indirect cost areas associated with PNES.

Pre-diagnosis costs

The average costs generated prior to the diagnosis of PNES in the US have been estimated to range from $8156 [52] to $15 000 [53]. Outpatient EEG examination is often a first step in the diagnostic process along with medical examination by a neurologist. Few studies provide information regarding the frequency of outpatient EEG monitoring [54]. CT and MRI scanning are standard parts of routine diagnostic procedures for the differential diagnosis of NES [54], and in some cases may be repeated during the course of the diagnostic workup [52, 55]. No large-scale study has systematically investigated these costs. However, studies of time-to-diagnosis can help provide a sense of the extra costs associated with the diagnosis of PNES. Table 3.1 highlights several recent studies that reported the time to diagnosis from initial seizure. Patients with PNES incur costs associated with an extended period prior to the definitive diagnosis of PNES. Moreover, Martin and colleagues [56] found the longer the pre-diagnosis period, the poorer the long-term prognosis, although this has not been consistently reported [42, 57].

Tertiary care

Reuber and colleagues [51] found that patients with PNES (n = 98) were comparable to those with ES in percentage treated in intensive care units (27.8% vs. 23.3%). Martin et al. [52] noted that 75% of their patients with PNES went to the emergency room (ER)

Table 3.2 Antiepileptic drug (AED) therapy among patients with PNES

Author	Year	Sample	AED use	Comments
Martin et al. [52]	1998	20 PNES	19/20 at time of diagnosis	
De Timary et al. [67]	2002	103 PNES	72% at time of diagnosis	
Reuber et al. [73]	2002	212 PNES	76% at time of diagnosis	
Oto et al. [54]	2005	184 PNES	99 (54%) at diagnosis 47 (26%) prior to hospitalization	Range 1 to 3 (1.4 mean) AEDs
Finlayson et al. [55]	2007	50 PNES	44/50 (88%)	
Binder & Salinsky [53]	2007	Not described	80%	25% taking > 1 AED
Hantke et al. [60]	2007	170 PNES 178 ES	1.5 (mean AEDs) 2.0 (mean AEDs)	
O'Sullivan et al. [70]	2007	20 PNES	3.0 (mean AEDs)	
Testa et al. [74]	2007	45 PNES 69 ES	0.94 (mean AED) at time of diagnosis 1.88 (mean AED)	
Duncan & Oto [71]	2008	263 PNES 25 PNES + learning disability	51% taking AED, only 15% >1 AED 80% taking AED, 40% > 1 AED	
Selkirk et al. [75]	2008	176 PNES	Patients reporting history of sexual abuse more commonly receiving 2+ AEDs compared to PNES with no abuse history	

PNES, psychogenic nonepileptic seizures; ES, epileptic seizures.

in the six-month period prior to PNES diagnosis. They found patients with PNES had an average of six ER visits with an estimated cost of $3400 per visit. Dworetzky and colleagues [58] found higher seizure frequency rates and more emergency services utilization for patients with PNES than those with ES. However, the group with PNES was also referred for inpatient VEEG monitoring sooner, thereby providing a quicker time to diagnosis (Table 3.2).

Few studies provide information regarding the frequency of outpatient EEG monitoring [59]. Neuroimaging expenses are a standard part of routine diagnostic procedures for the differential diagnosis of PNES. Magnetic resonance imaging and CT scans are commonly employed and in some cases may be repeated during the course of the diagnostic workup [55, 56]. However, like other direct cost areas no study has formally investigated these cost areas in a systematic fashion in a large patient sample.

Antiepileptic drug use

One of the most common costs incurred by patients with PNES is related to AEDs. A majority of patients with PNES are taking one or more AEDs at the time of diagnosis. Initial research suggests that patients with PNES have substantially higher non-AED medication use compared to patients with ES [60]. Whereas some studies find AED discontinuation after definitive diagnosis of PNES [52], others suggest that many patients with PNES continue to receive AEDs post-diagnosis [61]. Martin et al. [52] reported a 69% average reduction in total AED costs (dollar value) in the six-month period following diagnosis. Reuber and Elger [45] reviewed several studies on PNES outcome and found an average of 30% of patients with PNES only continued AEDs following diagnosis. In another study from their center, Reuber et al. [57] found that 40% of their patients with PNES (and without ES) continued to receive AEDs after diagnosis; some patients continued receiving AEDs up to ten years post-diagnosis. Further complicating the picture, many of the studies fail to specify whether the continued AED use is targeted toward seizures or psychiatric symptoms (i.e., used as mood stabilizers or for neuropathic pain control).

Comorbid medical and psychiatric conditions

Adding to the difficulty in establishing cost-of-illness estimates, comorbid medical conditions are often difficult to distinguish from costs related to the seizures. Moreover, in the PNES literature, studies describing comorbid medical conditions are often limited to psychiatric comorbidity [39, 62, 63]. In many cases, treatment may evolve from neurological care to psychiatric or other medical specialty care (in relation to other physical symptoms discussed earlier), but the economic implications of this transition are poorly understood. Specifically, the type, frequency or duration of psychiatric and medical treatments rendered after the diagnosis of PNES is made are not well documented.

Employment and financial assistance

Substantial numbers of patients with PNES are not in the workforce at the time of their diagnosis, thereby contributing to the indirect cost totals. This likely reflects a number of factors that may in part be similar to reasons that persons with ES have high rates of unemployment, including no longer being able to drive, workplace safety concerns, and discrimination. A few studies have also reported on the change in job status from the time of PNES onset to time of diagnosis. For example, Martin *et al.* [56] reported that at the time of PNES onset, 69% of patients were fully employed, whereas at the time of diagnosis of PNES, only 20% were in the workforce. Table 3.3 highlights employment and disability status in patients with PNES. The changes in employment status (i.e., from full-time to part-time work, restricted activity days, employment loss and reduction) have not been addressed within the PNES literature. Additionally, Binder and Salinsky [53] found an estimated $22 000 per year per patient with PNES in costs associated with lost work.

Prognosis

Reuber found that patients with PNES have poor long-term seizure cessation outcomes after diagnosis [64]. Specifically, 71% of patients with PNES in their review continued to have seizures at a mean of 11 years post-diagnosis. The literature continues to support these poor outcome statistics, and their implications for continuing high utilization of medical services [82]. Walczak and colleagues [66] found poor economic outcomes (i.e., return to employment) for patients with PNES.

Conclusions

Although the available evidence paints an incomplete picture, it is clear enough that the proportional costs of PNES are comparable to the costs associated with intractable epilepsy. Delayed diagnosis results in greater pre-diagnosis costs and seems to entrench patients in the sick role, as evidenced by a lower likelihood of post-diagnosis employment. Moreover, patients with PNES, relative to patients with ES, have increased costs associated with psychiatric and medical comorbidities. Though one might expect these costs to be offset relative to patients with ES by a reduction in both direct and indirect costs post-diagnosis, a substantial minority of patients with PNES only continue to be treated with AEDs and remain unemployed or underemployed.

The literature reveals a clear trend toward discarding historical and arbitrary distinctions among patients with MUS. The traditional framework for the somatoform disorders is beginning to yield to data indicating that pain disorder, somatization disorder, and conversion disorder cannot be meaningfully distinguished from one another. They share common demographic profiles and similar patterns of psychiatric comorbidity. The same is true for the functional somatic symptoms. Again, skirting the controversial issue of whether these conditions have an underlying pathophysiology, their demographic features and psychiatric comorbidities do not distinguish one from another. We believe that this trend should be carried further by acknowledging that persons with somatoform disorder or functional somatic syndromes and persons with PNES may be more alike than different.

The question of where PNES fits into this landscape is crucial for at least two reasons. The first has to do with its potential methodological significance. The primary impediment to research on medically unexplained signs and symptoms is the absence of a gold-standard criterion for distinguishing these complaints from complaints linked to demonstrable pathophysiology. Complaints like pain and fatigue are highly subjective and not closely linked to any biological markers, making them difficult to authenticate and leaving researchers with no reliable criterion measures. In contrast, ES are well correlated with fairly definitive objective biological markers (i.e., EEG patterns). Video-EEG and other medical tests to rule out neurological or cardiac causes of seizure-like events, in

Table 3.3 Employment status of patients with PNES

Author	Year	Country	Sample	Employment status
Walczak et al. [66]	1995	US	72 PNES	59% unemployed at diagnosis, 75% no employment status change at follow-up
Krawetz et al. [82]	2001	Canada	31 PNES	55% unemployed at diagnosis
Quigg et al. [26]	2002	US	30 PNES	33% received disability benefits 60% at follow-up
Dikel et al. [76]	2003	US	17 PNES 34 ES	41% not in labor force at diagnosis 29% not in labor force
Kuyk et al. [77]	2003	Netherlands	60 PNES 25 PNES + ES	20.7% receiving disability at diagnosis 60% unemployed at diagnosis 36% receiving disability at diagnosis
Martin et al. [56]	2003	US	84 PNES	69% working at seizure onset 20% working at time of diagnosis
Reuber et al. [45]	2003	Germany	98 PNES 63 ES	46.5% dependent at time of diagnosis 50.8% dependent at time of diagnosis
Reuber et al. [57]	2003	Germany	164 PNES	More than 50% patients with PNES receiving disability benefits up to 10 years post diagnosis
Marzooqi et al. [78]	2004	UK	97 PNES 97 ES	71% classified as unemployed at time of post-diagnosis interview (12–36 months) 67% classified as unemployed
Oto et al. [59]	2005	UK	160 PNES	70% receiving disability benefits
Reuber et al. [79]	2005	Germany	147 PNES	>40% not working/receiving benefits at time of post-diagnosis follow-up (mean 4 years)
Arain et al. [69]	2007	US	48 PNES	50% unemployed at 3-month follow-up post diagnosis
Finlayson et al. [55]	2007	Canada	50 PNES	36% classified as disabled at time of diagnosis. Additional, 12% unemployed
O'Sullivan et al. [70]	2007	Ireland	20 PNES 18 PNES + ES	80% unemployed at diagnosis 50% unemployed at diagnosis
Schramke et al. [80]	2007	US	51 PNES 57 ES	22% applying for disability at time of diagnosis 18% applying for disability
Duncan & Oto [71]	2008	Scotland, UK	263 PNES 25 PNES + LD history	57% receiving benefits at time of diagnosis 88% receiving benefits
Selkirk et al. [75]	2008	Scotland, UK	112 PNES – no sexual abuse history 64 PNES – positive abuse history	59% receiving government benefits 75% receiving government benefits
Kuyk et al. [81]	2008	Netherlands	22 PNES	64% employed at time of post-diagnosis follow-up. All receiving psychiatric treatment

PNES, psychogenic nonepileptic seizures; ES, epileptic seizures; LD, learning disability.

conjunction with psychiatric assessment, provide a reliable way of identifying patients with PNES. To the extent that the biopsychosocial process that leads to a vulnerability for PNES shares similarities with other expressions of medically unexplained signs and symptoms, it might be productive to adapt the findings of research on PNES to patients with MUS, and vice versa.

From a practical standpoint, we have emphasized that PNES resembles, and is comorbid with, a wide array of MUS, both neurological and beyond. Throughout the world, but particularly in the US, few research funding initiatives have been targeted toward understanding and treating chronic or multiple MUS, despite their huge financial and iatrogenic costs. Framing MUS, in their many manifestations, as a single medical problem would demonstrate the magnitude of the problem posed by these disorders and may help stimulate increased public and private research support.

References

1. American Psychiatric Association. *Diagnostic and Statistical Manual of Mental Disorders*, 4th edn., Text Revision (DSM-IV-TR). Washington, DC: American Psychiatric Association, 2000.
2. Marchetti RL, Kurcgant D, Neto JG, *et al.* Psychiatric diagnoses of patients with psychogenic non-epileptic seizures. *Seizure* 2008;**17**(3):247–53.
3. Simon GE, VonKorff M. Somatization and psychiatric disorder in the NIMH Epidemiologic Catchment Area study. *Am J Psychiatry* 1991;**148**(11):1494–500.
4. De Waal MWM, Arnold IA, Eekhof JAH, Van Hemert AM. Somatoform disorders in general practice: prevalence, functional impairment and comorbidity with anxiety and depressive disorders. *Br J Psychiatry* 2004;**184**(6):470–6.
5. Fink P, Hansen MS, Oxhoj M-L. The prevalence of somatoform disorders among internal medical inpatients. *J Psychosom Res* 2004;**56**(4):413–8.
6. Escobar JI, Waitzkin H, Silver RC, Gara M, Holman A. Abridged somatization: a study in primary care. *Psychosom Med* 1998;**60**(4):466–72.
7. Kroenke K, Spitzer RL, deGruy FV, III, *et al.* Multisomatoform disorder: an alternative to undifferentiated somatoform disorder for the somatizing patient in primary care. *Arch Gen Psychiatry* 1997;**54**:352–8.
8. Verhaak PFM, Meijer SA, Visser AP, Wolters G. Persistent presentation of medically unexplained symptoms in general practice. *Fam Pract* 2006;**23**(4):414–20.
9. Barsky AJ, Borus JF. Functional somatic syndromes. *Ann Intern Med* 1999;**130**(11):910–21.
10. Nimnuan C, Rabe-Hesketh S, Wessely S, Hotopf M. How many functional somatic syndromes? *J Psychosom Res* 2001;**51**(4):549–57.
11. Neumann L, Buskila D. Epidemiology of fibromyalgia. *Curr Pain Headache Rep* 2003;**7**(5):362–8.
12. Nimnuan C, Hotopf M, Wessely S. Medically unexplained symptoms: an epidemiological study in seven specialities. *J Psychosom Res* 2001;**51**(1):361–7.
13. Fliege H, Grimm A, Eckhardt-Henn A, *et al.* Frequency of ICD-10 factitious disorder: survey of senior hospital consultants and physicians in private practice. *Psychosomatics* 2007;**48**(1):60–4.
14. Feldman MD, Hamilton JC, Deemer HN. Factitious disorder. In: Phillips KA, ed. *Somatoform and Factitious Disorders*. Washington, DC: American Psychiatric Association. 2001; 129–66.
15. Lowe B, Mundt C, Herzog W, *et al.* Validity of current somatoform disorder diagnoses: perspectives for classification in DSM-V and ICD-11. *Psychopathology* 2008;**41**(1):4–9.
16. Katon W, Sullivan M, Walker E. Medical symptoms without identified pathology: relationship to psychiatric disorders, childhood and adult trauma, and personality traits. *Ann Intern Med* 2001;**134**(9 Pt 2):917–25.
17. Barsky AJ, Orav EJ, Bates DW. Somatization increases medical utilization and costs independent of psychiatric and medical comorbidity. *Arch Gen Psychiatry* 2005;**62**(8):903–10.
18. Fink P. Surgery and medical treatment in persistent somatizing patients. *J Psychosom Res* 1992;**36**(5): 439–47.
19. Fink P. The use of hospitalizations by persistent somatizing patients. *Psychol Med* 1992;**22**(1):173–80.
20. Cohen ME, Robins E, Purtell JJ, Altmann MW, Reid DE. Excessive surgery in hysteria; study of surgical procedures in 50 women with hysteria and 190 controls. *J Am Med Assoc* 1953;**151**(12):977–86.
21. Zimmerman J. Extraintestinal symptoms in irritable bowel syndrome and inflammatory bowel diseases: nature, severity, and relationship to gastrointestinal symptoms. *Dig Dis Sci* 2003;**48**(4):743–9.
22. Pace F, Molteni P, Bollani S, *et al.* Inflammatory bowel disease versus irritable bowel syndrome: a hospital-based, case-control study of disease impact on quality of life. *Scand J Gastroenterol* 2003;**38**(10):1031–8.
23. Walker EA, Gelfand AN, Gelfand MD, Katon WJ. Psychiatric diagnoses, sexual and physical

victimization, and disability in patients with irritable bowel syndrome or inflammatory bowel disease. *Psychol Med* 1995;**25**(6):1259–67.

24. Walker JG, Littlejohn GO. Measuring quality of life in rheumatic conditions. *Clin Rheumatol* 2007;**26**(5): 671–3.

25. Wolfe F, Michaud K. Severe rheumatoid arthritis (RA), worse outcomes, comorbid illness, and sociodemographic disadvantage characterize RA patients with fibromyalgia. *J Rheumatol* 2004;**31**(4): 695–700.

26. Krawetz P, Fleisher W, Pillay N, *et al.* Family functioning in subjects with pseudoseizures and epilepsy. *J Nerv Ment Dis* 2001;**189**(1): 38–43.

27. Carson AJ, Ringbauer B, Stone J, *et al.* Do medically unexplained symptoms matter? A prospective cohort study of 300 new referrals to neurology outpatient clinics. *J Neurol Neurosurg Psychiatry* 2000;**68**: 207–10.

28. Snijders TJ, de Leeuw FE, Klumpers UM, Kappelle LJ, van Gijn J. Prevalence and predictors of unexplained neurological symptoms in an academic neurology outpatient clinic–an observational study. *J Neurol* 2004;**251**(1):66–71.

29. Fink P, Steen HM, Sondergaard L. Somatoform disorders among first-time referrals to a neurology service. *Psychosomatics* 2005;**46**(6):540–8.

30. Perkin GD. An analysis of 7836 successive new outpatient referrals. *J Neurol Neurosurg Psychiatry* 1989;**52**(4):447–8.

31. Schiffer RB. Psychiatric aspects of clinical neurology. *Am J Psychiatry* 1983;**140**(2):205–7.

32. Marsden CD. Hysteria – a neurologist's view. *Psychol Med* 1986;**16**(2):277–88.

33. Lempert T, Dieterich M, Huppert D, Brandt T. Psychogenic disorders in neurology: frequency and clinical spectrum. *Acta Neurol Scand* 1990;**82**(5): 335–40.

34. Schofield A, Duane MM. Neurologic referrals to a psychiatric consultation-liaison service. A study of 199 patients. *Gen Hosp Psychiatry* 1987;**9**(4):280–6.

35. Parry AM, Murray B, Hart Y, Bass C. Audit of resource use in patients with non-organic disorders admitted to a UK neurology unit. *J Neurol Neurosurg Psychiatry* 2006;**77**:1200–1.

36. Mace CJ, Trimble MR. Ten-year prognosis of conversion disorder. *Br J Psychiatry* 1996;**169**(3): 282–8.

37. Carson AJ, Stone J, Warlow C, Sharpe M. Patients whom neurologists find difficult to help. *J Neurol Neurosurg Psychiatry* 2004;**75**(12):1776–8.

38. Ettinger AB, Devinsky O, Weisbrot DM, Goyal A, Shashikumar S. Headaches and other pain symptoms among patients with psychogenic non-epileptic seizures. *Seizure* 1999;**8**(7):424–6.

39. Benbadis SR. A spell in the epilepsy clinic and a history of "chronic pain" or "fibromyalgia" independently predict a diagnosis of psychogenic seizures. *Epilepsy Behav* 2005;**6**(2):264–5.

40. Lempert T, Schmidt D. Natural history and outcome of psychogenic seizures: a clinical study in 50 patients. *J Neurol* 1990;**237**(1):35–8.

41. Bowman ES, Markand ON. Psychodynamics and psychiatric diagnoses of pseudoseizure subjects. *Am J Psychiatry* 1996;**153**(1):57–63.

42. Meierkord H, Will B, Fish D, Shorvon S. The clinical features and prognosis of pseudoseizures diagnosed using video-EEG telemetry. *Neurology* 1991;**41**(10): 1643–6.

43. Pakalnis A, Paolicchi J. Frequency of secondary conversion symptoms in children with psychogenic nonepileptic seizures. *Epilepsy Behav* 2003;**4**(6): 753–6.

44. Crimlisk HL, Bhatia K, Cope H, *et al.* Slater revisited: 6 year follow up study of patients with medically unexplained motor symptoms. *BMJ* 1998;**316**(7131): 582–6.

45. Reuber M, Elger C. Psychogenic nonepileptic seizures: review and update. *Epilepsy Behav* 2003;**4**: 205–16.

46. Reuber M, Howlett S, Khan A, Grunewald RA. Non-epileptic seizures and other functional neurological symptoms: predisposing, precipitating, and perpetuating factors. *Psychosomatics* 2007;**48**(3): 230–8.

47. Benbadis SR, Allen HW, Hauser W. An estimate of the prevalence of psychogenic non-epileptic seizures. *Seizure* 2000;**9**(4):280–1.

48. Strzelczyk A, Reese JP, Dodel R, Hamer HM. Cost of epilepsy: a systematic review. *Pharmacoeconomics* 2008;**26**(6):463–76.

49. Begley CE, Beghi E. The economic cost of epilepsy: a review of the literature. *Epilepsia* 2002;**43** Suppl 4:3–9.

50. Begley C, Annegers J, Lairson D, Reynolds T, Hauser WA. Cost of epilepsy in the United States: a model based on incidence and prognosis. *Epilepsia* 1994; **35**(6):1230–43.

51. Reuber M, House A, Pukrop R, Bauer J, Elger C. Somatization, dissociation and general psychopathology in patients with psychogenic non-epileptic seizures. *Epilepsy Res* 2003;**57**:159–67.

52. Martin R, Gilliam F, Kilgore M, Faught E, Kuznicky R. Improved health care resource utilization following

video-EEG confirmed diagnosis of nonepileptic psychogenic seizures. *Seizure* 1998;7:385–90.
53. Binder L, Salinsky M. Psychogenic nonepileptic seizures. *Neuropsychol Rev* 2007;17:405–12.
54. Oto M, Espie C, Pelosi A, Selkirk M, Duncan R. The safety of antiepileptic drug withdrawal in patients with non-epileptic seizures. *J Neurol Neurosurg Psychiatry* 2005;76:1682–5.
55. Finlayson O, Mirsattari S, Derry P, et al. Economic impact of non-epileptic seizures on the health care system and the importance of their early diagnosis and treatment. *Epilepsia* 2007;46 Suppl 6:33 (abstract).
56. Martin R, Bell B, Hermann B, Mennemeyer S. Nonepileptic seizures and their costs: the role of neuropsychology. In: Prigatano G, Pliskin N, eds. *Clinical Neuropsychology and Cost Outcome Research*. New York: Psychology Press, Inc. 2003; 235–58.
57. Reuber M, Pukrop R, Bauer J, et al. Outcome in psychogenic nonepileptic seizures: 1 to 10-year follow-up in 164 patients. *Ann Neurol* 2003;53: 305–11.
58. Dworetzky B, Mortati K, Rossetti A, et al. Clinical characteristics of psychogenic nonepileptic seizure status in the long-term monitoring unit. *Epilepsy Behav* 2006;9:335–8.
59. Oto M, Conway P, McGonigal A, Russell A, Duncan R. Gender differences in psychogenic non-epileptic seizures. *Seizure* 2005;14:33–9.
60. Hantke N, Doherty M, Haltiner A. Medication use profiles in patients with psychogenic nonepileptic seizures. *Epilepsy Behav* 2007;10:333–5.
61. Bodde N, Janssen A, Theuns C, et al. Factors involved in the long-term prognosis of psychogenic nonepileptic seizures. *J Psychosom Res* 2007;62:545–51.
62. Marquez AV, Farias ST, Apperson M, et al. Psychogenic nonepileptic seizures are associated with an increased risk of obesity. *Epilepsy Behav* 2004;5(1):88–93.
63. Reilly J, Baker G, Rhodes J, Salmon P. The association of sexual and physical abuse with somatization: characteristics of patients presenting with irritable bowel syndrome and non-epileptic attack disorder. *Psychol Med* 1999;29(2):399–406.
64. Reuber M. Psychogenic nonepileptic seizures: answers and questions. *Epilepsy Behav* 2008;12:622–35.
65. So EL, Schauble BS. Ictal asomatognosia as a cause of epileptic falls: simultaneous video, EMG, and invasive EEG. *Neurology* 2004;63(11):2153–4.
66. Walczak T, Papacostas S, Williams D, Scheuer M, Notarfanscesco A. Outcome after diagnosis of psychogenic nonepileptic seizures. *Epilepsia* 1995;36:1131–7.
67. De Timary P, Fouchet P, Sylin M, et al. Non-epileptic seizures: delayed diagnosis in patients presenting with electroencephalographic (EEG) or clinical signs of epileptic seizures. *Seizure* 2002;11: 193–7.
68. D'Alessio L, Giagante B, Oddo S, et al. Psychiatric disorders in patients with psychogenic non-epileptic seizures, with and without comorbid epilepsy. *Seizure* 2006;15:333–9.
69. Arain A, Hamadani A, Islam S, Abou-Khalil B. Predictors of early seizure remission after diagnosis of psychogenic nonepileptic seizures. *Epilepsy Behav* 2007;11:409–12.
70. O'Sullivan S, Spillane J, McMahon E, et al. Clinical characteristics and outcome of patients diagnosed with psychogenic nonepileptic seizures: a 5-year review. *Epilepsy Behav* 2007;11:77–84.
71. Duncan R, Oto M. Psychogenic nonepileptic seizures in patients with learning disability: comparison with patients with no learning disability. *Epilepsy Behav* 2008;12:183–6.
72. Kuyk J, Siffels M, Bakvis B, Swinkels W. Psychological treatment of patients with psychogenic non-epileptic seizures: an outcome study. *Seizure* 2008;17(7): 595–603.
73. Reuber M, Fernandez G, Bauer J, Helmstaedter C, Elger C. Diagnostic delay in psychogenic nonepileptic seizures. *Neurology* 2002;58:493–5.
74. Testa S, Schefft B, Szaflarski J, Yeh H, Privitera M. Mood, personality and health-related quality of life in epileptic and psychogenic seizure disorders. *Epilepsia* 2007;48(5):973–8.
75. Selkirk M, Duncan R, Oto M, Pelosi A. Clinical differences between patients with nonepileptic seizures who report antecedent sexual abuse and those who do not. *Epilepsia* 2008;49(8):1446–50.
76. Dikel T, Fennell E, Gilmore R. Posttraumatic stress disorder, dissociation, and sexual abuse history in epileptic and nonepileptic seizure patients. *Epilepsy Behav* 2003;4:644–50.
77. Kuyk J, Swinkels WAM, Spinhoven P. Psychopathologies in patients with nonepileptic seizures with and without comorbid epilepsy: how different are they? *Epilepsy Behav* 2003;4(1): 13–8.
78. Marzooqi S, Baker G, Reilly J, Salmon P. The perceived health status of people with psychologically derived non-epileptic attack disorder and epilepsy: a comparative study. *Seizure* 2004;13(2):71–5.
79. Reuber M, Mitchell A, Howlett S, Elger C. Measuring outcome in psychogenic nonepileptic seizures: how relevant is seizure remission? *Epilepsia* 2005;46(11): 1788–95.

80. Schramke C, Valeri A, Valeriano J, Kelly K. Using the Minnesota Multiphasic Inventory 2, EEGs, and clinical data to predict nonepileptic events. *Epilepsy Behav* 2007;**11**:343–6.

81. Kuyk J, Siffels MC, Bakvis P, Swinkels WA. Psychological treatment of patients with psychogenic non-epileptic seizures: an outcome study. *Seizure* 2008;**17**(7):595–603.

82. Quigg M, Armstrong R, Farace E, Fountain N. Quality of life outcome is associated with cessation rather than reduction in psychogenic nonepileptic seizures. *Epilepsy Behav* 2002;**3**:455–9.

Section 1 Chapter 4

Recognition, diagnosis, and impact of nonepileptic seizures

Clinical features and the role of video-EEG monitoring

Selim R. Benbadis and W. Curt LaFrance, Jr.

The erroneous diagnosis of epilepsy is relatively common. At a typical epilepsy center, 20% to 40% of patients previously diagnosed with epilepsy and whose seizures are not responding to drugs are found to be misdiagnosed [1–4]. Most patients misdiagnosed with having epilepsy are eventually shown to have psychogenic nonepileptic seizures (PNES), or (more rarely) syncope or parasomnias [1]. Occasionally other paroxysmal conditions can be misdiagnosed as epilepsy, but they are uncommon in an epilepsy monitoring unit (EMU). Unfortunately, once the diagnosis of "seizures" is made, it is easily perpetuated without being questioned, which explains the usual diagnostic delay [5, 6] and associated cost [7–9] (see Chapter 3).

Generally, misdiagnosed patients present to the epilepsy center after carrying the wrong diagnosis of seizures for 7 to 10 years [5, 6], indicating that neurologists may not have a high enough index of suspicion when drugs fail to control symptoms. Some are referred by the general neurologist, and others are self-referred out of frustration of trying yet another medication regimen without success. The diagnosis of PNES can be suspected based on historical features, with a good predictive value, but after being clinically suspected, it should be confirmed with video-EEG (VEEG) recordings.

Since its inception [10, 11] VEEG monitoring has become widely available. In the US, most large referral medical centers now have an epilepsy program and an EMU, and many smaller hospitals are acquiring the equipment to perform VEEG. However, like any procedure, VEEG must be performed and interpreted correctly in order to avoid serious diagnostic errors. Consequently, it is performed better and more reliably at centers that perform high volumes and are exposed to high numbers of recordings that include epileptic seizures, PNES, and other physiological (i.e., nonepileptic and non-psychogenic) episodes. Stated more bluntly, combining an EEG with a video is not enough to "perform" VEEG. This chapter will review the diagnostic process of PNES with emphasis on VEEG.

Suspicion by history

Psychogenic nonepileptic seizures are initially suspected based on the history (see Table 4.1), so much so that in our experience, even by a telephone "screening," a good predictive value can be obtained. A number of "red flags" are clinically useful to raise the suspicion that "seizures" may be psychogenic rather than epileptic. Of course, resistance to antiepileptic drugs (AEDs) can be the first clue, and is usually the reason for referral to the epilepsy center. In fact most (about 80%) patients with PNES have been treated with AEDs for some time before the correct diagnosis is made [12]. A high frequency of events (e.g., daily episodes) that is completely unaffected by AEDs should also suggest the possibility of a psychogenic etiology. The presence of specific triggers that are unusual for epileptic seizures can be very suggestive of PNES, and this should be specifically asked about during history-taking. For example emotional triggers ("stress" or "getting upset") are commonly reported in PNES. Other triggers that suggest PNES can include pain, certain movements, sounds, lights, and more unusual ones (e.g., sexual activity, foods), and these should raise the suspicion, especially if they are alleged to *consistently* trigger a "seizure." Stress as a precipitant of seizures, however, is not pathognomonic of PNES. Stress has been shown to be a precipitant of epileptic seizures in a number of studies [13, 14].

The circumstances in which events occur can be very helpful. Psychogenic nonepileptic seizures (like

Gates and Rowan's Nonepileptic Seizures, 3rd edn. ed. Steven C. Schachter and W. Curt LaFrance, Jr. Published by Cambridge University Press. © S. Schachter and W. C. LaFrance, Jr. 2010.

Table 4.1 Historical aspects that can help distinguish psychogenic nonepileptic seizures from epileptic seizures

	Psychogenic nonepileptic seizures	Epileptic seizures
History		
Started < 10 years of age	Unusual	Common
Seizures in presence of doctors	Common	Unusual
Recurrent "status"	Common	Rare
Multiple unexplained physical symptoms, including a diagnosis of fibromyalgia or unexplained "chronic pain"	Common	Rare
Multiple operations/invasive tests	Common	Rare
Psychiatric treatment	Common	Rare
Sexual and physical abuse	Common	Rare

From Posner *et al.* [100]; modified from Reuber and Elger [101], with permission.

other psychogenic symptoms) tend to occur in the presence of an "audience." For example, occurrence in the physician's office or the waiting room is highly suggestive of PNES [15]. Similarly, while PNES can occur at night, they tend to not occur during physiological sleep, although they may seem to and be reported as doing so [16, 17]. Duncan *et al.* found that the prevalence of a history of sleep events is similar in PNES and epilepsy, and is of no value in discriminating between the two, although a history of events occurring exclusively during sleep does suggest epileptic seizures [18].

With a carefully obtained history and observant witnesses, the detailed description of the events often includes characteristics that are inconsistent with epileptic seizures. In particular, some characteristics of the motor ("convulsive") phenomena are associated with PNES (see below under "Video-EEG monitoring: ictal semiology"). However, witnesses' accounts are rarely detailed enough to describe these accurately, and, in fact, even seizures witnessed by physicians and thought to be epileptic often turn out to be PNES. Thus, although they can be sought by history, the actual ictal behaviors are best studied with video recordings, which nowadays include home videos and recordings with cell phones. The past medical history can be very useful, because the presence of poorly defined and "fashionable" (possibly psychogenic) conditions, such as "fibromyalgia" and chronic pain, has a high predictive value (~70–80%) for a diagnosis of PNES [15]. Other such suspicious diagnoses may include seronegative Lyme disease and chronic fatigue syndrome. Generally, an extensive review of systems, including lengthy written lists of symptoms or diagnoses, can suggest somatization [19]. A psychosocial history with evidence for maladaptive behaviors or associated psychiatric diagnoses should further raise the suspicion of PNES.

The examination, paying particular attention to mental status evaluation including the general demeanor and appropriate level of concern, overdramatization, or hysterical features, can be very telling. Lastly, the examination often uncovers histrionic behaviors such as give-way weakness or "tight-roping" on attempted tandem walking. Performing the examination can in itself act as an "activation" in suggestible patients (see below), making an event more likely to occur during the history taking or examination [15].

Routine EEG: because of its low sensitivity, routine EEG is not very helpful in making a diagnosis of PNES. However, the presence of repeatedly normal EEGs, especially in light of frequent events that resist medications, certainly can be viewed as a "red flag" [20].

Ambulatory EEG is increasingly used, is cost-effective, and can contribute to the diagnosis by recording the habitual episode and documenting the simultaneous absence of ictal EEG changes. However, because of the difficulties in conveying this diagnosis, it should always be confirmed by VEEG.

Home video recordings are also increasingly used, since they are now widely available, including on cellular phones. If the quality is sufficient, they could be extremely useful [21], and when they can be coupled with ambulatory EEG, they may become the way of the future.

Video-EEG monitoring

Simultaneous recording of the clinical manifestations (video) and EEG is the gold standard for diagnosis, and in fact is indicated in all patients who continue to have frequent seizures despite medications [22]. In the hands of experienced epileptologists, the combined electroclinical analysis of both the clinical semiology of the "ictus" and the ictal EEG findings allows a definitive diagnosis in nearly all cases. If an event is recorded, with a good neurological and psychiatric history and semiological assessment coupled with EEG, it is rare that this question (PNES vs. epileptic seizures) cannot be answered, and the diagnosis of PNES can be made with high confidence.

The principle of VEEG monitoring is to record an episode and demonstrate that (1) there is no epileptiform change in the EEG during the clinical event, and (2) the clinical event is not consistent with seizure types that can be unaccompanied by ictal EEG changes, i.e. making sure that the recorded event is not an epileptic seizure without epileptiform EEG changes. One of the greatest concerns voiced by neurologists and other clinicians is that of missing scalp "EEG negative" epilepsy. Fortunately there are only a few seizure types that are notoriously *unaccompanied* by scalp EEG changes (see "Limitations and pitfalls of VEEG monitoring" later in this chapter).

Ictal semiology

Analysis of the ictal semiology (i.e., using video) is at least as important as the ictal EEG, as it often shows behaviors that are obviously not associated with epileptic seizures or other known neurological conditions (see Table 4.2). It is critical to recognize that no single characteristic is pathognomonic of PNES. However, certain characteristics of the motor phenomena are strongly associated with PNES and rare in epileptic seizures, so that they are relatively specific. Since the typical PNES includes more than one of these behaviors, the diagnosis is usually not difficult. Behaviors or signs strongly suggestive of PNES include the following: a very gradual onset or termination; pseudosleep; and discontinuous (stop-and-go), irregular or asynchronous (out-of-phase) activity including side-to-side head movement, pelvic thrusting, opisthotonic posturing, stuttering, and weeping [23–30]. Ictal eye closure is associated with PNES [31], and although this has been questioned [32], eye closure, especially when prolonged and with complete unresponsiveness, is quite specific for PNES. Behaviors that are modified by an examiner, such as avoidance of a noxious stimulus (dropping the patient's hands onto the face), and nonanatomical progression of symptoms (various limbs moving at various times) can also help. Another useful sign is preserved awareness and ability to interact with the examiner during bilateral motor activity, which is relatively specific to PNES. Finally, "overdramatic" postictal responses such as whispering voice or partial motor responses have a strong association with PNES [33]. Some features of PNES may be slightly different between patients who report a history of sexual abuse and those who do not [34]. Those reporting sexual abuse may have earlier onset PNES and more features suggestive of epilepsy (convulsive and more severe attacks, nocturnal attacks, injuries, incontinence), more emotional triggers, prodromes, and flashbacks. They also may have more severe psychiatric diagnoses, more social security benefits and were less often in cohabiting relationships.

Observing what the patients bring into the EMU also has some value. One group found that of those admitted for monitoring, more patients with PNES brought a toy stuffed animal with them [35]. In their study, 381 patients with PNES were compared to 453 patients with epilepsy. Of 23 patients (2.5%) who had toy animals during admission, 20 were diagnosed with PNES, and 3 were diagnosed with epilepsy ($p < 0.001$). The three patients with epilepsy had a history of a psychiatric disorder. Sensitivity was 5.2% and specificity was 99.3%, with a positive predictive power of 87%, and a negative predictive power of 55%. The authors proposed that such behaviors may represent nonverbal expressions of attachment desires, dependency needs, or other psychological traits.

Certain symptoms, when present, argue in favor of epileptic seizures and should warrant caution when observed. These include ictal grasping and postictal behaviors, such as postictal nose rubbing and stertorous breathing. Ictal grasping is seen in frontal lobe seizures and some temporal lobe seizures [36, 37]. Stertorous breathing is quite specific for convulsive epileptic seizures [38, 39]. Postictal "confusion" is well known to follow most epileptic seizures; however, it is noted by many patients with PNES and its absence does not rule out epileptic seizures, as seen in certain frontal lobe seizures and in absence epilepsy. Postictal nose rubbing and cough are seen in temporal lobe epilepsy and not in PNES [40–42].

Contrary to the notion that certain common signs are specific to epilepsy, incontinence, significant injury, and tongue lacerations occur in both epileptic seizures and PNES [23–25, 43, 44]. At least one of the usual signs associated with generalized tonic-clonic seizures (tongue biting, falling or incontinence) was reported by 66% of patients with PNES [45]. Obviously documented incontinence or tongue biting are much more specific than *reported* incontinence or tongue biting. Lateral tongue biting is highly specific

Table 4.2 Ictal semiology that may help differentiate psychogenic nonepileptic seizures from epileptic seizures

Observation	Psychogenic nonepileptic seizures	Epileptic seizures
Situational onset	Occasional	Rare
Gradual onset	Common	Rare
Precipitated by stimuli (noise, light)	Occasional	Rare
Purposeful movements	Occasional	Very rare
Opisthotonus "*arc de cercle*"	Occasional	Very rare
Tongue biting (tip)	Occasional	Rare
Tongue biting (side)	Rare	Common
Prolonged ictal atonia	Occasional	Very rare
Vocalization during "tonic-clonic" phase	Occasional	Very rare
Reactivity during "unconsciousness"	Occasional	Very rare
Rapid postictal reorientation	Common	Unusual
Undulating motor activity	Common	Very rare
Asynchronous limb movements	Common	Rare
Rhythmic pelvic movements	Occasional	Rare
Side-to-side head shaking	Common	Rare
Ictal crying	Occasional	Very rare
Ictal stuttering	Occasional	Rare
Postictal whispering	Occasional	Not present
Closed mouth in "tonic phase"	Occasional	Very rare
Closed eyelids during seizure onset	Very common	Rare
Convulsion > 2 minutes	Common	Very rare
Resisted eyelid opening	Common	Very rare
Pupillary light reflex	Usually retained	Commonly absent
Lack of cyanosis	Common	Rare
Ictal grasping	Rare	Occurs in FLE and TLE
Postictal nose rubbing	Not present	Occurs in TLE
Stertorous breathing postictally	Not present	Common
Self-injury	May be present	May be present
Urinary incontinence	May be present	May be present

FLE, frontal lobe epilepsy; TLE, temporal lobe epilepsy.
From Posner et al. [100]; Modified from Reuber & Elger [101] and LaFrance [102], with permission.

to generalized tonic-clonic seizures [43], and thus is a very helpful sign for epileptic seizures when present; conversely, tip of the tongue biting is observed in PNES and syncope.

Data that described injuries in patients with PNES were largely based on patients' self-reports [46], however, longitudinal follow-up of patients with PNES reveals that approximately 60% had PNES-related injuries [47]. The authors have evaluated and cared for a number of patients with PNES only who have sustained significant fractures and cranial and bodily hematomas with their swooning events or from falls down stairs. Sometimes the *character* of the injury is helpful in distinguishing epileptic seizures from

PNES. The injuries from epileptic seizures are typically lacerations on bony edges. Conversely, Trimble has described "the rug-burn sign" seen in patients with PNES who sustain excoriations to cheeks or long bones while seizing [48].

Inductions

Provocative techniques, activation procedures, or "inductions" can be extremely useful for the diagnosis of PNES, particularly when the diagnosis remains uncertain and no spontaneous attacks occur during monitoring. Many epilepsy centers use some sort of provocative technique to aid in the diagnosis of PNES [49]. Traditionally, hypnosis and amobarbital have been used to distinguish epileptic from nonepileptic seizures [50, 51]. More recently, IV saline injection has been the most commonly used [49, 52–57], but various other techniques have been described [58–60]. In addition, false alarms from automated seizure detections often act as unintentional inductions and trigger PNES in suggestible patients.

There are many advantages to the use of provocative techniques. First, when carefully performed and using simultaneous EEG, their specificity approaches 100% [61]. Second, there are difficult situations in which the combination of semiology (video) and EEG does *not* allow one to conclude that an episode is psychogenic in origin. Two relatively common scenarios are (1) the ictal EEG is uninterpretable due to movement-related artifacts; and (2) the ictal EEG is normal but the symptoms are consistent with a "simple partial" seizure. In these situations, the very presence of suggestibility (i.e., suggestion triggers the episode in question) is the strongest argument to support a psychogenic etiology. Third, at least theoretically, nonepileptic is not quite synonymous with psychogenic. The combination of a recorded episode with normal ictal EEG makes the diagnosis of a nonepileptic event, but does not in itself categorize it as psychogenic. However, a positive induction does stamp the episode as psychogenic. Fourth, there is a strong economic argument for the use of these techniques: when spontaneous attacks do not occur in the allotted time for monitoring, the evaluation may be inconclusive. In this situation, provocative techniques often turn an inconclusive evaluation into a diagnostic one.

The main limitation of provocative techniques is that they may raise ethical concerns. Several valid ethical arguments against placebo induction have been raised and acknowledged [62, 63]. Of main concern is the fact that physicians cannot honestly disclose the content of the syringe (for IV saline), or cannot say that the maneuver (e.g., tuning fork or patch) induces seizures. Even if the term "seizures" is then used in a broader sense, encompassing PNES, a degree of disingenuousness persists. The problem is particularly acute when a placebo is used, which results in deceptive "beating around the bush." Thus, techniques that do not use placebo may be preferable, since they circumvent these ethical problems while retaining similar diagnostic value.

The best documented technique uses a combination of hyperventilation, photic stimulation, and strong verbal suggestion [64–66]. If hyperventilation is contraindicated or ill-advised, counting aloud with arms raised will work equally well. The sensitivity is comparable to other methods, ranging from 60% to 90%. One major advantage of this technique is that hyperventilation and photic stimulation truly induce seizures, so that deception is not inherent to the procedure. Indeed these maneuvers are performed during most EEGs, so that most patients will have undergone them previously. For this reason patients or their families are not intrigued by the induction technique and do not ask about it. In fact a comparable provocative technique using "psychiatric interview" was found not harmful and even useful by patients [56]. Provocative techniques should only be performed during VEEG. In many ways, such provocative techniques are similar to other clinical maneuvers performed during the neurological examination when non-neuroanatomic symptoms are suspected.

Short-term outpatient VEEG with activation

An extension of the use of inductions is that, when patients are strongly suspected to have PNES on clinical grounds, they can undergo outpatient short-term "EEG-video with activation" [67, 68]. This can be very efficient (shortening the wait time) and cost-effective while retaining the same specificity and a reasonably high sensitivity. Using hyperventilation + photic stimulation + suggestion, short-term outpatient VEEG with saline induction yields a diagnosis in 60% to 70% of patients, thus obviating the need for "long-term" VEEG monitoring [64–68] in patients who have only one seizure type and where there is no concern for mixed epileptic seizures and NES.

Difficult and special issues in diagnosis

Multiple seizure types

When taking the history, it is essential not just to ask for a description of "the seizure," but descriptions of *all* the types of seizures, if there are more than one. While most patients with PNES will have only one type and there is not a risk for both, i.e., mixed epileptic seizures/PNES (as described below), having a description of the other seizure type(s) aids in the diagnostic process. The EMU admission may require AED tapering in order to capture both the epileptic seizure type(s) and the PNES. Capturing all seizure types also may aid in treatment, in that showing the patient and their family which are due to epilepsy and will be treated with AEDs, and which are not and will require other interventions (see Section 5), is of great value to patients, their families and clinicians.

Previous abnormal EEG

This is a very common problem. Many patients with PNES seen at epilepsy centers have had previous EEGs interpreted as showing epileptiform abnormalities. A common error is that the episodic symptoms are not even suggestive of seizures, i.e., nonspecific symptoms like light-headedness, dizziness, and numbness, and the diagnosis of seizures is entirely based on the (over-interpreted) EEG. In this situation, it is essential to obtain and review the actual tracing previously read as abnormal because of epileptiform features, since no number of normal subsequent EEGs will "cancel" the previous abnormal one. When reviewed, the vast majority will turn out to show normal variants that were misread as epileptiform [69–71]. Unfortunately, obtaining prior EEGs can be difficult. First, records are not always available or accessible, and second, digital EEG systems are not compatible among each other. In this regard, software that allows one to read any digital EEG format is very valuable. By far the most common errors in EEG interpretation, and the main source of over-reading, are benign temporal sharp transients or "wicket spikes" [70]. In children, an additional issue is the frequently coexisting benign focal epileptiform discharges (BFEDC), which are often seen in asymptomatic children.

Coexisting epilepsy

There is a widely held belief that many or most patients with PNES also have epilepsy. A careful review of the literature shows that this belief is inaccurate. Reports that have found high percentages of patients with PNES to also have epileptic seizures are based on loose criteria (such as an "abnormal EEG"), whereas those that required definite evidence for coexisting epilepsy found percentages of coexistent epilepsy between 9% and 15% [72, 73] (see Chapter 5).

Coexisting neurological disease

A related phenomenon is that seizures are especially likely to be overdiagnosed in patients with other neurological diseases, e.g., multiple sclerosis, stroke, antecedent brain surgery [74], or a history of head injury. For example, among patients in one study with traumatic brain injury diagnosed with posttraumatic epilepsy, 30% had PNES instead of epilepsy [75]. Thus, as is the general rule, if seizures do not respond to AEDs, a diagnosis of PNES should be considered despite the coexistence of neurologic disease. Psychogenic nonepileptic seizures after some kind of head injury are particularly thorny because the patients are often involved in litigation.

PNES in the elderly

In general, psychogenic symptoms begin in young adulthood. However, late-onset PNES are not rare in patients evaluated at epilepsy centers [76, 77] (see Chapter 10).

PNES after epilepsy surgery

Psychogenic nonepileptic seizures may occur after epilepsy surgery and should always be considered if seizures recur and are somewhat different than preoperatively. Psychogenic nonepileptic seizures tend to occur within a month after surgery [76]. Risk factors include neurological dysfunction in the right hemisphere, seizure onset after adolescence, low IQ, serious preoperative psychopathological conditions, and major surgical complications [78–80].

Limitations and pitfalls of VEEG monitoring

In the majority of cases, the diagnosis of PNES with VEEG is clear cut and can be made with a high degree of confidence. There are limitations to VEEG monitoring, however, and it is important to be familiar with them in order to avoid serious diagnostic errors.

Ictal EEG has limitations because it may be negative in simple partial seizures [81, 82] and in some "complex partial" seizures, especially those of frontal lobe onset [67]. Ictal EEG may also be uninterpretable or difficult to read if movements generate excessive artifact. Knowledge of the types of clinical seizures that may be unaccompanied by ictal EEG changes, therefore, is critical. The most common seizures that are unaccompanied by ictal EEG changes are those without impairment of awareness, i.e., simple partial seizures. This includes all simple partial seizures with subjective phenomena, i.e., auras, which can involve any of the five senses as well as psychic or experiential sensations. Other simple partial seizures that are commonly unaccompanied by ictal EEG changes are brief tonic phenomena such as those typical of frontal lobe seizures. These are typically brief (5 to 30 seconds) and tonic and may be "hypermotor," but not usually as dramatically flailing or thrashing as PNES. In those situations, it can be impossible to "prove" that such episodes are psychogenic. For example, brief episodes of déjà vu or fear or tonic stiffening with no EEG changes can never be *proven* to be psychogenic. Weighing in favor of PNES is when the events never progress to clear seizures and if there is suggestibility (triggering them with placebo maneuvers).

This situation is similar to psychogenic movement disorders, where the diagnosis rests solely on phenomenology (i.e., there is no equivalent of the EEG), and response to placebo or suggestion is considered a diagnostic criterion for a *definite* psychogenic mechanism [68]. A very solid rule is that psychogenic events do not occur out of physiological sleep, so that attacks that arise out of EEG-verified sleep are always related to neurological disorders (epileptic seizures or parasomnias). Epileptic seizures with altered awareness and no EEG changes are very rare, and if the clinical events are strongly suggestive of seizures, it is best to err on the side of treating them as epileptic. More recently, video split-screen techniques have been shown to be helpful in diagnosing epileptic seizures [83].

Of course, lack of ictal EEG changes only indicates that the episodes are nonepileptic, and nonepileptic does not always mean psychogenic. Other diagnoses must be considered before making a diagnosis of PNES. The most common ones to consider are syncope for episodes that occur during waking, and parasomnias for episodes that occur in sleep.

A common myth is that a recorded episode with a negative EEG is all it takes to make a diagnosis of PNES. This is grossly inaccurate. A "negative" EEG can only be interpreted in the context of the semiology of the event in question. Thus, both the video and EEG must be available. (In fact the diagnosis would probably be more accurate with video alone than with EEG alone.)

Unlike the definitive diagnosis of brain tumors, the closest test to a "biopsy" for distinguishing epileptic seizures from PNES is intracranial monitoring. The risk and morbidity associated with craniotomy and grid or depth electrode placement outweighs their use in patients with a suspicion of PNES. In the absence of the definitive confirmation of the diagnosis, there is no way to "prove" that the PNES diagnosis is correct even when we have a high degree of certainty. Ramsay *et al.* described the limitations of scalp EEG and reported the use of depth electrodes on patients with scalp negative EEGs [84]. Subsequent EEG monitoring revealed patients with epilepsy were found to have an epileptic focus in either the mesial ($n = 8$) or inferior frontal ($n = 2$) areas. A study of the interrater reliability of the diagnosis by VEEG, sampling a group of epileptologists, only found a *good* interrater agreement for PNES [85], indicating that there is a certain component of subjective "artful" judgment. When used properly, VEEG allows the diagnosis of paroxysmal seizure-like events, and in particular the diagnosis of PNES, with a high degree of confidence.

Other tests

Postictal laboratory tests can be useful in clinical settings where VEEG is not readily available, but their sensitivity and specificity are not high enough compared to VEEG to be of great value [86]. They include prolactin (PRL), which peaks at 20 minutes post-seizure, and creatine kinase (CK), which peaks at 24 hours. Prolactin was the subject of a recent American Academy of Neurology (AAN) practice parameter [87], reporting a pooled sensitivity of 60% for diagnosis of generalized tonic-clonic seizures, a pooled sensitivity of 46% for complex partial seizures, and pooled specificity of 96%. The authors concluded that elevated serum PRL, when measured in the appropriate clinical setting at 10 to 20 minutes after a suspected event, is a useful adjunct for the differentiation of generalized tonic-clonic or complex partial seizures from PNES among adults and older children. Serum PRL assay, however, does not distinguish epileptic seizures from syncope and has not been established in the evaluation of status epilepticus, repetitive seizures, and neonatal seizures, demonstrating that it is not a definitive diagnostic tool.

Neuropsychological evaluation is of little value in establishing the diagnosis of PNES, again because sensitivity and specificity are mediocre for this purpose. This testing is, however, useful to define the patient's psychological profile and possibly to target treatment modalities [88].

Physiological nonepileptic events (nonepileptic nonpsychogenic episodes)

As mentioned above, nonepileptic does not equal psychogenic. Other conditions that can mimic seizures, however, are usually diagnosed without VEEG, so they are less likely to be encountered in an EMU. The two that are relatively commonly seen in the EMU, after PNES, are syncope and parasomnias. These differential diagnoses are covered briefly here, and more extensively in Chapters 6 and 7.

Syncope is common, and while it is a distant second to PNES in terms of conditions misdiagnosed as epilepsy at referral epilepsy centers (and thus encountered in the EMU), it may be more common in general neurology practices. The first reason that syncope is misdiagnosed as seizures is the erroneous belief that seizures can cause a flaccid motionless episode of loss of consciousness (LOC) for seconds to minutes. In reality, no seizure type does this. Generalized tonic-clonic seizures have obvious motor manifestations; myoclonic seizures are very short jerks with no detectable LOC; atonic seizures may cause abrupt falls but no prolonged LOC; and complex partial seizures or absence seizures cause alteration of awareness but not limp LOC. In general, episodes of LOC with eyes closed for several seconds to minutes are either psychogenic or syncopal, but not epileptic. The second reason for the misdiagnosis is the frequency with which syncopal events are "convulsive." While the conventional teaching is that syncopal episodes are limp, motionless events, they in fact frequently involve brief body jerks [1, 89–91]. Motor symptoms associated with convulsive syncope are clonic- or myoclonic-like, tend to last only a few seconds, and terminate once the patient is horizontal, in sharp contrast to the typical generalized tonic-clonic seizure duration of 30 to 90 seconds, and continuation irrespective of body position. Electroencephalography is very sensitive to decreased cerebral flow, and by the time LOC occurs in syncope, EEG changes are present. When syncope (convulsive or not) is recorded on VEEG, the EEG proceeds through a very stereotyped pattern of changes (delta slowing and voltage suppression due to lack of cerebral blood flow) [92, 93].

When an accurate description is missing (e.g., unwitnessed event), the distinction between syncope and seizures can at times be difficult, as it is based on history alone. However, several symptoms are helpful in pointing one way or the other. Among these are the circumstances of the attacks, since the most common mechanism for syncope (vasovagal response) is typically triggered by known precipitants (e.g., pain such as inflicted by medical procedures, emotions, cough, micturition, hot environment, prolonged standing, exercise). Other historical features that favor syncope include presyncopal prodromes (vertigo, dizziness, lightheadedness, nausea, chest pain) as well as advanced age and a history of cardiovascular disease. Historical features that favor seizures include biting, head turning, posturing, urinary incontinence, cyanosis, déjà vu, and postictal confusion [44, 94].

A related issue is that a high proportion of "syncope of unknown origin" is likely to be psychogenic, but probably never diagnosed because such patients see cardiologists rather than neurologists and are rarely sent for VEEG monitoring. When such patients are seen in the EMU, the diagnosis of psychogenic syncope is very straightforward to confirm since syncope shows a reliable series of EEG changes [92].

Parasomnias that are most likely to resemble seizures are the slow-wave parasomnias (somnambulism, somniloquy, and confusional arousal), and REM sleep behavior disorder (RBD). Parasomnias are the most likely sleep disorders to present a diagnostic challenge since they are by definition short-lived paroxysmal behaviors that occur out of sleep. In particular, the non-REM parasomnias (night terrors, sleepwalking, and confusional arousals) can superficially resemble seizures since they include complex behaviors and some degree of unresponsiveness and amnesia for the event. The non-REM parasomnias are most common between ages 4 and 12 years, and night terrors are particularly common. They are often familial and may be worsened by stress, sleep deprivation, and intercurrent illnesses.

Similarly, rhythmic movement disorder is a parasomnia typically seen at sleep transition or stage 1 sleep, which can also resemble partial seizures. One common example is head banging (*jactatio capitis*). Among REM sleep parasomnias, nightmares rarely present a diagnostic challenge, but RBD may, especially with violent and injurious behaviors during REM sleep. The diagnosis of RBD is usually easy as it affects older men and the description of acting out a dream is quite typical. Several historical features can help in differentiating parasomnias from seizures [95], but occasionally VEEG may be necessary, provided that the episodes are frequent enough. Video-EEG will usually confirm the absence of ictal EEG findings and usually shows that the behavior arises from a specific stage of sleep [96].

Occasionally, in the absence of ictal EEG changes, the differentiation between seizure and parasomnia can be difficult. Hypnic jerks or sleep starts are benign myoclonic jerks that everyone has experienced on occasion. While they resemble the jerks of myoclonic seizures, their occurrence only upon falling asleep stamps them as benign nonepileptic phenomena. They occur at all ages and can lead to evaluations for seizures, especially when the jerks are unusually violent. They are easily identified on VEEG by the fact that they occur in waking to stage 1 transition and have no EEG correlate associated with the jerks [97]. Restless legs syndrome and paroxysmal limb movements of sleep also may interfere with sleep, however, no ictal EEG changes are seen with these disorders.

Paroxysmal movement disorders can be difficult to differentiate from seizures and PNES. Tremors are not usually paroxysmal and rarely cause diagnostic difficulties. Paroxysmal dystonias, such as nocturnal paroxysmal dystonia, can be difficult to differentiate from seizures [83]. Another difficult situation is nonepileptic myoclonus, which of course has no EEG changes and is therefore diagnosed solely on the basis of the clinical data and VEEG. Hiccups and hypnic jerks are examples of normal nonepileptic myoclonus, but abnormal nonepileptic myoclonus can be seen in metabolic or toxic encephalopathies and neurodegenerative diseases. Since there is no EEG discharge in nonepileptic or "subcortical" myoclonus, differentiating it from psychogenic movements is fraught with the same challenges as purely subjective symptoms. Often the diagnosis of psychogenic myoclonic-like movements, like other psychogenic movement disorders [98], will rest on its response to suggestion and the company it keeps (other attacks or other symptoms).

Other conditions to be considered include migraine, narcolepsy, transient ischemic attacks (TIA), transient global amnesia (TGA), and panic attacks. In young children, other conditions include breath-holding spells and shudder attacks [1].

A recently identified entity that should be part of the differential diagnosis is abnormal movements in the intensive care unit (ICU). With the advent of digital videos available with any EEG machine, the differential diagnosis of seizures in the ICU can be more readily pursued. Many such movements are not epileptic, and do not really qualify as "psychogenic" either. Rather, they are abnormal nonepileptic movements related to the environment and discomfort [99].

Conclusion

In summary, VEEG is the gold standard for diagnosis of PNES and is useful in discerning the diagnosis in paroxysmal disorders. In experienced hands, it is highly reliable for the diagnosis of seizures and other paroxysmal events. Like any other test, it has limitations, so it should be used by knowledgeable physicians and in the proper context.

References

1. Benbadis SR. Differential diagnosis of epilepsy. *Continuum Lifelong Learning Neurol* 2007;**13**(4):48–70.
2. Benbadis SR, O'Neill E, Tatum IV, WO, Heriaud L. Outcome of prolonged video-EEG monitoring at a typical referral epilepsy center. *Epilepsia* 2004;**45**(9):1150–3.
3. Smith D, Defalla BA, Chadwick DW. The misdiagnosis of epilepsy and the management of refractory epilepsy in a specialist clinic. QJM 1999;**92**(1):15–23.
4. Scheepers B, Clough P, Pickles C. The misdiagnosis of epilepsy: findings of a population study. *Seizure* 1998;7(5):403–6.
5. Reuber M, Fernandez G, Bauer J, Helmstaedter C, Elger CE. Diagnostic delay in psychogenic nonepileptic seizures. *Neurology* 2002;**58**(3):493–5.
6. Carton S, Thompson PJ, Duncan JS. Non-epileptic seizures: patients' understanding and reaction to the diagnosis and impact on outcome. *Seizure* 2003;**12**(5):287–94.
7. Nowack WJ. Epilepsy: a costly misdiagnosis. *Clin Electroencephalogr* 1997;**28**(4):225–8.

8. Martin RC, Gilliam FG, Kilgore M, Faught E, Kuzniecky R. Improved health care resource utilization following video-EEG-confirmed diagnosis of nonepileptic psychogenic seizures. *Seizure* 1998;7(5):385–90.

9. LaFrance Jr WC, Alper K, Babcock D, et al. Nonepileptic seizures treatment workshop summary. *Epilepsy Behav* 2006;8(3):451–61.

10. Hunter J, Jasper HH. A method of analysis of seizure pattern and electroencephalogram: a cinematographic technique. *Electroencephalogr Clin Neurophysiol* 1949;1:113–14.

11. Penin H. Elektonische Patientenuberwachung in der Nervenklinik Bonn [Electronic patient monitoring in the neurologic hospital of Bonn]. *Umsschau in Wissenschaft und Technik* 1968;7:211–12.

12. Benbadis SR. How many patients with pseudoseizures receive antiepileptic drugs prior to diagnosis? *Eur Neurol* 1999;41(2):114–15.

13. Temkin NR, Davis GR. Stress as a risk factor for seizures among adults with epilepsy. *Epilepsia* 1984;25(4):450–6.

14. Frucht MM, Quigg M, Schwaner C, Fountain NB. Distribution of seizure precipitants among epilepsy syndromes. *Epilepsia* 2000;41(12):1534–9.

15. Benbadis SR. A spell in the epilepsy clinic and a history of "chronic pain" or "fibromyalgia" independently predict a diagnosis of psychogenic seizures. *Epilepsy Behav* 2005;6(2):264–5.

16. Benbadis SR, Lancman ME, King LM, Swanson SJ. Preictal pseudosleep: a new finding in psychogenic seizures. *Neurology* 1996;47(1):63–7.

17. Thacker K, Devinsky O, Perrine K, Alper K, Luciano D. Nonepileptic seizures during apparent sleep. *Ann Neurol* 1993;33(4):414–18.

18. Duncan R, Oto M, Russell AJC, Conway P. Pseudosleep events in patients with psychogenic non-epileptic seizures: prevalence and associations. *J Neurol Neurosurg Psychiatry* 2004;75(7):1009–12.

19. Benbadis SR. Hypergraphia and the diagnosis of psychogenic attacks. *Neurology* 2006;67(5):904.

20. Davis BJ. Predicting nonepileptic seizures utilizing seizure frequency, EEG, and response to medication. *Eur Neurol* 2004;51(3):153–6.

21. Stephenson J, Breningstall G, Steer C, et al. Anoxic-epileptic seizures: home video recordings of epileptic seizures induced by syncopes. *Epileptic Disord* 2004;6(1):15–19.

22. Benbadis SR, Tatum IV, WO, Vale FL. When drugs don't work: an algorithmic approach to medically intractable epilepsy. *Neurology* 2000;55(12):1780–4.

23. Desai BT, Porter RJ, Penry JK. Psychogenic seizures. A study of 42 attacks in six patients, with intensive monitoring. *Arch Neurol* 1982;39(4):202–9.

24. Guberman A. Psychogenic pseudoseizures in non-epileptic patients. *Can J Psychiatry* 1982;27(5):401–4.

25. Meierkord H, Will B, Fish D, Shorvon S. The clinical features and prognosis of pseudoseizures diagnosed using video-EEG telemetry. *Neurology* 1991;41(10):1643–6.

26. Gates JR, Ramani V, Whalen S, Loewenson R. Ictal characteristics of pseudoseizures. *Arch Neurol* 1985;42(12):1183–7.

27. Gulick TA, Spinks IP, King DW. Pseudoseizures: ictal phenomena. *Neurology* 1982;32(1):24–30.

28. Bergen D, Ristanovic R. Weeping as a common element of pseudoseizures. *Arch Neurol* 1993;50(10):1059–60.

29. Vossler DG, Haltiner AM, Schepp SK, et al. Ictal stuttering: a sign suggestive of psychogenic nonepileptic seizures. *Neurology* 2004;63(3):516–19.

30. O'Sullivan SS, Spillane JE, McMahon EM, et al. Clinical characteristics and outcome of patients diagnosed with psychogenic nonepileptic seizures: a 5-year review. *Epilepsy Behav* 2007;11(1):77–84.

31. Chung SS, Gerber P, Kirlin KA. Ictal eye closure is a reliable indicator for psychogenic nonepileptic seizures. *Neurology* 2006;66(11):1730–1.

32. Syed TU, Arozullah AM, Suciu GP, et al. Do observer and self-reports of ictal eye closure predict psychogenic nonepileptic seizures? *Epilepsia* 2008;49(5):898–904.

33. Chabolla DR, Shih JJ. Postictal behaviors associated with psychogenic nonepileptic seizures. *Epilepsy Behav* 2006;9(2):307–11.

34. Selkirk M, Duncan R, Oto M, Pelosi A. Clinical differences between patients with nonepileptic seizures who report antecedent sexual abuse and those who do not. *Epilepsia* 2008;49(8):1446–50.

35. Burneo JG, Martin R, Powell T, et al. Teddy bears: an observational finding in patients with non-epileptic events. *Neurology* 2003;61(5):714–15.

36. Gardella E, Rubboli G, Tassinari CA. Ictal grasping: prevalence and characteristics in seizures with different semiology. *Epilepsia* 2006;47 Suppl 5:59–63.

37. Gardella E, Rubboli G, Tassinari CA. Video-EEG analysis of ictal repetitive grasping in "frontal-hyperkinetic" seizures. *Epileptic Disord* 2006;8(4):267–73.

38. Sen A, Scott C, Sisodiya SM. Stertorous breathing is a reliably identified sign that helps in the differentiation

of epileptic from psychogenic non-epileptic convulsions: an audit. *Epilepsy Res* 2007;**77**(1):62–4.

39. Azar NJ, Tayah TF, Wang L, Song Y, Abou-Khalil BW. Postictal breathing pattern distinguishes epileptic from nonepileptic convulsive seizures. *Epilepsia* 2008;**49**(1):132–7.

40. Geyer JD, Payne TA, Faught E, Drury I. Postictal nose-rubbing in the diagnosis, lateralization, and localization of seizures. *Neurology* 1999;**52**(4):743–5.

41. Wennberg R. Electroclinical analysis of postictal noserubbing. *Can J Neurol Sci* 2000;**27**(2):131–6.

42. Wennberg R. Postictal coughing and noserubbing coexist in temporal lobe epilepsy. *Neurology* 2001;**56**(1):133–4.

43. Benbadis SR, Wolgamuth BR, Goren H, Brener S, Fouad-Tarazi F. Value of tongue biting in the diagnosis of seizures. *Arch Intern Med* 1995;**155**(21):2346–9.

44. Hoefnagels WA, Padberg GW, Overweg J, van der Velde EA, Roos RA. Transient loss of consciousness: the value of the history for distinguishing seizure from syncope. *J Neurol* 1991;**238**(1):39–43.

45. de Timary P, Fouchet P, Sylin M, *et al*. Non-epileptic seizures: delayed diagnosis in patients presenting with electroencephalographic (EEG) or clinical signs of epileptic seizures. *Seizure* 2002;**11**:193–7.

46. Peguero E, Abou-Khalil B, Fakhoury T, Mathews G. Self-injury and incontinence in psychogenic seizures. *Epilepsia* 1995;**36**(6):586–91.

47. Reuber M, Pukrop R, Bauer J, *et al*. Outcome in psychogenic nonepileptic seizures: 1 to 10-year follow-up in 164 patients. *Ann Neurol* 2003;**53**(3):305–11.

48. Trimble MR. Non-epileptic seizures. In: Halligan PW, Bass CM, Marshall JC, eds. *Contemporary Approaches to the Study of Hysteria: Clinical and Theoretical Perspectives*. Oxford, New York: Oxford University Press. 2001; 143–54.

49. Schachter SC, Brown F, Rowan AJ. Provocative testing for nonepileptic seizures: attitudes and practices in the United States among American Epilepsy Society members. *J Epilepsy* 1996;**9**(4):249–52.

50. Sumner JW, Jr, Cameron RR, Peterson DB. Hypnosis in differentiation of epileptic from convulsive-like seizures. *Neurology* 1952;**2**:395–402.

51. Lambert C, Rees WL. Intravenous barbiturates in the treatment of hysteria. *BMJ* 1944;**2**:70–3.

52. Stagno SJ, Smith ML. Use of induction in diagnosing psychogenic seizures. *J Epilepsy* 1996;**9**:153–8.

53. Walczak TS, Williams DT, Berten W. Utility and reliability of placebo infusion in the evaluation of patients with seizures. *Neurology* 1994;**44**(3 Pt 1):394–9.

54. Cohen RJ, Suter C. Hysterical seizures: suggestion as a provocative EEG test. *Ann Neurol* 1982;**11**(4):391–5.

55. Bazil CW, Kothari M, Luciano D, *et al*. Provocation of nonepileptic seizures by suggestion in a general seizure population. *Epilepsia* 1994;**35**(4):768–70.

56. Slater JD, Brown MC, Jacobs W, Ramsay RE. Induction of pseudoseizures with intravenous saline placebo. *Epilepsia* 1995;**36**(6):580–5.

57. Ribai P, Tugendhaft P, Legros B. Usefulness of prolonged video-EEG monitoring and provocative procedure with saline injection for the diagnosis of non epileptic seizures of psychogenic origin. *J Neurol* 2006;**253**(3):328–32.

58. Cohen LM, Howard III, GF, Bongar B. Provocation of pseudoseizures by psychiatric interview during EEG and video monitoring. *Int J Psychiatry Med* 1992;**22**(2):131–40.

59. Luther JS, McNamara JO, Carwile S, Miller P, Hope V. Pseudoepileptic seizures: methods and video analysis to aid diagnosis. *Ann Neurol* 1982;**12**(5):458–62.

60. Riley TL, Berndt T. The role of the EEG technologist in delineating pseudoseizures. *Am J EEG Technol* 1980;**20**:89–96.

61. Lancman ME, Asconape JJ, Craven WJ, Howard G, Penry JK. Predictive value of induction of psychogenic seizures by suggestion. *Ann Neurol* 1994;**35**(3):359–61.

62. Benbadis SR. Provocative techniques should be used for the diagnosis of psychogenic nonepileptic seizures. *Arch Neurol* 2001;**58**(12):2063–5.

63. Gates JR. Provocative testing should not be used for nonepileptic seizures. *Arch Neurol* 2001;**58**(12):2065–6.

64. Benbadis SR, Johnson K, Anthony K, *et al*. Induction of psychogenic nonepileptic seizures without placebo. *Neurology* 2000;**55**(12):1904–5.

65. Benbadis SR, Siegrist K, Tatum IV, WO, Heriaud L, Anthony K. Short-term outpatient EEG video with induction in the diagnosis of psychogenic seizures. *Neurology* 2004;**63**(9):1728–30.

66. Varela HL, Taylor DS, Benbadis SR. Short-term outpatient EEG-video monitoring with induction in a veterans administration population. *J Clin Neurophysiol* 2007;**24**(5):390–1.

67. Bhatia M, Sinha PK, Jain S, Padma MV, Maheshwari MC. Usefulness of short-term video EEG recording with saline induction in pseudoseizures. *Acta Neurol Scand* 1997;**95**(6):363–6.

68. McGonigal A, Oto M, Russell AJ, Greene J, Duncan R. Outpatient video EEG recording in the diagnosis of non-epileptic seizures: a randomised controlled trial of

simple suggestion techniques. *J Neurol Neurosurg Psychiatry* 2002;**72**(4):549–51.
69. Benbadis SR, Tatum IV, WO. Overinterpretation of EEGs and misdiagnosis of epilepsy. *J Clin Neurophysiol* 2003;**20**(1):42–4.
70. Benbadis SR, Lin K. Errors in EEG interpretation and misdiagnosis of epilepsy. Which EEG patterns are overread? *Eur Neurol* 2008;**59**(5):267–71.
71. Benbadis SR. Errors in EEGs and the misdiagnosis of epilepsy: importance, causes, consequences, and proposed remedies. *Epilepsy Behav* 2007;**11**(3): 257–62.
72. Benbadis SR, Agrawal V, Tatum IV, WO. How many patients with psychogenic nonepileptic seizures also have epilepsy? *Neurology* 2001;**57**(5):915–17.
73. Lesser RP, Lueders H, Dinner DS. Evidence for epilepsy is rare in patients with psychogenic seizures. *Neurology* 1983;**33**(4):502–4.
74. Reuber M, Kral T, Kurthen M, Elger CE. New-onset psychogenic seizures after intracranial neurosurgery. *Acta Neurochir (Wien)* 2002;**144**(9):901–7.
75. Hudak AM, Trivedi K, Harper CR, *et al.* Evaluation of seizure-like episodes in survivors of moderate and severe traumatic brain injury. *J Head Trauma Rehabil* 2004;**19**(4):290–5.
76. Duncan R, Oto M, Martin E, Pelosi A. Late onset psychogenic nonepileptic attacks. *Neurology* 2006; **66**(11):1644–7.
77. Behrouz R, Heriaud L, Benbadis SR. Late-onset psychogenic nonepileptic seizures. *Epilepsy Behav* 2006;**8**:649–50.
78. Davies KG, Blumer DP, Lobo S, *et al.* De novo nonepileptic seizures after cranial surgery for epilepsy: incidence and risk factors. *Epilepsy Behav* 2000;**1**: 436–43.
79. Glosser G, Roberts D, Glosser DS. Nonepileptic seizures after resective epilepsy surgery. *Epilepsia* 1999;**40**(12):1750–4.
80. Ney GC, Barr WB, Napolitano C, Decker R, Schaul N. New-onset psychogenic seizures after surgery for epilepsy. *Arch Neurol* 1998;**55**(5):726–30.
81. Devinsky O, Sato S, Kufta CV, *et al.* Electroencephalographic studies of simple partial seizures with subdural electrode recordings. *Neurology* 1989;**39**(4):527–33.
82. Sperling MR, O'Connor MJ. Auras and subclinical seizures: characteristics and prognostic significance. *Ann Neurol* 1990;**28**(3):320–8.
83. Tinuper P, Grassi C, Bisulli F, *et al.* Split-screen synchronized display. A useful video-EEG technique for studying paroxysmal phenomena. *Epileptic Disord* 2004;**6**(1):27–30.
84. Ramsay RE, Cohen A, Brown MC. Coexisting epilepsy and non-epileptic seizures. In: Rowan AJ, Gates JR, eds. *Non-Epileptic Seizures*, 1st edn. Stoneham, MA: Butterworth-Heinemann. 1993; 47–54.
85. Benbadis SR, LaFrance Jr WC, Lorabathina K, *et al.* Interrater reliability of EEG-video monitoring. *Neurology* 2009; in press.
86. Willert C, Spitzer C, Kusserow S, Runge U. Serum neuron-specific enolase, prolactin, and creatine kinase after epileptic and psychogenic non-epileptic seizures. *Acta Neurol Scand* 2004;**109**(5):318–23.
87. Sandstrom SA, Anschel DJ, Chen DK, So YT, Fisher RS. Use of serum prolactin in diagnosing epileptic seizures: report of the Therapeutics and Technology Assessment Subcommittee of the American Academy of Neurology. *Neurology* 2006;**67**(3):544–5.
88. Cragar DE, Berry DT, Fakhoury TA, Cibula JE, Schmitt FA. Performance of patients with epilepsy or psychogenic non-epileptic seizures on four measures of effort. *Clin Neuropsychol* 2006;**20**(3): 552–66.
89. Aminoff MJ, Goodin DS, Berg BO, Compton MN. Ambulatory EEG recordings in epileptic and nonepileptic children. *Neurology* 1988;**38**(4): 558–62.
90. Zaidi A, Clough P, Cooper P, Scheepers B, Fitzpatrick AP. Misdiagnosis of epilepsy: many seizure-like attacks have a cardiovascular cause. *J Am Coll Cardiol* 2000; **36**(1):181–4.
91. Lempert T, Bauer M, Schmidt D. Syncope: a videometric analysis of 56 episodes of transient cerebral hypoxia. *Ann Neurol* 1994;**36**(2):233–7.
92. Benbadis SR, Chichkova R. Psychogenic pseudosyncope: an underestimated and provable diagnosis. *Epilepsy Behav* 2006;**9**(1):106–10.
93. Sheldon RS, Koshman ML, Murphy WF. Electroencephalographic findings during presyncope and syncope induced by tilt table testing. *Can J Cardiol* 1998;**14**(6):811–6.
94. Sheldon R, Rose S, Ritchie D, *et al.* Historical criteria that distinguish syncope from seizures. *J Am Coll Cardiol* 2002;**40**(1):142–8.
95. Derry CP, Davey M, Johns M, *et al.* Distinguishing sleep disorders from seizures: diagnosing bumps in the night. *Arch Neurol* 2006;**63**(5):705–9.
96. Iranzo A, Santamaria J, Rye DB, *et al.* Characteristics of idiopathic REM sleep behavior disorder and that associated with MSA and PD. *Neurology* 2005;**65**(2): 247–52.
97. Montagna P, Liguori R, Zucconi M, *et al.* Physiological hypnic myoclonus. *Electroencephalogr Clin Neurophysiol* 1988;**70**(2):172–6.

98. Fahn S, Williams DT. Psychogenic dystonia. *Adv Neurol* 1988;**50**:431–55.
99. Benbadis SR, Chen S, Melo M. The differential diagnosis of seizures in the ICU: a video-EEG study. *Epilepsia* 2008;**49** Suppl 7:3.
100. Posner JB, Saper CB, Schiff N, Plum F. Psychogenic unresponsiveness. In: Posner JB, Saper CB, Schiff N, Plum F, eds. *Plum and Posner's Diagnosis of Stupor and Coma*, 4th edn. New York: Oxford University Press. 2007; 297–308.
101. Reuber M, Elger CE. Psychogenic nonepileptic seizures: review and update. *Epilepsy Behavior* 2003; 4(3):205–16.
102. LaFrance WC, Jr. Psychogenic nonepileptic seizures. *Curr Opin Neurol* 2008;**21**(2): 195–201.

Section 1 Chapter 5

Recognition, diagnosis, and impact of nonepileptic seizures

Comorbidity of epileptic and psychogenic nonepileptic seizures: diagnostic considerations

Peter Widdess-Walsh, Siddhartha Nadkarni, and Orrin Devinsky

Psychogenic nonepileptic seizures (PNES) are defined as "episodes of altered movement, sensation, or experience similar to epileptic seizures (ES), but caused by a psychological process and not associated with abnormal electrical discharges in the brain" [1]. In contrast, ES are spontaneous paroxysmal electrical discharges from an epileptogenic brain substrate usually causing transient physical manifestations. Psychogenic nonepileptic seizures and ES co-occur in 10% of patients with ES, which can present a challenging scenario for both physicians and caregivers [2]. Failure to recognize either comorbidity can result in diagnostic delay and inappropriate treatment.

The possibility of comorbid ES and PNES should be especially considered under several conditions, including medical intractability, changes in typical seizure semiology, psychosocial stressors, and in the setting of risk factors for PNES, especially a history of psychic or physical trauma. These disorders can coexist in many other settings where they may not be readily suspected (e.g., children, individuals with mental retardation, elderly).

The coexistence of PNES and ES was first reported in 1836 by Beau [3]. Esquirol [4] noted in 1838 "hysteric patients who are at the same time epileptics…with a little practice one could recognize very well, when the attacks are separate, to which of the two diseases the convulsions belong." The aim of this chapter is to aid in the differentiation of PNES and ES when both occur in the same patient.

Case examples

Case 1. A 21-year-old woman developed intractable left parieto-occipital partial epilepsy from an autoimmune encephalopathy. Her MRI revealed left posterior encephalomalacia and gliosis from prior prolonged status epilepticus and immune-mediated damage. She had interictal spikes on EEG in the left parieto-occipital region and daily seizures, recorded on video-EEG (VEEG) with right face sensory or motor clonic seizures. Subdural electrode implantation for epilepsy surgery was aborted due to postoperative optic neuropathy as well as focal right hemi-clonic status epilepticus with new MRI lesions. Several weeks later, her parents called to report frequent events of right-sided movements of her head, arm, and leg. Episodes continued despite upward titration of her antiepileptic drugs (AEDs). Repeat VEEG showed that the events, with non-clonic arm and jaw movements, head shaking, and unresponsiveness, were nonepileptic. Interictal left parieto-occipital spikes continued on EEG (Figure 5.1). A previous history of abuse was established, supporting the diagnosis of PNES. After several months of psychiatric treatment, PNES occurred rarely.

Case 2. A 24-year-old woman had staring spells and epilepsy diagnosed at age 9 years. She had a mild learning disability. Her mother had poorly controlled epilepsy and schizophrenia, and was on AEDs during her pregnancy. The staring spells returned at the age of 20 years and AED therapy was initiated. She began to have daily intractable events of agitated behavior with reduced responsiveness. The behavior was semi-purposeful, and at times violent such as throwing objects or furniture, turning the gas stove on, and hitting her relatives. There were also episodes of vomiting and incontinence without an identifiable medical or epileptic basis. The events typically occurred only in the evening after returning from her job in a childcare center. Her EEG showed generalized polyspikes and photic stimulation produced bursts of spikes and

Gates and Rowan's Nonepileptic Seizures, 3rd edn. ed. Steven C. Schachter and W. Curt LaFrance, Jr. Published by Cambridge University Press. © S. Schachter and W. C. LaFrance, Jr. 2010.

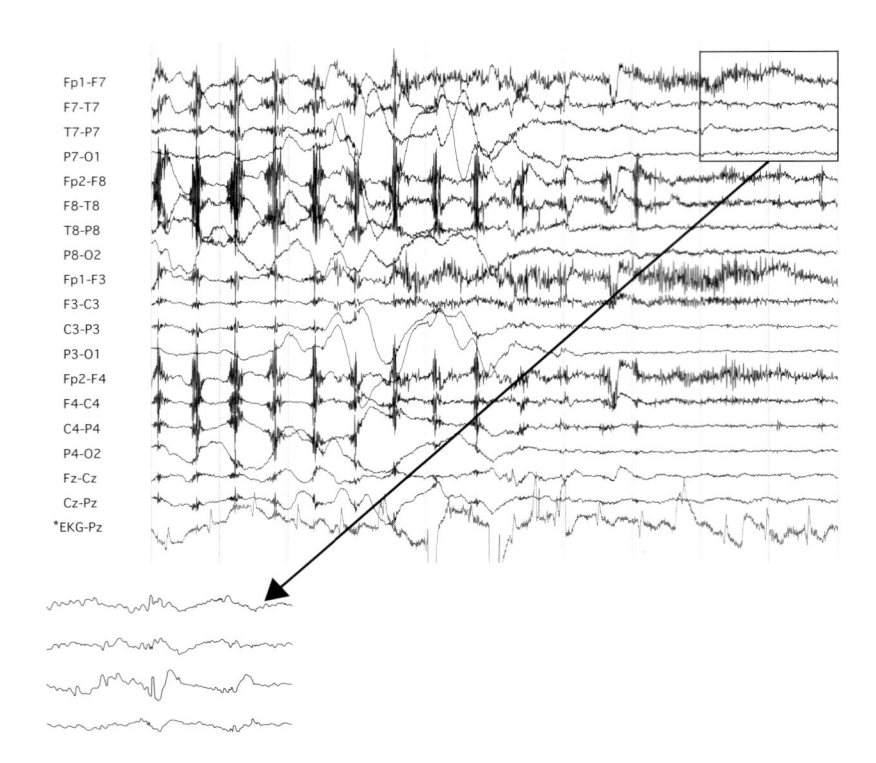

Figure 5.1. EEG showing rhythmic motion artifact from a psychogenic nonepileptic seizure in a patient with comorbid PNES and ES. Interictal epileptiform discharges are seen in the background (detail in insert).

myoclonic jerks. Ambulatory and VEEG monitoring captured the events and staring spells and confirmed them as nonepileptic. Photic stimulation also produced loss of responsiveness and pelvic thrusting without an epileptic seizure pattern on EEG. She was maintained on low-dose topiramate without clinical ES, although PNES persisted despite treatment.

Incidence and prevalence of comorbid ES and PNES

Patients with ES and PNES often come to attention at tertiary epilepsy centers. The reported prevalence of ES in patients with PNES varies widely, ranging between 5% and 50% [5–10] (Table 5.1). Reasons for the marked differences between studies are largely attributable to the rigor of the diagnosis of ES (e.g., clinical history, direct observation of events, presence of interictal discharges, and VEEG recordings). Slowing accounted for some of the "abnormal" EEGs in these studies, which is not specific for epilepsy. Also, inclusion of recently documented versus historically remote seizure events could affect the estimated prevalence of ES in patients with PNES. Finally, other confounding factors such as

Table 5.1 Percentage of ES in patients with PNES

Author	ES/total PNES	Definition of ES
Reuber et al. [11]	90/329 (27%)	History and EEG, 90 with abnormal EEG 55 with ictal epileptiform EEG
Muller et al. [6]	9/44 (20%)	History only in 3/9 patients
Benbadis et al. [7]	3/32 (9%)	Abnormal interictal EEG
Martin et al. [5]	29/514 (6%)	24 with ictal epileptiform EEG 5 with abnormal interictal EEG only
De Timary et al. [24]	53/103 (51%)	"Refractory epilepsy" and found to have PNES, 80% had abnormal interictal EEG
Kotsopoulos et al. [53]	3/63 (5%)	Abnormal interictal EEG
Lesser et al. [2]	5/50 (10%)	Abnormal interictal epileptiform EEG

PNES, psychogenic nonepileptic seizures; ES, epileptic seizures.

Table 5.2 Percentage of PNES and PNES/ES in patients referred for EEG monitoring (recent series)

Study	PNES	PNES and ES
Dodrill & Holmes [12]	14.8%	3.6%
Muller et al. [6]	13.6%	2.8%
Martin et al. [5]	25.6%	1.4%

PNES, psychogenic nonepileptic seizures; ES, epileptic seizures.

referral bias can significantly alter results. Based on more stringent criteria of epileptiform activity on EEG, an estimate of 10% of patients with PNES also have ES [2, 7].

In patients with mixed ES/PNES, there is often a delay in diagnosis, particularly of the PNES; the average delay in presentation of PNES for assessment at an epilepsy center was 7.2 years in one study [10]. There may be a "pseudoresistance" response to AEDs for suspected epilepsy, where the epilepsy may be well controlled, but PNES continue, leading to progressive escalation in the number and dosage of AEDs [5]. Among patients with "refractory seizures" presenting to epilepsy centers, the prevalence of PNES is reported to be 15% to 30% [6]. The average prevalence of comorbid ES and PNES in patients referred for VEEG monitoring is up to 5% (Table 5.2). An EEG with epileptiform discharges was found in 10% of PNES patients [6]. Almost all patients with both PNES and ES were treated for epilepsy before PNES was diagnosed; ES typically begin before PNES. Most patients with both PNES and ES have focal temporal lobe epilepsy [11], but ES in patients with PNES can be frontal in onset, from other partial foci, or idiopathic generalized.

Medical and social impact of comorbid ES and PNES

Quality of life (QOL) for patients with PNES is significantly impaired, even more than in patients with ES, largely due to the higher frequencies of depression and other psychiatric disorders [12, 13]. Impaired QOL in patients with ES correlates mainly with depression, but also with seizure activity [14, 15]. Comorbid PNES and ES can compound the impairment of QOL, assuming some additive impairment of QOL with both disorders (see Chapter 15).

Patients with uncontrolled PNES have a similar cost-utilization as patients with intractable ES; whether the PNES or the ES are persistent, the same implications exist for cost to society and to the patient [16] (see Chapter 3). As discussed in Chapter 4, VEEG provides the best tool to obtain the correct diagnosis and is cost-effective [17].

In patients with PNES, ES should be treated pharmacologically or even surgically [18]. In some cases, frequent ES may impair neurological function and contribute to the pathogenesis of PNES, as addressed below, although this is speculative. Comorbid ES may not receive the appropriate therapy if assumed to be PNES, and can cause accidents, injuries, or death. Likewise, undetected or untreated psychiatric morbidity can have devastating consequences to the patient and family.

Diagnosis of comorbid PNES and ES

History and examination

In patients with both PNES and ES, the onset of PNES is typically after ES onset [5, 11]. Most patients with mixed ES/PNES are female, similar to patients with PNES alone [19, 20]. There is often a family history of epilepsy *and* a family history of abuse [21]. A family history of epilepsy may predispose to PNES that imitates the ES suffered by other family members [22]. Patients reporting abuse often have a more severe "convulsive" form of PNES, which may include prodromes, nocturnal occurrence, incontinence, or injuries [23]. There is a longer time to diagnosis of PNES and use of more AEDs (mean number of AEDs 2.58 vs. 1.46) when ES are also present compared to PNES alone [24]. Predisposing factors for PNES in a recent series included emotional trauma (90%; 30% sexual), bereavement (56.7%), and family dysfunction (70%) [25], all of which may occur in patients with ES. In a comparison of patients with PNES to those with complex partial seizures (CPS), there was a significantly increased frequency of a history of sexual or physical abuse (32.4%) in those with PNES than the control patients with CPS (8.6%) [26]. A history of psychiatric issues and new bizarre seizure behavior in a patient with established ES suggests a diagnosis of comorbid ES and PNES.

"Typical" signs of ES such as tongue biting, incontinence, falls, and injuries are sometimes reported by patients with PNES, so they cannot be relied upon to fully distinguish ES from PNES [24]. Stereotypy of the events suggests epilepsy, but it is often helpful to confirm that both the clinical features and duration of episodes are fairly consistent from a reliable witness. Nocturnal occurrence supports an epileptic origin, although "apparent sleep" (i.e., eyes closed with wakefulness on EEG) may suggest that the event occurs from sleep to observers [27]. To further complicate the diagnostic morass, PNES may rarely emerge from EEG-verified sleep [28]. The occurrence of events in the office [29] or consistently around family or specific settings can suggest, but are not pathognomonic for, PNES.

Triggers such as stress or emotion also suggest PNES, but are very commonly reported among patients with ES [30]. In patients with epilepsy, stress can precipitate seizures. Even in persons with no previous history of seizures, stress can precipitate new-onset ES in those already predisposed either genetically or from a potentially epileptogenic lesion [31]. Patients with reflex epilepsy can seem to have "induced" seizures. Acute symptomatic seizures rather than ES may occur in patients with PNES, for example alcohol-induced or posttraumatic seizures, and should not be confused with comorbid ES and PNES.

Several groups compared clinical characteristics of patients with comorbid ES and PNES with those of patients who had either PNES or ES. Features that distinguished comorbid PNES/ES versus ES alone were impaired global neuropsychological scores, below average IQ, and impaired visual memory [5]. The impaired visual memory in this series and in other studies reporting an association of PNES with right hemisphere epilepsy [32] might suggest that comorbid PNES is a lateralizing sign for right hemisphere epilepsy. A reasonable hypothesis is that dysfunction from any cause in right hemisphere areas dominant for emotional expression and perception, frontal areas involved in inhibition and behavior, and limbic areas could predispose to the development of psychiatric or conversion symptoms. If the dysfunction also causes an epileptogenic region, then ES may also occur as part of the overall syndrome. However, right-sided lesions or seizures were not more common in other series [5].

Epilepsy is a risk factor for the development of PNES [11, 19]. More specifically, the high incidence of depression or other psychiatric disorders as well as brain dysfunction in epilepsy may be important risk factors for PNES. High rates of physical and/or sexual abuse, posttraumatic stress disorder, personality disorders, and major depression are reported in PNES [33]. Personality disorders are common in patients with both PNES and ES [33]. There may be other somatoform symptoms referable to other organ systems.

A conversation analysis approach of patients' historical seizure descriptions was used to determine whether seizures were ES or PNES, using a linguist blinded to the results of the VEEG diagnosis to analyze the patient interview [34]. The linguist made the correct diagnosis in all cases (five with ES, six with PNES). Patients with ES used great effort to describe their events, whereas patients with PNES provided less information about specific seizure descriptions and more about the circumstances in which they occurred. This method is more fully described in Chapter 8 and an example is provided on the accompanying DVD.

The physical and neurological examinations should seek evidence of ES risk factors such as focal neurological deficits, neurocutaneous signs, previous surgery or trauma, as well as evidence of psychiatric comorbidity and psychogenic findings such as functional signs or demeanor. However, since PNES and ES can coexist, no clinical feature is pathognomonic.

Temporal relationship of seizures in patients with both PNES and ES

Psychogenic nonepileptic seizures and ES usually occur at separate times, as either the ES or PNES may be in remission [35]. However, they may also occur closely together, which may be coincidental if one is more frequent. PNES may occur prior to an ES, during the premonitory phase or aura. Conversely, PNES have been reported after an ES, or as an ES evolving into PNES by seizure-induced psychological changes predisposing to conversion symptoms [36]. For example, epileptic orgasmia (female) may precipitate PNES due to recollection of a childhood sexual abuse episode [37]. Other epileptic sexual behaviors such as sexual manual automatisms or masturbation may be misinterpreted as being nonepileptic [38]. Analysis of movements on VEEG can distinguish one phase from another. In these cases it is possible that the strong emotional experience of the abuse was incorporated into the ictal experience – symptoms from ictal activation of limbic structures will depend partially on the patient's own limbic content. Patients with a sexual

Table 5.3 Medical, neurological, and psychiatric disorders confused with psychogenic nonepileptic seizures

Medical
Syncope
Gastroesophageal reflux (especially young children)
Neurological
Transient ischemic attack
Migraine
Myoclonus
Tics
Attention deficit disorder
Paroxysmal choreathetosis
Sleep disorders (e.g., parasomnias)
Psychiatric
Other somatoform disorders
Dissociative states
Impulse control disorder (motor agitation or anger)
Posttraumatic stress disorder
Panic disorder
Psychosis
Paroxysmal psychosensory phenomena in bipolar disorder and schizophrenia

Table 5.4 Ictal phenomena of PNES in patients with comorbid PNES and ES versus patients with PNES alone

	Group 1 ES/PNES (N = 38)		Group 2 PNES (N = 31)	
	(N)	(%)	(N)	(%)
Autonomic symptoms and signs*	9	23.7	16	51.6
Motor phenomena	7	18.4	12	38.7
Altered responsiveness	7	18.4	10	32.2
GTC-PNES	6	15.7	8	25.8
Atonia (flaccid fall)	2	5.3	4	12.9
Affective symptoms	9	23.7	5	16.1
Experiential phenomena	9	23.7	5	16.1
Somatosensory and sensorial phenomena	8	21	3	9.6
Vague feelings	8	21	3	9.6
Language disturbances	5	13.1	2	6.4

ES, epileptic seizures; PNES, psychogenic nonepileptic seizures; GTC-PNES, "generalized tonic-clonic" PNES.
*p = 0.03.
Adapted from Galimberti et al. [33], with permission from Springer.

component to their ES should be screened for a history of abuse, which would also put them at particular risk for PNES [38]. Sexual abuse is rarely associated with development of ES, sometimes as a result of physical trauma suffered in the abuse, or extreme stress in a susceptible individual.

Psychogenic nonepileptic seizures were recorded in some patients during depth recording of ES – the authors concluded that a predisposition to PNES, the stressful setting, and the ictal discharge (perhaps causing disinhibition or limbic activation) precipitated the events [39]. New-onset PNES were documented on VEEG during the recovery phase of status epilepticus [40]. NES can be exacerbated by AED toxicity, possibly from a state of disinhibition [41]. Withdrawal or reduction of AEDs from patients with PNES was associated with a reduction in the PNES [21, 41]. It is unclear whether this was an effect of the medication withdrawal, or due to the initiation of more appropriate PNES-orientated therapy or even disclosure of the diagnosis [42]. Early well controlled seizures may not be documented; when PNES develop and are diagnosed, withdrawal of AEDs can result in return of the ES, presenting as a new seizure type. This occurred in 2 of 78 patients with PNES in whom AEDs were discontinued [42].

The medical, neurological and psychiatric disorders that should be distinguished from PNES are summarized in Table 5.3.

Ictal semiology

There are limited data comparing the semiology of PNES in patients with both PNES and ES versus PNES alone. In one study, autonomic symptoms were more common in lone PNES [33] (Table 5.4). Another group found no semiological differences in motor, subjective or akinetic seizure components [8]. In 64% of these patients, the clinical manifestations of their ES and PNES were similar, making diagnoses more challenging. In another series, 40% of PNES were similar to the ES in comorbid PNES/ES [11]. Suggestion techniques are less likely to elicit PNES in PNES/ES patients than in patients with PNES alone [8].

Characteristics of PNES versus ES

The clinical features of nonepileptic seizures and ES have been reviewed [39–53] and are summarized throughout this book. Because verbal descriptions can be inaccurate, a first-hand witnessed account recorded shortly after the event or videotaped events should always be sought. VEEG recordings are the gold standard for diagnosis, as even experienced clinicians may have difficulty distinguishing ES from PNES in some cases based solely on video and audio recordings, and rarely, even with VEEG recordings. Assisting the family to recognize ES and PNES (for example, by showing them VEEG of the ES and the PNES) can help outpatient decision making according to seizure type.

Negative VEEG using scalp recordings in patients with ES and PNES

Frontal lobe partial seizures and epileptic auras (simple partial seizures) are notoriously difficult to differentiate from PNES as even VEEG can be negative due to limitations in scalp EEG recordings or obscuration by movement artifact. Turning to a prone position, short duration, nocturnal occurrence, and continuous monotonous (as opposed to emotional) vocalization occurred in frontal lobe-onset EG rather then PNES [54]. Supplementary motor ES differ from PNES by being of shorter duration, occurrence during sleep, a monotonous cry, and tonic posturing in an abducted position [55]. In one study, thrashing movements of the body occurred in both ES and PNES, but thrashing movements of the head and neck occurred only in PNES [44].

Pseudostatus and status epilepticus

Pseudostatus has been defined as "a series of pseudoseizures which had been misdiagnosed as status epilepticus and treated with repeated or continual parenteral administration of short-acting, sedative, antiepileptic drugs" [56].

Pseudostatus is common, occurring in between 18% and 77% of patients with PNES [56–59]. The incidence of pseudostatus in comorbid PNES/ES was 16.7% [11]. Intensive care admission for misdiagnosed pseudostatus was reported in 27% of patients with PNES [58]. Pseudostatus may be more common in younger patients, with a history of impulsivity or self-harm [58].

Reasons for the misdiagnosis of pseudostatus as status epilepticus include failure to recognize PNES by inexperienced physicians or a false previous diagnosis of epilepsy often due to overinterpretation of interictal EEGs. Pseudostatus is usually seen and managed by emergency room physicians rather than neurologists. Familiarity with the clinical characteristics of PNES can avoid misdiagnosis. Characteristics of pseudostatus (Table 5.5) may not always differentiate this con-

Table 5.5 Characteristics that distinguish status epilepticus from PNES status

PNES status	Status epilepticus
Multiple events	Single event
Semiology atypical for ES	Most typical for ES, stereotyped
Psychiatric/somatization history	
Port or IV access system	
Retention of consciousness/resistance to examination	
Normal creatine kinase (CK)	High CK
Rapid recovery	Slow recovery
Normal ictal EEG	Ictal, postictal and interictal EEG abnormal
Higher benzodiazepine requirement	

ES, epileptic seizures.
Howell et al. [56]; Dworetzky et al. [60].

dition from epileptic status, as urinary incontinence, tongue biting, cyanosis, or injuries were reported in pseudostatus and a control group of patients with convulsive status epilepticus [56]. A comparison of patients with PNES with and without pseudostatus found few differences; patients with pseudostatus were on fewer AEDs, and were more likely to have urgent admissions to the hospital for VEEG monitoring [60]. Early EEG is critical to differentiate between pseudostatus and epileptic status epilepticus.

Complications of pseudostatus are iatrogenic and include respiratory arrest, intubation, infection, central venous lines, venous cutdowns, and reinforcement of somatization behavior [56, 58]. Intubation is more common in pseudostatus rather than status epilepticus, due to the longer duration or recurrent nature of the events and lack of response to AEDs [59]. It may take high doses of sedative agents (e.g., benzodiazepines, barbiturates) to render the patient unconscious for the nonepileptic event to cease [57]. In contrast to status epilepticus, patients in pseudostatus are not at risk of metabolic or brain injury.

Neuropsychological evaluations

Neuropsychological testing can help identify patients at risk for comorbid PNES and ES. In one study comparing lone PNES, ES, and comorbid PNES and ES, patients with both ES and PNES had higher

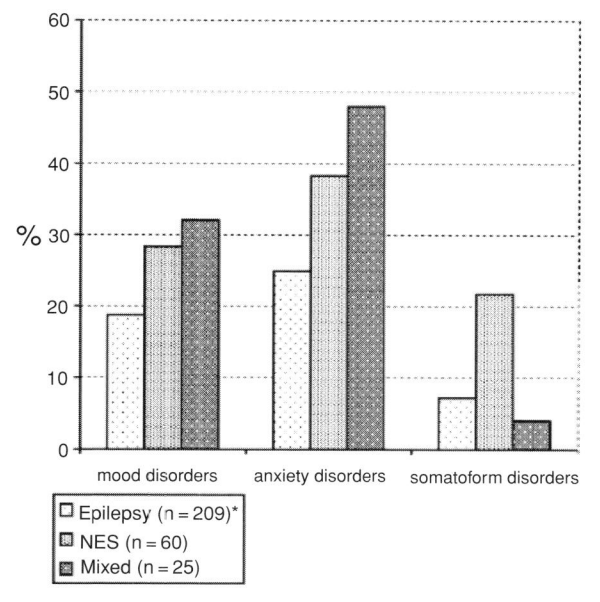

Figure 5.2. Prevalence of DSM-III R Axis I disorders in groups of patients with ES, PNES, and comorbid ES and PNES. Adapted from Kuyk et al. [19]. With permission from Elsevier.

psychological distress scales on the cognitive behavioral assessment compared to a matched control group of patients with only ES [33]. All patients with PNES with or without ES had a Diagnostic and Statistical Manual of Mental Disorders (DSM) Axis I or II disorder compared to 70% of patients with ES only. In patients with PNES and ES, 52% had somatoform disorders compared to 0% of patients with ES. Anxiety disorders and borderline personality trait were more common in the PNES/ES group. Obsessive-compulsive personality trait was seen in the PNES/ES and ES groups, and not in the lone PNES group. Mood disorders (often dysthymic disorder) were more common in the ES group. Another study found that somatoform disorders were more common in a PNES group compared to patients with both PNES and ES [19]. The patients with comorbid PNES and ES had more cluster C personality disorders (avoidant, dependent, and obsessive-compulsive) and mood disorders than those with only PNES (Figure 5.2).

The Minnesota Multiphasic Personality Inventory (MMPI) can help identify conversion or malingering symptoms, although hysteria scale questions could be consistent with symptoms of ES [61]. The MMPI anxiety scores were higher across a group of patients with PNES or comorbid PNES/ES versus ES alone [62].

Similar MMPI profiles were seen in the PNES/ES and lone PNES groups, with high hypochondriasis and hysteria subscores [63]. Somatization scores (involving neurological symptoms) were significantly higher in patients with PNES compared to those with PNES/ES or ES only [64].

Overall, evidence suggests that epilepsy influences the clinical manifestations of PNES in patients with both PNES and ES, as well as the psychopathology. Recognition of these profiles can assist in diagnosis and reduce the number of patients misdiagnosed.

EEG

An interictal EEG showing epileptiform discharges is insufficient to diagnose ES and to exclude PNES. Sharp waves or nonepileptiform transients resembling sharp waves such as normal variants occur in up to 8% of patients without epilepsy [65]. A higher percentage of patients with both PNES and ES will have sharp waves, but the frequency does not correlate with the cause of recent seizure activity (see cases above). PNES may be seen in association with "risk factors" for ES such as interictal EEG abnormalities [66], structural brain abnormalities [67], mesial temporal sclerosis [68], head trauma [69], and prior neurosurgery [70, 71].

VEEG

Video-EEG analysis of the typical events or seizures is the gold standard to diagnose PNES and ES, particularly in comorbid ES and PNES. Other similar studies such as short-term VEEG with induction [72], ambulatory EEG with or without video and analysis of home video recordings can also assist in the diagnosis. Inducibility by suggestion (sometimes combined with saline injections, hypnosis, or other methods) supports a diagnosis of PNES. There are concerns that these induced events may differ from spontaneous PNES and also that the induction procedures are ethically and consensually questionable [73]. If used, they should be utilized exceedingly sparingly, and only are useful if the patient's typical target event is captured behaviorally as well as on VEEG. Any other events captured are less useful in making a diagnosis, and only speak to a certain level of suggestibility, which is not uncommon in the population at large.

Video-EEG can establish the diagnosis of ES, although simple partial seizures and CPS with prominent movements may not produce ictal EEG changes that are detectable on scalp recordings. Rhythmic movement artifact has a stable, rather than evolving, frequency in PNES compared to ES [20]. There is no indication for the intracranial EEG diagnosis of PNES versus ES given the risks involved [74]. A repeat or better quality VEEG recording can often help confirm the diagnosis. Some centers have employed complementary techniques such as ictal or postictal SPECT imaging to detect ES-induced abnormalities in cerebral blood flow when the scalp EEG was not conclusive [75].

Even if VEEG recorded events are clearly nonepileptic, this does not mean that other events that the patient may experience are also nonepileptic unless they are also captured and excluded as epileptic. Antiepileptic drugs may reduce the detection of true interictal or ictal activity and should be discontinued in a controlled fashion where possible for VEEG; AED use occurs in up to 80% of patients with PNES [76].

Prolactin

A recent review and guideline from the American Academy of Neurology on the use of serum prolactin to diagnose ES concluded that there was class B evidence that prolactin measured within 10 to 20 minutes of the event and compared to baseline prolactin (before or at least six hours after the event) can help differentiate ES (generalized tonic-clonic and CPS) from nonepileptic events in adults and older children [77]. In the patient with comorbid ES/PNES, if one knows that there is a consistent increase in prolactin with ES rather than PNES, and other methods of differentiation are inadequate or not available, this approach may be helpful in distinguishing seizure types.

Epilepsy surgery and PNES

New-onset PNES can emerge after epilepsy surgery. The incidence of *de novo* PNES after epilepsy surgery varies from 1.8% to 3.6% [70, 78, 79]. Psychogenic nonepileptic seizures after epilepsy surgery were associated with a long duration of epilepsy, below-average IQ, and remission of the ES [78]. The recurrence of ES is always a concern in surgical patients, even in those with the best prognostic features. Most patients with PNES after surgery had a good outcome, and may have been under stress due to adjustment to a PNES more normalized life, and poor coping strategies and social skills on top of existing psychiatric disorders. PNES may be precipitated by stressful life events after surgery or major surgical complications (such as in case 1 above). Most patients had PNES within six months of surgery [70]. A majority of patients were female, had a right hemisphere focus, a later onset of epilepsy and had more frequent psychiatric disorders (usually mood instability) after surgery than a control group of surgical patients without PNES [70]. Patients can be just as disabled or depressed about their postoperative PNES as their preoperative ES.

Comorbid ES and PNES are not a contraindication for epilepsy surgery for treatment of the ES as long as it is confirmed that the ES are intractable and well localized. Psychiatric evaluation may assist in finding patients at risk for developing PNES postoperatively. Preventative measures should be taken including coping strategies, and development of social and vocational skills.

Developmental delay and comorbid PNES/ES

The developmentally delayed pediatric and adult populations have a high incidence of ES. A variety of nonepileptic events can also occur including PNES, behavioral outbursts, migraines, syncope, and movement disorders. In this population, VEEG is extremely valuable in making the diagnosis [80–85]. Further confounding the diagnosis, there is a higher rate in this population of sexual or physical abuse, inability to verbalize or communicate distress, and limited problem-solving skills that contribute to the development of PNES [81, 77, 85]

Summary

The neurologist, epileptologist, psychiatrist, and other healthcare professionals have a clear role in the diagnosis and management of comorbid ES and PNES by differentiating between events to direct the patient towards the appropriate avenue of treatment. The morbidity and mortality associated with mistaking one for the other in this unique population is exceedingly high. Recognition of PNES risk factors in patients with ES, psychological assessment, and seizure analysis by

VEEG are critical components of the evaluation and management of comorbid PNES and ES. Treatment needs to be multidisciplinary and is best carried out at a comprehensive epilepsy center with resources such as psychological and psychiatric assessment and treatment in addition to epileptologists. In these settings, the appropriate biopsychosocial models of treatment can be employed.

References

1. Lesser RP. Psychogenic seizures. *Neurology* 1996;**46**: 1499–507.
2. Lesser RP, Lüders H, Dinner DS. Evidence for epilepsy is rare in patients with psychogenic seizures. *Neurology* 1983;**33**.
3. Beau B. Récherches statisques pour servir a l'histoire de l'epilepsie et de l'hysterie. *Arch Gen Med* 1836;**11**: 328–52.
4. Esquirol E. *Des maladies mentales*. Vol. 1. Paris: J. S. Chaude. 1838;284.
5. Martin R, Burneo JG, Prasad A, *et al*. Frequency of epilepsy in patients with psychogenic seizures monitored by video-EEG. *Neurology* 2003;**61**: 1791–2.
6. Muller T, Merschhemke M, Dehnicke C, Sanders M, Meencke H-J. Improving diagnostic procedure and treatment in patients with non-epileptic seizures (NES). *Seizure* 2002;**11**:85–9.
7. Benbadis SR, Agrawal V, Tatum IV, WO. How many patients with psychogenic nonepileptic seizures also have epilepsy? *Neurology* 2001;**57**:915–17.
8. Mari F, Di Bonaventura C, Vanacore N, *et al*. Video-EEG study of psychogenic non-epileptic seizures: differential characteristics in patients with and without epilepsy. *Epilepsia* 2006;**47** Suppl 5:64–7.
9. Sigurdardottir KR, Olafsson E. Incidence of psychogenic seizures in adults: a population-based study in Iceland. *Epilepsia* 2005;**39**(7):749–52.
10. Reuber M, Fernández G, Bauer J, Helmstaedter C, Elger CE. Diagnostic delay in psychogenic nonepileptic seizures. *Neurology* 2002;**58**:493–5.
11. Reuber M, Qurishi A, Bauer J, *et al*. Are there physical risk factors for psychogenic non-epileptic seizures in patients with epilepsy? *Seizure* 2003;12(8):561–7.
12. Dodrill CB, Holmes MD. Psychological and neuropsychological evaluation of the patient with non-epileptic seizures. In: Gates JR, Rowan AJ, eds. *Non-Epileptic Seizures*, 2nd edn. Boston, MA: Butterworth-Heinemann. 2000; 169–81.
13. Szaflarski JP, Hughes C, Szaflarski M, *et al*. Quality of life in psychogenic nonepileptic seizures. *Epilepsia* 2003;**44**(2):236–42.
14. Boylan LS, Flint LA, Labovitz DL, *et al*. Depression but not seizure frequency predicts quality of life in treatment-resistant epilepsy. *Neurology* 2004;**62**: 258–61.
15. Devinsky O, Vickrey BG, Cramer J, *et al*. Development of the quality of life in epilepsy inventory. *Epilepsia* 1995;**36**:1089–104.
16. LaFrance WC, Jr, Benbadis SR. Avoiding the costs of unrecognized psychological nonepileptic seizures. *Neurology* 2006;**66**(11):1620–1.
17. Martin RC, Gilliam FG, Kilgore M, Faught E, Kuzniecky R. Improved health care resource utilization following video-EEG-confirmed diagnosis of nonepileptic psychogenic seizures. *Seizure* 1998;7:385–90.
18. Henry TR, Drury I. Non-epileptic seizures in temporal lobectomy candidates with medically refractory seizures. *Neurology* 1997;**48**:1374–82.
19. Kuyk J, Swinkels WAM, Spinhoven P. Psychopathologies in patients with non-epileptic seizures with and without comorbid epilepsy: how different are they? *Epilepsy Behav* 2003;4(1): 13–18.
20. Vinton A, Carino J, Vogrin S, *et al*. "Convulsive" nonepileptic seizures have a characteristic pattern of rhythmic artifact distinguishing them from epileptic seizures. *Epilepsia* 2004;**45**(11):1344–50.
21. Blumer D, Adamolekun B. Treatment of patients with co-existing nonepileptic and epileptic seizures. *Epilepsy Behav* 2006;**9**:498–502.
22. Ramani SV, Quesney LP, Olson D, Gumnit RJ. Diagnosis of hysterical seizures in epileptic patients. *Am J Psychiatry* 1980;**137**:705–9.
23. Selkirk M, Duncan R, Oto M, Pelosi A. Clinical differences between patients with nonepileptic seizures who report antecedent sexual abuse and those who do not. *Epilepsia* 2008;**49**:1446–50.
24. De Timary P, Fouchet P, Sylin M, *et al*. Non-epileptic seizures: delayed diagnosis in patients presenting with electroencephalographic (EEG) or clinical signs of epileptic seizures. *Seizure* 2002;**11**:193–7.
25. Reuber M, Howlett S, Khan A, Grünewald RA. Non-epileptic seizures and other functional neurological symptoms: predisposing, precipitating, and perpetuating factors. *Psychosomatics* 2007;**48**(3): 230–8.
26. Alper K, Devinsky O, Perrine K, Vazquez B, Luciano D. Nonepileptic seizures and childhood sexual and physical abuse. *Neurology* 1993;**43**:1950–3.

Section 1: Recognition, diagnosis, and impact

27. Thacker K, Devinsky O, Perrine K, *et al.* Nonepileptic seizures during apparent sleep. *Ann Neurol* 1993;**33**:414–18.
28. Orbach D, Ritaccio A, Devinsky O. Psychogenic, nonepileptic seizures associated with video-EEG-verified sleep. *Epilepsia* 2003;**44**:64–8.
29. Benbadis SR. A spell in the epilepsy clinic and a history of "chronic pain" or "fibromyalgia" independently predict a diagnosis of psychogenic seizures. *Epilepsy Behav* 2005;**6**:264–5.
30. Haut SR, Hall CB, Masur J, Lipton RB. Seizure occurrence: precipitants and prediction. *Neurology* 2007;**69**:1905–10.
31. Betts, T. Epilepsy and stress. *BMJ* 1992;**305**:378–9.
32. Devinsky O, Mesad S, Alper K. Nondominant hemisphere lesions and conversion nonepileptic seizures. *J Neuropsychiatry Clin Neurosci* 2001;**13**:367–73.
33. Galimberti CA, Ratti MT, Murelli R, *et al.* Patients with psychogenic non-epileptic seizures, alone or epilepsy-associated, share a psychological profile distinct from that of epilepsy patients. *J Neurol* 2003;**250**:338–46.
34. Schwabe M, Howell SJ, Reuber M. Differential diagnosis of seizure disorders: a conversation analytic approach. *Soc Sci Med* 2007;**65**:712–24.
35. Devinsky O, Sanchez-Villasenor F, Vasquez B, *et al.* Clinical profile of patients with epileptic and nonepileptic seizures. *Neurology* 1996;**46**:1530–3.
36. Devinsky O, Gordon E. Epileptic seizures progressing into nonepileptic conversion seizures. *Neurology* 1998;**51**(5):1293–6.
37. Greig E, Betts T. Epileptic seizures induced by sexual abuse. Pathogenic and pathoplastic factors. *Seizure* 1992;**1**:269–74.
38. Bancaud J, Favel P, Bovis A, *et al.* Paroxysmal sexual manifestations and temporal lobe epilepsy. *Electroencephalogr Clin Neurophysiol* 1971;**30**:368–74.
39. Kapur J, Pillai A, Henry TR. Psychogenic elaboration of simple partial seizures. *Epilepsia* 1995;**36**:1126–30.
40. Wilner AN, Bream PR. Status epilepticus and pseudostatus epilepticus. *Seizure* 1993;**2**:257–60.
41. Niedermayer E, Blumer D, Holscher E, *et al.* Classical hysterical seizures facilitated by anticonvulsant toxicity. *Psychiatr Clin (Basel)* 1970;**3**:71–84.
42. Oto M, Espie C, Pelosi A, Selkirk M, Duncan R. The safety of antiepileptic drug withdrawal in patients with non-epileptic seizures. *J Neurol Neurosurg Psychiatry* 2005;**76**(12):1682–5.
43. Gates JR, Ramani V, Whalen S, *et al.* Ictal characteristics of pseudoseizures. *Arch Neurol* 1985;**42**:1183–7.
44. Kanner AM, Morris HH, Lüders H, *et al.* Supplementary motor seizures mimicking pseudoseizures: some clinical differences. *Neurology* 1990;**40**:1404–7.
45. Chung SS, Gerber P, Kirlin KA. Ictal eye closure is a reliable indicator for psychogenic nonepileptic seizures. *Neurology* 2006;**66**:1730–1.
46. Ettinger AB, Weisbrot DM, Nolan E, Devinsky O. Postictal symptoms help distinguish patients with epileptic seizures from those with non-epileptic seizures. *Seizure* 1999;**8**:149–51.
47. D'Alessio L, Giagante B, Oddo S, *et al.* Psychiatric disorders in patients with psychogenic nonepileptic seizures with and without comorbid epilepsy. *Seizure* 2006;**15**:333–9.
48. Fuller G, Lindahl A. Silent witnesses in the diagnosis of epilepsy. *Pract Neurol* 2005;**5**:206–9.
49. Bergen D, Ristanovic R. Weeping as a common element of pseudoseizures. *Arch Neurol* 1993;**50**:1059–60.
50. Vossler DG, Haltiner AM, Schepp SK, *et al.* Ictal stuttering: a sign suggestive of psychogenic non-epileptic seizures. *Neurology* 2004;**63**:516–19.
51. Sen A, Scott C, Sisodiya S. Stertorous breathing is a reliably identified sign that helps in the differentiation of epileptic from psychogenic non-epileptic convulsions: an audit. *Epilepsy Res* 2007;**77**:62–4.
52. Opherk C, Hirsch L. Ictal heart rate differentiates epileptic from non-epileptic seizures. *Neurology* 2002;**58**:636–8.
53. Kotsopoulos IAW, de Krom CTFM, Kessels FGH, *et al.* The diagnosis of epileptic and non-epileptic seizures. *Epilepsy Res* 2003;**57**:59–67.
54. Saygi S, Katz A, Marks DA, Spencer SS. Frontal lobe partial seizures and psychogenic seizures: comparison of clinical and ictal characteristics. *Neurology* 1992;**42**:1274–7.
55. Morris III, HH, Dinner DS, Lüders H, Wyllie E, Kramer R. Supplementary motor seizures: clinical and electroencephalographic findings. *Neurology* 1988;**38**(7):1075–82.
56. Howell SJ, Owen L, Chadwick DW. Pseudostatus epilepticus. *Q J Med* 1989;**71**(266):507–19.
57. Holtkamp M, Othman J, Buchheim K, Meierkord H. Diagnosis of psychogenic nonepileptic status epilepticus in the emergency setting. *Neurology* 2006;**66**(11):1727–9.
58. Reuber M, Pukrop R, Mitchell AJ, Bauer J, Elger CE. Clinical significance of recurrent psychogenic nonepileptic seizure status. *J Neurol* 2003;**250**(11):1355–62.

59. Drake ME Jr, Pakalnis A, Phillips BB. Neuropsychological and psychiatric correlates of intractable pseudoseizures. *Seizure* 1992;**1**(1):11–13.

60. Dworetzky BA, Mortati KA, Rossetti AO, *et al*. Clinical characteristics of psychogenic nonepileptic seizure status in the long-term monitoring unit. *Epilepsy Behav* 2006;**9**(2):335–8.

61. Wilkus RJ, Dodrill CB. Factors affecting the outcome of MMPI and neuropsychological assessments of psychogenic and epileptic seizure patients. *Epilepsia* 1989;**30**(3):339–47.

62. Owczarek K. Anxiety as a differential factor in epileptic versus psychogenic pseudoepileptic seizures. *Epilepsy Res* 2003;**52**:227–32.

63. Owczarek K, Drzejezak J. Patients with coexistent psychogenic pseudoepileptic and epileptic seizures: a psychological profile. *Seizure* 2001;**10**(8):566–9.

64. Owczarek K. Somatization indexes as differential factors in psychogenic pseudoepileptic and epileptic seizures. *Seizure* 2003;**12**(3):178–81.

65. Sam MC, So EL. Significance of epileptiform discharges in patients without epilepsy in the community. *Epilepsia* 2001;**42**(10):1273–8.

66. Reuber M, Fernández G, Bauer J, Singh DD, Elger CE. Interictal EEG abnormalities in patients with psychogenic non-epileptic seizures. *Epilepsia* 2002;**43**:1013–20.

67. Reuber M, Fernández G, Helmstaedter C, Qurishi A, Elger CE. Evidence of brain abnormality in patients with psychogenic nonepileptic seizures. *Epilepsy Behav* 2002;**3**:246–8.

68. Benbadis SR, Tatum IV, WO, Murtagh R, Vale FL. MRI evidence of mesial temporal sclerosis in patients with psychogenic nonepileptic seizures. *Neurology* 2000;**55**:1061–2.

69. Westbrook LE, Devinsky O, Geocadin R. Nonepileptic seizures after head injury. *Epilepsia* 1998;**39**:978–82.

70. Glosser G, Robers D, Glosser DS. Nonepileptic seizures after resective epilepsy surgery. *Epilepsia* 1999;**12**:1750–4.

71. Reuber M, Kurthen M, Kral T, Elger CE. New-onset psychogenic seizures after intracranial neurosurgery. *Acta Neurochir (Wien)* 2002;**144**:901–8.

72. Benbadis SR, Siegrist K, Tatum IV, WO, Heriaud L, Anthony K. Short-term outpatient EEG video with induction in the diagnosis of psychogenic seizures. *Neurology* 2004;**63**:1728–30.

73. Devinsky O, Fisher R. Ethical use of placebos and provocative testing in diagnosing nonepileptic seizures. *Neurology* 1996;**47**:866–70.

74. Henry TR. Nonepileptic seizures and depth recording (Letter). *Neurology* 1998;**50**:832–3.

75. Blend M, De Leon O, Jobe T, *et al*. Cerebral perfusion SPECT imaging in epileptic and nonepileptic seizures. *Clin Nucl Med* 1997;**22**(6):363–8.

76. Benbadis SR. How many patients with pseudoseizures receive antiepileptic drugs prior to diagnosis? *Eur Neurol* 1999;**41**:114–15.

77. Chen DK, So YT, Fisher RS. Use of serum prolactin in diagnosing epileptic seizures: report of the Therapeutics and Technology Assessment Subcommittee of the American Academy of Neurology. *Neurology* 2005;**65**(5):668–75.

78. Krahn LE, Rummans TA, Sharbrough FW, Jowsey FG, Cascino GD. Pseudoseizures after epilepsy surgery. *Psychosomatics* 1995;**36**:487–93.

79. Parra J, Iriarte J, Kanner AM, Bergen DC. De novo psychogenic nonepileptic seizures after epilepsy surgery. *Epilepsia* 1998;**39**(5):474–7.

80. Krumholz A, Niedermeyer E. Psychogenic seizures: a clinical study with follow-up data. *Neurology* 1983;**33**:498–502.

81. Silver LB. Conversion disorder with pseudoseizures in adolescence: a stress reaction to unrecognized and untreated learning disabilities. *J Am Acad Child Psychiatry* 1982;**21**:508–12.

82. Devinsky O. What do you do when they grow up? Approaches to seizures in developmentally delayed adults. *Epilepsia* 2002;**43** Suppl 3:71–9.

83. DeToledo JC, Lowe MR, Haddad H. Behaviors mimicking seizures in institutionalized individuals with multiple disabilities and epilepsy: a video-EEG study. *Epilepsy Behav* 2002;**3**:242–4.

84. Cole AJ. Evaluation and treatment of epilepsy in multiply handicapped individuals. *Epilepsy Behav* 2002;**3**:S2–6.

85. Tharinger D, Horton CB, Millea S. Sexual abuse and exploitation of children and adults with mental retardation and other handicaps. *Child Abuse Negl* 1990;**14**(3):301–12.

Section 1 Chapter 6

Recognition, diagnosis, and impact of nonepileptic seizures

Nonepileptic paroxysmal neurological and cardiac events

Fergus J. Rugg-Gunn and Josemir W. Sander

A large number of neurological and cardiac conditions result in paroxysmal clinical events, with a single clinical feature often having many and varied underlying pathophysiological processes. This chapter surveys physiological nonepileptic events and focuses on the specific paroxysmal neurological and cardiac events that may be confused with epileptic seizures (ES) and psychogenic nonepileptic seizures (PNES) (Table 6.1).

An accurate clinical diagnosis requires differentiation between epilepsy and other causes of transient neurological disturbance and collapse, but the manifestations of ES are diverse and there are many imitators, ranging from convulsive syncope to parasomnias. Nevertheless, the diagnosis of epilepsy is frequently straightforward, particularly when precise and detailed personal and eye-witness accounts of the prodrome, onset, evolution, and recovery period after the event are obtained.

Misdiagnosis is common, however, and possibly affects up to 20% to 30% of adults with a diagnosis of epilepsy [1, 2]. A study reported on 184 consecutive patients referred to one consultant neurologist with a provisional diagnosis of epilepsy; 46 (25%) were believed to have been misdiagnosed, of whom 12 were referred with refractory, drug resistant, epilepsy. Nineteen had experienced significant and intrusive medication side effects, 12 had unnecessary driving restrictions, and 5 had considerable employment difficulties with 3 dependent on state benefits [2]. In another study, 74 patients previously diagnosed with epilepsy were investigated with tilt-table testing, prolonged EKG monitoring, blood pressure- and EEG-monitored carotid sinus massage, and an alternative, cardiological diagnosis was found in 31 (41.9%) patients, including 13 taking antiepileptic drugs (AEDs) [3].

These and other reports highlight the high rate of misdiagnosis of epilepsy, the cause of which is undoubtedly multifactorial. The reasons for misdiagnosis may include a deficiency of relevant semiological information obtained during the ascertainment of the clinical history, lack of understanding of the significance of specific clinical features, and over-reliance on the diagnostic value of routine investigations [4]. The attainment of a correct diagnosis is of paramount importance as an erroneous diagnosis of epilepsy has physical, psychosocial [5] and socioeconomic consequences for the patient, and economic implications for the health and welfare services [6].

Syncope

Transient loss of awareness is common, and may affect up to 50% of people at some stage of life [7–9]. It is also a significant burden on healthcare services, comprising 3% of all patients evaluated in emergency departments and 1% of hospital admissions [10]. Elucidating the etiological basis for an episode of loss of awareness is challenging. Typically, the episode is transient, patients are generally unable to provide an accurate description of the event, and there may be a lack of reliable witnesses, particularly in the elderly who, more frequently, live alone. Additionally, approximately 30% of elderly patients deny any loss of awareness due to transient retrograde amnesia [11]. The difficulty in establishing an accurate diagnosis is further hampered by medical and neurological examinations and subsequent investigations frequently being normal after an episode or between habitual attacks when the patient is seen in the hospital ward or clinic [12]. Where information regarding the episode is available, ideally

---

Gates and Rowan's Nonepileptic Seizures, 3rd edn. ed. Steven C. Schachter and W. Curt LaFrance, Jr. Published by Cambridge University Press. © S. Schachter and W. C. LaFrance, Jr. 2010.

Chapter 6: Nonpsychogenic nonepileptic seizures

Table 6.1 Nonepileptic paroxysmal neurological and cardiac events

Syncope
Neurocardiogenic (also known as vasovagal, reflex, vasodepressor syncope)
Cardiac
Structural
Cardiomyopathies (obstructive, dilated, restrictive, right ventricular dysplasia)
Valvular disease (mitral and aortic stenosis and mitral valve prolapse)
Other (atrial myxoma)
Arrhythmia
Inherited (long QT, Brugada and Wolff-Parkinson-White syndromes)
Acquired (SVT, VT, atrioventricular block, sinus node disease)
Orthostatic
Autonomic failure
Neuropathy
Complex autonomic failure (primary, multiple system atrophy)
Postural orthostatic tachycardia syndrome
Carotid sinus hypersensitivity
Situational
Tussive, micturition, swallowing
Neurological
Cerebrogenic cardiac arrhythmias

Drop attacks
Cardiac (as above)
Neurological
Cerebrospinal fluid dynamics
Colloid cyst of third ventricle, Arnold-Chiari malformation
Diencephalic attacks
Lower limb weakness
Brainstem and spinal cord lesions and lower motor neuron disorders
Cataplexy
Idiopathic drop attacks
Vertebrobasilar ischemia
Periodic hypo- and hyperkalemic paralyses

Transient hypermotor episodes
Myoclonus
Cortical, subcortical, brainstem, spinal cord, and lower motor neuron disorders
Tics
Dystonia
Tremor
Chorea
Paroxysmal dyskinesia
Kinesigenic, nonkinesigenic, exertion-induced, choreoathetosis with spasticity
Episodic ataxia
Type 1 and 2
Startle syndromes
Hyperekplexia
Culture-specific syndromes
Jumping Frenchmen of Maine, Latah, Myriachit
Acquired
Stiff-person syndrome, progressive encephalomyelitis with rigidity
Tonic spasms
Upper motor neuron disorders
Multiple sclerosis, cerebral palsy
Cerebral ischemia

Table 6.1 (cont.)

Transient focal sensory attacks
Migraine
Transient ischemic attacks
Lower motor neuron disorders
Radiculopathies, neuropathies
Vertigo
Ménière's disease, benign paroxysmal positional vertigo

Psychic experiences
Panic attacks
Loss of primary sense
Charles Bonnet syndrome
Post-amputation

Aggressive or vocal outbursts
Episodic dyscontrol syndrome

Episodic phenomena in sleep
Sleep-wake transition disorders
Hypnic jerks
Rhythmic movement disorders
Jactatio Capitis Nocturna
Restless legs syndrome
Periodic limb movements in sleep
Non-REM parasomnias
Somnambulism, night terrors, confusional arousals
REM parasomnias
Nightmares, sleep paralysis, REM sleep behavior disorder
Sleep apnea
Obstructive
Central

Prolonged confusional or fugue states
Encephalopathy
Neurological
Intracranial infection, ischemia, head injury
Systemic
Infection, hypoxia, hypercapnia, hypoglycemia, hypocalcemia, hyponatremia, hepatic and renal failure, drug and alcohol withdrawal or intoxication, endocrine dysfunction including thyroid disorders, pheochromocytoma, carcinoid
Transient global amnesia

from both the patient and a witness, careful examination of the prodrome, onset, course, and recovery is mandatory.

Transient loss of awareness has three main underlying mechanisms:

1. Transient global cerebral hypoperfusion, i.e., syncope
2. Epilepsy
3. Psychogenic nonepileptic seizures (PNES).

Epilepsy and PNES are important causes of transient loss of awareness; however, detailed discussion of these conditions is beyond the scope of this chapter and are discussed throughout much of this book.

Syncope, derived from the Greek "syn" meaning "with" and "kopto" meaning "I interrupt," may be defined as transient, self-limited loss of consciousness, usually leading to collapse, due to cerebral hypoperfusion [13]. Syncope is more prevalent than either epilepsy or PNES and is common across all age groups, with an overall incidence of 10.5% over a 17-year period [14]. Vasovagal syncope is most frequently encountered in adolescence, whereas syncope due to cardiac causes becomes increasingly prevalent with advancing age. The annual incidence of syncope in the elderly population in long-term care has been reported to be as high as 6% [9]. Recurrence is not unusual, occurring in approximately 30% of patients, typically within the first two years after symptom onset [15]. Recurrence is associated with increased morbidity, such as fractures, subdural hematomas and soft-tissue injuries [16], and impaired quality of life [13]. There are numerous causes of syncope, each resulting in inappropriate systemic hypotension and critical cerebral hypoperfusion. The causes can be divided into two main groups, cardiac and vascular.

Cardiac conditions that cause syncope may be either structural heart disease, such as aortic stenosis, hypertrophic cardiomyopathy, right ventricular dysplasia, some forms of congenital heart disease, severe ischemic cardiomyopathy, and left atrial myxoma, or arrhythmias, such as ventricular tachycardia, ventricular fibrillation, Brugada syndrome, long QT syndrome, supraventricular tachycardia, atrioventricular block, and sinus node disease causing bradyarrhythmia or asystole. Vascular causes include reflex syncope, such as neurocardiogenic or carotid sinus hypersensitivity, situational syncope, for example, during coughing [17] or micturition, and postural syncope, including orthostatic hypotension or postural orthostatic tachycardia syndrome (POTS).

Neurocardiogenic syncope is the most common cause of syncope [13] and has many synonyms including vasovagal, reflex, vasodepressor and neurally mediated hypotension. It arises through the provocation of inappropriate reflex hypotension, with a variable degree of bradycardia, or even transient asystole. The specific precipitant of the afferent arc of this reflex is unknown, but the efferent arc, which arises in the brainstem vasomotor and cardioinhibitory centers, results in an abrupt withdrawal of sympathetic outflow to resistance vessels, particularly in skeletal muscle, and as a result of the Bezold-Jarisch reflex, rapid vagal hypertonia [18]. This results in venous pooling and impaired cardiac filling, bradycardia, and subsequent cerebral hypoperfusion. There is often a precipitating cause such as prolonged standing in a warm environment or fright, for example, venipuncture or the sight of blood. There may be a family history of "fainting" or recent addition of vasoactive medication targeted at, for example, hypertension or ischemic heart disease.

A typical attack commences with prodromal symptoms of nausea, clammy sweating, blurring or greying visual impairment, lightheadedness, and ringing or roaring tinnitus. Occasionally, visual and auditory hallucinations can be more complex, and involve figures or scenes [19]. Many of these individual symptoms are difficult for patients to describe and their description may be vague, but collectively the cluster of symptoms is characteristic. Subsequently, the patient will look pale and be sweaty during the event. Mydriasis, tachypnea, bradycardia, and acral paresthesias may be present. Muscle tone is reduced, causing the eyes to roll up, and the patient to fall to the ground. In the horizontal position, skin color, pulse, and consciousness usually return within a few seconds, and while the patient may feel briefly unwell, confusion, amnesia, and drowsiness are not prolonged. Injury and incontinence are rare but may occur. Tongue biting in syncope of any cause is unusual, but frequently seen in epilepsy. Presyncope refers to less profound symptomatology, partial impairment of consciousness, and a near fall.

Orthostatic syncope is caused by autonomic failure rather than an exaggerated and inappropriate but essentially normal physiological response, as seen in neurocardiogenic syncope. Patients lose the normal vasoconstrictor response to standing, resulting in venous pooling and a postural fall in blood pressure, usually within seconds or minutes of becoming upright. Unlike in neurocardiogenic syncope, the skin stays warm and well perfused, the pulse rate is unchanged, and sweating is absent. The causes of autonomic dysfunction are varied and include autonomic neuropathy due to diabetes, alcohol, amyloidosis, genetic abnormalities, or complex autonomic failure, such as primary autonomic failure or multiple system atrophy. Medications such as antihypertensives, phenothiazines, tricyclic antidepressants, diuretics, and medication for Parkinson's disease may also be implicated.

Postural orthostatic tachycardia syndrome (POTS) is an autonomic disturbance characterized by symptoms of orthostatic intolerance, mainly lightheadedness, fatigue, sweating, tremor, anxiety, palpitation, exercise intolerance, and syncope or presyncope on upright posture [20]. Patients also have a heart rate greater than 120 beats per minute on standing or an increase in heart rate of 30 beats per minute from a resting heart rate after standing for 1 to 5 minutes, compared to an increase of only 15 beats per minute in heart rate in the first minute of standing in normal subjects. Postural orthostatic tachycardia syndrome is most common in females between the ages of 12 and 50 years and may follow surgery, pregnancy, sepsis, or trauma [21]. The pathophysiological basis of POTS is not well understood. Hypotheses include impaired vascular innervation, baroreceptor dysfunction, and high plasma norepinephrine concentrations, of which impaired innervation of the veins or their response to sympathetic stimulation is probably the most important [22].

Carotid sinus hypersensitivity (CSH) is an exaggerated response to carotid sinus baroreceptor stimulation. Even mild stimulation to the neck in affected patients results in presyncopal symptoms or syncope from marked bradycardia and a drop in blood pressure causing transiently reduced cerebral perfusion. Carotid sinus hypersensitivity is found in 0.5% to 9.0% of patients with recurrent syncope and is observed in up to 14% of elderly nursing home patients and 30% of elderly patients with unexplained syncope and drop attacks [23, 24]. It is more common in males and associated with an increased risk of falls, drop attacks, bodily injuries, and fractures in elderly patients, but rates of total mortality, sudden death, myocardial infarction, or stroke are similar to the general population. Thirty percent of cases are classified as cardioinhibitory where the predominant manifestations are sinus bradycardia, atrioventricular block, or asystole due to vagal action on sinus and atrioventricular nodes. Permanent pacemaker implantation is effective at reducing recurrence rate [25]. The vasodepressor type also comprises 30% of cases and results in a marked decrease in vasomotor tone without a change in heart rate. The remaining patients are of a mixed type [26]. Untreated symptomatic patients have a syncope recurrence rate as high as 62% within 4 years.

The diagnosis is established by performing carotid sinus massage with the patient supine, under EKG and blood pressure monitoring. The point of maximal carotid impulse is massaged for 5 seconds on both sides, with a 1-minute interval. A result is considered positive if either asystole exceeding 3 seconds (indicating cardioinhibitory CSH) or a reduction in systolic blood pressure exceeding 50 mm Hg (indicating vasodepressor CSH) is observed [23].

Cardiogenic syncope arises from either a rhythm disturbance or structural cardiac defects. The identification of a cardiac cause of syncope is of paramount importance because the prognosis is poor if untreated [12, 15, 27, 28]. A family history of sudden cardiac death may be present, indicating the possibility of Brugada syndrome, long QT syndrome, or an inherited cardiomyopathy, for example, hypertrophic cardiomyopathy, familial dilated cardiomyopathy, or arrhythmogenic right ventricular dysplasia. Typically, presyncopal symptoms will be absent, and the circumstances of the syncope may be important. Syncope *after* exercise is a manifestation of neurocardiogenic syncope, whereas syncope *during* exercise is more suggestive of cardiomyopathy or primary electrical disturbance such as Wolff-Parkinson-White syndrome or right ventricular dysplasia.

Tachyarrhythmias reduce cardiac output by shortening the time for diastolic ventricular filling. Supraventricular tachycardias, such as Wolff-Parkinson-White syndrome, which is manifest in between episodes of tachycardia as a delta wave and short PR interval on 12-lead EKG, result in rapid palpitations, but rarely syncope. Conversely, the long QT syndromes, such as Romano-Ward and Lange-Neilson syndromes, result in the potentially fatal ventricular tachycardia known as "torsade de pointes." These inherited channelopathies cause recurrent syncope, particularly on rising, and are associated with sudden death. Acquired QT interval changes may be due to medication, such as digoxin and antihistamines, and ischemic heart disease [29–31]. Bradyarrhythmias may be due to cardiac disease, CSH, exaggerated physiological reflexes, such as cough or swallowing syncope (typically associated with glossopharyngeal neuralgia), or neurological causes, such as ES or raised intracranial pressure.

Syncope as a result of structural cardiac disease is due to left ventricular outflow obstruction (aortic stenosis, hypertrophic obstructive cardiomyopathy), reduced ventricular filling (mitral stenosis, atrial myxoma), or cardiomyopathy (dilated or restrictive). These conditions may lead to reduced cardiac output or may induce increased vagal tone secondary to vigorous ventricular contractions. Hypertrophic obstructive cardiomyopathy (HOCM) is a relatively common autosomal dominant disorder, with an estimated prevalence of 0.2% in adults. Morphological evidence of disease is found in approximately 25% of first-degree relatives of patients with HOCM on echocardiography, consistent with a pattern of variable expressivity. The overall mortality rate is approximately 1% per year [32, 33]. Patients with HOCM may be asymptomatic and usually present with sudden death secondary to ventricular fibrillation, particularly during vigorous exertion. Patients may, however, complain of angina, palpitations, shortness of breath and dizziness, and syncope or presyncope secondary to inadequate cardiac output on exertion or from a cardiac tachy- or bradyarrhythmia [34].

Cerebrogenic cardiac dysfunction has also been observed. Arrhythmias, conduction block, and repolarization EKG abnormalities have been reported in up to 56% of ES. Abnormalities appear to be more common in nocturnal, prolonged, and generalized seizures than in focal seizures or those occurring during wakefulness [35–39]. Ictal tachycardia is almost universally observed during ES; however, ictal bradycardia has received more attention due to the potential progression to cardiac asystole and the intuitive but unproven association with sudden unexpected death in epilepsy (SUDEP). Ictal bradycardia is observed in <5% of recorded seizures [40–43] but may occur in a higher percentage of patients because a consistent cardiac response to each apparently electroclinically identical seizure is not seen [40]. Short periods of EEG/EKG monitoring may underestimate the prevalence of ictal asystole. In contrast, a study reported on 19 patients with refractory focal epilepsy who were implanted with an EKG loop recorder for up to 18 months in which over 220 000 patient hours of EKG recording were monitored [40]. Over this 18-month period, 3377 seizures (1897 complex partial or secondarily generalized tonic-clonic seizures and 1480 simple partial seizures) were reported by patients. Cardiac rhythm was captured on the implantable loop recorders in 377 seizures. Ictal bradycardia, defined as a rate of less than 40 beats per minute, was seen in 0.24% of all seizures over the study period and 2.1% of the recorded seizures. One patient developed supraventricular tachycardia (rate of 120 beats per minute), lasting approximately 30 seconds, during a complex partial seizure. Seven of the 19 patients experienced ictal bradycardia. Four of these had severe bradycardia or periods of asystole, which led to the insertion of a permanent pacemaker. Notably, only a small proportion of seizures for every patient were associated with significant cardiac events, despite identical seizure characteristics [40].

The presence of brief myoclonic jerks during a syncopal episode of any cause, observed in approximately 15% of patients [19, 44], is often overinterpreted by witnesses, and occasionally health professionals, leading to diagnostic confusion. Such myoclonic jerks are usually multifocal and are rarely rhythmic, prolonged, or of large amplitude. Videotelemetric monitoring shows that the myoclonic jerks rarely last longer than 15 to 20 seconds [19] and do not have an EEG correlate, unlike true epileptic myoclonus. Rarely, manual and orofacial automatisms may occur, even during the presyncopal stage [45]. If recovery from cerebral hypoperfusion is delayed, for example if the patient is held in an upright position, a secondary anoxic convulsive seizure may occur. These should not be classified as ES however.

Diagnostic accuracy following the first episode of loss of consciousness is low [46], but may be improved with the application of simple diagnostic criteria [44, 47]. In one study a questionnaire was administered to 671 patients referred for transient loss of consciousness [44]. It comprised 118 items pertaining to patient symptomatology, including provocative situations, peri-syncopal symptoms, seizure markers, witness derived information, and relevant medical history [48]. The patients had a range of etiologies including neurocardiogenic syncope (40%), epilepsy (15%), cardiac arrhythmias (23%), structural heart disease (22%), cough syncope (<1%), autonomic neuropathy, and hyperventilation. Despite undergoing a number of cardiological and neurological investigations, approximately 20% to 25% of patients remained undiagnosed, concordant with similar studies [49]. Patients with epilepsy had more episodes of loss of consciousness and a longer history than patients with syncope. The clinical features that were most strongly predictive of syncope of any cause versus seizures were a postural component, a prior history of presyncopal episodes with unpleasant situations, diaphoresis, dyspnea, chest pain, palpitations, a feeling of warmth, nausea, and vertigo. Patients were also more likely to have hypertension and ischemic heart disease. Epilepsy was predicted by the presence of tongue biting, urinary incontinence, prodromal déjà vu, postictal confusion, mood disturbance, muscle pain, headaches, witnessed convulsive movements, head turning, and cyanosis [44]. The application of the questionnaire resulted in a diagnostic accuracy of 86%, suggesting that the careful evaluation of the history from the patient and witness is of principal importance in attaining the correct diagnosis. It is important to note that syncope due to primary cardiac disease may present with sudden collapse and have a less well defined, or often completely absent, prodromal period compared to vasovagal syncope [19, 45, 50].

In patients with syncope, neurological and cardiological examinations are frequently unrevealing. Further investigations may be necessary and are dependent on the history obtained. Extensive investigation is not mandatory, however, in patients with, for example, a typical history of neurocardiogenic syncope. A 12-lead EKG should, however, be undertaken in all patients. Patients with an abnormal cardiological examination or 12-lead EKG or those patients with a family history of sudden cardiac death or a personal history that is atypical for neurocardiogenic syncope, for example, episodes during exercise, while lying flat, or with palpitations, warrant more extensive cardiac investigations including a transthoracic echocardiogram, prolonged EKG monitoring and, frequently, tilt-table testing. In conditions such as Brugada syndrome, the EKG abnormalities may be intermittent. Serial EKGs in undiagnosed syncope may, therefore, be helpful. In patients with infrequent episodes, 1- to 7-day prolonged, Holter type, EKG recordings have a yield of less than 1% [13] and implantable loop recorders, which can monitor cardiac rhythm for up to 18 months, are more appropriate, with a yield in unexplained syncope of up to 50% [51–53]. Autonomic function testing, and more specifically tilt-table testing (for example, 70° tilt for 45 minutes), also has high sensitivity, approaching 70%, for identifying patients with a syncopal tendency, particularly in patients over the age of 50 years with recurrent syncope and no structural cardiac pathology [49, 54], but reproducibility has been reported to be poor [55]. Measures to induce syncope, such as isoprenaline, provoke syncope more rapidly and provide additional sensitivity (10% to 15%), but at the expense of reduced specificity [56].

The prognosis and treatment of syncope is entirely dependent on the underlying etiology. Structural heart disease significantly increases the risk of death in patients with syncope [13]. For example, patients with syncope and severe left ventricular failure have a one-year mortality rate of 45% compared to a similar group of patients with cardiac failure but no syncope [12, 27, 28]. In contrast, patients with neurocardiogenic syncope, aged 45 years or less, without structural heart disease have no increase in mortality rate. Even patients who remain undiagnosed following extensive investigations have a good prognosis [12, 15]. It is therefore of paramount importance, from a prognostic and interventional point of view, to identify those patients with syncope due to an underlying cardiac cause.

Drop attacks

Neurological causes of sudden collapse other than epilepsy and autonomic dysfunction include intermittent obstructive hydrocephalus caused by, for example, a colloid cyst of the third ventricle or a craniocervical junction abnormality such as an Arnold-Chiari malformation. Colloid cysts present with syncope and sudden death, particularly with changes in posture, are readily identified on neuroimaging, and are amenable to neurosurgical intervention [57, 58].

Diencephalic attacks, as sequelae of diffuse brain injury, are extremely rare and manifest as autonomic dysfunction with diaphoresis, sinus tachycardia, collapse and intermittent hypertension [59].

Brainstem and spinal cord lesions or lower limb weakness of any cause may present with unexplained falls without impairment of consciousness. There are usually fixed neurological signs that will guide appropriate investigations, and the episodes are rarely confused with atonic or tonic seizures of epilepsy. Cataplexy usually occurs in association with the other features of narcolepsy: excessive daytime somnolence, hypnagogic hallucinations, and sleep paralysis although it may be the presenting feature. Cataplexy, meaning "to strike down with fear," is a brief and sudden loss of muscle tone due to REM intrusion during wakefulness, typically leading to falls. There is no loss of awareness with the attacks and often there is only loss of tone in the neck musculature, leading to brief slumping of the head, rather than complete falls. Narcolepsy is believed to result from abnormal immune modulation and aberrant neurotransmitter functioning and sensitivity, particularly of the muscarinic cholinergic pathways in the pontine reticular activating system and the meso-cortico-limbic dopaminergic system, on the background of a genetic predisposition. Narcolepsy is strongly associated with the HLA DR2 and DQB1*0602 alleles [60]. The close HLA association and postmortem finding of dramatically reduced hypocretin (orexin) neurons and low cerebrospinal fluid concentrations of hypocretin in patients with sporadic narcolepsy has led to the hypothesis that narcolepsy is caused by an autoimmune destruction of hypocretin cells in genetically susceptible individuals [61]. The connection with the limbic system may, at least partly, explain why cataplexy is often precipitated by emotion, in particular laughter. Treatment with tricyclic antidepressants, CNS stimulants, and selective serotonin reuptake inhibitors is frequently effective.

Idiopathic drop attacks are most commonly seen in middle-aged women. They take the form of a sudden fall without loss of consciousness, and patients frequently remember hitting the ground. Recovery is instantaneous but injury often occurs. Neurological, cardiac, and autonomic investigations are unrewarding.

It is likely that vertebrobasilar ischemia is overdiagnosed and probably accounts for only a small proportion of drop attacks. Typically, the attacks occur in the elderly, with evidence of vascular disease and cervical spondylosis, both commonly occurring conditions which frequently coexist in the elderly population. Furthermore there is clinical overlap with other more commonly occurring but benign conditions such as benign paroxysmal positional vertigo. The attacks may be precipitated by head turning or neck extension resulting in distortion of the vertebral arteries and hemodynamic ischemia, although embolic events are probably a more frequent cause. Drop attacks are accompanied by features of brainstem ischemia such as diplopia, vertigo, and bilateral facial and limb sensory and motor deficits [62].

Hyper- and hypokalemic periodic paralyses (PP) are rare autosomal dominant disorders of sodium and calcium ion channel dysfunction characterized by episodic flaccid weakness secondary to abnormal sarcolemmal excitability and rapid changes in serum potassium levels. Cranial musculature and respiratory muscles are usually spared. Attacks last from between minutes in hyperkalemic PP to hours and occasionally days in hypokalemic PP. Precipitants include fasting, alcohol, resting following exercise, stress (hyperkalemic PP), and a high carbohydrate meal, and cold and exertion the previous day (hypokalemic PP). Acute treatment is directed at supportive care and normalization of the serum potassium. Effective prophylaxis of hypokalemic PP, like many of the channelopathies, is with acetazolamide [63]. Thyrotoxicosis is the commonest cause of secondary periodic paralysis.

Convulsive movements and transient hypermotor episodes

Convulsive limb movements commonly accompany episodes with transient loss of awareness and, as previously discussed, are most commonly due to either epilepsy, syncope, or PNES. Transient, episodic limb movements without loss of awareness are also frequently misdiagnosed as epilepsy. There is often a degree of overlap with myoclonus as the clinical manifestation of a variety of pathophysiological processes embracing the subspecialty fields of both epilepsy and movement disorders. Epileptic myoclonus, which is cortical in origin, can be confused with other hyperkinetic movement disorders, including myoclonus originating from subcortical structures, brainstem, spinal cord or peripheral nerves, tics, chorea, dystonia, and tremor. Definitive localization of the myoclonic focus requires electrophysiology, specifically a time-locked back-averaged EEG. Careful neurological examination is also often helpful in this regard, for example, in identifying spinal cord pathology or evidence of a cortical process. Cortical myoclonus arises from a hyperexcitable focus within the sensorimotor cortex, and involves an arm, leg, or the face. In general, it is typically arrhythmic, although in the setting of epilepsia partialis continua jerks may appear rhythmic. Cortical myoclonus is triggered by action or intention, and is often stimulus-sensitive. Subcortical myoclonus refers to myoclonus without a preceding cortical discharge and arises from structures such as the thalamus, and is usually, although not exclusively, stimulus-insensitive. In practice, it is frequently difficult to differentiate cortical from subcortical myoclonus on clinical grounds, and neurophysiological investigation is required. Neuroimaging may also be helpful in this regard. Myoclonus arising from the brainstem (startle, palatal and reticular reflex myoclonus), spinal cord (segmental and propriospinal myoclonus), and peripheral nerves are usually recognized and differentiated from epilepsy without difficulty.

Among the hyperkinetic movement disorders, tremor is the entity most often confused with myoclonus and convulsive limb movements. Tremor is habitually rhythmic and oscillatory, and significantly slower than myoclonus; however, occasionally tremor may be jerky and irregular, mimicking clonic jerks to the degree that electrophysiological investigation is required to differentiate between them.

Like myoclonus, tics are also brief; however, they are typically preceded by an urge to perform the movement and can usually be temporarily suppressed, features not seen in myoclonus or simple partial seizures. Tics are usually stereotyped, repetitive, and often complex, involving multiple different noncontiguous muscle groups.

Chorea, a brief involuntary "'dance-like" movement, is usually easy to distinguish from myoclonus and epilepsy due to the characteristic flowing movements. Dystonia is an involuntary movement disorder characterized by repetitive, sustained movements that typically produce twisting postures. Dystonia rarely mimics myoclonus although it may be confused with epileptic tonic spasms or the dystonic posturing seen in partial seizures of frontal or temporal lobe origin. Many patients with dystonia possess a maneuver that attenuates the dystonia, termed a "geste antagoniste."

Paroxysmal dyskinesias are a genetically and clinically heterogeneous group of rare movement disorders characterized by episodic dystonic or choreiform movements. Paroxysmal kinesiogenic dyskinesia (PKD) is the most common type, although the precise prevalence is unknown. This condition is characterized by brief attacks of unilateral or bilateral limb dystonia or chorea, lasting less than one minute and with preserved consciousness, triggered by initiation of voluntary movements. An "aura," such as an unusual cephalic or epigastric sensation may precede the attacks, further adding to the diagnostic confusion [64]. Sporadic cases occur; however, PKD is considered to be an autosomal dominant condition with variable penetrance, linked to the pericentromeric region of chromosome 16 [65–67]. The underlying pathophysiological mechanism is thought to be a sodium channelopathy because the condition is highly responsive to carbamazepine and there is possibly some overlap with afebrile infantile convulsions and channelopathy-related epilepsies, such as autosomal dominant nocturnal frontal lobe epilepsy (ADNFLE). This condition was previously termed nocturnal hypnogenic paroxysmal dyskinesia before an epileptic basis was elucidated. Furthermore, a single case study reported an individual with ictal discharges arising from the supplementary sensorimotor cortex with concomitant discharges from the ipsilateral caudate nucleus, although there were a number of atypical clinical features [68]. A small case series failed to replicate these findings and an epileptic basis for paroxysmal dyskinesias is generally considered improbable [69]. Other paroxysmal dyskinesias may also be confused with epilepsy, for example, paroxysmal dystonic choreoathetosis, which is characterized by attacks of longer duration precipitated by alcohol, stress, and caffeine rather than movement.

A growing number of episodic human disorders are being recognized as disorders of ion channels. These include a number of epilepsies such as ADNFLE, generalized epilepsy with febrile seizures (GEFS+), and other conditions such as episodic ataxia (EA1 and EA2) and hyperekplexia, which have been clearly defined as channelopathies, and other conditions like PKD where despite no ion channel gene mutations being isolated, there are strong suspicions that this is likely to be the underlying basis. Episodic ataxias typically present in childhood or adolescence and manifest as ataxia and myokymia (type 1, potassium channelopathy) or vertigo, ataxia, and occasionally syncope (type 2, calcium channelopathy). These events are commonly diagnosed as epilepsy and EEG recordings can show sharp and slow waves. Moreover, true ES can occur, confounding the diagnosis further.

Painful tonic spasms of multiple sclerosis and other upper motor neuron disorders are involuntary, unilateral dystonic movements that are frequently precipitated by movement. The clinical history and neurological examination should usually provide sufficient evidence to differentiate between tonic spasms of, for example, multiple sclerosis, ES, and paroxysmal dyskinesias.

Startle syndromes are a heterogeneous group of disorders, comprising hyperekplexia, startle epilepsy, and neuropsychiatric syndromes, which are characterized by an abnormal motor response to startling events. Despite some clinical overlap, a carefully recorded history is frequently sufficient to accurately differentiate these entities [70]. Hyperekplexia is characterized by an exaggerated startle response consisting of forced closure of the eyes and an extension of the extremities followed by a generalized stiffness and collapse. It can be mistaken for cataplexy in patients with narcolepsy, or atonic or tonic ES. More minor forms of hyperekplexia display an exaggerated startle response without tonicity and collapse. Hyperekplexia may be hereditary, due to a genetic mutation in the alpha-1 subunit of the glycine receptor on chromosome 5, sporadic, or symptomatic, secondary to widespread cerebral or brainstem damage. Clonazepam may be helpful in reducing both the severity of the startle response and degree of tonicity [71]. There are a number of culture-specific startle syndromes, such as the Jumping Frenchmen of Maine, Latah from Indonesia and Myriachit from Siberia, which involve nonhabituating hyperstartling evoked by loud noises or unexpected tactile stimulation. After the startle reflex, other more unusual responses may be seen including "forced obedience" which typically involves violent or humiliating acts, echolalia, and echopraxia. There is a lack of consensus as to whether these disorders are primarily behavioral [72, 73], or whether they represent a group of hereditary neurological disorders with a phenotypic expression that is strongly amenable to local cultural influences [74]. Startle epilepsy usually manifests as an asymmetric tonic seizure, triggered by a sudden stimulus [75, 76]. Other ictal patterns such as absences, atonic seizures, or generalized seizures are less common. Electroencephalogram abnormalities during such seizures may be obscured by profuse electromyographic activity in the pericranial muscles, although occasionally, epileptiform activity over the vertex may be seen. Startle-provoked seizures usually become manifest after spontaneous ES of the same ictal phenotype have been present for a prolonged period with a high frequency, possibly due to a kindling-like phenomenon. In the majority of cases, both ictal phenotype and neuroimaging data suggest a seizure onset zone within the supplementary motor area. Other than hyperekplexia, startle-induced conditions which may be confused with reflex startle epilepsy include stiff-person syndrome [77] and progressive encephalomyelitis with rigidity and tetanus, although the presence and nature of concomitant neurological symptoms and signs readily distinguish these conditions from each other.

Transient focal sensory attacks

Migraine and epilepsy are both characterized by paroxysmal cerebral dysfunction, and a possible relationship between migraine and epilepsy has been postulated [78, 79]. Migraine is frequently confused for epilepsy, particularly in acephalgic migraine, when the headache is mild or absent. Epileptic seizures can be accompanied or followed by migraine-like headache [80–82], and attacks of migraine can lead to unconsciousness [83], particularly in basilar migraine [84], and acute confusional migraine [85, 86]. Migraine attacks can cause epileptiform EEG abnormalities [87–89], although the EEG changes are usually nonspecific. It has been suggested that episodes of migraine with aura may provoke seizures, in a condition termed "migralepsy" [90], although this has not been universally accepted [91]. Attacks of migraine and of epilepsy also have various precipitants in common, such as hormonal factors and sleep disturbance [79]. A migrainous aura may have visual, sensory, or motor features that may be suggestive of seizure activity, and alertness may be impaired. There are, however, a number of important semiological differences. Visual migraine auras are monochromatic, angulated, bright, and frequently scintillating. They commence in the center of the visual field and gradually evolve over several minutes towards the periphery of one hemi-field, often leaving a scotoma. They usually last between 30 and 60 minutes. In contrast, simple partial seizures arising from the occipital lobe are circular, amorphous, multicolored obscurations that develop rapidly within seconds, and are brief in duration (2 to 3 minutes). They often appear in the periphery of a temporal visual hemi-field, becoming larger and multiplying in the course of the seizure, while frequently moving horizontally towards the other side [92, 93]. Somatosensory migraine commences with unilateral paresthesias spreading from one area to another over 15 to 30 minutes, often resolving in the first area before becoming evident in the next. Epileptic sensory symptoms arise quickly and spread rapidly over seconds to involve other somatic areas in summation, often culminating in secondary generalization. Peripheral neuropathies or radiculopathies also cause sensory symptoms and may be transient if, for example, they are compressive or inflammatory in etiology. Neurological examination may reveal evidence of a fixed neurological deficit, and the circumstances in which the sensory symptoms develop and lack of associated epileptic semiology rarely result in diagnostic confusion. Transient ischemic attacks (TIAs) are broadly distinguished from seizures and migraine by their "negative" symptoms, that is, sensory loss, weakness, or visual impairment, with retained awareness. However, tingling and focal jerking may occur in association with local cerebral hypoperfusion and occasionally with severe bilateral carotid stenosis [94].

Vertigo with brief episodes of dysequilibrium is often misinterpreted as seizure activity. More commonly, the symptoms are due to disorders of the peripheral vestibular system, such as benign paroxysmal positional vertigo or Ménière's disease. Vertigo may occur as a feature of focal seizures, arising from the frontal or parietal regions and specifically the intraparietal sulcus, posterior superior temporal lobe, and the temporo-parietal border regions [95–98]. Vertigo observed in ES rarely occurs in isolation and other clinical manifestations of seizure activity, such as impaired awareness, are also usually present. Vertigo due to a peripheral vestibular disorder is often accompanied by nausea and vomiting and precipitated by head movement, such as rolling over in bed or on provocation with Hallpike's maneuver. Focal onset or generalized ES may be provoked by the same maneuvers in patients with "vestibular epilepsy," a subtype of the reflex epilepsies.

Psychic experiences

Focal seizures arising from the temporal lobe commonly involve psychic phenomena, including déjà vu, panic and fear, visual, olfactory or auditory hallucinations. Perception of the environment may be altered with derealization, micropsia, and macropsia, and interaction with others may be impaired by abnormal language function and altered thought patterns, seen most commonly in temporal and frontal lobe seizures. Panic attacks, which have a psychological rather than epileptic basis, are associated with feelings of fear and anxiety, hyperventilation, and palpitations. The diagnosis is usually clear as they are commonly situational rather than spontaneous, and have a protracted time course with a characteristic evolution. Simple partial seizures arising from the amygdala can, however, be difficult to differentiate from brief episodes of fear and anxiety [99, 100].

Hallucinations or illusions can occur in the context of loss of a primary sense. This is well recognized in limb amputees, with phantom limb pain and sensory disturbance. Similarly, patients with visual impairment may develop Charles Bonnet syndrome with visual hallucinations in the area of visual field loss. This results from damage to the visual system due to, for example, age-related macular degeneration or glaucoma, but it may also arise in patients with intracranial pathology and secondary deafferentation of the visual cortex [101].

Aggressive or vocal outbursts

Episodic dyscontrol syndrome (EDS) and its counterpart, intermittent explosive disorder (IED), are patterns of abnormal, episodic, and frequently violent and uncontrollable social behaviors often in the absence of significant provocation. These events are frequently attributed to epilepsy as they often arise seemingly out of character. Uncontrolled rage occurring in the context of ES is also unprovoked, however, the anger is usually undirected or reactive, the episodes occur in isolation, and other manifestations of a seizure disorder are frequently present. Additionally, routine interictal EEG recordings in EDS have not shown epileptiform activity [102]. Interestingly, however, a significant proportion of patients demonstrate non-specific diffuse or focal slowing not attributable to drowsiness or the effects of medication, there is neuroimaging evidence of frontolimbic involvement in the pathogenesis of EDS and IED and coexistent neurological and psychiatric conditions are frequently seen [103]. So although the rage attacks themselves may not have an epileptic basis, the two conditions may be pathogenetically linked.

Episodic phenomena in sleep

Epilepsy has a complex association with sleep. Seizures may be more common during sleep or show prominent diurnal variation. Occasionally, seizures may arise exclusively from sleep and can therefore be readily confused with parasomnias [104]. This is particularly true of frontal lobe seizures which can manifest as brief stereotypical abrupt arousals, complex stereotypical nocturnal movements and posturing, or episodic nocturnal wanderings with confusion [105].

Sleep-wake transition disorders may be confused with epilepsy. The most common is hypnic jerks, which are fragmentary physiological myoclonias occurring during REM and stages 1 and 2 of non-REM sleep. These are entirely benign and require no treatment. Excessive fragmentary myoclonus persisting into sleep stages 3 and 4 often indicates an underlying sleep disorder and should therefore be investigated appropriately. Rhythmic movement disorders are a collection of childhood conditions characterized by repetitive movements during sleep transition, the most dramatic of which is head banging or jactatio capitis nocturna. Persistence of these rhythmic movements beyond the age of 10 years is often associated with learning difficulties, autism, or emotional disturbance.

Restless legs syndrome is characterized by an unpleasant sensory disturbance akin to paresthesias, associated with an irresistible urge to move the legs, which temporarily relieves the discomfort. It is seen in approximately 5% of the population and may be familial or secondary to peripheral neuropathy, renal failure, iron deficiency, pregnancy, and spinal cord lesions.

The vast majority of patients with restless legs syndrome also have periodic limb movements in sleep (PLMS), but the converse is seen less frequently. Approximately 50% of patients over the age of 65 years have PLMS, which are brief, jerking flexion and extension movements of predominantly the legs, occurring every 20 to 40 seconds. Some parasomnias are specific for the stage of sleep.

Non-REM parasomnias, also called sleep arousal disorders, usually occur in slow-wave (stage 3–4) sleep between 30 minutes and 4 hours after going to sleep. Somnambulism is reported in 25% of children, with a peak age of 11 to 12 years. The condition is characterized by wanderings lasting a few minutes, often with associated complex behavior, such as carrying objects and eating. Patients may respond when spoken to, but their speech is often slow and monosyllabic. Brief, abortive attempts are commoner, involving sitting up in bed with fidgeting and shuffling, mimicking a complex partial seizure. Night terrors and confusional arousals are less frequent non-REM parasomnias. These conditions are benign and rarely require treatment, although if hazardous behavior is encountered, treatment with benzodiazepines, such as clonazepam, is usually effective [106].

In contrast, REM parasomnias usually occur in middle age or the elderly, and show a marked male predominance. Nightmares and sleep paralysis are relatively benign conditions which rarely require treatment. Of greater concern, however, is REM sleep behavior disorder, which results from the dissociation between REM sleep and axial atonia, resulting in the patient enacting their dreams. During REM sleep, patients may have an increase in the frequency or severity of fragmentary myoclonus, thrash about, and display directed violence or vocalize. The episodes may last several minutes. In approximately one-third of patients, REM sleep behavior disorders are symptomatic of an underlying neurological condition, such as multiple system atrophy, brainstem tumors, multiple sclerosis, subarachnoid hemorrhage, and cerebrovascular disease. In view of this, a history of possible REM sleep behavior disorder needs to be investigated by polysomnography, and if confirmed, then possible etiologies need to be investigated [106].

Sleep apnea may be obstructive or central in origin. Obstructive sleep apnea (OSA) is relatively common, occurring in approximately 2% of women and 4% of men. Predisposing factors include obesity, micrognathia, and large neck size. Patients with obstructive sleep apnea usually present with daytime hypersomnolence although the nocturnal apneic episodes may cause episodic grunting, flailing, or other restless activity suggestive of nocturnal epilepsy. Untreated, patients may develop pulmonary and systemic hypertension, cardiac failure, and stroke. Additionally, OSA may worsen seizure control in patients with epilepsy and effective assisted ventilation may reduce seizure frequency [107]. Polysomnography with oxygen saturation monitoring is the investigation of choice. Treatment options include nocturnal positive pressure ventilation, dental appliances to pull the jaw forward, and airway widening surgical procedures such as palatoplasty, adenoidectomy, and tonsillectomy.

Prolonged confusional or fugue states

Acute neurological conditions, such as nonconvulsive status epilepticus, intracranial infections, head injuries, ischemic events, and drug intoxication or withdrawal, may result in an acute confusional state. Episodes of acute encephalopathy and transient loss of consciousness may also arise due to systemic disorders such as renal or hepatic failure and endocrine and metabolic abnormalities, the most common of which is hypoglycemia related to insulin therapy in diabetes mellitus. Other precipitants of hypoglycemia include alcohol, insulinomas, rare inborn metabolic abnormalities, such as congenital deficiencies of gluconeogenic enzymes and renal or hepatic disease. The symptoms of hypoglycemia are protean, and include visual disturbance, diaphoresis, confusion, unconsciousness, and altered behavior including irritability and aggression. Peri-oral and acral paresthesias, ataxia, tremor, and dysarthria are common features, leading to diagnostic confusion unless an accurate history and appropriate laboratory investigations are performed. The rare disorders of pheochromocytoma, carcinoid syndrome, and hypocalcemia may also present with confusion, presyncope, or syncope and the hypocalcemic sensory disturbance may be mistaken as an epileptic aura [108].

Transient global amnesia (TGA) usually occurs in middle-aged or elderly people and is characterized by the abrupt onset of anterograde amnesia, accompanied by repetitive questioning [109]. With the exception of the amnesia, there are no neurological deficits. There is neither clouding of consciousness nor loss of personal identity. Attacks last between minutes and hours, with six hours being the average duration. The ability to lay down new memories gradually recovers, leaving only a dense amnesic gap for the duration of the episode and a variable degree of retrograde amnesia. The attacks are often associated with headache, dizziness, and nausea. The duration and number of attacks are important in distinguishing TGA from transient epileptic amnesia and transient ischemic events affecting mesial temporal lobe structures. Unlike the epileptic form of amnesia, TGA rarely lasts less than one hour, and recurrences occur in less than 10% of patients. The etiological basis of TGA is uncertain. Possible underlying mechanisms include cortical spreading depression or venous congestion. Most likely, however, TGA may refer to a single expression of several pathophysiological phenomena [109, 110].

Fugue states may also be psychogenic, as a dissociative state symptom. Inconsistencies in cognition and mental state are often elucidated if the patient is examined during an episode, which may be prolonged, lasting days or even weeks.

Summary

In conclusion, there are a large number of neurological and cardiac conditions that result in paroxysmal clinical events and although the causes are multiple and diverse, the clinical manifestations may be similar. The attainment of an accurate and detailed history from the patient and a witness is essential in differentiating these conditions. The application of appropriate investigations frequently increases clinical yield and directs apposite therapy. Nevertheless, misdiagnosis is common and may have profound physical, psychosocial, and socioeconomic consequences for the patient, and economic implications for the health and welfare services.

References

1. Chadwick D, Smith D. The misdiagnosis of epilepsy. *BMJ* 2002;**324**(7336):495–6.
2. Smith D, Defalla BA, Chadwick DW. The misdiagnosis of epilepsy and the management of refractory epilepsy in a specialist clinic. *QJM* 1999;**92**(1):15–23.
3. Zaidi A, Clough P, Cooper P, Scheepers B, Fitzpatrick AP. Misdiagnosis of epilepsy: many seizure-like attacks have a cardiovascular cause. *J Am Coll Cardiol* 2000;**36**(1):181–4.
4. Smith D, Bartolo R, Pickles RM, Tedman BM. Requests for electroencephalography in a district general hospital: retrospective and prospective audit. *BMJ* 2001;**322**(7292):954–7.
5. Jacoby A, Johnson A, Chadwick D. Psychosocial outcomes of antiepileptic drug discontinuation. The Medical Research Council Antiepileptic Drug Withdrawal Study Group. *Epilepsia* 1992;**33**(6):1123–31.
6. Cockerell OC, Hart YM, Sander JW, Shorvon SD. The cost of epilepsy in the United Kingdom: an estimation based on the results of two population-based studies. *Epilepsy Res* 1994;**18**(3):249–60.
7. Savage DD, Corwin L, McGee DL, Kannel WB, Wolf PA. Epidemiologic features of isolated syncope: the Framingham Study. *Stroke* 1985;**16**(4):626–9.
8. Dermksian G, Lamb LE. Syncope in a population of healthy young adults; incidence, mechanisms, and significance. *J Am Med Assoc* 1958;**168**(9):1200–7.
9. Lipsitz LA, Wei JY, Rowe JW. Syncope in an elderly, institutionalised population: prevalence, incidence, and associated risk. *Q J Med* 1985;**55**(216):45–54.
10. Silverstein MD, Singer DE, Mulley AG, Thibault GE, Barnett GO. Patients with syncope admitted to medical intensive care units. *JAMA* 1982;**248**(10):1185–9.
11. Benditt DG, Blanc JJ, Brignole M, Sutton B. *The Evaluation and Treatment of Syncope. A Handbook of Clinical Practice*. New York: Blackwell, 2003.
12. Kapoor WN, Karpf M, Wieand S, Peterson JR, Levey GS. A prospective evaluation and follow-up of patients with syncope. *N Engl J Med* 1983;**309**(4):197–204.
13. Brignole M, Alboni P, Benditt DG, et al. Guidelines on management (diagnosis and treatment) of syncope–update 2004. *Europace* 2004;**6**(6):467–537.
14. Soteriades ES, Evans JC, Larson MG, et al. Incidence and prognosis of syncope. *N Engl J Med* 2002;**347**(12):878–85.
15. Kapoor WN. Evaluation and outcome of patients with syncope. *Medicine (Baltimore)* 1990;**69**(3):160–75.
16. Kapoor WN, Peterson J, Wieand HS, Karpf M. Diagnostic and prognostic implications of recurrences in patients with syncope. *Am J Med* 1987;**83**(4):700–8.
17. Gelisse P, Genton P. Cough syncope misinterpreted as epileptic seizure. *Epileptic Disord* 2008;**10**(3):223–4.
18. Benditt DG, Ermis C, Lu Fei. Head-up tilt table testing. In: Zipes DP, Jalife J, eds. *Cardiac Electrophysiology. From Cell to Bedside*, 4th edn. Philadelphia: Saunders. 2004.
19. Lempert T, Bauer M, Schmidt D. Syncope: a videometric analysis of 56 episodes of transient cerebral hypoxia. *Ann Neurol* 1994;**36**(2):233–7.

20. Agarwal AK, Garg R, Ritch A, Sarkar P. Postural orthostatic tachycardia syndrome. *Postgrad Med J* 2007;**83**(981):478–80.

21. Kanjwal Y, Kosinski D, Grubb BP. The postural orthostatic tachycardia syndrome: definitions, diagnosis, and management. *Pacing Clin Electrophysiol* 2003;**26**(8):1747–57.

22. Goldstein DS, Eldadah B, Holmes C, *et al.* Neurocirculatory abnormalities in chronic orthostatic intolerance. *Circulation* 2005;**111**(7):839–45.

23. Kenny RA, Richardson DA, Steen N, *et al.* Carotid sinus syndrome: a modifiable risk factor for nonaccidental falls in older adults (SAFE PACE). *J Am Coll Cardiol* 2001;**38**(5):1491–6.

24. Kenny RA, Richardson DA. Carotid sinus syndrome and falls in older adults. *Am J Geriatr Cardiol* 2001; **10**(2):97–9.

25. Healey J, Connolly SJ, Morillo CA. The management of patients with carotid sinus syndrome: is pacing the answer? *Clin Auton Res* 2004;**14** Suppl 1:80–6.

26. McIntosh SJ, Lawson J, Kenny RA. Clinical characteristics of vasodepressor, cardioinhibitory, and mixed carotid sinus syndrome in the elderly. *Am J Med* 1993;**95**(2):203–8.

27. Middlekauff HR, Stevenson WG, Saxon LA. Prognosis after syncope: impact of left ventricular function. *Am Heart J* 1993;**125**(1):121–7.

28. Middlekauff HR, Stevenson WG, Stevenson LW, Saxon LA. Syncope in advanced heart failure: high risk of sudden death regardless of origin of syncope. *J Am Coll Cardiol* 1993;**21**(1):110–6.

29. Ritter JM. Drug-induced long QT syndrome and drug development. *Br J Clin Pharmacol* 2008;**66**(3):341–4.

30. Roden DM. Clinical practice. Long-QT syndrome. *N Engl J Med* 2008;**358**(2):169–76.

31. Sze E, Moss AJ, Goldenberg I, *et al.* Long QT syndrome in patients over 40 years of age: increased risk for LQTS-related cardiac events in patients with coronary disease. *Ann Noninvasive Electrocardiol* 2008;**13**(4):327–31.

32. Spirito P, Seidman CE, McKenna WJ, Maron BJ. The management of hypertrophic cardiomyopathy. *N Engl J Med* 1997;**336**(11):775–85.

33. Spirito P, Chiarella F, Carratino L, *et al.* Clinical course and prognosis of hypertrophic cardiomyopathy in an outpatient population. *N Engl J Med* 1989; **320**(12):749–55.

34. Fifer MA, Vlahakes GJ. Management of symptoms in hypertrophic cardiomyopathy. *Circulation* 2008; **117**(3):429–39.

35. Nei M, Ho RT, Sperling MR. EKG abnormalities during partial seizures in refractory epilepsy. *Epilepsia* 2000;**41**(5):542–8.

36. Nei M, Ho RT, Abou-Khalil BW, *et al.* EEG and ECG in sudden unexplained death in epilepsy. *Epilepsia* 2004;**45**(4):338–45.

37. Zijlmans M, Flanagan D, Gotman J. Heart rate changes and ECG abnormalities during epileptic seizures: prevalence and definition of an objective clinical sign. *Epilepsia* 2002;**43**(8):847–54.

38. Opherk C, Coromilas J, Hirsch LJ. Heart rate and EKG changes in 102 seizures: analysis of influencing factors. *Epilepsy Res* 2002;**52**(2):117–27.

39. Altenmuller DM, Zehender M, Schulze-Bonhage A. High-grade atrioventricular block triggered by spontaneous and stimulation-induced epileptic activity in the left temporal lobe. *Epilepsia* 2004;**45**(12):1640–4.

40. Rugg-Gunn FJ, Simister RJ, Squirrell M, Holdright DR, Duncan JS. Cardiac arrhythmias in focal epilepsy: a prospective long-term study. *Lancet* 2004;**364**(9452):2212–9.

41. Tinuper P, Bisulli F, Cerullo A, *et al.* Ictal bradycardia in partial epileptic seizures: autonomic investigation in three cases and literature review. *Brain* 2001;**124**(Pt 12):2361–71.

42. Smith PE, Howell SJ, Owen L, Blumhardt LD. Profiles of instant heart rate during partial seizures. *Electroencephalogr Clin Neurophysiol* 1989;**72**(3):207–17.

43. Leutmezer F, Schernthaner C, Lurger S, Potzelberger K, Baumgartner C. Electrocardiographic changes at the onset of epileptic seizures. *Epilepsia* 2003;**44**(3):348–54.

44. Sheldon R, Rose S, Ritchie D, *et al.* Historical criteria that distinguish syncope from seizures. *J Am Coll Cardiol* 2002;**40**(1):142–8.

45. Lempert T. Recognizing syncope: pitfalls and surprises. *J R Soc Med* 1996;**89**(7):372–5.

46. Hoefnagels WA, Padberg GW, Overweg J, Roos RA. Syncope or seizure? A matter of opinion. *Clin Neurol Neurosurg* 1992;**94**(2):153–6.

47. van Donselaar CA, Geerts AT, Meulstee J, Habbema JD, Staal A. Reliability of the diagnosis of a first seizure. *Neurology* 1989;**39**(2 Pt 1):267–71.

48. Calkins H, Shyr Y, Frumin H, Schork A, Morady F. The value of the clinical history in the differentiation of syncope due to ventricular tachycardia, atrioventricular block, and neurocardiogenic syncope. *Am J Med* 1995;**98**(4):365–73.

49. Mathias CJ, Deguchi K, Schatz I. Observations on recurrent syncope and presyncope in 641 patients. *Lancet* 2001;**357**(9253):348–53.

50. Benke T, Hochleitner M, Bauer G. Aura phenomena during syncope. *Eur Neurol* 1997;**37**(1):28–32.

51. Inamdar V, Mehta S, Juang G, Cohen T. The utility of implantable loop recorders for diagnosing unexplained syncope in 100 consecutive patients: five-year, single-center experience. *J Invasive Cardiol* 2006;**18**(7):313–15.

52. Krahn AD, Klein GJ, Skanes AC, Yee R. Insertable loop recorder use for detection of intermittent arrhythmias. *Pacing Clin Electrophysiol* 2004;**27**(5):657–64.

53. Krahn AD, Klein GJ, Yee R, Skanes AC. Randomized assessment of syncope trial: conventional diagnostic testing versus a prolonged monitoring strategy. *Circulation* 2001;**104**(1):46–51.

54. Fitzpatrick AP, Lee RJ, Epstein LM, et al. Effect of patient characteristics on the yield of prolonged baseline head-up tilt testing and the additional yield of drug provocation. *Heart* 1996;**76**(5):406–11.

55. Brooks R, Ruskin JN, Powell AC, et al. Prospective evaluation of day-to-day reproducibility of upright tilt-table testing in unexplained syncope. *Am J Cardiol* 1993;**71**(15):1289–92.

56. Sheldon R. Evaluation of a single-stage isoproterenol-tilt table test in patients with syncope. *J Am Coll Cardiol* 1993;**22**(1):114–18.

57. Jeffree RL, Besser M. Colloid cyst of the third ventricle: a clinical review of 39 cases. *J Clin Neurosci* 2001;**8**(4):328–31.

58. Spears RC. Colloid cyst headache. *Curr Pain Headache Rep* 2004;**8**(4):297–300.

59. Penfield W. Diencephalic autonomic epilepsy. *Arch Neurol Psychiatry* 1929;**22**:358–74.

60. Mignot E, Hayduk R, Black J, Grumet FC, Guilleminault C. HLA DQB1*0602 is associated with cataplexy in 509 narcoleptic patients. *Sleep* 1997;**20**(11):1012–20.

61. Bourgin P, Zeitzer JM, Mignot E. CSF hypocretin-1 assessment in sleep and neurological disorders. *Lancet Neurol* 2008;**7**(7):649–62.

62. Macleod D, McAuley D. Vertigo: clinical assessment and diagnosis. *Br J Hosp Med (Lond)* 2008;**69**(6):330–4.

63. Venance SL, Cannon SC, Fialho D, et al. The primary periodic paralyses: diagnosis, pathogenesis and treatment. *Brain* 2006;**129**(Pt 1):8–17.

64. Bruno MK, Hallett M, Gwinn-Hardy K, et al. Clinical evaluation of idiopathic paroxysmal kinesigenic dyskinesia: new diagnostic criteria. *Neurology* 2004;**63**(12):2280–7.

65. Bennett LB, Roach ES, Bowcock AM. A locus for paroxysmal kinesigenic dyskinesia maps to human chromosome 16. *Neurology* 2000;**54**(1):125–30.

66. Tomita H, Nagamitsu S, Wakui K, et al. Paroxysmal kinesigenic choreoathetosis locus maps to chromosome 16p11.2–q12.1. *Am J Hum Genet* 1999;**65**(6):1688–97.

67. Vidailhet M. Paroxysmal dyskinesias as a paradigm of paroxysmal movement disorders. *Curr Opin Neurol* 2000;**13**(4):457–62.

68. Lombroso CI. Paroxysmal choreoathetosis: an epileptic or non epileptic disorder? *Ital J Neurol* 1995;**16**(27):271–7.

69. Sadamatsu M, Masui A, Sakai T, et al. Familial paroxysmal kinesigenic choreoathetosis: an electrophysiologic and genotypic analysis. *Epilepsia* 1999;**40**(7):942–9.

70. Bakker MJ, van Dijk JG, van den Maagdenberg AM, Tijssen MA. Startle syndromes. *Lancet Neurol* 2006;**5**(6):513–24.

71. Zhou L, Chillag KL, Nigro MA. Hyperekplexia: a treatable neurogenetic disease. *Brain Dev* 2002;**24**(7):669–74.

72. Saint-Hilaire MH, Saint-Hilaire JM, Granger L. Jumping Frenchmen of Maine. *Neurology* 1986;**36**(9):1269–71.

73. Bartholomew RE. Disease, disorder, or deception? Latah as habit in a Malay extended family. *J Nerv Ment Dis* 1994;**182**(6):331–8.

74. Simons R. *Boo! Culture, Experience and the Startle Reflex*. Oxford: Oxford University Press, 1996.

75. Saenz-Lope E, Herranz FJ, Masdeu JC. Startle epilepsy: a clinical study. *Ann Neurol* 1984;**16**(1):78–81.

76. Manford MR, Fish DR, Shorvon SD. Startle provoked epileptic seizures: features in 19 patients. *J Neurol Neurosurg Psychiatry* 1996;**61**(2):151–6.

77. Khasani S, Becker K, Meinck HM. Hyperekplexia and stiff-man syndrome: abnormal brainstem reflexes suggest a physiological relationship. *J Neurol Neurosurg Psychiatry* 2004;**75**(9):1265–9.

78. Ottman R, Lipton RB. Comorbidity of migraine and epilepsy. *Neurology* 1994;**44**(11):2105–10.

79. Haut SR, Bigal ME, Lipton RB. Chronic disorders with episodic manifestations: focus on epilepsy and migraine. *Lancet Neurol* 2006;**5**(2):148–57.

80. Yankovsky AE, Andermann F, Mercho S, Dubeau F, Bernasconi A. Preictal headache in partial epilepsy. *Neurology* 2005;**65**(12):1979–81.

81. Yankovsky AE, Andermann F, Bernasconi A. Characteristics of headache associated with intractable partial epilepsy. *Epilepsia* 2005;**46**(8):1241–5.

82. Ito M, Adachi N, Nakamura F, *et al*. Characteristics of postictal headache in patients with partial epilepsy. *Cephalalgia* 2004;**24**(1):23–8.

83. Lees F, Watkins SM. Loss of consciousness in migraine. *Lancet* 1963;**2**(7309):647–9.

84. Bickerstaff ER. The basilar artery and the migraine epilepsy syndrome. *Proc R Soc Med* 1962;**55**:167–9.

85. Haan J, Ferrari MD, Brouwer OF. Acute confusional migraine. Case report and review of literature. *Clin Neurol Neurosurg* 1988;**90**(3):275–8.

86. Evans RW, Gladstein J. Confusional migraine or photoepilepsy? *Headache* 2003;**43**(5):506–8.

87. Sand T. EEG in migraine: a review of the literature. *Funct Neurol* 1991;**6**(1):7–22.

88. Bjork M, Sand T. Quantitative EEG power and asymmetry increase 36 h before a migraine attack. *Cephalalgia* 2008;**28**(9):960–8.

89. Hockaday JM, Whitty CW. Factors determining the electroencephalogram in migraine: a study of 560 patients, according to clinical type of migraine. *Brain* 1969;**92**(4):769–88.

90. Milligan TA, Bromfield E. A case of "migralepsy". *Epilepsia* 2005;**46** Suppl 10:2–6.

91. Panayiotopoulos CP. "Migralepsy" and the significance of differentiating occipital seizures from migraine. *Epilepsia* 2006;**47**(4):806–8.

92. Panayiotopoulos CP. Elementary visual hallucinations, blindness, and headache in idiopathic occipital epilepsy: differentiation from migraine. *J Neurol Neurosurg Psychiatry* 1999;**66**(4):536–40.

93. Panayiotopoulos CP. Visual phenomena and headache in occipital epilepsy: a review, a systematic study and differentiation from migraine. *Epileptic Disord* 1999;**1**(4):205–16.

94. Schulz UG, Rothwell PM. Transient ischaemic attacks mimicking focal motor seizures. *Postgrad Med J* 2002;**78**(918):246–7.

95. Penfield W, Jasper H. *Epilepsy and Functional Anatomy of the Human Brain*. Boston: Little, Brown, 1954.

96. Erbayat AE, Serdaroglu A, Gucuyener K, *et al*. Rotational vestibular epilepsy from the temporo-parieto-occipital junction. *Neurology* 2005;**65**(10):1675–6.

97. Fried I, Spencer DD, Spencer SS. The anatomy of epileptic auras: focal pathology and surgical outcome. *J Neurosurg* 1995;**83**(1):60–6.

98. Kluge M, Beyenburg S, Fernandez G, Elger CE. Epileptic vertigo: evidence for vestibular representation in human frontal cortex. *Neurology* 2000;**55**(12):1906–8.

99. Gallinat J, Stotz-Ingenlath G, Lang UE, Hegerl U. Panic attacks, spike-wave activity, and limbic dysfunction. A case report. *Pharmacopsychiatry* 2003;**36**(3):123–6.

100. Sazgar M, Carlen PL, Wennberg R. Panic attack semiology in right temporal lobe epilepsy. *Epileptic Disord* 2003;**5**(2):93–100.

101. Rovner BW. The Charles Bonnet syndrome: a review of recent research. *Curr Opin Ophthalmol* 2006;**17**(3):275–7.

102. Drake ME, Jr, Hietter SA, Pakalnis A. EEG and evoked potentials in episodic-dyscontrol syndrome. *Neuropsychobiology* 1992;**26**(3):125–8.

103. Tebartz Van Elst L, Baeumer D, Lemieux L, *et al*. Amygdala pathology in psychosis of epilepsy: a magnetic resonance imaging study in patients with temporal lobe epilepsy. *Brain* 2002;**125**(Pt 1):140–9.

104. Malow BA. Paroxysmal events in sleep. *J Clin Neurophysiol* 2002;**19**(6):522–34.

105. Derry CP, Duncan JS, Berkovic SF. Paroxysmal motor disorders of sleep: the clinical spectrum and differentiation from epilepsy. *Epilepsia* 2006;**47**(11):1775–91.

106. Wills L, Garcia J. Parasomnias: epidemiology and management. *CNS Drugs* 2002;**16**(12):803–10.

107. Malow BA, Weatherwax KJ, Chervin RD, *et al*. Identification and treatment of obstructive sleep apnea in adults and children with epilepsy: a prospective pilot study. *Sleep Med* 2003;**4**(6):509–15.

108. Riggs JE. Neurologic manifestations of electrolyte disturbances. *Neurol Clin* 2002;**20**(1):227–39, vii.

109. Quinette P, Guillery-Girard B, Dayan J, *et al*. What does transient global amnesia really mean? Review of the literature and thorough study of 142 cases. *Brain* 2006;**129**(Pt 7):1640–58.

110. Zeman A, Hodges J. Transient global amnesia and transient epileptic amnesia. In: Berrios G, Hodges J, eds. *Memory Disorders in Psychiatric Practice*. Cambridge: Cambridge University Press, 2000; 187–203.

Section 1 Chapter 7

Recognition, diagnosis, and impact of nonepileptic seizures

Parasomnias: epileptic/nonepileptic parasomnia interface

Roderick Duncan and Aline Russell

The diagnosis of events that occur during sleep can be difficult and often requires video review with overnight polysomnography (PSG) to assess sleep architecture and clinical events [1]. However, the problem can usefully be restricted to a small proportion of patients at the stage of initial clinical assessment by remembering the obvious: some manifestations of narcolepsy aside, sleep disorders manifest only during sleep, while a "during sleep only" pattern is only rarely reported by patients with psychogenic nonepileptic seizures (PNES) [2].

Nonetheless, a proportion of patients with PNES, possibly as many as half, report that some of their events occur during sleep [2]. In most such patients, eyewitnesses will support the story, stating that the event arises when the patient appears asleep. When PNES have been recorded during what appears to be sleep with video-EEG (VEEG) monitoring [3], the EEG recording shows that they are in fact awake. In a small number of patients, PNES do appear to occur immediately on awakening [4].

When a patient with a suspected or established diagnosis of PNES gives a history that suggests that some events arise during sleep, there is often concern that the patient has both epileptic seizures (ES) and PNES. Such a dual diagnosis occurs probably in only 10% to 15% of patients with PNES [5, 6], rather fewer than was once thought. An exception occurs in patients with both learning disability and PNES, among which up to 30% also have ES [7].

Sleep disorders are grouped into eight major categories; the insomnias, sleep-related breathing disorders, hypersomnias of central origin, circadian rhythm sleep disorders, parasomnias, sleep-related movement disorders, isolated symptoms, and normal variants [8]. The parasomnias and sleep-related movement disorders are the most likely to cause diagnostic confusion.

Parasomnias

Parasomnias are motor and/or experiential events that occur during wake-sleep transition, within different stages of sleep, or during arousals from sleep. These behaviors can be complex and appear purposeful, but may not be associated with awareness. Parasomnias fall into a number of categories.

Sleep transition parasomnias

Sleep transition parasomnias include hypnic jerks, sensory starts, and propriospinal myoclonus. Hypnic jerks or sleep starts are a common normal experience on falling asleep. They may be associated with sensory symptoms (sensory starts), which may be dramatic explosive auditory or visual sensations (exploding head syndrome), and can then be frightening [9, 10].

A severe form of hypnic jerks that may prevent sleep onset, called excessive fragmentary hypnic myoclonus [11], may cause confusion with epilepsy and possibly with PNES. Propriospinal myoclonus is characterized by quasiperiodic axial jerks or unpleasant sensorimotor symptoms which prevent sleep, and similarly may cause diagnostic difficulty, particularly as the jerks may be distractible [12]. At sleep onset or offset, REM sleep can intrude into wakefulness, resulting in sleep paralysis from persistent atonia. Hallucinations, hypnagogic when occurring at sleep onset and hypnopompic at sleep offset, are a common normal experience, but can be associated with narcolepsy [13].

Nonrapid eye movement (NREM)-related parasomnias

Nonrapid eye movement-related parasomnias are disorders of arousal from slow-wave sleep. These tend to

Gates and Rowan's Nonepileptic Seizures, 3rd edn. ed. Steven C. Schachter and W. Curt LaFrance, Jr. Published by Cambridge University Press. © S. Schachter and W. C. LaFrance, Jr. 2010.

occur about one hour into sleep during the first and longest episode of slow-wave sleep and include the spectrum of confusional arousals, sleep terrors, and sleepwalking [14]. These parasomnias are relatively common in children but can persist into adulthood or arise secondarily to other factors. A UK telephone-based adult sleep survey found a prevalence of 4% for confusional arousals, 2% for sleepwalking, and 2% for sleep terrors [15]. The subject appears to be awake but is characteristically amnesic for the event. Electroencephalography may continue to show the pattern of slow-wave sleep or a mixture of wake and sleep rhythms. Confusional arousals are associated with little motor change, but confusion and disorientation last several minutes, occasionally hours. Sleepwalking is associated with complex motor activity including dressing, cooking, eating, and even driving, and may result in falls and life-threatening injuries [16]. Closely related to sleepwalking is nocturnal sleep-related eating disorder (SRED) which is characterized by recurrent and bizarre eating-related behavior during partial arousals from NREM sleep [17]. With night or sleep terrors, marked autonomic activity predominates including tachycardia, tachypnea, flushing, sweating, mydriasis, and increased muscle tone. The subject suddenly sits up in bed, often screaming, terrified and is unresponsive. If "awakened," they remain confused and disoriented.

Nocturnal panic attacks also arise from deep NREM sleep. The subject wakes 1 to 3 hours after sleep onset or on entering deep sleep, with non-specific extreme fear, palpitations, tingling, choking, and breathlessness. In 44% to 71% of patients, daytime panic attacks are also reported [18]. It is unusual for more than one episode a night to occur. Subjects wake fully, are not amnesic, and may have difficulty returning to sleep. They may also have difficulty falling asleep, with prolonged sleep latencies of two or more hours [19]. Sudden awakening with visual hallucinations that disappear if a light is put on can occur in the elderly or severely visually impaired [20].

Rapid eye movement (REM)-related parasomnias

Rapid eye movement sleep behavior disorder (RBD) results from the loss of atonia during REM sleep, resulting in the acting out of dreams [21]. The episodes consist of motor activity and vocalizations that are sometimes violent and vigorous, causing injury to partners. They occur during the second half of sleep periods, when most REM sleep occurs. Rapid eye movement sleep behavior disorder usually occurs after the age of 50, and is associated with neurodegenerative conditions such as Parkinson's disease [22]. Over 80% of patients are men [23]. The episodes can be confused with postictal behavior, and may be thought to be psychogenic or deliberate because of the seemingly directed nature of violent behavior in some cases. The manifestations of REM-related parasomnias are unlike those of PNES, and of course occur only during sleep, making PNES an unlikely diagnosis.

Nonstate dependent parasomnias

Nonstate dependent parasomnias occur in any stage of sleep. Sleep talking usually occurs during light NREM sleep, but can occur during arousals from deeper NREM sleep and occasionally REM sleep. This is common in childhood, and often familial [24, 25], and may be associated with body movements. In catathrenia, or nocturnal groaning, recurrent vocalization [26] lasting between 2 and 20 seconds occurs in clusters for up to an hour. This may occur in both stages 2 NREM and REM sleep. In some cases this may be a form of sleep disordered breathing rather than a true parasomnia [27].

Sleep-related movement disorders

Sleep-related movement disorders are characterized by simple, stereotypic movements that disturb sleep, with or without awareness. They include periodic limb movement disorder, and sleep-related rhythmic movement disorder. Subjects often report excessive daytime sleepiness from the frequent arousals that cause sleep fragmentation. Typically partners are also significantly disturbed.

Periodic limb movement disorder

Periodic limb movement disorder occurs during light NREM sleep. The movements occur every 20 to 40 seconds and usually involve the distal lower limbs, with toe and ankle dorsiflexion, but can involve the upper limbs and head. It is commoner in older patients, may be familial, and is associated with restless legs syndrome [28, 29].

Rhythmic movement disorder

Rhythmic movement disorder (RMD) consists of brief stereotyped repetitive movements such as head banging, side-to-side head rolling, or body rocking that occur at sleep onset, stage 1 NREM sleep, during short arousals in light sleep [30], or very rarely confined to REM sleep [31]. Onset is usually in childhood as with the NREM parasomnias, so it is unusual in adults [32].

Other sleep-related movement disorders include sleep-related bruxism (tooth grinding), excessive fragmentary hypnic myoclonus, and faciomandibular myoclonus [33–35].

Pseudoparasomnias are rarely reported in the literature and are behavioral episodes apparently resembling true parasomnias but during which PSG records a normal awake state [36–38]. These can be regarded as a variant of PNES occurring in apparent sleep. There may also be elaboration of normal sleep phenomena, e.g. RMD and arousal parasomnia.

In summary, the common parasomnias, i.e. confusional arousals, sleepwalking, sleep terrors, sleep talking, and the RMDs typically have onsets in early childhood and are often familial. When appearing in or continuing into adulthood, the timing, duration, rhythmicity, if present, and recurrence through sleep should alert one to the likelihood of a parasomnia or a sleep-related movement disorder. Rapid eye movement sleep behavior disorder can also rarely occur in childhood, especially as an overlap disorder with narcolepsy but the older onset male predominance is more typical and the occurrence in the later stages of sleep timing and dream recall should be diagnostic.

Clinical features of PNES during "pseudosleep"

The semiology of PNES falls into three main clinical types, often termed "convulsive," "swoon," and "pseudo-absence" [39]. Convulsive events are the commonest in most series, and for obvious reasons are the only ones to be reported to occur during sleep [2]. They consist of low frequency high amplitude tremors (sometimes termed "alternating movements") of the limbs and trunk and head (usually side-to-side) with variable loss of responsiveness. Occasionally, limb movements may be "thrashing" or "struggling," and might seem rather like those in RBD or NREM arousal parasomnia, especially through the "filter" of an eyewitness account.

Nocturnal epileptic seizures

Most epilepsies manifest as seizures during waking, or during both waking and sleep. A purely nocturnal pattern is associated with frontal lobe epilepsies [40]. This pattern is rare in PNES [2], so the differential diagnosis is with sleep disorders rather than with PNES. In some cases, the seizures are tonic-clonic, and therefore are not usually confused with a sleep disorder where an eyewitness is available. Even if no eyewitness is available, patients may complain of having bitten the tongue or inside of the cheek, headache or myalgia, which are not features that could readily be explained by a sleep disorder. Where attacks occur during both sleep and waking, the possibility of PNES remains.

Complex partial seizures may occur during sleep [41] and may be more difficult to identify correctly on clinical grounds. Symptoms the next day may be less helpful, in that the patients may be less unwell, and of course features such as tongue biting and myalgia are absent. The "motionless stare" phase may not wake a partner and for the eyewitness, therefore, the seizure may consist of a period of confused behavior. This can be confused with sleep disorders such as RBD, but is not usually mistaken for PNES.

Frontal lobe epilepsies may manifest as hypermotor events, and these events may superficially resemble some PNES, with high amplitude movements of the limbs that might be described as "thrashing." However, if a few points are borne in mind, there should seldom be real diagnostic difficulty. First, PNES are common, while hypermotor frontal lobe seizures are rather rare, probably even in epilepsy practice. Second, hypermotor frontal lobe seizures are short, with durations of seconds or tens of seconds at most, whereas the great majority of PNES last minutes [42, 43]. Third, while "thrashing" movements may occur in PNES, the great majority of patients with PNES have movements that are effectively low frequency high amplitude tremors, sometimes termed alternating movements. These are quite unlike the proximal semi-coordinated automatic movements associated with hypermotor frontal lobe seizures, though care has to be taken to make the distinction through an eyewitness account. Last, patients with nocturnal frontal lobe epilepsy (NFLE) have a tendency to give an account suggesting preserved consciousness during attacks, uncommon in PNES (see accompanying DVD).

It is important to stress the clinical distinction of hypermotor frontal lobe seizures from other types of events, especially because EEG changes may be absent or obscured by muscle artifact. The clinical distinction of NFLE from parasomnias has been reviewed recently, and the usefulness of a scoring system of key clinical features assessed [44, 45].

Conclusion

As in most diagnostic situations, the crux of identifying events during sleep is a good clinical history. An initial clinical assessment should sort patients into groups presenting two differential diagnoses. If events occur only during sleep, then PNES becomes an unlikely diagnosis, and the main differential lies between nocturnal epilepsy, usually frontal lobe, and a sleep disorder. If events are reported to occur during both sleep and waking, then a sleep disorder becomes unlikely, and the differential diagnosis lies between epilepsy and PNES.

As with any "rule" there are caveats. Although narcolepsy is a sleep disorder, it may present with events during the day that mimic complex partial seizures (dream-like states intruding into wakefulness). While the focus of this chapter has been the distinction between epilepsy, PNES, and sleep disorders, in some patients other diagnoses that are mainly in the differential diagnosis of epilepsy (such as hypoglycemia or cardiac dysrhythmia) need to be considered when attacks occur partly or exclusively during sleep.

References

1. Aldrich MS, Jahnke B. Diagnostic value of video-EEG polysomnography. *Neurology* 1991;**41**(7):1060–6.
2. Duncan R, Oto M, Russell AJC, Conway P. Pseudosleep events in patients with psychogenic non epileptic seizures: prevalence and associations. *J Neurol Neurosurg Psychiatry* 2004;**75**:1009–12.
3. Benbadis SM, Lancman ME, King LM, Swanson SJ. Preictal pseudosleep: a new finding in psychogenic seizures. *Neurology* 1996;**47**:63–7.
4. Orbach D, Ritaccio A, Devinsky O. Psychogenic nonepileptic seizures associated with video EEG verified sleep. *Epilepsia* 2003;**44**:64–8.
5. Benbadis SR, Agrawal V, Tatum IV WO. How many patients with psychogenic non-epileptic seizures also have epilepsy? *Neurology* 2001;**57**:915–17.
6. Duncan R, Oto M, Martin E, Pelosi A. Late onset psychogenic nonepileptic attacks. *Neurology* 2006;**66**:1644–7.
7. Duncan R, Oto M. Psychogenic non-epileptic seizures in patients with learning disability: comparison with patients with no learning disability. *Epilepsy Behav* 2008;**12**:183–6.
8. American Academy of Sleep Medicine. *The International Classification of Sleep Disorders: Diagnostic and Coding Manual*, 2nd edn. Westchester, Ill: American Academy of Sleep Medicine, 2005.
9. Sander HW, Geisse H, Quinto C, Sachdeo R, Chokroverty S. Sensory sleep starts. *J Neurol Neurosurg Psychiatry* 1998;**64**:690.
10. Pearce JM. Clinical features of the exploding head syndrome. *J Neurol Neurosurg Psychiatry* 1989;**52**:907–10.
11. Broughton R, Tolentino MA, Krelina M. Excessive fragmentary myoclonus in NREM sleep: a report of 38 cases. *Electroencephalogr Clin Neurophysiol* 1985;**61**:123–33.
12. Montagna P, Provini F, Vetrugno R. Propriospinal myoclonus at sleep onset. *Neurophysiol Clin* 2006;**5**:351–5.
13. Ohayon MM, Priest RG, Caulet M, Guilleminault C. Hypnagogic and hypnopompic hallucinations: pathological phenomena? *Br J Psychiatry* 1996;**169**:459–67.
14. Mahowald MW, Schenck CH. NREM sleep parasomnias. *Neurol Clin* 1996;**14**:675–96.
15. Ohayon MM, Guilleminault C, Priest RG. Night terrors, sleepwalking, and confusional arousals in the general population: their frequency and relationship to other sleep and mental disorders. *J Clin Psychiatry* 1999;**60**:268–76.
16. Schenck CH, Mahowald MW. A polysomnographically documented case of adult somnambulism with long-distance automobile driving and frequent nocturnal violence: parasomnia with continuing danger as a noninsane automatism? *Sleep* 1995;**18**:765–72.
17. Howell MJ, Schenck CH, Crow SJ. A review of nighttime eating disorders. *Sleep Med Rev* 2009;**13**(1):23–34. Epub 2008 Sep 25.
18. Craske MG, Tsao JC. Assessment and treatment of nocturnal panic attacks. *Sleep Med Rev* 2005;**9**:173–84.
19. Hauri PJ, Friedman M, Ravaris CL. Sleep in patients with spontaneous panic attacks. *Sleep* 1989;**12**:323–37.
20. Silber MH, Hansen MR, Girish M. Complex nocturnal visual hallucinations. *Sleep Med* 2005;**6**:363–6.
21. Schenck CH, Bundlie SR, Ettinger MG, Mahowald MW. Chronic behavioral disorders of human REM sleep: a new category of parasomnia. *Sleep* 1986;**9**:293–308.

22. Schenck CH, Mahowald MW. REM sleep behavior disorder: clinical, developmental, and neuroscience perspectives 16 years after its formal identification in SLEEP. *Sleep* 2002;**25**:120–38.

23. Schenck CH, Hurwitz TD, Mahowald MW. Symposium: Normal and abnormal REM sleep regulation: REM sleep behaviour disorder: an update on a series of 96 patients and a review of the world literature. *J Sleep Res* 1993;**2**:224–31.

24. Abe K, Amatomi M, Oda N. Sleepwalking and recurrent sleeptalking in children of childhood sleepwalkers. *Am J Psychiatry* 1984;**141**:800–1.

25. Petit D, Touchette E, Tremblay RE, Boivin M, Montplaisir J. Dyssomnias and parasomnias in early childhood. *Pediatrics* 2007;**119**:1016–25.

26. Vetrugno R, Provini F, Plazzi G, *et al*. Catathrenia (nocturnal groaning): a new type of parasomnia. *Neurology* 2001;**56**(5):681–3.

27. Guilleminault C, Hagen CC, Khaja AM. Catathrenia: parasomnia or uncommon feature of sleep disordered breathing? *Sleep* 2008;**31**:132–9.

28. Ohayon MM, Roth T. Prevalence of restless legs syndrome and periodic limb movement disorder in the general population. *J Psychosom Res* 2002;**53**:547–54.

29. Montplaisir J, Boucher S, Poirier G, *et al*. Clinical, polysomnographic, and genetic characteristics of restless legs syndrome: a study of 133 patients diagnosed with new standard criteria. *Mov Disord* 1997;**12**:61–5.

30. Dyken ME, Rodnitzky RL. Periodic, aperiodic, and rhythmic motor disorders of sleep. *Neurology* 1992;**42** Suppl 6:68–74.

31. Manni R, Terzaghi M. Rhythmic movements during sleep: a physiological and pathological profile. *Neurol Sci* 2005;**26** Suppl 3:181–5.

32. Stepanova I, Nevsimalova S, Hanusova J. Rhythmic movement disorder in sleep persisting into childhood and adulthood. *Sleep* 2005;**28**:851–7

33. Lavigne GJ, Kato T, Kolta A, Sessle BJ. Neurobiological mechanisms involved in sleep bruxism. *Crit Rev Oral Biol Med* 2003;**14**:30–46.

34. Vetrugno R, Plazzi G, Provini F, *et al*. Excessive fragmentary hypnic myoclonus: clinical and neurophysiological findings. *Sleep Med* 2002;**3**:73–6.

35. Loi D, Provini F, Vetrugno R, *et al*. Sleep-related faciomandibular myoclonus: a sleep-related movement disorder different from bruxism. *Mov Disord* 2007;**22**:1819–22.

36. Molaie M, Deutsch GK. Psychogenic events presenting as parasomnia. *Sleep* 1997;**20**:402–5.

37. Hicks JA, Shapiro CM. Pseudo-narcolepsy: case report. *J Psychiatry Neurosci* 1999;**24**:348–50.

38. Williams DR, Cowey M, Tuck K, Day B. Psychogenic propriospinal myoclonus. *Mov Disord* 2008;**23**:1312–13.

39. Reuber M, Elger CE. Psychogenic non-epileptic seizures: review and update. *Epilepsy Behav* 2003;**4**:205–16.

40. Provini F, Plazzi G, Tinuper P, *et al*. Nocturnal frontal lobe epilepsy: a clinical and polygraphic overview of 100 consecutive cases. *Brain* 1999;**122**:1017–31.

41. Chokroverty S, Quinto C. In: Chokroverty S, ed. *Sleep Disorders Medicine*. Boston: Butterworth-Heinemann. 1998; 697–727.

42. Kanner AM, Morris HH, Luders H, *et al*. Supplementary motor seizures mimicking pseudoseizures: some clinical differences. *Neurology* 1990;**40**:1404–7.

43. Saygi S, Katz A, Marks DA, Spenser SS. Frontal lobe partial seizures and psychogenic seizures: comparison of clinical characteristics. *Neurology* 1992;**42**:1274–7.

44. Derry CP, Duncan JS, Berkovic SF. Paroxysmal motor disorders of sleep: the clinical spectrum and differentiation from epilepsy. *Epilepsia*. 2006;**47**(11):1775–91.

45. Manni R, Terzaghi M, Repetto A. The FLEP scale in diagnosing nocturnal frontal lobe epilepsy, NREM and REM parasomnias: Data from a tertiary sleep and epilepsy unit. *Epilepsia* 2008;**49**(9):1581–5. Epub 2008 Apr 10. [doi 10.1111/J.1528–1167.2008.01602]

Section 1 Chapter 8

Recognition, diagnosis, and impact of nonepileptic seizures

The use of hypnosis and linguistic analysis to discriminate between patients with psychogenic nonepileptic seizures and patients with epilepsy

John J. Barry and Markus Reuber

The frequency of psychogenic nonepileptic seizures (PNES) ranges from 1.4 to 4.6 per 100 000 in samples from the general population, up to 5% to 20% from epilepsy outpatient clinics, and up to nearly 50% of inpatients being evaluated by video-EEG (VEEG) monitoring [1]. In a review of 18 studies, the frequency of comorbid epileptic seizures (ES) and PNES was estimated to be between 10% and 18% [2]. An erroneous diagnosis of ES can result in the inappropriate use of antiepileptic drugs (AEDs) with resultant toxicity and even intubation for presumed status epilepticus. The use of VEEG as the gold standard in the diagnosis of epilepsy requires that a "typical" seizure take place during the evaluation. In previous chapters in this text, useful diagnostic clinical signs and symptoms have been outlined to help increase the clinician's awareness of the presence of possible PNES. In this chapter the authors describe two interventions that may additionally help in this process. The first is the use of hypnosis to induce a typical event. This process is presented in detail and the sensitivity and specificity of the procedure are also described. The second is the use of linguistic analysis to help discriminate patients with PNES from those with ES. This involves the application of microanalytic sociolinguistic analysis of the interaction between patient and physician in their first clinical encounter.

Diagnosing patients with PNES by hypnosis

John J. Barry

History

The use of hypnosis dates back to antiquity. Hypnosis has been used for many purposes, including healing as well as the induction of convulsions and altered motoric functioning [3]. The eighteenth century brought the "healer" Franz Anton Mesmer and the use of magnetism [4]. He was discredited later by the Benjamin Franklin commission. It was not until Charcot that hypnosis became utilized in the scientific world with any seriousness. In 1880, Freud and Breuer, in their clinical finding in the case of Anna O., coined the term "conversion" to describe the somatic manifestations of unconscious conflicts. The use of hypnosis was critical in the treatment of Anna O. and was also a central concept in *Studies In Hysteria* [5, 6].

Charcot, Gilles de la Tourette, and Fredrick Myers introduced the concept of "dissociation" as a fragmentation of the psyche [3]. Janet emphasized the role of trauma in this process and also the concept of posttraumatic stress disorder (PTSD). In addition, trauma has a pleomorphic effect on the central nervous system including potential psychobiological and neurohormonal effects. Neuroanatomical changes have also been documented with trauma including effects on amygdala activity and hippocampal volumes. Psychogenic tremors and hyperkinesis were seen during World War II in soldiers under continued stress [5–8] (see accompanying DVD).

Pathophysiology of the hypnotic state

Hypnosis has also been studied to determine its physiological basis. From the time of Charcot, hypnosis has been used to induce PNES, then referred to as hystero-epilepsy. A specific signature on the EEG has not been seen with hypnosis but in those patients who are highly hypnotizable, EEG changes have been noted in the hypnotic state [9, 10]. Event-related potentials offer a more specific marker for the hypnotic state and may lend credence to the trait hypothesis of hypnotizability [11–13]. Positron emission tomography (PET) has shown possible physiological commonality between hypnosis and hysteria, implicating the anterior cingulate cortex in particular but also the orbitofrontal, prefrontal, and dorsolateral regions [14–17]. The cingulate plays an important role in affective disorders, coupled with its connections to other important anatomical areas modulating behavior such as the amygdala, orbitofrontal and anterior insular cortices as well as the periaqueductal grey [18, 19]. It has been postulated that corticofugal inhibition of somatosensory processing may be an explanation of the symptoms seen in patients with hysterical somatic complaints or perhaps for the disconnection of awareness [19].

Hypnosis and psychopathology

Since there appears to be a connection between trauma and dissociation, it is reasonable to postulate that hypnotic ability could differentiate different psychopathological states [20]. This was confirmed by Frischholz et al., who found that higher scores on the Hypnotic Induction Profile (HIP) and the Stanford Hypnotic Susceptibility Scale Form C were noted for patients with dissociative disorders compared to those with schizophrenia [21]. This has been debated by others, but elevated hypnotic ability does appear to be present in patients with dissociative identity disorder (DID) [20].

This fact is particularly important since trauma may lead to memory processing fragmentation and the use and persistence of dissociation as a defense mechanism. It would therefore be expected that those patients experiencing high degrees of trauma would have higher levels of dissociability and that this would be associated with increased levels of hypnotizability. In patients with DID, the use of autohypnosis has been postulated [20]. These concepts are in keeping with the original ideas of Janet, with trauma coming from not only childhood episodes [22–25], but also other clinical sources including burn injuries [26], combat experiences [27], and other episodes of stress [28]. It is also important to realize that the occurrence of stress can be very individualized and must be interpreted as an idiosyncratic process.

Use of hypnosis as an induction procedure in the diagnosis of PNES

Charcot used the term hystero-epilepsy for seizures felt to be of psychological etiology and was responsible for a provocative test which could induce and terminate events [3]. Janet also used hypnosis to explore dissociative phenomena. Peterson et al. used hypnosis coupled with a recall technique to discriminate between PNES and ES [29]. Under hypnosis, patients were asked to recall events surrounding their "seizures." It was postulated that only those patients with PNES would retain recall of events occurring during seizure activity. Sixty-five patients were evaluated. Of the 30 patients with ES, 20 were hypnotizable and amnestic for details of their events. In contrast, of the 35 patients with PNES, 25 were hypnotizable and all recalled detail during their seizures (one patient with an abnormal EEG did have recall but was diagnosed with PNES). In a study with similar methodology, Kuyk et al. examined 13 subjects, with data on 9 of them eventually used for analysis [30]. The resolution of amnesia under hypnosis was a statistically significant factor differentiating between ES and PNES (although the numbers are very small). Schwarz et al. used hypnosis to attempt seizure induction in 26 patients. Sixteen of the patients had histories of ES confirmed by EEG changes and none of these subjects experienced seizure induction. In the 10 patients with PNES, events were induced but without simultaneous EEG changes [31].

The use of hypnosis as a diagnostic tool has been further investigated with a study conducted at Stanford. The HIP was used to measure the level of hypnotic ability, as described in Table 8.1. The technique itself was developed by Spiegel and Spiegel and more fully described in *Trance and Treatment* [32].

Table 8.1 Aspects of the Hypnotic Induction Profile (HIP)

1. Measure of hypnotizability
2. Combines a measure of the patient's innate ability to be hypnotized, as measured by the eye roll sign with a measure of hypnotic expression, the induction score
3. Scores range from 0 (not hypnotizable) to 10 (very hypnotizable)
4. Hypnotic potential without hypnotizability = Decrement profile (decrement profile is defined as showing a potential for a trance but an inability to experience it) [32]

Barry and Atzmon [58].

Table 8.2 Hypnosis and seizure induction

1. Patient is hypnotized and taught self-relaxation
2. Split screen technique is employed
3. Patient is asked to recall the last seizure experienced and the extent of memory for the event is determined
4. Seizure induction ensues
5. Patients are taught the technique and can often self-induce and terminate PNES

Barry and Atzmon [58].

Table 8.3 HIP and diagnosis by seizure induction

Group	N	Hypnotic Induction Profile scores Mean	SD	Diagnosis by seizure induction Sensitivity	Specificity
EE	22	5.18[a,b]	3.31		
NEE	36	6.80[a]	3.14		
EE/NEE	11	6.92[a]	1.99		
NEE + EE/NEE	47	6.83[b]	2.87		
All patients	69			77%	95%

EE, epileptic events; NEE, nonepileptic events.
[a] Means are not different statistically ($p = 0.117$).
[b] Means are statistically significant ($p = 0.038$).
Barry et al. [33]

The level of hypnotizability can in itself have diagnostic implications [19] and one would expect that patients with PNES would score higher on this evaluation tool. With the HIP score calculated, the subject is then hypnotized in the manner described in Table 8.2.

The use of hypnosis for PNES induction is demonstrated on the DVD that accompanies this book.

The hypothesis that hypnosis can be utilized successfully to differentiate patients with PNES from those with ES was evaluated in a study conducted at the Stanford Comprehensive Epilepsy Center involving 82 patients, with 62 meeting criteria for the study [33], including 22 patients with localization-related epilepsy, 36 patients with PNES, and 11 subjects with both PNES and ES. Results are listed in Table 8.3 [1, 33].

When the patients with ES were compared with the PNES and the mixed PNES/ES groups, the HIP scores differentiated between the groups. In addition, the sensitivity of seizure induction via hypnosis to differentiate between the two disorders was 77% with a specificity of 95%. It should be noted that one patient with both PNES and ES had an ES during the hypnotic induction, but she was not hypnotizable as measured by the HIP, had several seizures the day of the test, and was unable to have PNES induced despite multiple attempts. However, the subject did have an ES during the induction procedure and thus the specificity was calculated at 95% [33]. It is also critical to remember the importance of determining whether the induced events are "typical." As can be seen above, some patients with only ES were also hypnotizable. Although ES were not induced in these patients, atypical mild events may be experienced that do not represent the subjects' usual experiences. Hypnosis-provoked PNES have also been induced in children [34] and has been discussed in a single case report [35].

Comparisons with other induction procedures

There are other induction procedures that have been discussed in the literature. Walczak et al. used a placebo infusion technique in 68 subjects, which resulted in 82% of the patients with PNES having a psychogenic event and two patients with ES experiencing an ES [36]. Lancman et al. used an alcohol patch technique with 93 patients with PNES and 20 with ES and found that the procedure had a sensitivity of 77.4% and a specificity of 100% [37]. However, there is concern about the possibility of deception with these two procedures [38, 39]. In addition, psychogenic status epilepticus has been reported in patients undergoing induction with saline infusion [40]. This contrasts with hypnotic induction where the procedure and its goal are entirely discussed with the patient in advance of the procedure. In the authors' experience, no adverse side effects have resulted from this procedure. Likewise, Walczak et al. have reported no ill effects from their technique [41]. Persinger has commented on the biological basis of suggestibility and hypothesized that there is an association between "hypnotizability" and complex partial epileptic-like signs in patients who have not yet developed a full clinical picture of complex partial-like seizure activity [42]. However, much more research in this area must be done to validate this opinion.

The use of hypnosis in the diagnosis of PNES is both sensitive and specific. In addition, it is a very useful treatment in itself and an ideal introduction to individual and group therapy (see Chapter 30). It fosters a therapeutic alliance and can be administered without deception. Patients can be easily trained to use the procedure to start and stop their events. Overall, therefore, hypnosis can be a useful tool in the diagnosis and management of patients with PNES.

Diagnosing patients with PNES by linguistic analysis

Markus Reuber

That patients with medically unexplained neurological symptoms (formerly given the label "hysteria") interact in a characteristic way with their doctor has been known for centuries and was well summarized by Freud, who wrote in 1905:

I can only wonder, how the smooth and exact case reports on hysteria have been written. In reality, these patients are incapable of providing such reports on themselves. Although they may be able to give satisfactory and cohesive reports on this or that period of their lives, this is followed by long periods, in which their reports become sparse, reveal gaps and mysteries, the coherences are mostly torn. The sequence of various events uncertain (. . .). The patient's inability to present their biography in an ordered way, to the extent that this relates to the history of their illness, is characteristic for the (hysterical) neurosis [43].

More recently, Freud's insights have been enlarged upon with a number of studies using different microanalytical sociolinguistic approaches to transcripts of encounters between doctors and patients with PNES. Three of these studies will be described and are based on the same dataset – video recordings and verbatim transcripts of first encounters of patients with a neurologist (one of the authors; MR). All patients were undergoing VEEG because their referring neurologist was uncertain about the nature of their seizure disorder. The interview procedure is described in Table 8.4 (for a more detailed discussion see [44]).

Table 8.4 Interview procedure

Interview phase	Inquiries	Approximate duration
'Open' phase	What were your expectations when you came to the hospital?	10 mins
Elicited seizure episode accounts	Can you tell me about the first seizure you can remember? Can you tell me about the last seizure you can remember? Can you tell me about the worst seizure you can remember?	10 mins
'Challenge' phase	Inquiry or inquiries challenging the patient's description	5 mins
Topic shift	Can you tell me about things which you enjoy doing?	5 mins

Doctor's instructions

- Avoid introducing new topics
- Tolerate silence
- Use continuers (*mmm*, *right*, etc.) to indicate continued attention
- Repeat what the patient has said to encourage elaboration

Adapted from [52].

Twenty patients were included in the first study, and one extra patient in the second and third studies. All patients had seizures involving loss of consciousness, and "gold standard" diagnoses (the observation of a typical attack by VEEG) were made in all cases. The transcripts were analyzed by linguists who were blinded to all additional information (including the results of the VEEG monitoring).

Conversation analysis

The first study examined interactional phenomena in the encounter between patient and doctor. It was based on the established qualitative methodology of conversation analysis and focused especially on *how* patients with ES and patients with PNES talk to their doctor about seizures [45–48]. This research was inspired by the findings of an interdisciplinary research group in Bielefeld, which suggested that patients with PNES and

Table 8.5 Summary of the most important interactional, topical, and linguistic differential diagnostic features

Feature	Patients with ES	Patients with PNES
Subjective seizure symptoms	Typically volunteered, discussed in detail	Avoided, discussed sparingly
Formulation work (e.g., pauses, reformulation attempts, hesitations, restarts)	Extensive, large amount of detail	Practically absent, very little detailing efforts
Seizures as a topic of discussion	Initiated by the patient	Initiated by interviewer
Focus on seizure description	Easy	Difficult or impossible
Spontaneous reference to attempted seizure suppression	Often made	Rarely made
Seizure description by negation (I don't know, I can't hear, I can't remember)	Rarely, negation is usually contextualized ("I can remember this but I can't recall that")	Common and absolute (e.g., "I feel nothing", "I do not know anything has happened")
Description of periods of reduced consciousness or self-control	- Intensive formulation work - Aiming at a precise, detailed description - Attempts to reconstruct gap in consciousness - Precise placement of period of lost consciousness in the seizure process - Display of willingness to know what precisely happened during periods of unconsciousness - Degree of unconsciousness can be challenged interactively	- "Holistic" description of unconsciousness ("I know nothing", "I can't recall anything") - No differentiation of unconsciousness (e.g., less likely than patients with epilepsy to volunteer without questioning "I could see people but not respond") - Pointing out inability to remember anything or take in anything - No self-initiated detailed description - Presentation of gaps as most dominant element of the disorder - Completeness of unconsciousness cannot be challenged

PNES, psychogenic nonepileptic seizures; ES, epileptic seizures.
Adapted from Schwabe et al. [49].

those with ES have quite distinct interactional and linguistic profiles (for an overview of the findings, see Table 8.5) [49].

The most prominent "positive" features suggesting a diagnosis of PNES were termed "detailing block" and "focusing resistance." Detailing block refers to the paucity of volunteered information about subjective seizure symptoms and the incomplete seizure narratives often presented by patients with PNES. Focusing resistance is characterized by the patient's inability or unwillingness to "topicalize" seizure symptoms (rather than the situations in which seizures occur or their consequences) and the signs of avoidance or interactional misalignment which become apparent when they are prompted to speak about particular seizure episodes [50, 51]. It is beyond the scope of this chapter to give illustrative examples but the linguistic pointers to the diagnosis of PNES and the typical interactional differences between patients with PNES and those with ES have been characterized in detail in an exemplary case comparison published previously [52].

Having demonstrated that the observations made in German patients with seizures could be replicated in English speakers [53], we set out to prove the diagnostic potential of these findings. First, we produced a linguistic scoring form based on an operationalization of the features of potential discriminating value. Next, two linguists blinded to VEEG results were asked independently to rate each interview on each feature, to produce a total score, and to generate a diagnostic hypothesis. One linguist correctly predicted the VEEG-based diagnosis in 17/20 patients, the other in 18/20. This is quite an achievement considering that two-thirds of the patients carried an incorrect clinical diagnosis prior to their admission (Reuber et al., unpublished observations).

Table 8.6 Metaphoric conceptualization of seizures [54]

Category	Seizure as an agent/force	Seizure as an event/situation	Seizure as a space/place	Other
Grammatical subject	Seizure	Seizure	Patient	Variable
Semantic agency	With the seizure	Variable	With the patient	Variable
Examples	Seizures come, go, come in, come on, come up, creep up on you, get you, try to do things, set off, are sent in, are straight there, are fought, ccunteracted, contained, are let pass, wear off	Seizures happen, occur, take place, are due, start, finish, go on, carry on, develop, are experienced, witnessed, handled, controlled, stopped, avoided/put off, are brought on, run their course	Drifting off, being off somewhere else, going, going off, being gone, coming back, coming round, coming to, going down, being down, not being there, being out into seizures, in seizures, out of seizures, within seizures, through seizures	Seizures are started up, are fixed, like an electrical charge, like the lights are on but nobody's at home, like something going off, like shutting a computer off, like cold or hot water on the top of your head, are as if your head carries on without you

From Plug et al. [54].

Metaphoric conceptualizations

Inspired by a German study focusing on the use of seizure metaphors by patients with ES and those with PNES [51], we also examined the metaphoric conceptualizations of seizures used by patients in their interactions with the doctor [54]. Using the definition of metaphor by Lakoff and Johnson [55], a linguist blinded to the medical diagnosis identified all seizure metaphors in the transcripts. He then categorized the metaphors into different conceptualizations. Seizures were most frequently described as an agent/force, event/situation or space/place (see Table 8.6). Of 382 metaphors identified, 80.8% belonged to one of these categories. Most patients used metaphors from all categories, but the profile of metaphor choice differed significantly between the ES and PNES groups (Figure 8.1). Patients with ES preferred metaphors depicting the seizure as an agent/force or event/situation. By contrast, patients with PNES more often used metaphors of space/place. Logistic regression analyses correctly predicted the diagnosis of PNES or ES in 81.0% of cases.

Seizure labels

Struck by the difficulties some patients appear to have with naming their problem, we also analyzed patients' use of diagnostic labels [56]. The label most commonly used in the 21 transcripts was "seizure" (132 uses), followed by "attack" (66), "fit" (42) and "blackout" (22). Patients made fine lexical distinctions between the various diagnostic labels they use to describe their experiences. Whereas "fit" and "blackout" were represented as lay terminology, the term "seizure" was typically only used for attacks which had been diagnosed as such by a health professional. Patients with PNES used fewer symptom labels than patients with epilepsy (Figure 8.2). Although the term "seizure" seemed to be preferred to other label options (and was used by 8/13 patients with PNES), many patients displayed a degree of resistance towards this "medical" term. Apart from the failure to use the term "seizure" altogether, this resistance could become evident by patients only talking of "seizures" after prompting by the doctor, by hesitations (Pat: "I seem to have, erm, two different sorts of [0.9 sec pause] seizures happening"), the use of comments expressing a lack of commitment to the term (Betty: "during the seizure or whatever it is I've had"), or by self-repairs (i.e., rapid communication maneuvers which correct something the speaker has said or was going to say):

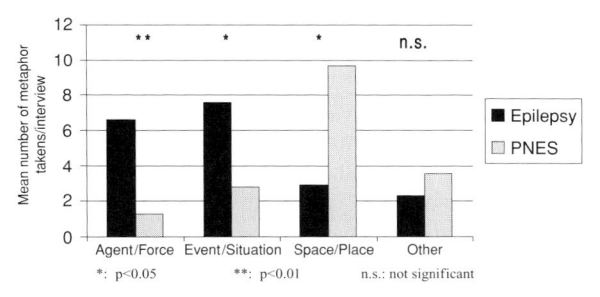

Figure 8.1. Preference of metaphoric conceptualizations by patients with ES or PNES. From Plug et al. [54].

*: $p<0.05$ **: $p<0.01$ n.s.: not significant

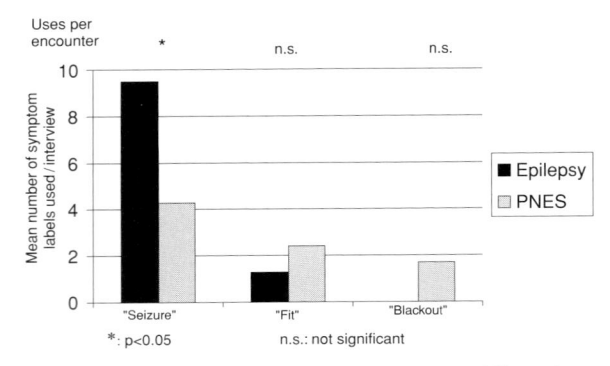

Figure 8.2. Patients with ES and patients with PNES differ in their preferences of symptom labels. From Plug et al. [56].

Doctor: "Is this related to (.) to the seizures er er not waking up from a seizure or just not (.) waking up?"

Tallulah: "Not waking up from (0.3) a sei- er having a fit."

Note: This material was transcribed as spoken – nonlexical utterances and pauses are included. "(.)" denotes a brief but audible pause, "(0.3)" a pause of 0.3 seconds duration.

The display of resistance towards the term "seizure" may have differential diagnostic value: 10/13 patients with PNES but only 1/8 with ES showed such resistance ($\chi^2 = 8.24$, $p = 0.004$).

Therapeutic potential of linguistic analysis

Linguistic analysis does not just facilitate the diagnostic process but also has therapeutic potential. We have previously shown the difficulty of engaging patients with PNES (or other functional neurological symptoms) with psychological treatment programs [57]. Physicians who have received their patients' subtle messages through linguistic analysis are in a better position to explain the nature of PNES and to engage them in psychological treatment.

More specifically, detailing block, focusing resistance, and the other discriminating interactional observations communicate aspects of the psychopathology that underpins PNES. Although further research is needed in this area, the memory gaps, sudden topic shifts, and interactive avoidance of the ictal first person perspective or of detailed symptom descriptions are likely to be related to the ego-structural deficits, dissociative tendencies, attachment difficulties, and unhelpful coping preferences that put patients at risk of developing PNES in the first place or which maintain the seizure disorder. Feeding back interactional observations to patients can be a particularly effective way of making links between seizures and (suboptimal) emotional processing ("When you talk about your seizures you seem to find it easy to tell me where different seizures have happened and what problems they caused you but you have great difficulty in telling me how you feel in the attacks").

Our study of seizure metaphors showed that ES are described (and probably experienced) as a more external, self-directed entity which does something to the patient or is witnessed by the patient. Patients with PNES on the other hand are more likely to experience their seizure as a state or place they go into. Patients may feel better understood by physicians who pay attention to their preferred seizure metaphors and who conceptualize the seizures like they do.

In the same way, the observation of patients' resistance to the "medical" term "seizure" is not only useful as a pointer to the diagnosis of PNES but also communicates an important message to the doctor. Some patients may be in doubt about the "medical" (or physical) etiology of their seizures and are ready for the physician to propose a psychological model. Alternatively, this kind of resistance may be a manifestation of misalignment (or discord) with the physician, suggesting that the physician has to take particular care not to push his/her own etiological model of the patient's seizures too rapidly or forcefully. The use of conversation analysis for PNES is described in a slide show on the DVD that accompanies this book.

Conclusion

Psychogenic nonepileptic seizures are a common phenomenon in patients seen at comprehensive epilepsy centers. Correct diagnosis is imperative to avoid the unnecessary treatment that is so common with this disorder. This chapter has outlined two different approaches to ascertaining a diagnosis of PNES. Hypnosis can be utilized to induce a typical event while the patient is being monitored by VEEG and thus facilitate the diagnosis. It can also be a helpful tool in treatment as well. Linguistic analysis may also help the clinician to make a diagnosis of PNES and may facilitate the treatment of the disorder.

References

1. Barry JJ. Nonepileptic seizures. *CNS Spectr* 2001;**6**(12):956–62.

2. Krumholz A, Ting T. Coexisting epilepsy and nonepileptic seizures. In: Kaplan PW, Fisher RS, eds. *Imitators of Epilepsy*, 2nd edn. New York, NY: Demos Medical Publishing, Inc. 2005; 261–76.

3. Barry JJ. Hypnosis and psychogenic movement disorders. In: Hallett M, Fahn S, Jankovic J, et al. eds. *Psychogenic Movement Disorders. Neurology and Neuropsychiatry*. Philadelphia: Lippincott Williams & Wilkins. 2006; 241–8.

4. Raz A, Shapiro T. Hypnosis and neuroscience: a cross talk between clinical and cognitive research. *Arch Gen Psychiatry* 2002;**59**(1):85–90.

5. Spiegel H, Greenleaf M, Spiegel D. Hypnosis. In: Sadock VA, ed. *Comprehensive Textbook of Psychiatry*. New York: Lippincott Williams & Wilkins. 2000; 2128–45.

6. Spanos NP, Chaves JF. History and historiography of hypnosis. In: Lynn SJ, Rhue JW, eds. *Theories of Hypnosis-Current Models and Perspectives*. New York: Guilford Press. 1991; 43–78.

7. Van der Kolk BA. The body keeps the score: approaches to the psychobiology of posttraumatic stress disorder. In: Van der Kolk BA, McFarlane AC, Weisaeth L, eds. *Traumatic Stress: the Effects of Overwhelming Experience on Mind, Body, and Society*. New York: Guilford Press. 1996; 242–78.

8. Kardiner A, Spiegel H. *War Stress and Neurotic Illness*. New York: Paul B. Hoeber, Inc. 1947; 428.

9. Sabourin ME, Cutcomb SD, Crawford HJ, et al. EEG correlates of hypnotic susceptibility and trance: spectral analysis and coherence. *Int J Psychophysiol* 1990;**10**(2):125–42.

10. Williams JD, Gruzelier JH. Differentiation of hypnosis and relaxation by analysis of narrow band theta and alpha frequencies. *Int J Clin Exp Hypn* 2001;**49**(3):185–206.

11. Jensen SM, Barabasz A, Barabasz M, et al. EEG P300 event-related markers of hypnosis. *Am J Clin Hypn* 2001;**44**(2):127–39.

12. De Pascalis V, Carboni G. P300 event-related-potential amplitudes and evoked cardiac responses during hypnotic alteration of somatosensory pereption. *Int J Neurosci* 1997;**92**(3–4):187–208.

13. Barabasz A, Barabasz M, Jensen S, et al. Cortical event-related potentials show the structure of hypnotic suggestions is crucial. *Int J Clin Exp Hypn* 1999;**47**(1):5–22.

14. Rainville P, Bushnell MC. Hypnosis modulates activity in brain structures involved in the regulation of consciousness. *J Cogn Neurosci* 2002:**14**; 887–901.

15. Rainville P, Hofbauer RK, Paus T, et al. Cerebral mechanisms of hypnotic induction and suggestion. *J Cogn Neurosci* 1999;**11**:110–25.

16. Halligan PW, Athwal BS, Oakley DA, et al. Imagining hypnotic paralysis: implications for conversion hysteria. *Lancet* 2000;**355**:986–7.

17. Marshall JC, Halligan PW, Fink GR, et al. The functional anatomy of a hysterical paralysis. *Cognition* 1997;**64**:B1–B8.

18. Devinsky O, Morrell MJ, Vogt BA. Contributions of anterior cingulated cortex to behavior. *Brain* 1995;**118**: 279–306.

19. Black DN, Taber KH, Hurley RA. Conversion hysteria: lesions from functional imaging. *J Neuropsychiatry Clin Neurosci* 2004;**16**(3):246–51.

20. Nash MR. Hypnosis, psychopathology, and psychological regression. In: Fromm E, Nash MR, eds. *Contemporary Hypnosis Research*. New York: Guilford Press. 1992; 149–72.

21. Frischholz EJ, Lipman LS, Braun BG, et al. Psychopathology, hypnotizability, and dissociation. *Am J Psychiatry* 1992;**149**(11):1521–5.

22. Butler LD, Duran REF, Jasiukaitis P, et al. Hypnotizability and traumatic experience: a diathesis-stress model of dissociative symptomatology. *Am J Psychiatry* 1996;**153**(7):42–63.

23. Ganaway GK. Hypnosis, childhood trauma, and dissociative identity disorder. *Int J Clin Exp Hypn* 1995;**53**(2):127–44.

24. Chu JA, Ganzel BL, Matthews JA. Memories of childhood abuse: dissociation, amnesia, and collaboration. *Am J Psychiatry* 1999;**156**(5):749–55.

25. Roelofs K, Keijsers GPF, Hoogduin KAL, et al. Childhood abuse in patients with conversion disorder. *Am J Psychiatry* 2002;**159**(11):1908–13.

26. DuHamel KN, Difede J, Foley F, et al. Hypnotizability and trauma symptoms after burn injury. *Int J Clin Exp Hypn* 2002;**50**(1):33–50.

27. Brown P, van der Hart O, Graafland M. Trauma-induced dissociative amnesia in World War II. Treatment dimensions. *Aust N Z J Psychiatry* 1999;**33**: 392–8.

28. Bryant RA, Guthrie RM, Moulds ML. Hypnotizability in acute stress disorder. *Am J Psychiatry* 2001;**158**: 600–4.

29. Peterson DB, Sumner JW, Jones GA. Role of hypnosis in differentiation of epileptic from convulsive like seizures. *Am J Psychiatry* 1950;**107**:428–32.

30. Kuyk J, Jacobs LD, Aldenkamp AP, *et al.* Pseudo-epileptic seizures: hypnosis as a diagnostic tool. *Seizure* 1995;**4**(2):123–8.
31. Schwarz BE, Bickford RG, Rasmussen WC. Hypnotic phenomena, including hypnotic activated seizures, studied with electroencephalogram. *J Nerv Ment Dis* 1955;**122**:564–74.
32. Spiegel H, Spiegel D. *Trance and Treatment*. New York: Basic Books Inc, 1978.
33. Barry JJ, Atzmon O, Morrell MJ. Discriminating between epileptic and nonepileptic events: the utility of hypnotic seizure induction. *Epilepsia* 2000;**41**(1):81–4.
34. Olson DM, Howard N, Shaw RJ. Hypnosis-provoked nonepileptic events in children. *Epilepsy Behav* 2007;**12**:456–9.
35. Zalsman G, Dror S, Gadoth N. Hypnosis provoked pseudoseizures: a case report and literature review. *Am J Clin Hypn* **2002**;45(1):47–53.
36. Walczak TS, Williams DT, Berten W. Utility and reliability of placebo infusion in the evaluation of patients with seizures. *Neurology* 1994;**44**:394–9.
37. Lancman ME, Asconape JJ, Craven WJ, *et al.* Predictive value of induction of psychogenic seizures by suggestion. *Ann Neurol* 1994;**35**:359–61.
38. Stagno SJ, Smith ML. the use of placebo in diagnosing psychogenic seizures: who is deceived? *Semin Neurol* 1997;**17**(3):213–18.
39. Devinsky O, Fisher R. Ethical use of placebos and provocative testing in diagnosing nonepileptic seizures. *Neurology* 1996;**47**(4):866–70.
40. Ney GC, Zimmerman C, Schaul N. Psychogenic status epilepticus induced by a provocative technique. *Neurology* 1996;**46**:546–7.
41. Walczak TS, Papacostas S, Williams DT, *et al.* Outcome after diagnosis of psychogenic nonepileptic seizures. *Epilepsia* 1995;**36**:1131–7.
42. Persinger MA. Seizure suggestibility may not be an exclusive differential indicator between psychogenic and partial complex seizures: the presence of a third factor. *Seizure* 1994;**3**(3):215–19.
43. Freud S. Bruchstück einer Hysterie-Analyse. In: Freud S, ed. *Gesammelte Werke*. London: Imago Publishing Co., Ltd. 1942; 161–286.
44. Plug L, Reuber M. Making the diagnosis in patients with blackouts: it's all in the history. *Pract Neurol* 2009;**9**(1):4–15.
45. Peräkylä A. Conversation analysis: a new model of research in doctor-patient communication. *J R Soc Med* 1997;**90**:205–8.
46. Drew P, Collins S, Chatwin J. Conversation analysis: a method for research into interaction between patients and healthcare professionals. *Health Expect* 2001;**4**:58–70.
47. Barnes R. Conversation analysis: a practical resource in the health care setting. *Med Educ* 2005;**39**:113–15.
48. Maynard DW, Heritage J. Conversation analysis, doctor-patient interaction and medical communication. *Med Educ* 2005;**39**:428–35.
49. Schwabe M, Reuber M, Schöndienst M, Gülich E. Listening to people with seizures: how can conversation analysis help in the differential diagnosis of seizure disorders? *Commun Med* 2008;**5**:59–71.
50. Kallmeyer W. "Frau Erle" und ihr Arzt. Zur gesprächtrhetorischen Analyse eines Arzt-Patienten Gesprächs. *Psychother Soz* 2002;**4**:301–10.
51. Surmann V. Anfallsbilder. Metaphorische Konzepte im Sprechen anfallskranker Menschen. Würzburg: Königshausen & Neumann, 2005.
52. Plug L, Sharrack B, Reuber M. Conversation analysis can help to distinguish between epilepsy and non-epileptic seizure disorders: a case comparison. *Seizure* 2009;**18**(1):43–50.
53. Schwabe M, Howell SJ, Reuber M. Differential diagnosis of seizure disorders: a conversation analytic approach. *Soc Sci Med* 2007;**65**:712–24.
54. Plug L, Sharrack B, Reuber M. Seizure metaphors differ in patients' accounts of epileptic and psychogenic nonepileptic seizures. *Epilepsia* 2009;**50**:994–1000.
55. Lakoff G, Johnson M. *Metaphors We Live By*. Chicago: University of Chicago Press, 1980.
56. Plug L, Sharrack B, Reuber M. Seizure, fit or attack? The use of diagnostic labels by patients with epileptic and non-epileptic seizures. *Appl Linguistics*, in press.
57. Howlett S, Grünewald R, Khan A, Reuber M. Engagement in psychological treatment for functional neurological symptoms – barriers and solutions. *Psychother Theory Res Pract Train* 2007;**44**:354–60.
58. Barry JJ, Atzmon O. Use of hypnosis to discriminate epileptic from nonepileptic events. In: Gates JR, Rowan JA, eds. *Non-Epileptic Seizures*. Boston, MA: Butterworth-Heinemann. 2000; 285–304.

Section 1 Chapter 9

Recognition, diagnosis, and impact of nonepileptic seizures

Diagnostic issues in children

Tobias Loddenkemper and Elaine Wyllie

Paroxysmal nonepileptic spells in children can frequently be mistaken for epileptic seizures (ES). Events may mimic ES due to discrete onset, ending and return to baseline, duration, frequency as well as clinical presentation resembling ES. Nonepileptic events can often be suspected based on a thorough history, although seizures should be ruled out by further investigations if the history is not clear. This chapter aims to outline the diagnostic approach to children with suspected nonepileptic events and subsequently lists child-specific nonepileptic spells resembling ES.

Diagnostic approach

Clinical suspicion and risk factors

Clinical event description

Several clinical tools may be helpful in determining the nature of the events. The most important is a detailed description of the event. This description should ideally be obtained from a person, i.e. a parent, caretaker, or teacher, who actually witnessed the event. It is also important to identify the person providing details on the spells and to determine who first noted these spells, as parents might be more likely than teachers to pick up ES [1]. Additionally, an attempt should be made to obtain a description of the episode from the patient, although this is, at times, limited in pediatric patients. Especially in older children, description of the actual event by the child may add important clues. Similar to ES, a description of age of onset, time of onset and state at baseline, clinical manifestations, duration, frequency, motor and oculomotor manifestations, recollection of the event, possible response to testing, possible response to medications, description of the period after the event, as well as associated features such as incontinence and tongue bite can provide important information.

Video documentation of events in question can also provide further clues. Parents are frequently able to provide a home video recording of the events in question that sometimes allows immediate diagnosis in the office without further testing. During staring spells, patients with nonepileptic staring events do not present with eye-fluttering, lip-smacking, and hand movements as are occasionally seen in patients with absence seizures [2]. Epileptic seizures and absences were more likely when automatisms were observed, or urinary incontinence was seen [1]. Additional features suggestive of nonepileptic seizures include responsiveness to touch during the event, lack of interruption of baseline activity, as well as identification of the event by a teacher or healthcare provider (and not by a parent) [1]. Semiological features alone may therefore assist in making the diagnosis. Even associated clinical features on video may be helpful: although not unusual in children, the presence of teddy bears and toy animals on video in adolescents indicated a higher likelihood of nonepileptic seizures [3], possibly as a marker of certain psychiatric conditions.

Clinical clues and risk factors from the history

Especially in the very young or developmentally delayed child, diagnosis is challenging due to lack of verbal skills. Additionally, specific age groups present with particular nonepileptic spells that are only seen during a certain time window of development and this can be one of the most important clues in the differential diagnosis. Diurnal patterns and relationship to daily activities and triggers, such as feeding, movement, or emotional excitation, may also add further information. State at baseline, i.e. sleep or wakefulness, may limit the differential diagnosis further. Other

Gates and Rowan's Nonepileptic Seizures, 3rd edn. ed. Steven C. Schachter and W. Curt LaFrance, Jr. Published by Cambridge University Press. © S. Schachter and W. C. LaFrance, Jr. 2010.

clinical features from the history potentially indicating nonepileptic paroxysmal events include cognitive impairment, developmental delay and mental retardation, lack of response to anticonvulsive medication, and underlying systemic condition suggesting other events, such as psychiatric, cardiological or gastroenterological disorders [4–6].

A thorough history may also elicit important features of the past medical history, such as history of gastroesophageal reflux, constipation, or heart murmurs. Furthermore, characterization of developmental delay or mental retardation; family history of other conditions, such as migraine, narcolepsy, movement disorder, psychiatric disease; or social determinants indicating possible parental drug abuse, Munchausen by proxy syndrome, or child abuse can provide further details.

Examination including a general pediatric and a complete neurological examination can rule out systemic conditions, major intracranial structural lesions, and related underlying neurological diseases. This may also involve, under appropriate circumstances, observation of reported triggers, i.e. observation of parents' feeding techniques, or repetition of certain stimuli, such as exercise, movements, hyperventilation, and others.

Narrowing down potential nonepileptic differential diagnoses

Due to the broad range of nonepileptic events that occur in children, the usual approach of distinguishing ES and psychogenic nonepileptic seizures (PNES) frequently applied in adults cannot easily be transferred to pediatric patients. Psychogenic nonepileptic seizures are not seen in patients under 5 to 6 years old. Only in late adolescence does the frequency and clinical presentation of PNES slowly reach the level of adults. In order to narrow down this broader differential diagnosis in pediatric patients with a frequently more limited history due to nonverbal or less articulate patients, several clinical features can be particularly helpful. Consideration of age at presentation (Table 9.1), clinical pathophysiological presentation (Table 9.2), occurrence out of sleep or wakefulness (Tables 9.1 and 9.3), and possible suspected underlying etiology or pathophysiological mechanism based on related medical conditions and additional information from the history (Table 9.3) are crucial. All these pieces of information are readily available during the first clinic visit and will assist in ruling out differential diagnoses. These tables do not claim to be a complete list of possible events. Separation into certain age, semiological, and pathophysiological categories is somewhat subjective and may be a matter of debate and may have significant overlap amongst each other. Nevertheless these categories may provide a simple orientation for clinicians evaluating children with nonepileptic events.

Although this chapter focuses on nonepileptic seizures in children, ES should never be left out of the differential diagnosis for these events, and therefore questions regarding clinical signs that make epilepsy more likely should always be included, i.e., inquiry about incontinence, tongue bite or postictal obtundation. However, none of these clinical signs is diagnostic, and similar symptoms may also occur during nonepileptic events. Additionally, coexistence of epileptic and nonepileptic events is also frequently seen in children and occurs in up to 30% of patients. Onset of a new type of spell in children with known nonepileptic events and/or epilepsy therefore warrants further investigations.

Confirmatory tests
Routine EEG

Once a nonepileptic event is suspected, the diagnosis should be confirmed. In patients with frequent events or events that can be easily reproduced and triggered, admission to the inpatient video-EEG (VEEG) monitoring unit may be avoided and diagnosis can be made on a routine, prolonged outpatient, or ambulatory EEG with video. Annotations by the technicians, notes by the parents during ambulatory EEGs as well as provocation maneuvers such as hyperventilation and photic stimulation are routinely used. In addition, an attempt should be made to record sleep. Additional known triggers of events in question may also be applied.

Simultaneous VEEG recording and polysomnography

The most important tool in the armamentarium of pediatric neurologists and epileptologists is VEEG recording [7]. Although a routine EEG may pick up spikes, slowing, and very rarely an event, targeting of the event and proof of the absence of associated ictal EEG changes during the event is the current gold standard to rule out ES. Simultaneous recording of EEG during suspicious events identified by

Chapter 9: Diagnostic issues in children

Table 9.1 Clinical presentation of paroxysmal events in children by age and clinical manifestations

Age	Generalized paroxysmal events	Motor manifestations	Oculomotor manifestations	Events during sleep
Neonates (birth to 8 weeks)	Apnea/ALTE	Jitteriness Hyperekplexia	Paroxysmal tonic upward gaze	Benign neonatal sleep myoclonus
Infants (2 months to 2 years)	Shuddering attacks Breath-holding spells (cyanotic and pallid)	Movement disorders - Dystonic choreoathetosis - Torticollis Sandifer syndrome Rumination Benign myoclonus of infancy Stereotypies Alternating hemiplegia Torticollis and dystonia Stool withholding Masturbation Spasmus nutans	Paroxysmal tonic upward gaze Opsoclonus Benign paroxysmal vertigo	Sleep myoclonus/hypnic jerks Rhythmic movement disorder of sleep
Children (2 years to 12 years)	Breath-holding spells Hyperventilation tetany Syncope Daydreaming Migraine and variants - Recurrent abdominal pain - Cyclic vomiting Benign paroxysmal vertigo Psychogenic nonepileptic seizures	Movement disorders including tics, paroxysmal torticollis, paroxysmal kinesiogenic choreoathetosis, paroxysmal dystonic choreoathetosis, dystonic drug reaction, episodic ataxia Stereotypies Sandifer syndrome Withholding activity Hyperekplexia Masturbation Munchausen by proxy Rage attacks	Benign paroxysmal vertigo	Parasomnias - Somnambulism - Somniloquy - Rhythmic movement disorder of sleep Pavor nocturnus Nightmares
Adolescents (12 years to 18 years)	Syncope Migraine and variants - Transient global amnesia Psychogenic nonepileptic seizures	Movement disorders including tics, paroxysmal torticollis, paroxysmal kinesiogenic choreoathetosis, paroxysmal dystonic choreoathetosis, paroxysmal hereditary ataxias - Tremors, dystonic drug reaction		Hypnic jerks Narcolepsy Somnambulism Somniloquy

ALTE, acute life-threatening event.
Table modified after Obeid and Mikati [5], with permission.

parents and family and by video review can rule out ES [7]. Polysomnography, possibly combined with VEEG analysis, may be helpful in differentiating sleep disorders from epilepsy, especially in the characterization of nocturnal events.

Additional workup regarding the underlying cause of nonepileptic events is warranted based on age and clinical presentation, and may in selected cases include some of the following tests and consultations: brain MRI, routine and multi-hour EKG, echocardiography, pH probe testing, other laboratory blood tests, genetic testing, as well as consultation of ancillary services, i.e., pediatric cardiology, pediatric gastroenterology, child and adolescent psychiatry, neuropsychology, and other services.

Types of paroxysmal events

There are several ways to classify paroxysmal events in children as outlined in the approach to differential diagnosis (Tables 9.1–9.3). One of the most useful approaches utilizes the age of the child because this information is usually readily available and gives the clinician important clues about the type of event. Besides age, time of day of the event and occurrence out of sleep or wakefulness, clinical presentation with motor- or oculomotor manifestations and loss of responsiveness, relationship to medication intake or feedings, and other clinical features are important. Subsequently, we will outline common mimickers of ES in neonates, infants, children, and adolescents by

Table 9.2 Nonepileptic paroxysmal events in children by pathophysiological mechanism

Cardiovascular
    Breath-holding spells (cyanotic and pallid)
    Syncope
    Tetspells

Movement disorder
    Neonatal jitteriness
    Paroxysmal dyskinesia and choreoathetosis
    Tremor
    Hyperekplexia
    Shuddering attacks
    Stereotypies
    Nonepileptic myoclonus
    Tics
    Miscellaneous
        Spasmus nutans
        Opsoclonus
        Infantile masturbation

Psychological and psychiatric mechanisms
    Psychogenic nonepileptic seizures
    Daydreaming
    Hyperventilation tetany
    Malingering
    Munchausen syndrome by proxy
    Panic attacks

Sleep disorders
    Arousal disorders
        Sleepwalking
        Sleep terrors
        Confusional arousals
    Sleep-wake transition disorders
        Hypnic jerks
        Somniloquy
        Rhythmic movement disorder
    Rapid eye movement sleep behavior disorder
        Nightmares
        Sleep paralysis
    Other
        Bruxism
        Enuresis
        Benign neonatal sleep myoclonus
        Narcolepsy and cataplexy

Gastrointestinal
    Sandifer syndrome (gastroesophageal reflux disease [GERD])
    Withholding activity (constipation)

Migraine and channelopathies
    Migraine headaches
    Possible migraine variants
        Cyclic vomiting
        Transient global amnesia
        Benign paroxysmal vertigo of infancy
    Alternating hemiplegia
    Episodic ataxia

Toxic and metabolic disorders
    Dystonic drug reactions
    Inherited disorders of metabolism
    Urea cycle disorders
    Aminoacidurias

Table modified after Bleasel and Kotagal [50], with permission.

age group. Although this categorization is not complete and includes some overlap it may give clinicians a rough estimate of what clinical syndrome to consider. More detailed outlines of many of these conditions in adults are available throughout this book. Although some of these conditions may also occur in adults, the presentation may be different because some typical diagnostic clues may be missing or may differ.

Neonatal period (birth to 8 weeks)

Apnea and Acute life-threatening event (ALTE)

In the 1986 National Institutes of Health Consensus Panel on infantile apnea and home monitoring, ALTE was defined as "an episode that is frightening to the observer and is characterized by some combination of apnea (central or occasionally obstructive), color change (usually cyanotic or pallid but occasionally erythematous or plethoric), marked change in muscle tone (usually marked limpness), choking, or gagging. In some cases the observer fears that the infant has died." [8]. A pathological apnea was defined as "apnea lasting 20 seconds or more and accompanied by bradycardia, cyanosis, hypotonia, or other signs of compromise." [8]. Reported incidence ranges from 0.05% to 6% [9, 10]. Depending on the mechanism and etiology, ALTE – the neonatal and infantile correlate of adult syncope – may be followed by a generalized tonic-clonic seizure, if cerebral hypoxia or hypoglycemia occurs.

Etiologies include idiopathic (50%) and symptomatic causes (50%). Symptomatic ALTE can be related to gastroenterological (40%), neurological (30%), respiratory (20%), cardiac (5%), or metabolic causes; child abuse and other less common causes such as anaphylaxis or medication-induced ALTE (5% or less) [9, 11]. Gastroenterological conditions may include gastroesophageal reflux, gastric volvulus, intussusception, swallowing abnormalities, and other gastrointestinal abnormalities. Neurological etiologies besides seizures encompass intracranial hemorrhage and other causes of increased intracranial pressure such as hydrocephalus, stroke, ventriculoperitoneal shunt malfunction or intracranial tumor, Chiari syndrome, malformation of the brainstem, meningitis, and encephalitis as well as vasovagal syncope. A rare cause of respiratory arrest during sleep is congenital central hypoventilation syndrome (Ondine's curse) due to mutations in the PHOX2B gene. Respiratory causes include conditions affecting

Table 9.3 Description of nonepileptic paroxysmal events mimicking similar epileptic seizure types

Nonepileptic event	Peak age	Tonic	Clonic	Tonic-Clonic	Myo-clonic	CPX motor	Auto-motor	Akinetic	Hypo-motor	Fluctuating consciousness	Atonic	Aura	Auto-nomic
ALTE	Neonate, infant	+	+	+					+	+	+		+
Jitteriness and startle	Neonate, infant	+	+		+								
Hereditary hyperekplexia	Neonate, infant	+			+								
Paroxysmal tonic upward gaze	Neonate, infant	+											
Benign neonatal sleep myoclonus	Neonate		+		+								
Shuddering attacks	Infant, child	+	+	+									
Breath-holding spells	Infant, child		+	+	+				+	+	+		+
Benign paroxysmal vertigo	Infant, child, adolescent		+									+	
Movement disorders	Infant, child, adolescent	+	+		+	+						+	
Sandifer syndrome	Infant	+							+				
Rumination	Infant						+						
Benign myoclonus of infancy	Infant	+	+	+	+								
Infantile masturbation	Infant	+	+		+	+							+
Spasmus nutans	Infant	+	+										
Opsoclonus	Infant		+		+								
Rhythmic movement disorder of sleep	Infant, child	+	+			+							
Alternating hemiplegia	Child, infant							+					
Stereotypies	Child, infant					+				+		+	
Stool withholding	Child, infant	+			+								
Hyperventilation	Child, adolescent	+		+						+		+	+
Daydreaming	Child									+			
Parasomnias	Child					+				+		+	
Pavor nocturnus	Child					+				+		+	+

(cont.)

Table 9.3 (cont.)

Nonepileptic event	Peak age	Tonic	Clonic	Tonic-Clonic	Myo-clonic	CPX motor	Auto-motor	Akinetic	Hypo-motor	Fluctuating consciousness	Atonic	Aura	Auto-nomic
Nightmares	Child	*				+				+		+	+
Munchausen syndrome by proxy	Child, infant	*	*	*	*	*	*	*	*	*	*	*	*
Migraine and variants	Adolescent, child, infant									+		+	+
Syncope	Adolescent, child			+						+	+	+	+
Psychogenic nonepileptic seizures	Adolescent, child	+	+	+	+	+	+	+	+	+	+	+	+
Narcolepsy/Cataplexy	Adolescent, child									+	+		
Hallucinations	Adolescent, child									+		+	+
Normal behavior or sensation mistaken for seizure	All age groups	+	+	+	+	+	+	+	+	+	+	+	+

CPX, complex

central respiratory control such as prematurity as well as peripheral respiratory causes including obstructive sleep apnea, vocal cord abnormalities, laryngotracheomalacia, foreign body aspirations, and infections of the respiratory tract (respiratory syncytial virus, pertussis, croup, and others). Cardiac etiologies consist of arrhythmia, congenital heart disease, and cardiomyopathy. Other etiologies include endocrine causes, electrolyte abnormalities, inborn errors of metabolism, infection, and allergic reaction. Child abuse and Munchausen by proxy syndrome always have to be considered in the differential diagnosis of ALTE [9, 11].

Jitteriness and startle response (hyperekplexia)

These conditions are frequently seen in infants and present in up to 44% of full-term neonates [12]. Clinical presentation consists of forward and backward movements of the same duration and extent in each phase. These movements are often triggered by touch or noise, but can also occur spontaneously [12]. Clinical differentiation from ES is supported by decrease in movement with stimulus reduction, and the equal biphasic movement as compared to epileptic clonus. Epileptic clonus is usually biphasic with different phase length, and myoclonic ES are usually shorter.

Etiologies are variable and may include, among others, hypoglycemia [13], hypocalcemia [14], hyperthyroidism [15], hypoxic-ischemic encephalopathies [16], and drug withdrawal [12, 17].

Hereditary hyperekplexia

This condition is a familial disease presenting with stiffness immediately after birth, an increased startle response to unexpected stimuli, especially noises and sounds, and a brief period of generalized stiffness after the startle response in the major form. The minor form presents with excessive startle reactions without stiffness. Severe episodes may cause apnea, cyanosis and bradycardia. Tapping of the root of the nose or the middle portion of the upper lip may lead to the head-retraction reflex with brisk extension of the head and neck [18].

To date five genes have been described in association with hereditary hyperekplexia. The most frequent gene is GLRA1, which encodes a glycine receptor subunit alpha 1 and accounts for 80% of cases. Other genes include genes for glycine receptor subunit beta (GLRB), glycinergic clustering molecule (GPHN), presynaptic glycine transporter 2 (GlyT2) and a gene encoding collybistin (ARHGEF9) [18].

Paroxysmal tonic upward gaze

This entity was first described in 1988 and presents in infants under one year of age [19]. Clinically, episodes consist of sustained conjugate upward deviation of both eyes with neck flexion, normal horizontal eye movements, and downbeating saccades with attempted downgaze [19, 20]. Symptoms eventually improve over time with resolution around the age of 5 years in almost all patients. There is fluctuation of symptoms during the day, with some relief by sleep. In some cases ataxia was noted during episodes and associated learning disabilities were noted later [19, 20].

The etiology is still uncertain. Some cases may be explained by a structural lesion in the upper dorsal brainstem. Additionally, familial cases with apparently dominant and recessive modes of inheritance have been described. In an 18-month-old child with the disorder who was killed in a motor vehicle accident, no pathological abnormalities were found [20].

Benign neonatal sleep myoclonus

This is a phenomenon that frequently manifests during the first two weeks after birth, and presents with myoclonic jerks during sleep, predominantly during quiet sleep [21, 22]. Episodes are clinically characterized by uni- or bilateral, repetitive, synchronous jerks of finger, wrist, and elbow muscles. Less frequently, ankles or all limbs are involved. Events may last up to 20 seconds and frequently recur in intervals [23]. Myoclonic jerks usually resolve by the age of 2 to 4 months, but may persist during the first years of life [24].

Clinical examination, EEG, and neuroimaging are usually normal. Interestingly, head-to-toe crib rocking during EEG recordings has been reported as a provocative maneuver for benign neonatal sleep myoclonus [25]. Another easy to perform confirmatory test is waking the child. Unlike seizures, benign neonatal sleep myoclonus can be interrupted and stops during wakefulness.

The underlying etiology is not known, but relationships to the maturation of the serotonergic system [22] as well as changes in the reticular activating system in the brainstem [21] are suspected.

Infancy (2 months to 2 years)

Shuddering attacks

These spells are characterized by a rapid tremor involving the head, arms, trunk, and occasionally legs. Arms are usually adducted and either flexed in the elbow joint or extended. Episodes usually last only a few seconds and may occur up to 100 times per day [26]. Onset has occasionally been observed around age 3 months and events may persist until the age of 10 years. Clinical examination and investigations including EEG and neuroimaging are in general normal.

Some authors consider shuddering attacks as an early form of essential tremor [27]. Neurological localization of the lesion has been suspected in the thalamus [28]. This is supported by an increased incidence of essential tremor in families of children with shuddering attacks [27, 29]. Additionally, a case report indicates beneficial effects from propranolol [30].

Breath-holding spells

These episodes are clinically characterized by "a stereotyped sequence beginning with a stimulus or provocation leading to crying followed by a noiseless state of expiration accompanied by color change and subsequent loss of consciousness" [31, 32]. In severe breath-holding spells, loss of consciousness may be followed by change in postural tone, a few myoclonic or clonic jerks, and then an inspiratory gasp [33]. Evolution into tonic and clonic clinical presentation may be seen in up to 55% of cases [31, 33, 34]. Consciousness returns after one to two minutes. Triggering stimulus might be fear, being startled, a confrontational situation, or a traumatic event. This triggering stimulus is the clue to making the diagnosis. Family history of breath-holding spells is seen in up to 35% of cases [31, 34].

Based on the child's skin coloration, two clinical types have been suggested by Lombroso and Lerman [32]: pallid and cyanotic breath-holding spells. Pallid breath-holding spells are more frequent than cyanotic breath-holding spells (20% to 30%) [33]. In up to 20% of children both types can occur. Age of onset of cyanotic breath-holding spells is usually earlier (0 to 18 months) as compared to pallid breath-holding spells (12 to 24 months) [33].

The prognosis of breath-holding spells is benign. In 50% of cases, breath-holding spells remit by the age of 3 years and in 90% by the age of 6 years [34]. Anemia may worsen breath-holding spells [34]. In patients with frequent generalized seizures triggered by anoxia, treatment with anticonvulsants may be warranted. Clinical examination and investigations are usually normal, although EEG during spells can reveal slowing and occasional seizures in association with hypoxia.

The suspected underlying mechanism of breath-holding spells is autonomic dysregulation in part mediated by parasympathetic dysregulation and vagal nerve efferents that leads to slowing of the heart rate and possible asystole in pallid breath-holding spells due to hypersensitivity of cardioinhibitory reflexes [35]. Additionally, there may be more widespread peripheral vasomotor response. Especially in younger infants, inappropriate stimulation of a normal pulmonary reflex may also lead to prolonged apnea, hypoxemia, and cyanosis [35]. Immaturity of the autonomic system may have underlying genetic components. If other symptoms of dysautonomia in addition to breath-holding spells are present, Riley Day syndrome, an autosomal recessive familial dysautonomia, should be ruled out.

Benign paroxysmal vertigo

This condition is characterized by sudden episodes of vertigo lasting seconds to minutes. Clinical signs include nystagmus and inability to stand. Because of the recurrent and paroxysmal presentation, events can be mistaken for ES, in particular if the child is too young to describe the symptoms in detail [36]. There is no loss of consciousness or postictal obtundation.

The presumed mechanism is related to otoliths, calcium carbonate particles, which are usually attached to hair cells on a membrane inside the utricle and saccule and which are displaced into the semicircular canals. Otoliths are then free-floating in the semicircular canals, most frequently the posterior canal, and changes of head movement cause movement of otoliths and endolymph causing stimulation of the cupula with subsequent nystagmus and vertigo. Head maneuvers may disperse the otoliths rendering them progressively less effective in producing symptoms [37].

Paroxysmal dyskinesia

This disorder consists of involuntary, rapid, brief, abrupt, jerky, and irregular movements of proximal extremities, face, and tongue that present as chorea and slower, involuntary writhing movements of distal extremities presenting as athetosis. These movements may be mistaken for ES, and may also occur in conjunction with epilepsy [38]. Episodes can occur spontaneously, or may be kinesiogenic or exercise induced [39]. Examination between episodes is normal.

Although most dyskinesias are idiopathic, several symptomatic presentations have been identified, including patients with cerebral infarctions, multiple sclerosis, hypoxic ischemic encephalopathy, and endocrine abnormalities such as hyperthyroidism and diabetes mellitus as well as hypoparathyroidism [38]. Multiple gene locations for paroxysmal dyskinesias have been described, and some of them have also been described in conjunction with generalized epilepsy [38, 40]. Phenytoin and carbamazepine may be helpful in selected forms.

Benign paroxysmal torticollis of infancy

This disorder results in involuntary contractions of neck muscles leading to an abnormal posture of the head. Presentation can involve retrocollis, laterocollis, or torticollis, and may be triggered by repositioning of the infant. Lateralization can vary [41]. It can be observed with vomiting, sweating, ataxia, pallor, or drowsiness. Duration may be minutes to days. Neurological examination between episodes as well as investigations are usually normal [41].

The etiology of benign paroxysmal torticollis is unknown. Some authors suspect a migraine variant, vestibular dysfunction, or labyrinthitis [41]. Torticollis in older children may also have multiple other different underlying causes, including congenital and acquired conditions. Congenital torticollis may be related to birth trauma resulting in injury of the sternocleidomastoid muscle and subsequent fibrosis. Acquired torticollis can be related to muscle injury or spasm, a regional lesion in the neck, a cervical spine process, focal dystonia or dystonic drug reaction, or posterior fossa pathology and Arnold Chiari malformation [42]. Head tilt may also occur as compensation for diplopia, nystagmus or tremor. Sandifer syndrome, tonic posturing events due to gastroesophageal reflux, is described in the following paragraph and can also present with torticollis [42].

Sandifer syndrome

Sandifer syndrome presents with paroxysmal arching of the back, rigid, dystonia-like posturing of the back, neck and arms, and occasional paroxysmal torticollis. Rotation of the head and neck, neck extension, as well as writhing limb movements have been described [43–45]. Episodes usually occur shortly after feeding.

Duration of posturing is one to three minutes. During episodes, infants and young children may become quiet, fussy, or cry. Physical examination is normal. Sandifer syndrome in older children is more likely to occur in the setting of mental impairment. The syndrome was named by Sutcliffe after the British neurologist Paul Sandifer [45], but was first described by Kinsbourne in 1964 [44, 46].

Suspected etiology of Sandifer syndrome is gastroesophageal reflux and dysmotility of the esophagus with or without underlying hiatal hernia [44, 46]. Treatment with head elevation after feeding and proton pump inhibitors or H2-blockers usually leads to resolution of symptoms.

Rumination

Rumination refers to regurgitation of partially digested food that is then subsequently either re-swallowed or expelled [47]. This is associated with repetitive swallowing, chewing, and tongue movements and can be mistaken for ES. Gastric contents reach the oropharynx usually without retching [47]. The infant is usually alert during episodes, and occasionally derives pleasure from regurgitation. Rumination occurs within minutes of feeding and can occur as early as two months of age and usually during the first year of life [48]. It can go along with weight loss, failure to thrive, and even aspiration, choking and death. In older children and adolescents, rumination can also be seen in the setting of psychiatric disease, in particular developmental delay and eating disorders [49].

The etiology of rumination is unknown, but several theories have attempted to explain this phenomenon, including abnormal mother–infant relationship, boredom, pleasure produced by rumination, gastroesophageal reflux, esophageal and gastrointestinal motility disorders, psychiatric disorders, and genetic factors, among others [47, 48].

Benign myoclonus of infancy (Benign nonepileptic infantile spasms)

This disorder presents with brief myoclonic jerks that occur between 3 and 8 months of age and spontaneously disappear within weeks to months. Development and neurological examination are normal. The condition remits by the age of 2 years [50, 51]. In order to differentiate patients from cases with benign myoclonic epilepsy of infancy and other early epileptic encephalopathies, Dravet *et al.* emphasized the nonepileptic character of this condition and suggested the term "benign nonepileptic infantile spasms" [52]. There may be overlap with shuddering spells [28]. Etiology is unknown.

Stereotypies

Stereotypies are involuntary, repetitive, rhythmic movements with a predictable pattern and location that can be suppressed with distraction and that seem purposeful in character but unusual in presentation [53]. Clinical examples include hand and arm flapping movements, body rocking and head nodding, as well as finger wiggling, hand rotating, and others [54]. Stereotypies may present in the setting of preexisting conditions including mental retardation, autistic spectrum disorder, and specific syndromes such as Rett syndrome but are also seen in otherwise healthy children [54].

The etiology of stereotypies is unknown, with explanations ranging from neurobiological and chemical abnormalities to neuropsychological theories [54]. Theories involve dopamine receptor activation, a defect in the fronto-striatal circuit, and possibly a genetic defect considering the predominance of affected first-degree relatives [55].

Spasmus nutans

This condition presents with horizontal, vertical or pendular nystagmus, head nodding, and head tilting (torticollis) [56–58]. Several authors consider head tilt and nodding as adaptive responses to the nystagmus [56]. Onset of symptoms is usually between 4 and 12 months of age. Episodes may fluctuate throughout the day. Symptoms usually remit spontaneously within months to years.

True spasmus nutans is usually idiopathic, and no etiology is found on imaging and ophthalmological examination. However, neuroimaging may be warranted to rule out intracranial lesions such as chiasmal gliomas, third ventricle tumors, or an arachnoid cyst [57]. Neuroblastoma can rarely mimic spasmus nutans and may be diagnosed by abdominal CT and urine catecholamines.

Infantile masturbation

Genital self-stimulation usually starts between 3 months and 3 years [59]. Common features include rocking or rhythmic movements, stereotypic posture, tightening of the thighs leading to pressure in the pubic and suprapubic area, vocalizations with quiet grunting, and no alteration of consciousness. Associated symptoms may include irregular breathing, flushing and other autonomic symptoms [60–62]. In infants, no manual genital stimulation is seen. Episodes may last minutes to hours. Whereas infants are easily distractible, masturbation in older, developmentally delayed children can be associated with decreased distractibility during events [62].

The underlying etiology and motivating factor is pleasure derived from stimulation of the genital area. The condition is benign and self-limiting in infants [59]. Reassurance and counseling should be provided. In older children with developmental delay or autism behavior, modification by behavioral therapy and medications may be helpful [63]. The authors have found the term "gratification behavior" at times more helpful during counseling because parents are occasionally taken aback by the term masturbation.

Opsoclonus

Opsoclonus can be seen in association with myoclonus and ataxia (Kinsbourne triad) [64]. This triad presents with continuous and unpredictable involuntary, rapid, conjugate eye movements in all directions (opsoclonus); brief, repeated myoclonic jerks of arms, legs or the whole body; and ataxic movements [64].

Etiology in 50% is a paraneoplastic syndrome in the setting of neuroblastoma [65]. The exact underlying pathophysiology of opsoclonus remains unclear, but disinhibition of the fastigial nucleus of the cerebellum has been described [66, 67] and antibodies against cerebellar granular cells were found in children with opsoclonus [68]. Viral encephalitis, i.e. due to Coxsackievirus, poliovirus, or St. Louis encephalitis virus, has also been described. It can also be seen in the setting of intoxication, medication effect, or multiple sclerosis.

Rhythmic movement disorder of sleep (RMD)

This movement disorder is classified as a parasomnia and consists of repetitive and stereotyped movements of large muscles, usually involving the head and neck, at the transition from wakefulness to light sleep or shortly after arousal [50]. Subtypes include jactatio capitis nocturna, headbanging, headrolling, body rocking, and rhythmie du sommeil [50]. Rhythmic movements occur in up to 58% of children at one year of age [69], and may persist into adolescence in 3% [70]. Some forms are more frequently seen in developmentally delayed and retarded children. Episodes usually last 10 to 30 minutes, but may also present only with a single jerk [71].

The etiology of RMD is unclear. Explanations include vestibular self-stimulation, possible attempts to maintain vigilance or to bring on sleep, or dysfunction of a central motor pattern generator [72].

Children (2 years to 12 years)

Alternating hemiplegia of childhood

This is a rare disorder presenting with episodic hemiplegia as well as emesis, headache, paroxysmal cranial nerve palsies, choreoathetosis, autonomic dysfunction, and mental retardation [73]. Episodes usually start after 18 months of age although earlier events have been reported [73], occur at least monthly, and may last minutes to hours and even days [74].

The underlying mechanism of these events is unknown. An autosomal dominant inherited presentation with mutations in the ATP1A2 gene has been found in some cases [75, 76]. A calcium channel blocker, flunarizine, reportedly reduced the frequency of recurrence [77, 78].

Stool withholding activity

This condition may present with brief paroxysmal staring and fluctuating responsiveness, behavioral arrest, trunk flexion, leg stiffening or scissoring mimicking ES [79–81]. Episodes can occur daily or multiple times per day lasting minutes. Events can be preceded by abdominal discomfort related to constipation and mimicking an abdominal aura [80]. Events are occasionally associated with encopresis or soiling of underwear and chronic abdominal pain. General examination may reveal palpable stool on abdominal examination as well as occasional anal fissures. Neurological examination is normal. Neurological investigations are usually normal and may be obviated by thorough clinical evaluation.

The underlying etiology is constipation and associated discomfort of passing hard stools. Treatment with laxatives and high fiber diet usually leads to resolution of events [80, 82].

Hyperventilation

Hyperventilation presents with circumoral and acral paresthesias as well as muscle cramps with stiffness, myalgia, and clumsiness. Forced thumb adduction with flexion of the metacarpophalangeal joints and wrist as well as finger extension can be seen. This may lead to carpopedal spasms, laryngospasm, potentially cyanosis, and occasionally also generalized or focal ES [83, 84]. Clinical examination reveals Trousseau's sign (carpopedal spasms after inflation of a manometer above systolic blood pressure) and Chvostek's sign (facial muscle contraction after tapping of the facial nerve).

Etiology is relative hypocalcemia due to respiratory alkalosis. This leads to increased calcium-binding of ionized calcium and subsequent hypocalcemia. Hypocalcemia leads to increased excitability of peripheral neurons due to changes in the resting membrane potential [85, 86]. Re-breathing of carbon dioxide, i.e., by breathing into a paper bag, can resolve symptoms.

Daydreaming

Daydreaming and staring occurs frequently in children with attention deficit disorder and may mimic absence seizures [87]. Distractibility and responsiveness to tactile stimulation, lack of interruption of playing, and initial identification by a teacher or health professional may be important to differentiate these episodes from ES [1]. Duration of episodes is seconds to minutes, and events may occur more frequently or may be reported more often in certain situations, such as school lessons, while watching TV, or shortly before bedtime. Daydreaming may be associated with inattention and trouble focusing, distractibility, disorganization, poor concentration, lack of following through with assignments, and poor attention to detail. Daydreaming never presents with automatisms, myoclonus, eyelid twitching, or other minor motor features frequently seen in patients with absence seizures [88]. Hyperventilation, i.e. by asking the child to blow a pinwheel, under EEG surveillance can help to provoke potential absence seizures and can differentiate absence seizures from daydreaming. However, concomitant EEG surveillance is necessary as nonepileptic events consisting of staring can also be brought on by hyperventilation [89].

The etiology of daydreaming is unclear. Recent research suggests that the tendency of the human mind to wander is a default network of cortical regions that are active when the brain is presumably resting [90]. Underlying ADHD, fatigue, or medication effect should also be considered.

Dyskinesias

Dyskinesias or hyperkinetic movement disorders potentially mimicking seizures include chorea, dystonia, athetosis, tics, tremors, and ballism. Overlap and confusion with ES occurs when dyskinesias are paroxysmal and episodic. Recognition of a geste antagoniste can be useful in differentiation and identification of dystonias.

Several forms of paroxysmal dyskinesias have been described in children [39, 91]. Paroxysmal kinesiogenic dyskinesia is triggered by movement and can present with dystonia and/or choreoathetosis lasting less than one minute. Children may have nonspecific warnings prior to attacks. Similar attacks of dystonia lasting minutes to days can occur without triggers and are termed paroxysmal nonkinesiogenic dyskinesia. Brief episodes of paroxysmal exercise-induced dystonia lasting minutes can be triggered by strenuous exercise. These remit slowly after discontinuation of exercise. Additionally, paroxysmal hypnogenic dyskinesias may occur during or shortly after arousal [39, 92].

Paroxysmal dyskinesias may be familial, sporadic, or secondary to an underlying intracranial lesion such as multiple sclerosis, stroke, or traumatic brain injury. Kinesiogenic dyskinesias tend to respond well to carbamazepine and phenytoin. Exercise-induced dyskinesias may be treated with acetazolamide.

Tics

Tics present with rapid, sudden, brief, repetitive, arrhythmic, intermittent stereotyped movements involving discrete muscle groups or with sounds and vocalization. Examples are eye blinking or throat clearing [93]. Based on clinical presentation, motor and vocal or phonic tics are distinguished, and these can be either simple or complex [94]. Occasionally, they can also present more slowly with a sustained muscle contraction. Duration is usually seconds. Unlike ES, tics can be voluntarily suppressed, but patients experience a premonitory feeling that is relieved upon completion of the tic. Confusion may arise with brief myoclonic seizures, i.e., in patients with juvenile myoclonic epilepsy, but not with tics.

The cause of tics is unknown. They can present in the setting of other comorbidities and associated disorders such as Tourette's syndrome, obsessive compulsive disorder, or attention deficit disorder [95]. Genetic predisposition is likely. Neurotransmitter defects, in particular of the dopaminergic system, are suspected [95].

Rage attacks (also called episodic dyscontrol or intermittent explosive disorder)

These events present with rapid onset of violent behavior and rage followed by remorse and fatigue. Unlike in ES, violent behavior in rage attacks is frequently directed and often has a trigger. Episodes occur in adolescents and older children. Tourette syndrome may be associated including impulse control problems, exhibition of obscene language or gestures, and inappropriate obsessions in addition to rage attacks [96, 97]. Electroencephology in patients with rage attacks may show nonspecific slowing [98] and brainstem auditory evoked response potentials (BAEP) may demonstrate increased interpeak latencies [99].

The etiology is unknown. Rage attacks have been described in the setting of head trauma or Tourette's syndrome, medication side effects, anxiety, sensory integration disorder, obsessive compulsive disorder, and posttraumatic stress disorder [100, 101].

Episodic ataxia

This diagnosis encompasses a heterogeneous group of seven different syndromes with only few well described subtypes. In hereditary episodic ataxia type 1, episodes of ataxia last for approximately two minutes, and may be accompanied by dysarthria and dystonia. Between episodes, myokymia can be observed [102]. Type 2 presents with longer lasting episodes up to several hours, and symptoms may be associated with vertigo and headache [103].

Underlying etiology in type 1 is a mutation in the voltage-gated potassium channel gene KCNA1 for Kv1.1 on chromosome 12p13 [104] and may respond to phenytoin. Mutations in the voltage-gated calcium channel gene CACNA1A on chromosome 19 cause type 2 [103] and these events usually respond to acetazolamide.

Munchausen syndrome by proxy

Also called pediatric condition falsification, this syndrome is diagnosed when a caretaker, usually a parent, provides a false history about the child's symptoms or induces symptoms in a child [105] (see also Chapter 20). This leads to unnecessary and potentially harmful evaluations by the physician. Diagnostic criteria include intentional fabrication of symptoms in another person who is under the individual's care, and the motivation by the caretaker to assume the sick role, by proxy. External incentives, such as financial gain, are usually not important [106]. Younger children, especially between the age of 6 months and 6 years, are at higher risk. Presenting symptoms are frequently seizure descriptions or ALTE among multiple other presentations. The perpetrator is frequently the mother [107]. Final diagnosis can be made by an observation protocol and use of hidden cameras. The etiology is an underlying psychiatric condition in the caretaker [107].

Pavor nocturnus (night terror)

Pavor nocturnus presents with sudden arousal from slow-wave sleep, gasping, moaning, agitation, crying, fear and temporary inability to gain full consciousness. Autonomic features such as mydriasis, tachycardia, and diaphoresis can be seen. It is frequently very difficult to arouse a child during an episode, and episodes may last from a few minutes to hours occurring usually one to three times per month. Events start most frequently between the age of 18 months and 6 years old, with a peak prevalence around 5 to 7 years. Resolution occurs in early adolescence. Night terrors may occur in up to 15% of children [108]. Episodes usually occur within the first half of the night, but after the first hour of sleep. Events are usually less stereotyped, longer, and less frequent than nocturnal seizures that may occur several times per night.

A higher incidence of sleep disordered breathing has been described in patients with pavor nocturnus. Genetic factors also appear to play a role. It is unclear whether genetic factors directly influence sleep terror and sleepwalking or instead influence other disorders that fragment sleep and lead to confusional and partial arousals [109]. Stress during the previous day and fever tend to trigger episodes. Episodes may also be triggered by stimulants or sedatives [50]. Sleep terror may also occur in the same individual as somnambulism and may therefore be part of the same spectrum of conditions.

Somnambulism (sleepwalking)

This is a non-REM sleep arousal disorder occurring in 15% to 20% of children between the age of 5 and 12 years [71]. Clinically, the eyes may be open, with a blank facial expression, decreased responsiveness as well as usually clumsy and purposeless movements [71, 110]. Like sleep terrors, somnambulism occurs in the first third of the night. It can be difficult to distinguish sleep walking from postictal confusion and wandering after nocturnal seizures. Suspected etiologies of somnambulism are similar to pavor nocturnus.

Nightmares

Nightmares present with a sudden awakening from REM sleep associated with confusion, fear, agitation, as well as some undirected motor activity. Crying and vocalization is frequently observed. Duration of episodes is usually a few minutes. Children are consolable.

The etiology is unclear. Medications influencing norepinephrine, serotonin, and dopamine neurotransmitters are associated with nightmares. Additionally, immune modifying medications and agents affecting GABA, histamine, and acetylcholine have been suspected [111].

Adolescents (12 years to 18 years)
Migraine

Migraine in children may mimic epileptic auras with unilateral visual symptoms, vertigo, nausea, auditory features, or painful sensations [112, 113]. Clinical presentation can assist in the differentiation of seizures from migraine. Overall, migrainous auras evolve over several minutes. Visual auras in migraine often present binocular, move or spread more slowly, and produce linear forms more frequently (zigzag lines) compared to occipital lobe onset seizures. Auditory auras in migraine tend to be more monotonous and less stereotyped. Vomiting during migraine can be mistaken for ictal emesis. Alice-in-Wonderland syndrome and "the rushes" with the perception of spatial and temporal distortions can resemble complex visuospatial auras [114–117]. Hemiplegic migraine can present like akinetic or aphasic seizures and can also mimic ictal nystagmus [118]. Finally, basilar artery migraine can present with syncope and loss of consciousness in childhood [119]. Certain types of epilepsy, in particular occipital lobe epilepsy, and migraine headaches appear to be related and may occur together [120–124].

Several pathophysiological mechanisms of migraine headaches have been suggested, including involvement of the trigeminal vascular system, cortical spreading depression, as well as involvement of serotonin, calcitonin gene-related peptide [125], and others. A definite genetic mutation has been described in familial hemiplegic migraine and several genes encoding for transmembrane ion channels (CACNA1A, ATP1A2, and SCN1A) [126]. Additional genes are suspected in common migraine [126].

Psychogenic nonepileptic seizures

Psychogenic nonepileptic seizures due to underlying psychological or psychiatric disorders can present with a variety of clinical symptoms such as subjective visual, sensory, olfactory, gustatory, and auditory symptoms as well as a variety of motor features [127]. Clinical signs that assist in the differentiation from ES include suggestibility of events, known psychological stress, fluctuating loss of consciousness longer than three minutes, side-to-side head movements, back arching, gradual onset, asymmetric flailing limb movements, variation between different episodes, lack of injury or tongue bite, and lack of postictal period. Occasionally, the termination of an episode can also be suggested. The value of ictal eye closure in differentiating epileptic from nonepileptic events has been debated [128]. Duration may be seconds to hours and days with multiple events per day.

Psychiatric etiologies of PNES are heterogeneous, including underlying possible somatoform disorder, i.e. conversion or somatization disorder. The typical history of psychological trauma or abuse, depression, anxiety disorder, posttraumatic stress symptoms, dissociative disorder, and psychosis found in adults differs from the psychopathology seen in children, where school, social, and learning disorders, occur more often [129]. PNES can also occur as an adjustment disorder in response to an acute stressful situation. Pediatric patients less frequently have insight into events and fabricate symptoms less frequently than adults, although malingering has been described in adolescents.

Syncope

Syncope is a brief period of sudden and transient loss of tone and consciousness followed by spontaneous recovery without residual neurological sequelae [130, 131]. Loss of consciousness can be preceded by lightheadedness, visual changes ("black curtain coming down," double vision, blurred vision), dizziness, nausea, pallor, and diaphoresis. Triggers of vasovagal syncope in children include prolonged standing, hair grooming, or micturition. Shock, coma, seizures, and other states of altered awareness are usually excluded by this term. However, prolonged syncope can be followed by seizures due to interruption of energy supply and oxygen to cerebral neurons.

The cause of syncope is usually global cerebral hypoperfusion and temporary hypoxia or hypoglycemia [130]. In 50% of children with syncope, the etiology is related to vasovagal reflex, and decreases in vasomotor tone and heart rate [131–133]. This leads to decrease in systemic vascular resistance and can also be seen in autonomic failure [131, 132]. Hypovolemia, anemia, vasodilators and other medications decreasing cardiac output and vascular tone, or electrolyte imbalance may also be predisposing or causative. Cardiac causes include electrical disturbances, conduction defects, and arrhythmias, as seen in Brugada syndrome, long QT syndrome, short QT syndrome, ventricular tachycardia, and pre-excitation syndromes. Structural defects such as hypertrophic and dilated cardiomyopathies, myocarditis, valvular and coronary artery anomalies, as well as pulmonary hypertension can lead to syncope [134]. Syncope can also be seen in patients with severe metabolic derangements, i.e., hypoglycemia or hyponatremia [135].

Tetspells may present with syncope or presyncopal symptoms in pediatric patients with tetralogy of Fallot. During these events, patients become cyanotic, remain still, and squat down. Younger children turn cyanotic, pass out, and may even die. The etiology is unclear, but it is suspected that spells are caused by a temporary increase in resistance of blood flow to the lungs and subsequently increased flow of desaturated blood to the body. Squatting down cuts off circulation to the legs and thereby improves blood flow to the brain.

Psychiatric disorders

A variety of psychiatric disorders may mimic a wide range of ES symptoms. In particular, differentiation of hallucinations and auras may be difficult, especially when the description of events is vague. Similar to epileptic auras, hallucinations can present with somatosensory, auditory, visual, or olfactory symptoms. Panic attacks may present with variable duration of minutes to hours, and can be accompanied by a sense of impending doom, palpitation, dyspnea, presyncope, hyperventilation, diaphoresis, and tremor. Autonomic symptoms, feeling of panic and impending doom as well as partial responsiveness during events may be misinterpreted as an epileptic aura or seizure.

The etiologies include schizophrenia, psychotic depression, anxiety disorder, medication withdrawal and abuse, intoxication, and structural brain lesions, among others. Interestingly, conversion disorder is only seen in children >5 years old and its frequency increases with age, becoming the most frequent cause of paroxysmal nonepileptic events among adolescents. In adolescents, conversion disorder is more common in females, whereas males predominate in the school-aged group [4].

Narcolepsy

This sleep disorder presents with four cardinal symptoms, namely excessive daytime sleep, cataplexy, sleep paralysis, and hypnagogic hallucinations. Sleep attacks may even occur during activities such as driving or talking. Cataplexy, the sudden loss of tone frequently triggered by an emotional event, may mimic atonic seizures. Sleep paralysis, the inability to move upon awakening, may last minutes. Hypnagogic hallucinations, usually visual but other modalities have also been described, may mimic epileptic auras. If these symptoms occur in isolation and the diagnosis of narcolepsy is not considered, clinical presentation may be misinterpreted as epilepsy [136]. Multi-sleep-latency test can assist in the diagnosis making.

According to current theories, narcolepsy may be caused by a combination of genetic predisposition, abnormal neurotransmitter functioning and sensitivity, and abnormal immune modulation. Stimulants may relieve symptoms.

Other conditions mimicking seizures in children

Many other events may mimic seizures and this list is by no means complete. Cerebrovascular insults, including strokes and transient ischemic attacks, frequently due to an embolus, can also occur in children and clinical symptoms depend on the location of the ischemia. Transient global amnesia, a temporary loss of memory presumably due to hypoperfusion of the hippocampus, has been described in adolescents. Increased intracranial pressure in children with ventriculoperitoneal shunts may present with seizures or with seizure-like episodes, such as dystonia or hydrocephalic attacks with tonic or opisthotonic presentation [6].

Conclusion

The selection and categorization of the nonepileptic events in children discussed in this chapter is by no means complete or exhaustive. Descriptions and categorizations may serve clinicians as an overview and initial guide and approach to differential diagnosis in children with nonepileptic events. Unless typical events are recorded on simultaneous VEEG, ES cannot be definitively ruled out. The diagnostic approach to children differs significantly from adults. Although several types of nonepileptic spells can occur in adults, the main focus is to rule out psychogenic events versus ES in older patients. As compared to adults, a broader spectrum of nonpsychogenic events is seen in children. Clinical characterization involving age of the patient at presentation, semiological presentation of events and possible triggers, diurnal and nocturnal patterns as well as concomitant conditions and diseases can assist in the approach to nonepileptic events in infants, children, and adolescents. Confirmatory VEEG, polysomnography, and further laboratory and imaging workup can provide complementary information.

Diagnostic challenges remain in children with abnormal EEGs and nonepileptic events, concomitant presentation of mixed nonepileptic and epileptic seizures, a structural intracranial lesion, or presurgical workup in patients with epilepsy and nonepileptic seizures.

References

1. Rosenow F, Wyllie E, Kotagal P, et al. Staring spells in children: descriptive features distinguishing epileptic and nonepileptic events. *J Pediatr* 1998;**133**(5):660–3.
2. Duchowny MS, Resnick TJ, Deray MJ, Alvarez LA. Video EEG diagnosis of repetitive behavior in early childhood and its relationship to seizures. *Pediatr Neurol* 1988;**4**(3):162–4.
3. Burneo JG, Martin R, Powell T, et al. Teddy bears: an observational finding in patients with non-epileptic events. *Neurology* 2003;**61**(5):714–15.
4. Kotagal P, Costa M, Wyllie E, Wolgamuth B. Paroxysmal nonepileptic events in children and adolescents. *Pediatrics* 2002;**110**(4):e46.
5. Obeid M, Mikati MA. Expanding spectrum of paroxysmal events in children: potential mimickers of epilepsy. *Pediatr Neurol* 2007;**37**(5):309–16.
6. Pellock JM. Other nonepileptic paroxysmal disorders. In: Wyllie E, Gupta A, Lachhwani DK, eds. *The Treatment of Epilepsy. Principles and Practice.* Philadelphia: Lippincott Williams & Wilkins. 2004; 631–42.
7. Watemberg N, Tziperman B, Dabby R, et al. Adding video recording increases the diagnostic yield of routine electroencephalograms in children with

frequent paroxysmal events. *Epilepsia* 2005;**46**(5):716–19.

8. Infantile Apnea and Home monitoring. NIH Consensus Statement Online 1986. http://consensus.nih.gov/1986/1986InfantApneaMonitoring058html.htm, 6, 1–10. 1986.

9. Brooks JG. Apparent life-threatening events and apnea of infancy. *Clin Perinatol* 1992;**19**(4):809–38.

10. Carroll JL. Apparent Life Threatening Event (ALTE) assessment. *Pediatr Pulmonol Suppl* 2004;**26**:108–9.

11. Hall KL, Zalman B. Evaluation and management of apparent life-threatening events in children. *Am Fam Physician* 2005;**71**(12):2301–8.

12. Parker S, Zuckerman B, Bauchner H, *et al.* Jitteriness in full-term neonates: prevalence and correlates. *Pediatrics* 1990;**85**(1):17–23.

13. Singhal PK, Singh M, Paul VK, *et al.* Neonatal hypoglycemia–clinical profile and glucose requirements. *Indian Pediatr* 1992;**29**(2):167–71.

14. Porcelli PJ, Jr, Oh W. Effects of single dose calcium gluconate infusion in hypocalcemic preterm infants. *Am J Perinatol* 1995;**12**(1):18–21.

15. Watkins MG, Dejkhamron P, Huo J, Vazquez DM, Menon RK. Persistent neonatal thyrotoxicosis in a neonate secondary to a rare thyroid-stimulating hormone receptor activating mutation: case report and literature review. *Endocr Pract* 2008;**14**(4):479–83.

16. Osredkar D, Derganc M, Paro-Panjan D, Neubauer D. Amplitude-integrated electroencephalography in full-term newborns without severe hypoxic-ischemic encephalopathy: case series. *Croat Med J* 2006;**47**(2):285–91.

17. Blumenthal I, Lindsay S. Neonatal barbiturate withdrawal. *Postgrad Med J* 1977;**53**(617):157–8.

18. Bakker MJ, van Dijk JG, van den Maagdenberg AM, Tijssen MA. Startle syndromes. *Lancet Neurol* 2006;**5**(6):513–24.

19. Ouvrier RA, Billson F. Benign paroxysmal tonic upgaze of childhood. *J Child Neurol* 1988;**3**(3):177–80.

20. Ouvrier R, Billson F. Paroxysmal tonic upgaze of childhood–a review. *Brain Dev* 2005;**27**(3):185–8.

21. Coulter DL, Allen RJ. Benign neonatal sleep myoclonus. *Arch Neurol* 1982;**39**(3):191–2.

22. Resnick TJ, Moshe SL, Perotta L, Chambers HJ. Benign neonatal sleep myoclonus. Relationship to sleep states. *Arch Neurol* 1986;**43**(3):266–8.

23. Montagna P. Sleep-related non epileptic motor disorders. *J Neurol* 2004;**251**(7):781–94.

24. Di Capua M, Fusco L, Ricci S, Vigevano F. Benign neonatal sleep myoclonus: clinical features and video-polygraphic recordings. *Mov Disord* 1993;**8**(2):191–4.

25. Alfonso I, Papazian O, Aicardi J, Jeffries HE. A simple maneuver to provoke benign neonatal sleep myoclonus. *Pediatrics* 1995;**96**(6):1161–3.

26. Tibussek D, Karenfort M, Mayatepek E, Assmann B. Clinical reasoning: shuddering attacks in infancy. *Neurology* 2008;**70**(13):e38–41.

27. Vanasse M, Bedard P, Andermann F. Shuddering attacks in children: an early clinical manifestation of essential tremor. *Neurology* 1976;**26**(11):1027–30.

28. Kanazawa O. Shuddering attacks-report of four children. *Pediatr Neurol* 2000;**23**(5):421–4.

29. Holmes GL, Russman BS. Shuddering attacks. Evaluation using electroencephalographic frequency modulation radiotelemetry and videotape monitoring. *Am J Dis Child* 1986;**140**(1):72–3.

30. Barron TF, Younkin DP. Propranolol therapy for shuddering attacks. *Neurology* 1992;**42**(1):258–9.

31. DiMario FJ, Jr. Prospective study of children with cyanotic and pallid breathholding spells. *Pediatrics* 2001;**107**(2):265–9.

32. Lombroso CT, Lerman P. Breathholding spells (cyanotic and pallid infantile syncope). *Pediatrics* 1967;**39**(4):563–81.

33. DiMario FJ, Jr. Breath-holding spells in childhood. *Am J Dis Child* 1992;**146**(1):125–31.

34. DiMario FJ, Jr. Breathholding spells in childhood. *Curr Probl Pediatr* 1999;**29**(10):281–99.

35. DiMario FJ, Jr, Bauer L, Baxter D. Respiratory sinus arrhythmia in children with severe cyanotic and pallid breath-holding spells. *J Child Neurol* 1998;**13**(9):440–2.

36. Paolicchi JM. The spectrum of nonepileptic events in children. *Epilepsia* 2002;**43** Suppl 3:60–4.

37. Marcelli V, Piazza F, Pisani F, Marciano E. Neuro-otological features of benign paroxysmal vertigo and benign paroxysmal positioning vertigo in children: a follow-up study. *Brain Dev* 2006;**28**(2):80–4.

38. Guerrini R. Idiopathic epilepsy and paroxysmal dyskinesia. *Epilepsia* 2001;**42** Suppl 3:36–41.

39. Demirkiran M, Jankovic J. Paroxysmal dyskinesias: clinical features and classification. *Ann Neurol* 1995;**38**(4):571–9.

40. Guerrini R, Parmeggiani L, Casari G. Epilepsy and paroxysmal dyskinesia: co-occurrence and differential diagnosis. *Adv Neurol* 2002;**89**:433–41.

41. Drigo P, Carli G, Laverda AM. Benign paroxysmal torticollis of infancy. *Brain Dev* 2000;**22**(3):169–72.

42. Herman MJ. Torticollis in infants and children: common and unusual causes. *Instr Course Lect* 2006;**55**:647–53.

43. Kostakis A, Manjunatha NP, Kumar A, Moreland ES. Abnormal head posture in a patient with normal ocular motility: Sandifer syndrome. *J Pediatr Ophthalmol Strabismus* 2008;**45**(1):57–8.

44. Kinsbourne M. Hiatus hernia with contortions of the neck. *Lancet* 1964;**1**(7342):1058–61.

45. Sutcliffe J. Torsion spasms and abnormal postures in children with hiatus hernia: Sandifer's syndrome. *Prog Pediatr Radiol* 1969;**2**:190–7.

46. Lehwald N, Krausch M, Franke C, *et al*. Sandifer syndrome–a multidisciplinary diagnostic and therapeutic challenge. *Eur J Pediatr Surg* 2007;**17**(3):203–6.

47. Olden KW. Rumination. *Curr Treat Options Gastroenterol* 2001;**4**(4):351–8.

48. Hyman PE, Milla PJ, Benninga MA, *et al*. Childhood functional gastrointestinal disorders: neonate/toddler. *Gastroenterology* 2006;**130**(5):1519–26.

49. Chial HJ, Camilleri M, Williams DE, Litzinger K, Perrault J. Rumination syndrome in children and adolescents: diagnosis, treatment, and prognosis. *Pediatrics* 2003;**111**(1):158–62.

50. Bleasel A, Kotagal P. Paroxysmal nonepileptic disorders in children and adolescents. *Semin Neurol* 1995;**15**(2):203–17.

51. Lombroso CT, Fejerman N. Benign myoclonus of early infancy. *Ann Neurol* 1977;**1**(2):138–43.

52. Dravet C, Giraud N, Bureau M, *et al*. Benign myoclonus of early infancy or benign non-epileptic infantile spasms. *Neuropediatrics* 1986;**17**(1):33–8.

53. Jankovic J. Stereotypies. In: Marsden C, Fahn S, eds. *Movement Disorders 3*. Oxford: Butterworth-Heinemann. 1994; 501–17.

54. Wolf DS, Singer HS. Pediatric movement disorders: an update. *Curr Opin Neurol* 2008;**21**(4):491–6.

55. Harris KM, Mahone EM, Singer HS. Nonautistic motor stereotypies: clinical features and longitudinal follow-up. *Pediatr Neurol* 2008;**38**(4):267–72.

56. Spaide RF, Klara PM, Restuccia RD. Spasmus nutans as a presenting sign of an arachnoid cyst. *Pediatr Neurosci* 1985;**12**(6):311–14.

57. Kiblinger GD, Wallace BS, Hines M, Siatkowski RM. Spasmus nutans-like nystagmus is often associated with underlying ocular, intracranial, or systemic abnormalities. *J Neuroophthalmol* 2007;**27**(2):118–22.

58. Newman SA, Hedges TR, Wall M, Sedwick LA. Spasmus nutans–or is it? *Surv Ophthalmol* 1990;**34**(6):453–456.

59. Yang ML, Fullwood E, Goldstein J, Mink JW. Masturbation in infancy and early childhood presenting as a movement disorder: 12 cases and a review of the literature. *Pediatrics* 2005;**116**(6):1427–32.

60. Omran MS, Ghofrani M, Juibary AG. Infantile masturbation and paroxysmal disorders. *Indian J Pediatr* 2008;**75**(2):183–5.

61. Casteels K, Wouters C, Van Geet C, Devlieger H. Video reveals self-stimulation in infancy. *Acta Paediatr* 2004;**93**(6):844–6.

62. Nechay A, Ross LM, Stephenson JB, O'Regan M. Gratification disorder ("infantile masturbation"): a review. *Arch Dis Child* 2004;**89**(3):225–6.

63. Albertini G, Polito E, Sara M, Di Gennaro G, Onorati P. Compulsive masturbation in infantile autism treated by mirtazapine. *Pediatr Neurol* 2006;**34**(5):417–18.

64. Dalmau J, Rosenfeld MR. Paraneoplastic syndromes of the CNS. *Lancet Neurol* 2008;**7**(4):327–40.

65. Raffaghello L, Conte M, De Grandis E, Pistoia V. Immunological mechanisms in opsoclonus-myoclonus associated neuroblastoma. *Eur J Paediatr Neurol* 2009;**13**(3):219–23.

66. Wong AM, Musallam S, Tomlinson RD, Shannon P, Sharpe JA. Opsoclonus in three dimensions: oculographic, neuropathologic and modelling correlates. *J Neurol Sci* 2001;**189**(1–2):71–81.

67. Helmchen C, Rambold H, Sprenger A, Erdmann C, Binkofski F. Cerebellar activation in opsoclonus: an fMRI study. *Neurology* 2003;**61**(3):412–15.

68. Blaes F, Fuhlhuber V, Korfei M, *et al*. Surface-binding autoantibodies to cerebellar neurons in opsoclonus syndrome. *Ann Neurol* 2005;**58**(2):313–17.

69. Klackenberg G. Incidence of parasomnias in children in a general population. In: Guilleminault C, ed. *Sleep and its Disorders in Children*. New York: Raven Press. 1987; 99–113.

70. Laberge L, Tremblay RE, Vitaro F, Montplaisir J. Development of parasomnias from childhood to early adolescence. *Pediatrics* 2000;**106**(1 Pt 1):67–74.

71. Derry CP, Duncan JS, Berkovic SF. Paroxysmal motor disorders of sleep: the clinical spectrum and differentiation from epilepsy. *Epilepsia* 2006;**47**(11):1775–91.

72. Manni R, Terzaghi M. Rhythmic movements during sleep: a physiological and pathological profile. *Neurol Sci* 2005;**26** Suppl 3:s181–5.

73. Mikati MA, Kramer U, Zupanc ML, Shanahan RJ. Alternating hemiplegia of childhood: clinical manifestations and long-term outcome. *Pediatr Neurol* 2000;**23**(2):134–41.

74. Bourgeois M, Aicardi J, Goutieres F. Alternating hemiplegia of childhood. *J Pediatr* 1993;**122**(5 Pt 1):673–9.
75. Kanavakis E, Xaidara A, Papathanasiou-Klontza D, *et al*. Alternating hemiplegia of childhood: a syndrome inherited with an autosomal dominant trait. *Dev Med Child Neurol* 2003;**45**(12):833–6.
76. Mikati MA, Maguire H, Barlow CF, *et al*. A syndrome of autosomal dominant alternating hemiplegia: clinical presentation mimicking intractable epilepsy; chromosomal studies; and physiological investigations. *Neurology* 1992;**42**(12):2251–7.
77. Neville BG, Ninan M. The treatment and management of alternating hemiplegia of childhood. *Dev Med Child Neurol* 2007;**49**(10):777–80.
78. Sasaki M, Sakuragawa N, Osawa M. Long-term effect of flunarizine on patients with alternating hemiplegia of childhood in Japan. *Brain Dev* 2001;**23**(5):303–5.
79. Cohn A. Stool withholding presenting as a cause of non-epileptic seizures. *Dev Med Child Neurol* 2005;**47**(10):703–5.
80. Loddenkemper T, Wyllie E, Kaplan B, Lachhwani DK. Stool-withholding activity mimicking epilepsy. *Neurology* 2003;**61**(10):1454–5.
81. Fernando del Rosario J, Orenstein SR, Crumrine P. Stool withholding masquerading as seizure disorder. *Clin Pediatr (Phila)* 1998;**37**(3):201–3.
82. Biggs WS, Dery WH. Evaluation and treatment of constipation in infants and children. *Am Fam Physician* 2006;**73**(3):469–77.
83. Rowland LP. Cramps, spasms and muscle stiffness. *Rev Neurol (Paris)* 1985;**141**(4):261–73.
84. Macefield G, Burke D. Paraesthesiae and tetany induced by voluntary hyperventilation. Increased excitability of human cutaneous and motor axons. *Brain* 1991;**114**(Pt 1B):527–40.
85. Fehlinger R, Seidel K. The hyperventilation syndrome: a neurosis or a manifestation of magnesium imbalance? *Magnesium* 1985;**4**(2–3):129–36.
86. Kukumberg P, Benetin J, Kuchar M. Changes of motor evoked potential amplitudes following magnetic stimulation after hyperventilation. *Electromyogr Clin Neurophysiol* 1996;**36**(5):271–3.
87. Murphy JV, Dehkharghani F. Diagnosis of childhood seizure disorders. *Epilepsia* 1994;**35** Suppl 2:S7–17.
88. Penry JK, Porter RJ, Dreifuss RE. Simultaneous recording of absence seizures with video tape and electroencephalography. A study of 374 seizures in 48 patients. *Brain* 1975;**98**(3):427–40.
89. North KN, Ouvrier RA, Nugent M. Pseudoseizures caused by hyperventilation resembling absence epilepsy. *J Child Neurol* 1990;**5**(4):288–94.
90. Mason MF, Norton MI, Van Horn JD, *et al*. Wandering minds: the default network and stimulus-independent thought. *Science* 2007;**315**(5810):393–5.
91. Bruno MK, Hallett M, Gwinn-Hardy K, *et al*. Clinical evaluation of idiopathic paroxysmal kinesigenic dyskinesia: new diagnostic criteria. *Neurology* 2004;**63**(12):2280–7.
92. Lotze T, Jankovic J. Paroxysmal kinesigenic dyskinesias. *Semin Pediatr Neurol* 2003;**10**(1):68–79.
93. Leckman JF, Bloch MH, King RA, Scahill L. Phenomenology of tics and natural history of tic disorders. *Adv Neurol* 2006;**99**:1–16.
94. Evidente VG. Is it a tic or Tourette's? Clues for differentiating simple from more complex tic disorders. *Postgrad Med* 2000;**108**(5):175–82.
95. Singer HS, Walkup JT. Tourette syndrome and other tic disorders. Diagnosis, pathophysiology, and treatment. *Medicine (Baltimore)* 1991;**70**(1):15–32.
96. Budman CL, Bruun RD, Park KS, Olson ME. Rage attacks in children and adolescents with Tourette's disorder: a pilot study. *J Clin Psychiatry* 1998;**59**(11):576–80.
97. Kano Y, Ohta M, Nagai Y, Spector I, Budman C. Rage attacks and aggressive symptoms in Japanese adolescents with Tourette syndrome. *CNS Spectr* 2008;**13**(4):325–32.
98. Riley TL. The electroencephalogram in patients with rage attacks or episodic violent behavior. *Mil Med* 1979;**144**(8):515–17.
99. Cannon PA, Drake ME, Jr. EEG and brainstem auditory evoked potentials in brain-injured patients with rage attacks and self-injurious behavior. *Clin Electroencephalogr* 1986;**17**(4):169–72.
100. Basson MD, Guinn JE, McElligott J, *et al*. Behavioral disturbances in children after trauma. *J Trauma* 1991;**31**(10):1363–8.
101. Budman CL, Rockmore L, Stokes J, Sossin M. Clinical phenomenology of episodic rage in children with Tourette syndrome. *J Psychosom Res* 2003;**55**(1):59–65.
102. Brunt ER, van Weerden TW. Familial paroxysmal kinesigenic ataxia and continuous myokymia. *Brain* 1990;**113**(Pt 5):1361–82.
103. Jodice C, Mantuano E, Veneziano L, *et al*. Episodic ataxia type 2 (EA2) and spinocerebellar ataxia type 6 (SCA6) due to CAG repeat expansion in the CACNA1A gene on chromosome 19p. *Hum Mol Genet* 1997;**6**(11):1973–8.

104. Browne DL, Gancher ST, Nutt JG, *et al.* Episodic ataxia/myokymia syndrome is associated with point mutations in the human potassium channel gene, KCNA1. *Nat Genet* 1994;**8**(2):136–40.

105. Meadow R. Munchausen syndrome by proxy. The hinterland of child abuse. *Lancet* 1977;**2**(8033):343–5.

106. Barber MA, Davis PM. Fits, faints, or fatal fantasy? Fabricated seizures and child abuse. *Arch Dis Child* 2002;**86**(4):230–3.

107. Alexander R, Smith W, Stevenson R. Serial Munchausen syndrome by proxy. *Pediatrics* 1990;**86**(4):581–5.

108. Mason TB, Pack AI. Sleep terrors in childhood. *J Pediatr* 2005;**147**(3):388–92.

109. Guilleminault C, Palombini L, Pelayo R, Chervin RD. Sleepwalking and sleep terrors in prepubertal children: what triggers them? *Pediatrics* 2003;**111**(1):e17–25.

110. Plazzi G, Vetrugno R, Provini F, Montagna P. Sleepwalking and other ambulatory behaviours during sleep. *Neurol Sci* 2005;**26** Suppl 3:s193–8.

111. Pagel JF, Helfter P. Drug induced nightmares–an etiology based review. *Hum Psychopharmacol* 2003;**18**(1):59–67.

112. Winner P, Hershey AD. Diagnosing migraine in the pediatric population. *Curr Pain Headache Rep* 2006;**10**(5):363–9.

113. Pakalnis A. Pediatric migraine: new diagnostic strategies and treatment options. *Expert Rev Neurother* 2006;**6**(3):291–6.

114. Evans RW. Case studies of uncommon headaches. *Neurol Clin* 2006;**24**(2):347–62.

115. Zwijnenburg PJ, Wennink JM, Laman DM, Linssen WH. Alice in Wonderland syndrome: a clinical presentation of frontal lobe epilepsy. *Neuropediatrics* 2002;**33**(1):53–5.

116. Dooley J, Gordon K, Camfield P. "The rushes." A migraine variant with hallucinations of time. *Clin Pediatr (Phila)* 1990;**29**(9):536–8.

117. Golden GS. The Alice in Wonderland syndrome in juvenile migraine. *Pediatrics* 1979;**63**(4):517–19.

118. Thomsen LL, Eriksen MK, Roemer SF, *et al.* A population-based study of familial hemiplegic migraine suggests revised diagnostic criteria. *Brain* 2002;**125**(Pt 6):1379–91.

119. Hockaday JM. Basilar migraine in childhood. *Dev Med Child Neurol* 1979;**21**(4):455–63.

120. Lebas A, Guyant-Marechal L, Hannequin D, *et al.* Severe attacks of familial hemiplegic migraine, childhood epilepsy and ATP1A2 mutation. *Cephalalgia* 2008;**28**(7):774–7.

121. Bernard G, Shevell MI. Channelopathies: a review. *Pediatr Neurol* 2008;**38**(2):73–85.

122. Parisi P, Villa MP, Pelliccia A, *et al.* Panayiotopoulos syndrome: diagnosis and management. *Neurol Sci* 2007;**28**(2):72–9.

123. Gargus JJ, Tournay A. Novel mutation confirms seizure locus SCN1A is also familial hemiplegic migraine locus FHM3. *Pediatr Neurol* 2007;**37**(6):407–10.

124. Caraballo RH, Cersosimo RO, Fejerman N. Childhood occipital epilepsy of Gastaut: a study of 33 patients. *Epilepsia* 2008;**49**(2):288–97.

125. Durham PL. Inhibition of calcitonin gene-related peptide function: a promising strategy for treating migraine. *Headache* 2008;**48**(8):1269–75.

126. Montagna P. Migraine genetics. *Expert Rev Neurother* 2008;**8**(9):1321–30.

127. Bhatia MS. Pseudoseizures. *Indian Pediatr* 2004;**41**(7):673–9.

128. Chung SS, Gerber P, Kirlin KA. Ictal eye closure is a reliable indicator for psychogenic nonepileptic seizures. *Neurology* 2006;**66**(11):1730–1.

129. Wyllie E, Glazer JP, Benbadis S, Kotagal P, Wolgamuth B. Psychiatric features of children and adolescents with pseudoseizures. *Arch Pediatr Adolesc Med* 1999;**153**(3):244–8.

130. Kapoor WN. Syncope. *N Engl J Med* 2000;**343**(25):1856–62.

131. Johnsrude CL. Current approach to pediatric syncope. *Pediatr Cardiol* 2000;**21**(6):522–31.

132. Narchi H. The child who passes out. *Pediatr Rev* 2000;**21**(11):384–8.

133. Braden DS, Gaymes CH. The diagnosis and management of syncope in children and adolescents. *Pediatr Ann* 1997;**26**(7):422–6.

134. Gutgesell HP, Barst RJ, Humes RA, Franklin WH, Shaddy RE. Common cardiovascular problems in the young: Part I. Murmurs, chest pain, syncope and irregular rhythms. *Am Fam Physician* 1997;**56**(7):1825–30.

135. Tavintharan S, Mukherjee JJ. A rare cause of syncope in a patient with diabetes mellitus – a case report. *Ann Acad Med Singapore* 2001;**30**(4):436–9.

136. Macleod S, Ferrie C, Zuberi SM. Symptoms of narcolepsy in children misinterpreted as epilepsy. *Epileptic Disord* 2005;**7**(1):13–17.

Section 1 Chapter 10

Recognition, diagnosis, and impact of nonepileptic seizures

Diagnostic issues in the elderly

Christoph Kellinghaus and Gabriel Möddel

Nonepileptic seizures (NES) are a well known diagnostic problem. The term NES is used for a diverse group of disorders characterized by paroxysmal events or attacks that may be confused with epileptic seizures (ES). Most epileptologists prefer the term NES instead of other terms such as "pseudo-seizures" or "hysterical seizures" – terms that are associated with stigma or are inaccurate regarding the underlying pathophysiology [1, 2]. From a neurological point of view, one may distinguish between physiological NES and psychogenic NES (PNES). Physiological NES include events caused by pathophysiologically identifiable disorders such as syncope, stroke, sleep disorders, or movement disorders. Psychogenic nonepileptic seizures include symptoms of psychiatric disorders such as panic disorder, dissociative disorder or conversion disorder [1, 3].

Although the diagnosis of NES may be difficult in all age groups, there are certain age-specific problems that have to be kept in mind when dealing with elderly patients. There are no significant age-specific semiological features of ES that occur independent of the epilepsy localization and etiology [4]. However, it is well established that the epilepsy etiology, and with it, the localization of the epileptogenic zone is different in the older age group [5, 6]. Thus, semiology may be different from what is seen in young or middle-aged patients. Moreover, the incidence and prevalence of disorders that may cause physiological NES are much higher in the elderly. Therefore, the proportion of these types of NES in patients presenting to an epilepsy clinic are considerably higher than in younger adults [7]. Finally, the incidence and prevalence of psychiatric diseases underlying PNES also differ between age groups. All these factors contribute to the specific features and thus specific diagnostic and therapeutic issues regarding NES in the elderly.

Epidemiology

Epidemiological data regarding NES in the elderly are scarce. There are very few reports regarding the population-based incidence and/or prevalence of PNES. A study from Iceland reported the annual incidence of PNES in patients older than 15 years to be 1.4/100 000. However, only 14 patients could be identified in the total population of 1 million persons, and none of them was above 55 years old [8]. Another population-based study performed in a US Midwest county found a mean annual incidence of 3.03/100 000 during a 4-year period. The incidence for the age-group older than 65 years was only 0.63/100 000 [9]. Again, only a very small total number (three) of patients in this age group were identified with PNES. In a community-based prevalence study from Brazil, there were 156 persons out of a sample of 908 interviewed persons who had at least one NES during their lifetime [10]. However, age distribution was not reported.

In contrast to the relatively low numbers from community-based studies, the percentage of NES among elderly patients presenting to clinical settings seems to be considerably higher. The percentage of patients with NES presenting to a neurological outpatient clinic is estimated to be approximately 5% [11]. Valid data regarding the elderly are not available. However, there is more solid information regarding the percentage of elderly people with NES among patients admitted to tertiary epilepsy centers for long-term video-EEG (VEEG) monitoring. Four studies [7, 12–14] found that almost 60% of the elderly patients admitted to long-term VEEG monitoring had NES. Three other studies found slightly lower percentages (40% to 50%) among their patients [15–17]. Studies including all age groups report lower numbers, ranging from 13% to 30% [18–20].

Gates and Rowan's Nonepileptic Seizures, 3rd edn. ed. Steven C. Schachter and W. Curt LaFrance, Jr. Published by Cambridge University Press. © S. Schachter and W. C. LaFrance, Jr. 2010.

Therefore, NES seem to have a high prevalence among elderly patients being monitored in epilepsy centers. This is in contrast to the low incidence and prevalence in population-based studies. One reason could be that paroxysmal events in the elderly are less easily classified using standard diagnostic tools. On the other hand, the low percentage of NES in the elderly in population-based studies could be caused by low awareness for these events in the community.

There is a significant group of elderly patients suffering from both ES and NES. The numbers from epilepsy center-based studies range from 5% to 30% [12–17]. This range is similar to cohorts of younger adults [7], children, and adolescents [21].

Specific problems/approach to the elderly patient

There are many relevant neurological and other diseases that have an incidence and prevalence that significantly increase with age. The incidence of stroke and its major risk factors such as hypertension, diabetes mellitus, and hyperlipidemia is much higher in persons aged 60 years and above compared to younger adults [22]. The same applies to syncope [23], Parkinson's disease [24], restless legs syndrome [25], REM sleep-associated parasomnias [26], and obstructive sleep apnea [27]. In contrast to that, migraine auras that may be mistaken for epileptic auras are much less frequent in elderly patients, and first occurrence of migraine after the age of 40 years is rare [28]. All these disorders may mimic ES, thus the age-specific differences regarding comorbidity have to be considered when paroxysmal events cannot be classified easily in elderly patients.

Neurodegenerative processes like dementia, as well as metabolic disorders that cause severe encephalopathy, are seen almost exclusively in elderly persons. Spontaneous or triggered fluctuations of these conditions are sometimes not easily distinguished from ES or nonconvulsive status epilepticus.

In addition, psychiatric diseases occur with age-specific prevalences as well. In Germany, the one-month prevalence of posttraumatic stress disorder has been found to be significantly higher in persons above the age of 60 years (3.4%) than in younger age groups (1.3% to 1.9%) [29]. Depression and other mood disorders also have a high prevalence in the elderly. In contrast to that, schizophrenia or personality disorder rarely develop *de novo* after the age of 50 years [30]. Therefore, the presentation of elderly patients with PNES may be different.

Diagnostic steps and problems

The first step of the diagnostic process is taking a thorough history of the events in question. A valid history may be difficult to obtain because of memory problems and dementia. A potential problem is the tendency of elderly people to spend more time being alone. Therefore, eyewitnesses of paroxysmal events may be more difficult to find. As in all patients with paroxysmal events, the time course of the seizure symptomatology should be analyzed, placing special emphasis on the beginning. During the interview, particular care should be taken to be nonsuggestive, to use open questions where possible, or at least to give the patient several alternatives when focusing on a specific sign or symptom. In the elderly, the age-related comorbidity has to be kept in mind. Vascular disease and therefore transient ischemic attacks (TIAs), cardiac arrhythmias, and autonomic insufficiency are much more frequent than in younger adults or adolescents. In addition, movement disorders play an important role in this age group. On the other hand, migraine is less frequently seen. Ideally, the interviewer should have expertise not only with epilepsy and seizure symptoms, but also with the range of signs and symptoms seen with the major disorders of elderly patients.

Clinical examination of elderly patients with paroxysmal events should include a thorough neurological as well as cardiovascular examination. Clinical abnormalities can be important clues to the diagnosis. For example, hypertonia may point to Parkinson's disease and thus to neurocardiogenic syncope due to autonomic insufficiency. Irregular pulse suggests cardiac arrhythmia and thus cardiovascular events. However, mild neurological deficits, such as decreased vibration sense in the feet as well as strength or reflex asymmetries, are common findings, as are cardiovascular abnormalities, in many elderly patients with ES as well. Therefore, it is not always easy to assess whether these abnormalities are related to the events in question. In the elderly, it is even more important to collect all diagnostic information and evaluate it regarding potential discordant clues.

Electroencephalography is still the standard routine diagnostic procedure in patients with paroxysmal attacks of unknown origin. However, there are several EEG changes and normal variants that are more frequently found in elderly patients that may be mistakenly reported as abnormal or even epileptiform. Whereas the background frequency does not change significantly with age alone [31], bilateral or even unilateral slowing is frequently seen in healthy elderly persons [32, 31] and may be mistaken as indicative of a structural lesion suggesting a vulnerability to epilepsy. Small sharp spikes or wicket spikes may occur in all adult age groups, whereas subclinical rhythmic electrographic discharges of adulthood (SREDA) seem to be much more frequent in elderly patients [32, 33].

In elderly patients in whom the diagnosis of epilepsy was eventually made, the routine EEG showed interictal epileptiform abnormalities in only 20% to 35% [5, 34], with a slightly better yield in those patients with higher seizure frequency. The diagnostic yield of EEG in epilepsy patients of all age groups is commonly found to be 30% to 55% [35–37], and even higher (60%) in young people with epilepsy [38]. Thus, a negative EEG may be even less significant in the elderly in the diagnosis of epilepsy.

By contrast, the specificity of epileptiform discharges on the EEG is relatively high. In community-based studies, epileptiform discharges are found in less than 5% of the probands, with most studies reporting only 0.2% to 0.5% [39]. However, epileptiform discharges can be found in a variety of conditions not associated with epilepsy, such as metabolic encephalopathy [40], hypoglycemia [41], and severe renal insufficiency [42], as well as in association with psychotropic drugs such as lithium [43], antidepressants, or neuroleptics [44]. These conditions are found more frequently in the elderly, thus presenting important potential pitfalls for a correct interpretation of epileptiform EEG findings. According to studies focussing on younger adults, epileptiform discharges during routine EEG may be seen in up to 10% to 15% of patients with PNES and no evidence for epilepsy or other neurological diseases [45–47]. In contrast to that, only 1 of 17 elderly patients with NES and without evidence for additional ES had epileptic discharges – this being a single sharp wave during routine EEG in a patient with no epileptiform discharges during long-term VEEG monitoring [7].

The gold standard for diagnosis of NES is long-term VEEG monitoring. A number of studies have shown the feasibility and practicability of this method also in elderly patients [7, 12–17, 48]. If a typical event can be recorded, which usually happens within 2 days after admission [49], a definite diagnosis can be made in almost all of the cases. However, in 20% to 30% of the patients no event occurs during VEEG (see Table 10.1, [49]). In addition, in patients suspected to have both epilepsy and NES (see Table 10.1), recording a single event may not be sufficient.

Although there are some reports emphasizing an age-specific semiology of ES in elderly patients, such as longer loss of responsiveness, longer postictal phase, and less distinct seizure semiology [50, 51] potentially obstructing correct diagnosis, there are no solid data to support that notion. Differences between age groups – if any – are mainly caused by different predominant location of the epileptogenic zone due to different predominant etiologies. Kellinghaus *et al.* failed to find significant differences in seizure semiology between elderly and younger adults matched for location of the epileptogenic zone [4].

Imaging studies should aim to identify both a potentially epileptogenic lesion and morphological signs of potential causes for physiological NES – such as remote stroke, intracranial hemorrhage, microangiopathy, or significant atrophy. In general, just like in younger patients, MRI constitutes the gold standard for lesion demarcation. It has to be considered, however, that there may be a higher percentage of patients with MRI contraindications in the elderly population, e.g., due to cardiac pacemakers, artificial cardiac valves of the first generation, artificial joints, or other metal implants. Furthermore, MRI is highly susceptible to movement artifact, which may be of relevance in elderly patients with dementia and/or other severe comorbidity in whom sedation for the procedure is problematic. In these cases, as well as in emergency diagnostics, CT scans have their place. Magnetic resonance or CT angiography may reveal extra- or intracranial arterial stenoses as a potential underlying cause of recurrent transient ischemic attacks. Functional imaging methods such as PET or SPECT are of minor importance, but may complement morphological studies, e.g. in the differential diagnosis of movement disorders.

Cardiovascular diagnostic methods are particularly important in elderly patients with paroxysmal loss of consciousness. Long-term EKG can document cardiac arrhythmias, and echocardiography may detect myocardial insufficiency. The tilt-table test ideally is performed with video and EEG documentation and helps to distinguish convulsive syncope from brief tonic ES.

Table 10.1 Video-EEG monitoring in elderly patients

	Number of patients total (m/f)	Mean age (range)	Number (%) of patients with NES	Number (%) of patients with both epilepsy and NES	Number (%) of patients with psychogenic NES	Etiology of psychogenic NES	Predominant seizure symptoms	Number (%) of patients with physiological NES	Etiology of physiological NES	Psychiatric comorbidity	Non-psychiatric comorbidity in psychogenic NES
Abubakr 2005 [12]	58 (m:32/f: 26)	NA (60–91)	26 (45%)	2 (3%)	6 (10%)	No data	Motor symptoms 5, abdominal spasm 1	20 (34%)	Confusion/altered mental status (14), agitation (2), TIA (2), syncope (3), tremor (3), drop attack (2)	No data	No data
Kawai et al. 2007 [48]	71 (m:67/f:4) Only 34 with events evaluated	68 (60–?)	22 (65%)	No data	12 (35%)	No data	Simple/complex movements 7, sensory symptoms 1, altered consciousness 6	10 (29%)	No data	No data	No data
Kipervasser et al. 2007 [14]	16 (m:9/f:7)	68 (60–82)	10 (63%)	1 (6%)	7 (44%)	Depression, anxiety disorder, PTSD, conversion disorder (no numbers)	Unresponsiveness 3, speech arrest 1, motor symptoms 3	3 (19%)	No data	No data	Mild cognitive decline 1, tremor/rigor 1
Kellinghaus et al 2004 [7]	39 (m:21/f:18)	66 (60–86)	23 (59%)	5 (12%)	13 (33%)	Anxiety disorder 3, somatoform disorder 8, mood disorder 1, reinforced behavior pattern 1	Simple motor 5, complex motor 3, unresponsiveness 4, sensory 1	10 (26%)	Stroke 3, syncope 3, movement disorder 2, sleep disorder 2	Mood disorder 6, anxiety disorder 5, conversion disorder 9	Movement disorder, vascular disease
Lancman et al. 1996 [16]	20 (m:9/f:11)	68 (61–92)	5 (25%)	None	2 (10%)	No data	Convulsion 1, vomiting 1	3 (15%)	Syncope 1, obstructive sleep apnea 2	No data	No data
Keränen et al 2002 [15]	36 (m:16/f:20) Only 16 with events evaluated	NA (60–83)	9 (56%)	1 (6%)	3 (19%)	No data	No data	6 (38%)	TIA 1, syncope 1, sleep apnea 1, encephalopathy 3	No data	No data
McBride et al. 2002 [17]	99 (m:37/f:62) only 64 with events evaluated	70 (60–94)	27 (42%)	4 (6%)	13 (20%)	No data	No data	14 (22%)	Cataplexy 1, syncope 1, nocturnal confusion 1, episodic vomiting 1, encephalopathy 2, TIA 2, unknown 6	No data	No data
Drury et al. 1999 [13]	18	69.5 (60–90)	10 (56%)	2 (11%)	No data	No data	No data	No data	No data	No data	No data

Psychogenic NES of the elderly

Psychogenic nonepileptic seizures include a variety of conditions that fall into the diagnostic categories of the Diagnostic and Statistical Manual of Mental Disorders, Fourth Edition (DSM-IV) and International Classification of Diseases, Tenth Edition (ICD-10) Chapter F, respectively. Onset of PNES in the majority of affected elderly patients is at an age of 60 years or above [17, 52], i.e., within 2 years before presentation to VEEG [17].

The ictal presentation of PNES in the elderly seems not to differ significantly from younger adults. Between 50% and 70% of all adult patients present with predominant motor symptoms, and between 20% and 40% with predominant loss of responsiveness or falls [53]. Similar rates are found in the elderly [7, 12, 14, 48] (see Table 10.1). Kellinghaus et al. compared the features of 27 seizures recorded in 13 elderly patients with PNES with those of 56 seizures in 19 younger adult patients [7]. They found no difference regarding the presence of simple motor or complex motor symptoms or loss or decrease of responsiveness. However, younger patients tended to report subjective seizure symptoms more frequently than the elderly.

Cluster analysis of PNES in younger adults has shown that there are three different semiological clusters [54]: the first cluster ("psychogenic motor seizure") consists of clonic or motor movements, pelvic thrusting, and/or head movements. The second cluster ("psychogenic trembling seizure") presents with predominant trembling of the extremities, and the third cluster ("psychogenic atonic seizure") is characterized by falling and loss of consciousness. Although reproducing this finding in elderly patients has not yet been attempted, available data [7, 12, 14] suggest that this differentiation of symptom clusters may also apply to the elderly.

There are very few data regarding etiology and association with psychiatric disorders in elderly patients with PNES. If there is a relationship between the seizure symptoms and stressful events, problems or needs of the patients, PNES can be diagnosed as a subgroup of conversion disorders in ICD-10. Therefore, this diagnosis is most common also among elderly patients [7, 52]. Mood disorders and anxiety disorders can be diagnosed in a relevant number of elderly patients as well. When compared to a control group of younger adults with PNES, there was no difference between elderly and younger persons regarding etiology and psychiatric comorbidity [7, 52].

Physiological NES of the elderly

Nonepileptic, nonpsychogenic paroxysmal events may be due to neurological or systemic medical conditions such as ischemic events, syncope, movement disorders, sleep disorders, or encephalopathy of various etiologies.

Ischemic events

Transient ischemic attacks may be associated with negative neurological symptoms such as hemiparesis, aphasia, or hemianopia, or with positive symptoms such as paresthesias. Both can be mistaken for ES, especially if stereotypic symptoms occur transiently and repetitively, as may be the case in patients with stenosis of the internal carotid artery or the middle cerebral artery. The distinction between ES and recurrent TIAs is especially critical in patients after a first stroke, as both a potentially epileptogenic lesion and increased risk of recurrent stroke are combined in the same individual [55–57].

Syncope

Elderly patients are highly susceptible to syncope due to age-related increase in cardiovascular morbidity, neurodegenerative disease associated with autonomic dysfunction, and other chronic illnesses. In patients older than 70 years, a lifetime incidence for syncope of close to 30% is reported [58]. Etiological factors include cardiac arrhythmias (such as atrioventricular block, asystole, ventricular or supraventricular tachycardia), congestive heart failure, aortic valve stenosis, and conditions associated with impairment of the sympathetic nervous system (such as diabetes, amyloid neuropathy, Parkinson's disease, multiple system atrophy, or Shy-Drager syndrome). In addition, medication effects should be considered, as elderly patients are frequently treated with multiple drugs affecting cardiac or vascular functions, such as antihypertensive or antiarrhythmic agents.

Diagnostic challenges in elderly patients arise from multimorbidity (i.e., presence of more than one attributable diagnosis), polypharmacy with multiple drug–drug interactions, and frequent lack of detailed semiological description, as many elderly patients live alone.

Hypoglycemia

Hypoglycemia may be caused by fasting, endogenous hyperinsulinism, or postprandial exuberant insulin secretion (e.g., caused by rapid food passage from the stomach to the small intestine in patients following stomach surgery). However, most cases of hypoglycemia are the result of insulin or oral antidiabetic drug overdose, or interaction of the antidiabetic therapy with other substances, such as alcohol. With a prevalence of over 20% in subjects over 65 years [59], diabetes mellitus is among the most common of all diseases in the elderly population in Europe and North America. Hypoglycemia is usually preceded by typical prodromal symptoms such as palpitation, sweating, and hunger. However, these warning symptoms are often diminished in elderly patients with autonomic neuropathy, β-blocker co-medication, or exaggeratedly strict long-term insulin treatment ("hypoglycemia unawareness"), leading to more or less sudden alteration of consciousness. Neuroglycopenic symptoms such as behavioral change, confusion, or coma suggest the differential diagnosis of nonconvulsive status epilepticus. The diagnostic situation is complicated by the fact that hypoglycemia can indeed also cause generalized tonic-clonic ES. In addition, some of the typical prodromal symptoms such as anxiety, paresthesia, or tremor may resemble epileptic auras or focal seizures.

Movement disorders

Hyperkinetic symptoms such as chorea, athetosis, ballism, and dystonia may be confused with tonic, clonic, or myoclonic ES. Chorea in elderly patients may be due to primary CNS diseases such as stroke, intracerebral hemorrhage, or tumor affecting the basal ganglia. However, choreatic symptoms in the elderly may also be associated with systemic conditions such as hyperosmolar hyperglycemia, hyperthyroidism, or polycythemia vera [60–65]. Even more importantly, choreatic hyperkinesias are a common side effect of long-term neuroleptic treatment, acute neuroleptic intoxication, as well as dopaminergic drug overdose, e.g., in patients with Parkinson's disease. Other drugs that have been reported to induce choreoathetosis include the anticonvulsant drugs phenytoin, valproate, gabapentin, and lamotrigine. Medications can cause diagnostic difficulties in elderly patients with epilepsy, as there is a high likelihood of comorbidity and drug interactions.

Sleep disorders

Sleep attacks during daytime can raise the differential diagnosis of ES, especially if they occur suddenly and cannot be controlled by the patient, or if history-taking is impaired, e.g., due to dementia. Disruption of night sleep is a common cause and may be related to sleep apnea, restless legs syndrome, painful dysesthesias in patients with diabetic or other polyneuropathy, or inability of patients with Parkinson's disease to turn around in their bed at night. Whereas obstructive sleep apnea is mostly associated with obesity or neuromuscular disease, central sleep apnea is frequently due to lower brainstem lesions, with medullary infarcts, anoxic encephalopathy, and multiple system atrophy being common etiologies in the elderly. Other reasons for daytime sleepiness in the elderly include hypercapnia (e.g., due to pulmonary disease), hypothyroidism, and medication side effects. Restless legs syndrome and periodic limb movements during sleep are usually easily distinguished from nocturnal motor seizures on the basis of the patient's or bedmate's description. However, diagnostic difficulties can arise in elderly patients with dementia or otherwise impaired ability to deliver a history, or in those living alone.

Rapid eye movement sleep behavior disorder is a parasomnia characterized by paroxysmal violent proximal limb motor activity and vocalization during REM sleep, resembling ES of frontal lobe origin. The attacks can be accompanied by vivid dreams, and involve a considerable risk of self-injury and injury of the bedmate. The disorder mostly affects elderly men, and there is a reported association with neurodegenerative disease such as Parkinson's [66, 67].

Encephalopathy

Encephalopathy is characterized by a more or less severe alteration of consciousness, ranging from somnolence to coma, due to diffuse impairment of brain function. The underlying cause may be primarily neurological, as in diffuse hypoxic brain injury, or systemic, such as metabolic (hepatic or uremic) derangement, electrolyte disturbance, or intoxication. If the onset of symptoms is (sub-)acute or unknown, nonconvulsive status epilepticus has to be ruled out with EEG. The differential diagnosis can be especially difficult if the EEG shows no unequivocal epileptiform pattern, but reveals diffuse rhythmic or periodic slowing, as those can be associated with both long-lasting status and encephalopathy. The situation is complicated by the fact that many conditions leading to encephalopathy, including hyponatremia and diffuse hypoxia, are also associated with ES and/or status epilepticus.

Alzheimer's dementia constitutes an encephalopathy in the broader sense, and is associated with both fluctuating vigilance and increased susceptibility to seizures [68, 69]. As history-taking is especially difficult in these patients, episodic alteration of consciousness should yield careful diagnostic workup including VEEG, if available, in order to distinguish nonconvulsive seizures from nonepileptic events.

Treatment and outcome

Treatment of NES of the elderly has to take into account the problems specific to this age group. First, mobility of elderly patients is frequently diminished, causing transport difficulties in the outpatient setting, as well as nursing problems upon admission for inpatient treatment. For treatment of PNES, decreased cognitive abilities due to neurodegenerative processes may pose problems for psychotherapeutic approaches used in younger persons. In addition, traumatic events may have occurred several decades before therapy onset and thus would be less accessible to psychotherapy. Supporting pharmacotherapy may be limited due to age-specific pharmacokinetic changes.

Therefore, treatment experiences and outcome data from younger adults may not be easily transferred to elderly patients with PNES. There are very limited data regarding treatment outcome in elderly patients with PNES. Kipervasser and coworkers [14] report complete cessation of PNES after diagnosis and tapering of anticonvulsant drugs in three of seven patients, relevant decrease of frequency in two patients, and no change or increase of frequency in two patients. However, they do not give details about duration of follow-up and the kind of treatment started.

For physiological NES, treatment is directed at the underlying etiology. Hence, careful history and diagnostic workup are the keys for successful therapy.

Conclusion

Nonepileptic seizures are frequently observed in elderly patients, but valid data about incidence and prevalence in healthy populations or even in general medicine or neurology settings remain scarce. Because of the age-specific morbidity of the elderly, NES and ES may easily be confused. VEEG monitoring has proven to be a valuable diagnostic tool that seems to be underused in elderly persons with refractory ES or suspected NES. Whereas treatment and outcome of nonpsychogenic NES and their underlying diseases have been studied more intensively, success rates and factors of the treatment of PNES remain to be elucidated. Prospective treatment studies using VEEG monitoring as diagnostic standard for inclusion should be initiated. This seems of particular importance because data derived from younger cohorts most likely are not comparable due to the age-specific problems of elderly patients.

References

1. Gates JR. Non-epileptic seizures: classification, coexistence with epilepsy, diagnosis, therapeutic approaches, and consensus. *Epilepsy Behav* 2002;**3**:28–33.
2. Schachter SC, Brown F, Rowan AJ. Provocative testing for nonepileptic seizures: attitudes and practices in the United States among American Epilepsy Society members. *J Epilepsy* 1996;**9**:249–52.
3. Gates JR, Luciano D, Devinsky O. The classification and treatment of non-epileptic events. In: Devinsky O, Theodore WH, eds. *Epilepsy and Behavior*. New York: Wiley-Liss. 1991; 251–63.
4. Kellinghaus C, Loddenkemper T, Dinner DS, Lachhwani D, Lüders HO. Seizure semiology in the elderly: a video analysis. *Epilepsia* 2004;**45**: 263–7.
5. Ramsay RE, Pryor F. Epilepsy in the elderly. *Neurology* 2000;**55**:S9–14.
6. Thomas RJ. Seizures and epilepsy in the elderly. *Arch Intern Med* 1997;**157**:605–17.
7. Kellinghaus C, Loddenkemper T, Dinner DS, Lachhwani D, Lüders HO. Non-epileptic seizures of the elderly. *J Neurol* 2004;**251**:704–9.
8. Sigurdardottir KR, Olafsson E. Incidence of psychogenic seizures in adults: a population-based study in Iceland. *Epilepsia* 1998;**39**:749–52.
9. Szaflarski JP, Ficker DM, Cahill WT, Privitera MD. Four-year incidence of psychogenic nonepileptic seizures in adults in Hamilton County, OH. *Neurology* 2000;**55**:1561–3.
10. Gomes MM, Kropf LA, Beeck ES, Figueira IL. Inferences from a community study about non-epileptic events. *Arq Neuropsiquiatr* 2002;**60**: 712–16.
11. Scott DF. Recognition and diagnostic aspects of nonepileptic seizures. In: Riley TL, Roy A, eds. *Pseudoseizures*. Baltimore: Williams & Wilkins. 2000; 21–4.

12. Abubakr A, Wambacq I. Seizures in the elderly: Video/EEG monitoring analysis. *Epilepsy Behav* 2005;**7**:447–50.
13. Drury I, Selwa LM, Schuh LA, *et al*. Value of inpatient diagnostic CCTV-EEG monitoring in the elderly. *Epilepsia* 1999;**40**:1100–2.
14. Kipervasser S, Neufeld MY. Video-EEG monitoring of paroxysmal events in the elderly. *Acta Neurol Scand* 2007;**116**:221–5.
15. Keränen T, Rainesalo S, Peltola J. The usefulness of video-EEG monitoring in elderly patients with seizure disorders. *Seizure* 2002;**11**:269–72.
16. Lancman ME, O'Donovan C, Dinner D, Coelho M, Lüders HO. Usefulness of prolonged video-EEG monitoring in the elderly. *J Neurol Sci* 1996;**142**:54–8.
17. McBride AE, Shih TT, Hirsch LJ. Video-EEG monitoring in the elderly: a review of 94 patients. *Epilepsia* 2002;**43**:165–9.
18. Gates JR, Ramani V, Whalen S, Loewenson R. Ictal characteristics of pseudoseizures. *Arch Neurol* 1985;**42**:1183–7.
19. King DW, Gallagher BB, Murvin AJ, *et al*. Pseudoseizures: diagnostic evaluation. *Neurology* 1982;**32**:18–23.
20. Müller T, Merschhemke M, Dehnicke C, Sanders M, Meencke HJ. Improving diagnostic procedure and treatment in patients with non-epileptic seizures (NES). *Seizure* 2002;**11**:85–9.
21. Kotagal P, Costa M, Wyllie E, Wolgamuth B. Paroxysmal nonepileptic events in children and adolescents. *Pediatrics* 2002;**110**:e46.
22. Ebrahim S, Harwood R. *Stroke – Epidemiology, Evidence, and Clinical Practice*, 2nd edn. Oxford: Oxford University Press, 1999.
23. Koeppen S, Pfefferkorn T. Syncope and orthostatic intolerance [in German]. In: Brandt T, Dichgans J, Diener HC, eds. *Therapy and Course of Neurological Disorders* [in German], 5th edn. Stuttgart: Kohlhammer. 2007; 239–58.
24. Bower JH, Maraganore DM, McDonnell SK, Rocca WA. Incidence and distribution of parkinsonism in Olmsted County, Minnesota, 1976–1990. *Neurology* 1999;**52**:1214–20.
25. Phillips BA. Restless legs syndrome: what is it? *Hosp Pract (Minneap)* 2001;**36**:53–6.
26. Schenck CH, Mahowald MW. REM sleep parasomnias. *Neurol Clin* 1996;**14**:697–720.
27. Redline S, Young T. Epidemiology and natural history of obstructive sleep apnea. *Ear Nose Throat J* 1993;**72**:20–6.
28. Stewart W, Wood C, Reed M, Roy J, Lipton R. Cumulative lifetime migraine incidence in women and men. *Cephalalgia* 2008;**28**:1170–80.
29. Maercker A, Forstmeier S, Enzler A, *et al*. Adjustment disorders, posttraumatic stress disorder, and depressive disorders in old age: findings from a community survey. *Compr Psychiatry* 2008;**49**:113–20.
30. Kessler RC, Wang PS. The descriptive epidemiology of commonly occurring mental disorders in the United States. *Annu Rev Public Health* 2008;**29**:115–29.
31. Torres F, Faoro A, Loewenson R, Johnson E. The electroencephalogram of elderly subjects revisited. *Electroencephalogr Clin Neurophysiol* 1983;**56**:391–8.
32. Lee KS, Pedley TA. Electroencephalography and seizures in the elderly. In: Rowan AJ, Ramsay RE, eds. *Seizures and Epilepsy in the Elderly*. Boston: Butterworth-Heinemann. 1997; 139–58.
33. Westmoreland BF, Klass DW. Unusual variants of subclinical rhythmic electrographic discharge of adults (SREDA). *Electroencephalogr Clin Neurophysiol* 1997;**102**:1–4.
34. Drury I, Beydoun A. Interictal epileptiform activity in elderly patients with epilepsy. *Electroencephalogr Clin Neurophysiol* 1998;**106**:369–73.
35. Goodin DS, Aminoff MJ, Laxer KD. Detection of epileptiform activity by different noninvasive EEG methods in complex partial epilepsy. *Ann Neurol* 1990;**27**:330–4.
36. Salinsky M, Kanter R, Dasheiff RM. Effectiveness of multiple EEGs in supporting the diagnosis of epilepsy: an operational curve. *Epilepsia* 1987;**28**:331–4.
37. Zivin L, Marsan CA. Incidence and prognostic significance of "epileptiform" activity in the EEG of non-epileptic subjects. *Brain* 1968;**91**:751–78.
38. Leach JP, Stephen LJ, Salveta C, Brodie MJ. Which electroencephalography (EEG) for epilepsy? The relative usefulness of different EEG protocols in patients with possible epilepsy. *J Neurol Neurosurg Psychiatry* 2006;**77**:1040–2.
39. Sam MC, So EL. Significance of epileptiform discharges in patients without epilepsy in the community. *Epilepsia* 2001;**42**:1273–8.
40. Chokroverty S, Gandhi V. Electroencephalograms in patients with progressive dialytic encephalopathy. *Clin Electroencephalogr* 1982;**13**:122–7.
41. Niedermeyer E. *Epilepsy Guide: Diagnosis and Treatment of Epileptic Seizure Disorders*. Baltimore: Urban & Schwarzenberg, 1983.
42. Noriega-Sanchez A, Martinez-Maldonado M, Haiffe RM. Clinical and electroencephalographic changes in progressive uremic encephalopathy. *Neurology* 1978;**28**:667–9.

43. Helmchen H, Kanowski S. EEG changes under lithium (Li) treatment. *Electroencephalogr Clin Neurophysiol* 1971;**30**:269.
44. Bauer G, Bauer R. EEG, drug effects, and central nervous system poisoning. In: Niedermeyer E, Lopes da Silva F, eds. *Electroencephalography. Basic Principles, Clinical Applications and Related Fields*, 4th edn. Philadelphia: Lippincott Williams & Wilkins. 1999; 671–91.
45. de Timary P, Fouchet P, Sylin M, *et al*. Non-epileptic seizures: delayed diagnosis in patients presenting with electroencephalographic (EEG) or clinical signs of epileptic seizures. *Seizure* 2002;**11**:193–7.
46. Krumholz A, Niedermeyer E. Psychogenic seizures: a clinical study with follow-up data. *Neurology* 1983;**33**:498–502.
47. Reuber M, Fernández G, Bauer J, Singh DD, Elger CE. Interictal EEG abnormalities in patients with psychogenic nonepileptic seizures. *Epilepsia* 2002;**43**:1013–20.
48. Kawai M, Hrachovy RA, Franklin PJ, Foreman PJ. Video-EEG monitoring in a geriatric veteran population. *J Clin Neurophysiol* 2007;**24**:429–32.
49. Lobello K, Morgenlander JC, Radtke RA, Bushnell CD. Video/EEG monitoring in the evaluation of paroxysmal behavioral events: duration, effectiveness, and limitations. *Epilepsy Behav* 2006;**8**:261–6.
50. Godfrey JB. Misleading presentation of epilepsy in elderly people. *Age Ageing* 1989;**18**:17–20.
51. Norris JW, Hachinski VC. Misdiagnosis of stroke. *Lancet* 1982;**1**:328–31.
52. Behrouz R, Heriaud L, Benbadis SR. Late-onset psychogenic nonepileptic seizures. *Epilepsy Behav* 2006;**8**:649–50.
53. Meierkord H, Will B, Fish D, Shorvon S. The clinical features and prognosis of pseudoseizures diagnosed using video-EEG telemetry. *Neurology* 1991;**41**:1643–6.
54. Gröppel G, Kapitany T, Baumgartner C. Cluster analysis of clinical seizure semiology of psychogenic nonepileptic seizures. *Epilepsia* 2000;**41**:610–14.
55. Burn J, Dennis M, Bamford J, *et al*. Epileptic seizures after a first stroke: the Oxfordshire Community Stroke Project. *BMJ* 1997;**315**:1582–7.
56. Fisch BJ, Tatemichi TK, Prohovnik I. Transient ischemic attacks resembling simple partial motor seizures. *Neurology* 1988;**38**:264.
57. Szaflarski JP, Rackley AY, Kleindorfer DO, *et al*. Incidence of seizures in the acute phase of stroke: a population-based study. *Epilepsia* 2008;**49**:974–81.
58. Kenny RA. Syncope in the elderly: diagnosis, evaluation, and treatment. *J Cardiovasc Electrophysiol* 2003;**14**:S74–7.
59. Seidell JC. Obesity, insulin resistance and diabetes–a worldwide epidemic. *Br J Nutr* 2000;**83** Suppl 1:S5–8.
60. Ahronheim JC. Hyperthyroid chorea in an elderly woman associated with sole elevation of T3. *J Am Geriatr Soc* 1988;**36**:242–4.
61. Chang CV, Felicio AC, Godeiro CO, Jr., *et al*. Chorea-ballism as a manifestation of decompensated type 2 diabetes mellitus. *Am J Med Sci* 2007;**333**:175–7.
62. Mas JL, Gueguen B, Bouche P, *et al*. Chorea and polycythaemia. *J Neurol* 1985;**232**:169–71.
63. Midi I, Dib H, Koseoglu M, Afsar N, Gunal DI. Hemichorea associated with polycythaemia vera. *Neurol Sci* 2006;**27**:439–41.
64. Oh SH, Lee KY, Im JH, Lee MS. Chorea associated with non-ketotic hyperglycemia and hyperintensity basal ganglia lesion on T1-weighted brain MRI study: a meta-analysis of 53 cases including four present cases. *J Neurol Sci* 2002;**200**:57–62.
65. Ristic AJ, Svetel M, Dragasevic N, *et al*. Bilateral chorea-ballism associated with hyperthyroidism. *Mov Disord* 2004;**19**:982–3.
66. Gjerstad MD, Boeve B, Wentzel-Larsen T, Aarsland D, Larsen JP. Occurrence and clinical correlates of REM sleep behaviour disorder in patients with Parkinson's disease over time. *J Neurol Neurosurg Psychiatry* 2008;**79**:387–91.
67. Kumru H, Santamaria J, Tolosa E, Iranzo A. Relation between subtype of Parkinson's disease and REM sleep behavior disorder. *Sleep Med* 2007;**8**:779–783.
68. Amatniek JC, Hauser WA, DelCastillo-Castaneda C, *et al*. Incidence and predictors of seizures in patients with Alzheimer's disease. *Epilepsia* 2006;**47**:867–72.
69. Lozsadi DA, Larner AJ. Prevalence and causes of seizures at the time of diagnosis of probable Alzheimer's disease. *Dement Geriatr Cogn Disord* 2006;**22**:121–4.

Section 2: Nonepileptic seizures: culture, cognition, and personality clusters

Section 2 Chapter 11

Nonepileptic seizures: culture, cognition, and personality clusters

Cultural aspects of psychogenic nonepileptic seizures

Alfonso Martínez-Taboas, Roberto Lewis-Fernández, Vedat Sar, and Arun Lata Agarwal

Although there is abundant clinical information on psychogenic nonepileptic seizures (PNES), there are very scant data on their cultural aspects. In fact, a recent exhaustive literature review on PNES [1] does not present any data on this topic. Our electronic and manual search of articles on "culture" and "PNES" corroborated this general absence of data. Recognizing the need to examine the cross-cultural aspects of PNES, a section of the international multidisciplinary NES Treatment Workshop was devoted to the subject, and a discussion of *ataques de nervios* (attack of nerves) was led by Dr. Roberto Lewis-Fernández [2].

In contrast to the lack of literature on cross-cultural aspects of PNES, some investigators have conducted culturally sensitive research on conversion and somatoform disorders that include a high proportion of PNES-like phenomena. Research of this kind in Turkey, India, and among Puerto Rican communities is summarized in this chapter in order to help stimulate more focused work on cultural aspects of PNES. As background, we first present a brief theoretical discussion on the role of culture in psychiatric phenomenology, with an emphasis on PNES.

Theoretical background

Research conducted mostly in the US and Western Europe has shown that PNES are strongly associated with exposure to trauma and other stressful life events [3]. In his recent review on PNES, Reuber [1] concluded that nearly 90% of patients with PNES report past traumatic events. Once physical, sexual, and psychological abuse exposure was aggregated, 75% of PNES patients reported some form of abuse, compared with 42% of patients with epilepsy [4]. In a prospective study, patients with PNES had significantly more stressful life events in the year that preceded their first episode than controls with epilepsy [5]. In addition, patients with PNES consistently reported diverse family conflicts and dysfunctions [6].

Given this apparent relationship between PNES and family and personal adversity, what role do cultural factors play in the prevalence and specific characteristics of these somatic manifestations? It is now clear that the sociocultural environment affects psychopathological phenomena in multiple ways [7]. Cultural factors may be even more salient in dissociative and somatoform manifestations of distress than in other forms of psychopathology [8]. As there is extensive evidence that PNES are comprised of dissociative and somatoform phenomena [9, 10], cultural factors are likely to affect the frequency and form of PNES differently as a function of different cultural settings, and, in turn, the manifestations of PNES may be viewed differently in different cultures. For example, the core symptoms of PNES, such as impairment of consciousness, excessive bodily movements, stiffness, and atonia, may be seen as culturally embodied metaphors that have familial, social, and political meanings and consequences that are specific to particular cultures. Likewise, among patients with somatoform disorders in the US and Western Europe, traumatic and abusive experiences may be the main gateway to PNES because PNES is a permissive idiom of distress in which powerlessness, terror, and distress are expressed in indirect ways, rife with connotation and therefore prone to cultural particularities of meaning.

Research conducted in Turkey, India, Puerto Rico, and among Puerto Rican communities in the US provides examples for various cultural effects on PNES-type manifestations. For example, prevalence rates for PNES in these societies and social groups (3% to 4%) appear to be greater by orders of magnitude than in the US general population (0.002% to 0.03%) [11].

Gates and Rowan's Nonepileptic Seizures, 3rd edn. ed. Steven C. Schachter and W. Curt LaFrance, Jr. Published by Cambridge University Press. © S. Schachter and W. C. LaFrance, Jr. 2010.

This enormous cross-national difference in rates itself points to a culturally shaped phenomenon. Differences in childrearing practices, family and gender roles, rates of traumatic exposure in childhood and adulthood, culturally shaped patterns for interpreting and expressing psychological issues, and degrees of personal and interpersonal tolerance for PNES-like symptoms may contribute to cross-cultural differences in PNES epidemiology and clinical characteristics.

Turkey

Epidemiology

Psychogenic nonepileptic seizures are the most prevalent form of conversion disorder in Turkish clinical populations. Approximately 41% to 71% of psychiatric outpatients [12, 13] and 31.7% to 44.1% of inpatients [14, 15] with conversion disorder have PNES as their leading symptom. Inpatients in India (43.2%) and Oman (71.4%) [16, 17] show a similar prevalence range, suggesting cross-national similarities across Middle Eastern and South Asian settings. Among primary care outpatients in a semi-rural area of central Turkey, the prevalence of conversion symptoms in the preceding month was 27.2% and the lifetime prevalence was 48.2% [18]. A survey of consecutive admissions to a medical emergency center in a northern Turkish city over one year [19] revealed that conversion disorder was the most prevalent cause of admittance, being observed in 62.6% of women and 45.9% of men among admissions due to a psychiatric reason. As a type of PNES, the prevalence of fainting spells was 48.1%. These combined data suggest elevated prevalence rates of PNES in Turkey, as well as other non-Western societies.

An epidemiological study conducted in western Turkey found a lifetime prevalence of 5.6% for Diagnostic and Statistical Manual of Mental Disorders, Fourth Edition (DSM-IV)-defined conversion disorder [20], which was equal across genders. Among these subjects, 65.6% had fainting spells, suggesting a lifetime prevalence of 3.7% for PNES [21]. In another recent epidemiological study on a representative sample of women in central Turkey, the lifetime prevalence of PNES was 3.8% [22].

Clinical phenomenology

Seizures resembling tonic-clonic convulsions are a hallmark of PNES in Turkey. Affected patients demonstrate tremors, shaking, and convulsions; most report hearing conversations during the episode without being able to speak [23]. However, seizures resulting in injury or urinary incontinence are uncommon [23]. The duration of the episode is typically 5 to 10 minutes to several hours, longer than an epileptic seizure. Screaming and aggressive or self-mutilative behavior may accompany the episode, while crying spells may occur during recovery [23].

Psychopathogenesis
Special role in the family

Many Turkish patients with conversion disorder, including PNES, describe a special familial role granted by parents and adopted by the patient, such as being the most favorite child usually combined with "complaisant overadjustment" by the potential patient, which continues throughout adulthood [24]. Complaisant overadjustment is defined as an enduring attitude aimed to please others despite being overburdened by duties (e.g., being in the service of family members, self-sacrifice for others' interests). This attitude usually serves to maintain a given role in the family supposed to be for the subject's own good. Similar observations have been made about "good" children with conversion disorder in Australia [25]. The potential patient tries to please family members by being "perfect" in his or her role. This submissive attitude has been conceptualized as a sequel of early traumatization [26] that leads to a special attachment to the perpetrator. Research with children and adolescents with a conversion symptom suggests the importance of early birth order [27, 28]. In accordance with this subtle dynamic, first-degree relatives of patients with complex dissociative disorders describe a special type of family that may predispose to dissociative and trauma-laden psychopathology [29]. These "apparently normal" families are characterized by affect dysregulation leading to angry outbursts in some members with resulting chronic traumatization of their relatives. Members of this type of family report childhood trauma more frequently than controls, suggesting transgenerational transmission of trauma-related psychopathology [25].

Insecure attachment

Insecure attachment has been reported as a culturally relevant etiological factor for dissociative disorders [30] as well as somatization [31]. Underlining the role of insecure attachment, Sar [23] underscores reports of maternal rejection common among patients in Turkey with PNES. Attachment is a circular construct: particular attachment strategies emerge in the context of information processing about the self in relation to an attachment figure, and behavioral expression of attachment strategies involves, in turn, further interactions with that attachment figure [25].

Childhood trauma and dissociation

As in the US and Western Europe, Turkish patients with PNES report more childhood trauma than patients with epilepsy [32]. Among patients with conversion disorder (most with PNES), 47.4% meet lifetime criteria for a dissociative disorder. In a study of male soldiers with conversion disorder in Turkey, those with PNES had higher mean Dissociative Experiences Scale (DES) scores than those without PNES [33].

Medically unexplained somatic symptoms, including PNES, can differentiate complex dissociative patients from other psychiatric diagnostic groups in Turkey [34]. Interestingly, there is no difference in somatic complaints between Turkish and Dutch patients with dissociative disorder except for the prevalence of PNES, which is higher in Turkey. Compared to patients with conversion without a dissociative disorder, those who also met criteria for a dissociative disorder had more comorbid psychiatric disorders, childhood trauma, suicide attempts, and self-mutilating behaviors. In a similar study among inpatients with conversion disorder in a university clinic in eastern Turkey, all of the subjects with a concurrent dissociative disorder reported sexual abuse or emotional neglect during childhood or adolescence [15].

Disadvantageous effects of exaggerated gender roles

Psychogenic nonepileptic seizures are more prevalent among women than men in both clinical [16, 23] and non-clinical Turkish samples [21]. Although there has been tremendous social change over the past few decades in Turkey, women still are in a disadvantageous position, especially in families with conservative attitudes in which women are restricted in their opportunities for self-expression. Arranged marriages during early adolescence, premature cessation of education, and quasi-religious gender oppression due to limited interpretation of Islamic practices are common in rural areas, or in towns among social strata emerging from a rural or semi-rural background. For these social groups, PNES may be a way of taking some form of control in family crises when a more direct channel is blocked for conflict expression and resolution. The dramatic phenomenology of PNES usually stops the hostility toward the patient and often creates a more supportive attitude among family members.

Difficulty in self-perception and self-expression (alexithymia)

Among Turkish men with alcohol abuse or dependence, dissociation may be related to difficulties identifying feelings, a dimension of alexithymia worsened by trait anxiety [35]. Conversion disorder (including PNES) can be understood as an implicit form of communication conditioned by cultural blocks to more explicit forms of communication. These blocks are usually enforced by the family as the agent of culture by means of shame-based practices.

Precipitating factors

In most Turkish patients (88.9%), psychosocial stress factors are observed during the first or last episodes of the conversion disorder [12]. Dysfunctional intrafamilial and intimate/marital relationships among women and conflicts in work among men have been observed as precipitating factors for PNES in central Turkey [16]. Problems related to migration from rural areas to mostly low-income towns appear to be an additional risk factor in eastern Turkey [12].

Comorbidity and variability in clinical course

Suggesting a high rate of psychiatric comorbidity, conversion symptoms are more frequent in patients with an International Classification of Diseases, Tenth Edition (ICD-10) diagnosis of major depression, generalized anxiety disorder, and neurasthenia [18]. Nearly two-thirds (64.5%) of the patients with PNES do not have seizures at one-year follow-up [36]. Reuber et al. [37] showed that only one in three patients with PNES remained seizure-free in a European sample follow-up. Longitudinal studies examining the recurrence of PNES in Turkish patients have been conducted as well. Overall, they reported that PNES tends to be less persistent among Turkish patients over time. Another study of outpatients with conversion disorder in Turkey (including 89.5% with PNES), found that nearly 90% still met Structural Clinical Interview for the DSM-IV Axis I Disorders (SCID-I) criteria for a psychiatric disorder other than conversion disorder after one year, while conversion disorder disappeared [13]. A 4-year follow-up of children and adolescents revealed that PNES had ceased in 85%; however 35% of the patients still met criteria for a mood or anxiety disorder [38]. These findings suggest that PNES may present transiently over the course of a long-lasting psychopathological syndrome that displays protean manifestations over time. An alternative theory is that patients with various psychiatric disorders may develop PNES superimposed onto their primary psychiatric disorder partly due to the effect of cultural factors, which channel distress into a behavioral "final common pathway."

Puerto Rican communities

Epidemiology

The prevalence of PNES in Puerto Rican communities appears elevated, both on the Island of Puerto Rico and among Puerto Rican emigrants to the US, relative to the US general population. Most of this work, however, has not been conducted on PNES directly, but rather on a culturally patterned syndrome labeled *ataque de nervios*. Community-based studies reveal the lifetime presence of *ataque* in 13.8% of adults and 8.9% of children in Puerto Rico [39, 40]. Outpatient psychiatric samples show lifetime prevalence rates of 52% to 55% among Puerto Rican adults in Boston and Puerto Rico and 25% among children in Puerto Rico [40, 41]. Although *ataque* is phenomenologically heterogeneous, PNES presentations make up approximately 15% of *ataques* in adult psychiatric samples [42]. In adult community-based studies, convulsions, loss of consciousness, and seizure-like episodes characterize about 30% of *ataque* episodes [43]. Taken together, these rates suggest gross lifetime estimates of approximately 3% to 4% for community-based and 4% to 8% for psychiatric clinic-based PNES manifestations among Puerto Rican children and adults.

Risk factors for *ataque* span a range of social and demographic characteristics. People reporting an *ataque de nervios* in Puerto Rico (including the PNES subtype) are more likely to be female, over the age of 45, with less than a high school education, formerly married (i.e., divorced, widowed, or separated), and out of the labor force [39]. However, 10% of the men in the sample reported an *ataque de nervios*, which indicates that some men do express their distress through this culturally related syndrome.

Clinical phenomenology

The phenomenology of many *ataques* resembles that of PNES-like conversion disorder episodes in Turkey. Guarnaccia and colleagues [43] surveyed a representative community sample of Puerto Rico residents (n = 912) for the presence of *ataque de nervios*. Qualitative coding of general descriptions of the syndrome among a subsample of 77 *ataque* sufferers yielded four domains of *ataque* experience. These were: emotional expressions, bodily sensations, action dimensions, and alterations in consciousness.

Although the specific *ataque* phenomenology differs across sufferers, it is nearly always characterized by an intense affective storm (e.g., fear, anger, grief) and a sense of loss of control (emotional expressions). These are accompanied by bodily sensations, which in PNES-like presentations include trembling, difficulty moving limbs, faintness, and dizziness. Action dimensions include striking out at others or at self, falling to the ground, shaking with convulsive movements, or lying "as if dead." Cessation may be abrupt or gradual, with return of ordinary consciousness and reported exhaustion. The attack is frequently followed by partial or total amnesia for the events of the episode, and descriptions of the following for the acute attack: loss of consciousness, depersonalization, mind going blank, and/or general unawareness of surroundings (alterations in consciousness) [43]. However, some *ataques* appear not to involve alterations in consciousness or other PNES-like symptoms. These *ataques* are manifested instead by uncontrolled fits of emotionality (e.g., screaming, crying) but without convulsions or syncopal-like episodes. Likewise, certain dissociative NES do not involve a motor component and may share similarities with these nonconvulsive *ataques*.

Psychopathogenesis

Childhood trauma

Studies in psychiatric samples of the relationship between childhood trauma exposure and presence of *ataques* have yielded conflicting results [44, 45]. In one study [45], childhood traumatic exposure was high across Puerto Rican psychiatric outpatients regardless of *ataque* status, suggesting that, in a clinical sample, factors in addition to childhood trauma account for the syndrome.

Relationship to dissociation

As with PNES presentations in North America, *ataque* is strongly associated with a dissociative experience. Severity of *ataques*, assessed as lifetime number of episodes, is positively and independently related to self-reported dissociative symptoms, measured with the Dissociative Experiences Scale (DES), and to clinician-diagnosed dissociative disorders, assessed with the Structured Clinical Interview for DSM-IV (SCID) [45]. Further evidence of the relationship between *ataque de nervios* and dissociation comes from the significant correlation between *ataque* and other Latino idioms of distress that are also related to higher dissociative capacity on the DES. These idioms are characterized by "pseudo-hallucinations" in several sensory modalities – hearing voices or noises, seeing shadows (*celajes*), and feeling presences when alone – that are popularly attributed to spiritual influences. Endorsement of a scale measuring the frequency of these idioms is strongly correlated to DES scores [8].

Cultural predispositions

Aspects of Caribbean Latino culture may promote the observed association between *ataque de nervios* and dissociation, since the appearance of dissociation during the *ataque* may be enhanced by the cultural perception that a mature social actor needs to be always in control of his/her emotions. Dissociation may be particularly promoted by the popular view that when out of control the person is no longer "him or herself" ("*ése no era yo* [that was not me]"). The uncontrolled behavior is disavowed as not being part of the self [46]. This may facilitate the emergence of dissociative splits that allows the person to distance him/herself from the moral consequences of the *ataque* episode.

Gender roles

Community rates of *ataque* show a 2:1 female-to-male ratio [39]. As in Turkey, this has been attributed in part to traditional gender roles requiring women in Puerto Rican communities to display a more restricted range of emotions in social situations, especially around sexual, aggressive, or assertive needs [47]. The gender-specific cultural directive to remain "in control" may predispose women to express suppressed feelings in situations of interpersonal conflict as acute paroxysms of emotionality and uncontrolled behavior, which can later be disavowed as unwilled or even ego-alien [46]. However, although women are more likely to seek psychiatric help, once a man overcomes the gender barrier and presents for psychiatric care, he shows the same lifetime rates of *ataque* as female patients [41].

Precipitating factors

Prototypically, *ataque de nervios* is linked by sufferers to an acute precipitating event or to the summation of many life episodes of suffering brought to a head by a trigger that overwhelmed the person's coping ability [43]. In a Puerto Rico community sample, the first experience of an *ataque* was closely tied to a precipitating event [39]. In 92% of cases, the *ataque* was directly provoked by a distressing situation, and 73% of the time it began within minutes or hours of the event. A majority of first *ataques* (81%) occurred in the presence of others, as opposed to when the sufferer was alone and usually led to the person receiving help (67%). This suggests that one function of the *ataque* may be to rally the person's social network, including reversing the current interpersonal arrangement in favor of the sufferer [41].

Specific precipitants are varied, but typically consist of acutely stressful experiences resulting in feelings of loss, grief, anger, or fear. Generally, the most frequent triggers identified by the Puerto Rico epidemiological study included arguments with a spouse or other close relatives, drunkenness of a family member, an accident which threatened the life of a person close to the subject, death of a close family member, natural disaster, or another stressful event that produced unexpected sudden fear [39]. Certain precipitants were obviously traumatic and were correlated with globally elevated prevalence rates in exposed subpopulations. For example, this survey showed a higher prevalence of *ataques* among those severely affected by a recent natural disaster (19%) than among non-exposed individuals (14%), and intermediate rates among subjects only moderately affected (16%).

Comorbidity and variability in clinical course

Psychiatric evaluations of *ataque* sufferers have usually revealed the presence of some form of psychopathology. The combined findings of these studies support a strong relationship between *ataques de nervios* and mood and anxiety disorders in children and adults, as well as disruptive disorders in children and dissociative disorders in adults [39, 40, 45]. These studies also suggest that different characteristics of *ataque* profiles are associated with different psychiatric diagnoses [48]. Of particular concern is the strong relationship between *ataque* (including its PNES convulsive/motoric subtype) with suicidal ideation (odds ratio [OR] = 6.22) and attempts (OR = 8.08) [39]. During *ataque* episodes, sufferers may make goal-directed or ill-formed attempts at self-harm, increasing the morbidity (and occasional mortality) of the syndrome. Although *ataques* with PNES convulsive-like phenomenology have not been studied separately from other types of *ataques*, anecdotal evidence suggests that this *ataque* subtype may be more strongly associated with dissociative symptoms than other *ataque* variants.

In a study of patients with *ataques de nervios*, the frequency of *ataque* shows a bimodal distribution, with the largest number of sufferers (28%) reporting only one lifetime episode and 23% describing more than five episodes. Two lifetime *ataques* were experienced by 13%, three by 8%, four by 9%, five by 4%, and 15% were unsure about the total [41].

India

Epidemiology

A meta-analysis of major Indian epidemiological studies computed a national prevalence rate for hysteria, subsumed in ICD-10 under the Dissociative (Conversion) Disorders, to be between 0.25% and 1.7%, with a median of 0.33 and a rural-to-urban ratio of over 2-fold (100:44) [49].

Numerous hospital-based Indian studies published in the last five decades have reported PNES to be the commonest presentation of hysteria, not only in adults [50–54] but also in children and adolescents [55–62]. The reported prevalence of PNES varies from around 25% to 85% of conversion phenomena. This wide variation in diagnosis is due to differences in the clinician's skill, clinic setting, diagnostic practices, and modes of classifying presentations; for example, fainting spells are often listed separately.

There is a substantial preponderance of women amongst Indian patients with PNES and other dissociative/conversion symptoms [50–62], although clinical presentation in males is qualitatively similar to females [50]. The gender difference in prevalence appears after puberty, though one study reported somewhat higher rates in males among prepubertal children with dissociative disorder [61]. Moreover, these problems are not uncommon in Indian children, in contrast to data from Western countries [55–63].

Almost all patients come from lower and middle socioeconomic groups, which could be a reporting bias. Most of the patients are educated, though not graduates [50–62]. All religious groups and faiths are proportionately represented.

An important caveat with Indian data is that only a small minority of patients with PNES seek clinical help while a large majority seek help from faith healers and quasi-religious treatment centers [64–66], which remain superficially studied.

Clinical phenomenology

Psychiatrists have prototypically reported movements resembling tonic-clonic convulsions ranging from an isolated limb to generalized seizures, and even Jacksonian march [50–54, 67, 68]. In contrast, neurologists, pediatricians and epileptologists have reported more diverse forms of PNES presentations [58, 61–63, 69].

Psychogenic nonepileptic seizures are usually accompanied by few other symptoms, but longitudinally such patients often display other types of conversion/dissociative features, such as possession states, dissociative identity alterations, obsessions, and paralysis [50–62, 67, 68, 70].

Psychopathogenesis

Indian studies have uniformly reported a negligible proportion of patients with complex personality issues in their dissociative disorder population. Almost all such patients seek help from a traditional faith healer prior to formal medical treatment or concurrently with it. The popularity of faith healers is thought to be due to their easy approachability, similarity with patients' cultural background, and healers' personality. Surprisingly, such help-seeking behavior is usually not related to patients' educational level, religion, or socioeconomic status [64–66]. Previous psychiatric explanations of PNES in India as due to cognitive inability to recognize or formulate emotional anguish in words (alexithymia) have been superseded by the view that

Chapter 11: Cultural aspects of PNES

Table 11.1 Characteristics of individuals presenting psychogenic nonepileptic seizures

Variable	Turkey	Puerto Rican Communities	India
Gender	More common in women	More common in women; 2:1	More common in women
Community prevalence	4% lifetime	3–4% lifetime	0.33% lifetime
Duration	Longer than epileptic seizures	No data	No data
Phenomenology	Fainting spells; tonic-clonic movements; amnesia may or may not occur; unable to speak but can listen; crying during recovery	Intense emotionality; trembling, difficulty moving limbs, faintness, dizziness, convulsive movements, striking out at others or self, fainting spells, amnesia, depersonalization	Tonic-clonic movements; Jacksonian march; fainting spells
Family or social characteristics	Special role given in the family; patient presents submissive attitudes and behaviors; pressure on patient in extended family	More prevalent in women with disruptive marital relations and from lower sociodemographic backgrounds	More prevalent in young unmarried women, with conflicts with society's prohibitions against college education or conflict with family members, and problems in romantic affairs
Trauma or abuse	Common	Inconsistent findings	Found in a minority of cases
Comorbidity	47% with dissociative disorders: this subgroup has comorbidity with mood, anxiety, somatization, and borderline personality disorder alongside self-mutilative and suicidal behavior	Strongly associated with dissociative experiences; also with mood and anxiety disorders. Accompanied by suicidal ideation or attempt in 25% of first episodes	Associated with possession states, dissociative disorders, depression, and anxiety
Precipitating factors	Very common	Very common; associated with a precipitating distressing event in 92% of cases	Very common

somatic symptoms are a culturally acceptable idiom of distress. This idiom may be used to convey psychological problems when other channels of expression are thwarted, allowing the message to be conveyed without loss of face.

Precipitating factors

In PNES presentations in India, as in other settings, the presence of acute and/or chronic stress is the norm. However, the direct relationship between PNES and traumatic-level stressors is not found. Commonly reported precipitants in children and adolescents are usually related to family or school stresses [55–62]. In young unmarried women, conflicts with society's prohibitions against college education or conflict with family members, and problems in romantic affairs, are common [69]. In young males, frustration arising due to repeated failure in obtaining jobs is the usual stressor [50–54]. Conflicts between a bride and her mother-in-law are a much maligned source of stress for married Indian women, but were not verified in a controlled study [69]. Marital conflict and previous abuse, physical or sexual, have been found to account for PNES in a small minority of patients [50–62, 64, 67–69].

Comorbidity and variability of clinical course

Psychiatric comorbidity is seen in less than one-third of patients and its presence may signal a poor prognosis. Common psychiatric morbidities reported in patients with PNES include depressive, anxiety, and somatization disorders, though these are also reported in schizophrenia and various neuropsychiatric syndromes, including the epilepsies [50–52, 55–57, 59–61].

Patients with dissociative disorder are usually successfully treated in both outpatient and inpatient settings in a relatively short time span [50–62, 67–69, 70]. Many types of psychotherapies are reportedly successful, including behavioral approaches [71], family therapy, and others. Most therapists concentrate on the apparent stressor and not on unconscious conflicts. Psycho-education and counseling of patients and family members form the mainstay of treatment along with use of medications.

Conclusion

As a clinical syndrome, PNES is exquisitely attuned to stressors that are environmentally, socially, and culturally shaped. A wide variety of abusive experiences, distressing familial relationships, gender-specific inequalities, and cultural scripts in the expression and management of distressing emotions are all related to PNES. Cultural factors are thus an important feature of the etiology, manifestation, clinical course, and treatment of the syndrome.

The effects of culture may be seen in the wide variation in epidemiological rates of PNES across societies and in the role of local bodily idioms of distress in linking PNES with particular symptom clusters. Culture also patterns the communicative role PNES plays in family settings in response to a range of interpersonal and communal situations. From a cultural perspective, PNES offers an emotional outlet for the effects of marginalization among disadvantaged social groups, such as women, ethno-racial minorities, and traumatized people.

Future work on PNES should expand on the following five findings from cross-cultural research (see Table 11.1). First, prevalence rates of PNES differ markedly between North Atlantic societies and other cultural settings. Second, cross-culturally, PNES appears deeply embedded in family structures and dynamics. Third, PNES is intrinsically connected to specific meanings and idioms of distress in different cultural milieus. Fourth, PNES has consistently been associated with childhood trauma, disturbed attachments, and dependent relationships, especially among women and other disadvantaged social groups. Fifth, PNES is frequently comorbid with dissociative, somatoform, and affective disorders. How the five findings relate to specific treatments is also an area of potential future research.

As PNES is usually examined from more universalistic biomedical and psychological perspectives, its cultural aspects and meanings are often understudied. This may hinder the development of culturally appropriate evidence-based treatments for this syndrome, since preventive and therapeutic interventions must clearly be attuned to the social construction of the patient's illness narrative [72]. Much more research is needed on the cultural aspects of PNES in order to develop clinical guidelines that are appropriate cross-culturally and that incorporate the multilayered cultural meanings of this syndrome.

References

1. Reuber M. Psychogenic nonepileptic seizures: answers and questions. *Epilepsy Behav* 2008;**12**:622–35.
2. LaFrance Jr WC, Alper K, Babcock D, *et al.* Nonepileptic seizures treatment workshop summary. *Epilepsy Behav* 2006;**8**:451–61.
3. Tojek TM, Lumley M, Barkley G, Mahr G, Thomas A. Stress and other psychosocial characteristics of patients with psychogenic nonepileptic seizures. *Psychosomatics* 2000;**41**:221–6.
4. Cragar DE, Berry DTR, Fakhoury TA, Cibula JE, Schmiditt FA. A review of diagnostic techniques in the differential diagnosis of epileptic and nonepileptic seizures. *Neuropsychol Rev* 2002;**12**:31–64.
5. Binzer M, Stone J, Sharpe M. Recent onset pseudoseizures: clues to aetiology. *Seizure* 2004;**13**:146–55.
6. Krawetz P, Fleisher W, Pillay N, *et al.* Family functioning in subjects with pseudoseizures and epilepsy. *J Nerv Ment Dis* 2001;**189**:38–43.
7. Tseng W-S. Culture and psychopathology: general view. In: Bhugra D, Bhui K, eds. *Textbook of Cultural Psychiatry*. New York: Cambridge University Press. 2007; 95–112.
8. Lewis-Fernández R, Martínez-Taboas A, Sar V, Patel S, Boatin A. The cross-cultural assessment of dissociation. In: Wilson JP, Tang CS, eds. *Cross-Cultural Assessment of Psychological Trauma and PTSD*. New York: Springer. 2007; 279–318.
9. Bowman ES. Why conversion seizures should be classified as a dissociative disorder. *Psychiatr Clin North Am* 2006;**29**:185–212.
10. Brown RJ. Epilepsy, dissociation and nonepileptic seizures. In: Trimble M, Schmitz B, eds. *The Neuropsychiatry of Epilepsy*. New York: Cambridge University Press. 2002; 189–209.
11. Benbadis SR, Hauser WA. An estimate of the prevalence of psychogenic non-epileptic seizures. *Seizure* 2000;**9**:280–1.
12. Kuloglu M, Atmaca M, Tezcan E, Gecici O, Bulut S. Sociodemographic and clinical characteristics of patients with conversion disorder in Eastern Turkey. *Soc Psychiatry Psychiatr Epidemiol* 2003;**38**:88–93.
13. Sar V, Akyuz G, Kundakci T, Kiziltan E, Dogan O. Childhood trauma, dissociation, and psychiatric comorbidity in patients with conversion disorder. *Am J Psychiatry* 2004;**161**:2271–6.

14. Sar I, Sar V. Symptom frequencies of conversion disorder. *J Uludag Univ Fac Med* 1990;**17**:67–74.
15. Tezcan E, Atmaca M, Kuloglu M, et al. Dissociative disorders in Turkish inpatients with conversion disorder. *Compr Psychiatry* 2003;**44**:324–330.
16. Deka K, Chaudhury PK, Bora K, Kalita P. A study of clinical correlates and socio-demographic profile in conversion disorder. *Indian J Psychiatry* 2007;**49**:205–7.
17. Chand SP, Al-Hussaini AA, Martin R, et al. Dissociative disorders in the Sultanate of Oman. *Acta Psychiatr Scand* 2000;**102**:185–7.
18. Sagduyu A, Rezaki M, Kaplan I, Özgen G, Gürsoy-Rezaki B. Prevalence of conversion symptoms in a primary health care center. *Turkish J Psychiatry* 1997;**8**:161–9.
19. Aker S, Böke Ö, Peksen, Y. Evaluation of psychiatric disorders among admittances to (112) emergency services in Samsun – 2004. *Anatolian J Psychiatry* 2006;**7**:211–17.
20. American Psychiatric Association. *Diagnostic and Statistical Manual of Mental Disorders*, 4th edn. (DSM-IV). Washington, DC: American Psychiatric Association, 1994.
21. Deveci A, Taskin O, Dinc G, et al. Prevalence of pseudoneurologic conversion disorder in an urban community in Manisa, Turkey. *Soc Psychiatry Psychiatr Epidemiol*, 2007;**42**:857–64.
22. Sar V, Akyüz G, Doǵan O, Öztü E. The prevalence of conversion symptoms in women from a general Turkish population. *Psychosomatics* 2009;**50**(1):50–8.
23. Sar I. A retrospective investigation of inpatients diagnosed as "hysteria" in Hacettepe University Psychiatric Clinic between 1970–1980. *Dissertation*, Hacettepe University, Ankara, 1983.
24. Öztürk M, Öztürk OM. The intra-family role patterns of children with conversion hysterias. *Med J Soc Psychiatry* 1981;**2**:81–7.
25. Kozlowska K. Intergenerational processes, attachment and unexplained medical symptoms. *ANZJFT*, 2007;**28**:88–99.
26. Sar I, Savasir Y. Orality in hysteria and its importance in Turkey. *Proceedings of the Turkish National Psychiatry Conference*. Bursa: Meteksan Matbaasi, 1984; 30.
27. Öztürk M. The special familial role of children with symptoms of hysteria. *Cocuk Sagligi ve Hastaliklari Dergisi* 1976;**19**:93–107.
28. Sar I, Sar V. Early birth order in hysteria. *Med Bull Sisli Etfal Hosp* 1991;**25**:114–22.
29. Öztürk E, Sar V. "Apparently normal" family: a contemporary agent of transgenerational trauma and dissociation. *J Trauma Prac* 2005;**4**:287–303.
30. Liotti G. Disorganized/disoriented attachment in the etiology of the dissociative disorders. *Dissociation* 1992;**5**:196–204.
31. Waldinger RJ, Schulz MS, Barsky AJ, Ahern DK. Mapping the road from childhood trauma to adult somatization: the role of attachment. *Psychosom Med* 2006;**68**:129–35.
32. Akyuz G, Kugu N, Akyuz A, Dogan O. Dissociation and childhood abuse history in epileptic and pseudoseizure patients. *Epileptic Disord* 2004;**6**:187–92.
33. Evren C, Can S. Clinical correlates of dissociative tendencies in male soldiers with conversion disorder. *Isr J Psychiatry Relat Sci* 2007;**44**:33–9.
34. Sar V, Kundakci T, Kiziltan E, Bakim B, Bozkurt O. Differentiating dissociative disorders from other diagnostic groups through somatoform dissociation in Turkey. *J Trauma Dissociation* 2000;**1**:67–80.
35. Evren C, Sar V, Evren B, et al. Dissociation and alexithymia among men with alcoholism. *Psychiatry Clin Neurosci* 2008;**62**:40–7.
36. Tütüncü R, Türkçapar MH. One year follow up of conversion disorder patients with pseudoepileptic seizures. *Klinik Psikiyatri* 2003;**6**:76–9.
37. Reuber M, Pukrob R, Bauer J, et al. Outcome in psychogenic nonepileptic seizures: 1 to 10-year follow-up in 164 patients. *Ann Neurol* 2003;**53**(3):305–11.
38. Pehlivantürk B, Ünal F. Conversion disorder in children and adolescents: a 4-year follow-up study. *J Psychosom Res* 2002;**52**:187–91.
39. Guarnaccia PJ, Canino G, Rubio-Stipec M, Bravo M. The prevalence of *ataques de nervios* in the Puerto Rico Disaster Study. *J Nerv Ment Dis* 1993;**181**:157–65.
40. Guarnaccia PJ, Martínez I, Ramírez R, Canino G. Are ataques de nervios in Puerto Rican children associated with psychiatric disorder? *J Am Acad Child Adolesc Psychiatry* 2005;**44**:1184–92.
41. Lewis-Fernández R, Guarnaccia PJ, Patel S, Lizardi D, Díaz N. *Ataque de nervios*: anthropological, epidemiological, and clinical dimensions of a cultural syndrome. In: Georgiopoulos AM, Rosenbaum JF, eds. *Perspectives in Cross-Cultural Psychiatry*. Philadelphia: Lippincott Williams & Wilkins. 2005; 63–85.
42. Lewis-Fernández R, Guarnaccia PJ, Martínez IE, et al. Comparative phenomenology of *ataques de nervios*, panic attacks, and panic disorder. *Cult Med Psychiatry* 2002;**26**:199–223.

43. Guarnaccia PJ, Rivera M, Franco F, Neighbors C. The experiences of *ataques de nervios*: towards an anthropology of emotions in Puerto Rico. *Cul Med Psychiatry* 1996;**2**:343–67.

44. Schechter DS, Marshall R, Salmán E, et al. *Ataque de nervios* and history of childhood trauma. *J Trauma Stress* 2000;**13**:529–34.

45. Lewis-Fernández, R, Garrido-Castillo P, Bennasar MC, et al. Dissociation, childhood trauma, and *ataque de nervios* among Puerto Rican psychiatric outpatients. *Am J Psychiatry* 2002;**159**:1603–5.

46. Lewis-Fernández R. "That was not in me ... I couldn't control myself": control, identity, and emotion in Puerto Rican communities. *Revista Ciencias Sociales* 1998;**4**:268–99.

47. Koss-Chioino J. *Women as Healers, Women as Patients: Mental Health Care and Traditional Healing in Puerto Rico*. Boulder, Co: Westview Press, 1992.

48. Salmán E, Liebowitz MR, Guarnaccia PJ, et al. Subtypes of *ataques de nervios*: the influence of coexisting psychiatric diagnoses. *Cult Med Psychiatry* 1998;**22**:231–44.

49. Ganguli HC. Epidemiological findings on prevalence of mental disorders in India. *Indian J Psychiatry* 2000;**42**(1):14–20.

50. Ray SD, Mathur SB. Patterns of hysteria observed at psychiatric clinic Irwin hospital, New Delhi. *Indian J Psychiatry* 1966;**8**(1):32–6.

51. Vyas JN, Bhardwaj PK. A study of hysteria: an analysis. *Indian J Psychiatry* 1977;**19**(4);71–4.

52. Subramanium D, Subramanium K, Devaky MN, Verghese A. A clinical study of 276 patients diagnosed as suffering from hysteria. *Indian J Psychiatry* 1980;**22**:63–8.

53. Jain A, Verma KK, Solanki RK. Is hysteria still prevailing: a retrospective study. *Indian J Psychiatry* 2000;**42** Suppl:14

54. Deka K, Chaudhary PK, Bora K, Kalita P. A study of clinical correlates and socio-demographic profile in conversion disorder. *Indian J Psychiatry* 2007; **49**(3):205–7.

55. Somasundram O, Raghavan GV, Krishnan G. Hysteria in children and adolescents. *Indian J Psychiatry* 1974;**16**(4):274–82.

56. Sharma SN, Bhatt VK, Sengupta J. Neurotic disorders in children: a psychosocial study. *Indian J Psychiatry* 1980;**22**(40):362–5.

57. Trivedi JK, Singh H, Sinha PK. A clinical study of hysteria in children and adolescents. *Indian J Psychiatry* 1982;**24**(1):70–4.

58. Tamer SK. The pediatric non-epileptic seizure. *Indian J Pediatr* 1997;**64**:671–6.

59. Bhatia MS. Pseudoseizures. *Indian Pediatr* 2004; **41**(7):673–9.

60. Prabhuswamy M, Jairam R, Srinath S, Girimaji S, Seshadri SP. A systematic chart review of inpatient population with childhood dissociative disorder. *J Indian Assoc Child Adolesc Ment Health* 2006;**2**(3): 72–7.

61. Ghosh JK, Majumdar P, Pant P, Dutta R, Bhatia BD. Clinical profile and outcome of conversion disorder in children in a tertiary hospital of northern India. *J Trop Pediatr* 2007;**53**(3):213–14.

62. Chinta SS, Malhi P, Singhi P, Prabhakar S. Clinical and psychosocial characteristics of children with nonepileptic seizures. *Ann Indian Acad Neurol* 2008;**11**:159–63.

63. Srikumar G, Bhatia M, Jain S, Maheshwari MC. Usefulness of short term video-EEG monitoring in children with frequent intractable episodes. *Neurol India* 2000;**48**:29–32.

64. Trivedi JK, Sethi BB. A psychiatric study of traditional healers in Lucknow city. *Indian J Psychiatry* 1979;**21**:133–7.

65. Raghuram R, Venkateswaran A, Ramakrishna J, Weiss MG. Traditional community resources for mental health: a report of temple healing from India. *BMJ* 2002;**325**:38–40.

66. Gupta SK, Agarwal AL, Jiloha RC. To study the pathways to psychiatric care in patients attending psychiatry outpatient department of a referral hospital. Delhi University 2008: Thesis submitted

67. Agrawal S, Lata A, Mago R, Trivedi JK. A case of pseudoepileptic seizures with Jacksonian march. *Indian J Psychiatry* 1993;**33**(4):318–20.

68. Jhingan HP, Aggarwal N, Saxena S, Gupta DK. Multiple personality disorder following conversion and dissociative disorder NOS: a case report. *Indian J Psychiatry* 2000;**42**(1):98–100.

69. Dhanraj M, Rangaraj R, Arulmozhi T, Vengatesan A. Nonepileptic attack among married women. *Neurol India* 2005;**53**(2):174–7.

70. Agarwal AL. Compulsive symptoms in dissociative (conversion) disorder. *Indian J Psychiatry* 2006; **48**:198–200.

71. Bhattacharya DD, Singh R. Behaviour therapy of hysterical fits: *Am J Psychiatry* 1971;**128**(5):602–6.

72. Miranda J, Bernal G, Lau A, et al. State of the science on psychosocial interventions for ethnic minorities. *Annu Rev Clin Psychol* 2005;**1**:113–42.

Section 2 Chapter 12

Nonepileptic seizures: culture, cognition, and personality clusters

Psychogenic nonepileptic seizures: why women?

Bettina Schmitz

Gender differences are relevant for many medical disorders. Neurological disorders which are more common in women than men include migraine, multiple sclerosis, pseudotumor cerebri, Alzheimer's disease, and temporal arteritis. With respect to psychiatric disorders, the spectrum of affective disorders is more common in women, while schizophrenia, drug abuse, and aggressive behavior disorders are more common in men [1].

Epilepsy in general is slightly more prevalent in men, which is largely explained by the higher rate of brain injuries in males [2]. There are also gender differences in genetically determined epileptic syndromes. For example, a female preponderance is described in juvenile myoclonic epilepsy and photosensitivity [3, 4].

There is no disorder – neither in neurology, psychiatry nor general medicine – with a female preponderance as striking as in somatoform/dissociative disorders, including psychogenic nonepileptic seizures (PNES). Epidemiological data suggest a ratio of at least 3:1 favoring women. It is remarkable that despite this striking link between female sex and PNES, research in this field has so far done very little to explore this relationship in more detail. About a century ago, Sigmund Freud was among the first in modern medicine to suggest a link between hysteria and (female) sexuality. According to Freud's psychodynamic concept, hysteria is a consequence of suppressed sexuality in women, with unfulfilled sexual desires or subconscious, unresolved Oedipal conflicts which are reactivated during adult relationships. Sociological explanations refer to female discrimination in most societies: frustration and suppressed aggression leads to a dissociative reaction towards helplessness and anger.

It has also been noted that one reason for the female preponderance of PNES is that hysterical behavior in general is socially better accepted in women than in men. Men tend to respond to stress with other behaviors, such as aggression and drug abuse. When men develop somatoform symptomatologies, these are often medical complaints that are socially better accepted, such as atypical chest pain or back pain [5].

Effects of sex hormones on mood have been increasingly studied recently. The different central effects of estrogens and progesterone are relevant for perimenstrual-, pregnancy- and menopause-related affective disorders [6]. Interestingly, little is known about the relationship between menarche, menstruation cycle, and menopause and the incidence of PNES. A personal impression of the author is that it is not rare that *de-novo* PNES manifest during pregnancy, but there are no reliable data on these issues in the literature.

Unfortunately, many studies looking at risk factors for PNES control for gender as if this was simply a confounding factor. Although there is little doubt that there are both biological and psychological reasons for an increased liability for PNES in women, the exact nature of this relationship is poorly understood. Future research should aim to disentangle the gender-related biological determinants and psychodynamic mechanisms of PNES.

History

The belief that the occurrence of PNES is largely restricted to women goes back to the ancient Greeks (see Chapter 2). Hippocrates' concept of hysteria related to a dysfunctional uterus. He observed that particularly widows and virgins were affected and explained this by neurotoxic effects of a frustrated uterus. ("The sexually frustrated uterus wanders through the body in search of semen, and finally settles in the brain, and eats the white matter as a substitute

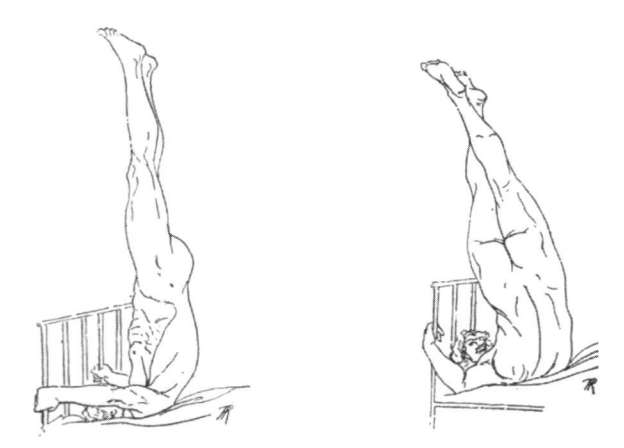

Figure 12.1. Even at the Salpetrière there was the exceptional male patient presenting with "hystero-epilepsy". From Charcot and Richer [24].

for semen. This results in fever, sweating, crisis and screaming" [5].

In medieval times Paracelsus (1493–1541) offered a first, yet simple, psychological explanation for hysterical seizures in women: "Women behave like this, because they want to either tease or shock their husbands" [5].

The atmosphere at the Salpetrière in Paris where Jean Marie Charcot invested much of his scientific enthusiasm into studies on hysteria at the turn of the nineteenth century (Figure 12.1) was well captured in a novel on Marie Curie and Blanche Wittman, one of Charcot's "star" patients [7].

> If you crossed the square ... you would come to the quarters of those suffering from nervous diseases, epilepsy and hysteria. That was where the famous Professor Charcot ruled over these lewd and menacing women. The most extraordinary among them, those whose experiments attracted the greatest interest, were the women who were called hysterics and who urgently worked to become "stars among the rats".
>
> It was said that during Prof. Charcot's performances and treatments the patients would seize every opportunity to attract attention through extravagant contortions, arcs-de-ciel, various acrobatic exercises, and guttural shrieks of despair, joy or relief.

Charcot's semiological obsession with the manifestations of hysteria and his conclusions about the relationship between female reproductive organs and hysteria, including the description of hysterogenic zones and ictal changes in vaginal secretion, were later criticized by Sigmund Freud. Freud studied at the Salpetrière between 1885 and 1886 (originally for a thesis on infantile cerebral palsy). According to Freud, seizure symptomatology was closely related to the nature of the underlying suppressed conflict: "...If you perform psychoanalysis in a hysteric you are easily convinced that these fits are nothing but pantomimically interpreted phantasies, translated into the motor system, projected into motility" [8].

It is certainly relevant for the specific patient–doctor relationship in hysteria that doctors until the beginning of the twentieth century were exclusively male. As an indication of a gradual change in society during Freud's days allowing more and more women to qualify in medicine, his early lectures were opened with "Meine Herren" ("Gentlemen"), and only in his later lectures did he also refer to women in the audience. Freud described and analyzed hysteria initially in female patients, but not exclusively. It is reported that when Freud commented in one of his public lectures that hysteria can also occur in men, this was considered as a provocation and caused a scandal in Viennese society [9]. Freud proposed a different psychodynamic background in males with hysterical seizures. He observed more aggressive and autoaggressive behaviors in his male patients with hysterical fits, which appeared to him as a re-enactment of childhood fights between boys [8].

Epidemiological data and the role of age

In most case series of PNES, women are affected 3 to 4 times more often than men. Most studies agree that the majority of patients are young adults with approximately 50% of reported patients being between 15 and 25 years old. In patients presenting in a tertiary center for difficult-to-treat or -diagnose PNES, the incidence peak can be attributed to the years around puberty (Figure 12.2), suggesting that hormonal and/or biographical changes associated with puberty may play an important etiological role [10].

It is likely that PNES in younger and older age groups are underdiagnosed. Benign events in young children that are clearly identified as psychogenic by parents and pediatricians (e.g., breath-holding spells) are usually not considered in epidemiological studies. It is interesting to note that a gender difference in pediatric studies is described only by those authors who included children after puberty. For example, Wyllie et al. [11] studied children up to the age of 18 years and confirmed a female preponderance.

Table 12.1 Gender preference in subtypes of PNES

Female preponderance	Equal sex distribution	Male preponderance
• Adult patients with PNES in the context of somatoform/dissociative disorders, depression, and anxiety disorders • Munchausen by proxy	• Children before puberty • Elderly patients • Patients with epilepsy plus PNES	• Malingering • Munchausen syndrome

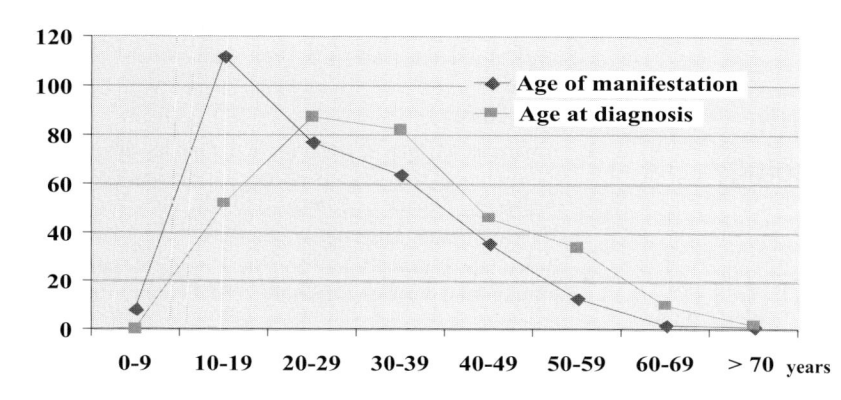

Figure 12.2. Age distribution with respect to the manifestation and diagnosis of PNES in a tertiary center. From Reuber et al. [10].

There was no gender difference among children with clinically relevant PNES before the age of 12 years in a study by Bhatia and Sapra [12]. In this study, school phobia and the fear of examinations were the most common precipitating factors for PNES.

Older patients with PNES are often not included in case series from epilepsy centers, because they are rarely referred for video-EEG monitoring. Interestingly, in elderly patients there is no gender difference, which suggests a different etiology. Psychogenic nonepileptic seizures in the elderly are often related to recent health-related traumatic experiences [13].

Subtypes of PNES and gender

While there is a female preponderance in young adults with PNES, a gender difference favoring women has not been confirmed in all semiological variants of PNES. In addition to very young and very old patients, there is also no female preponderance in patients with epilepsy plus PNES [14] possibly suggesting a different etiology in patients with mixed epilepsy/PNES. PNES in patients with epilepsy are often reactive towards psychosocial stress. In many patients the underlying psychology may aid in the etiological understanding, particularly in patients with learning disability. A common trigger is unprepared seizure freedom with the associated "burden of normality" and need for "personal reconceptualization," which may well be more stressful for men than for women.

There are also variants of psychiatric disorders presenting with PNES that are more common in men. Malingering, for example, is much more prevalent in men. While autodestructive behaviors in general (including self-injuring and factitious disorders) are twice as common in women as men, the gender preference is reversed in Munchausen syndrome, which occurs with a ratio of 2:1 in men compared to women [15]. On the other hand, in Munchausen by proxy (which often presents with seizures), mothers are perpetrators in about 75% of cases [16] (Table 12.1).

PNES and sexual trauma

Many studies have suggested a link between the increased occurrence of PNES after sexual abuse during childhood or adulthood. It is interesting to note, however, that several studies failed to find differences in the prevalence of sexual abuse comparing epilepsy and patients with dissociative disorders, highlighting both the frequency of sexual abuse in women in general and also the methodological difficulty in reliably identifying sexual abuse in retrospective studies [17].

Psychogenic nonepileptic seizures are often associated with posttraumatic stress disorder (PTSD) (see Chapter 22), which is more common in women than men. According to an epidemiological study across six European countries, rape is a traumatic event with the highest risk of consequent PTSD. Traumatic events in general are equally common in men and women, and the lower frequency of PTSD in men does not necessarily imply that men tolerate traumatic events better than women. It is more likely that men tend to express their distress more through behavioral than emotional/dissociative disorders [18].

Gender-related differences with respect to seizure symptomatology and prognosis

Remarkably, there are only limited data on clinical differences between men and women in terms of the phenomenology of PNES. As mentioned already, Freud pointed out that PNES in men more often include self-mutilating/autoaggressive behavioral elements which reminded Freud of fights among boys. In a study by van Merode *et al.* [19], of 62 patients with PNES, the phenomenology of events was divided into tonic-clonic type and complex partial type. Males tended to suffer especially from tonic-clonic type seizures (80% of cases), while in women as many tonic-clonic type as complex partial type events were observed. The authors concluded that the clinically more impressive nature of a tonic-clonic type event, which is more easily suspected to be "real," might make this type of seizure a more male form of acting out.

Whether gender is a predictor for outcome is not clear. The results from four studies looking at gender as a potential predictor for prognosis with respect to seizure freedom are inconsistent. In children, one study suggested that female sex is a positive predictor [20]. In adults, there was one positive [21], one negative [22], and one inconclusive study [23].

Conclusions

Although the close relationship between female gender and PNES has been confirmed by numerous epidemiological studies from different parts of the world, the exact nature of this relationship is not well understood. When looking at different subgroups of patients with PNES, it becomes obvious that a female preponderance does not apply to all subtypes and age groups, suggesting that the links are complex and heterogeneous. While there is no doubt that psychodynamic mechanisms including the experience of sexual and physical traumatic events play a major role in the pathogenesis of PNES in women, there are also important biological factors related to female gender. Recently discovered links between female sex hormones and the predisposition for several neuropsychiatric and other medical disorders suggest that there are biologically determined stress-related vulnerabilities in women that deserve further exploration.

References

1. Amatniek JC, Frey LC, Hauser WA. Gender differences in diseases of the nervous system. In: Kaplan PW, ed. *Neurologic Disease in Women*, 2nd edn. New York: Demos Medical Publishing, Inc. 2006; 3–14.
2. Bruns J, Jr, Hauser WA. The epidemiology of traumatic brain injury: a review. *Epilepsia* 2003;**44** Suppl 10:2–10.
3. Lu Y, Waltz S, Stenzel K, Muhle H, Stephani U. Photosensitivity in epileptic syndromes of childhood and adolescence. *Epileptic Disord* 2008;**10**(2):136–43.
4. Janz D. Epilepsy with impulsive petit mal (juvenile myoclonic epilepsy). *Acta Neurol Scand* 1985;**72**(5): 449–59.
5. Israël L. L'hystéerique, le sexe et le médicin. Paris: Masson, 1983.
6. Steiner M, Dunn E, Born L. Hormones and mood: from menarche to menopause and beyond. *J Affect Disord* 2003;**74**(1):67–83.
7. Enquist, PO. *The Book on Blanche and Marie*. London: Harvill Secker, 2006.
8. Freud S, Breuer J. *Studies in Hysteria*. London: Penguin Classics, 2004.
9. Weizsäcker V. v. Gesammelte Schriften 6: Körpergeschehen und Neurose. Suhrkamp Verlag, Frankfurt a. Main. 1986.
10. Reuber M, Fernandez G, Bauer J, Helmstaedter C, Elger CE. Diagnostic delay in psychogenic nonepileptic seizures. *Neurology* 2002;**58**:493–5.
11. Wyllie E, Glazer JP, Benbadis S, Kotagal P, Wolgamuth B. Psychiatric features of children and adolescents with pseudoseizures. *Arch Pediatr Adolesc Med* 1999;**153**: 244–8.
12. Bhatia MS, Sapra S. Pseudoseizures in children: a profile of 50 cases. *Clin Pediatr (Phila)* 2005;**44**(7): 617–21.
13. Duncan R, Oto M, Martin E, Pelosi A. Late onset psychogenic non epileptic attacks. *Neurology* 2006; **66**:1644–7.

14. Devinsky O, Gordon E. Epileptic seizures progressing into nonepileptic conversion seizures. *Neurology* 1998; **51**:1293–6.
15. Kocalevent RD, Fliege H, Rose M, *et al.* Autodestructive syndromes. *Psychother Psychosom* 2005;**74**:202–11.
16. Sheridan MS. The deceit continues: an updated literature review of Munchausen Syndrome by Proxy. *Child Abuse Negl* 2003;**27**:431–51.
17. Sharpe D, Faye C. Non-epileptic seizures and child sexual abuse: a critical review of the literature. *Clin Psychol Rev* 2006;**26**(8):1020–40. Epub 2006 Feb 10.
18. Darves-Bornoz JM, Alonso J, de Girolamo G, *et al.* ESEMeD/MHEDEA 2000 Investigators. Main traumatic events in Europe: PTSD in the European study of the epidemiology of mental disorders survey. *J Trauma Stress* 2008;**21**:455–62.
19. van Merode T, de Krom MC, Knottnerus JA. Gender-related differences in non-epileptic attacks: a study of patients' cases in the literature. *Seizure* 1997; **6**(4):311–6.
20. Gudmundsson O, Prendergast M, Foreman D, Cowley S. Outcome of pseudoseizures in children and adolescents: a 6-year symptom survival analysis. *Dev Med Child Neurol* 2001;**43**(8):547–51.
21. Meierkord H, Will B, Fish D, Shorvon S. The clinical features and prognosis of pseudoseizures diagnosed using video-EEG telemetry. *Neurology* 1991;**41**: 1643–46.
22. Ljungberg L. Hysteria, a clinical, prognostic and genetic study. *Acta Psychiatr Neurol Scand* 1957; 32 Suppl: 112.
23. Reuber M, Elger CE. Psychogenic nonepileptic seizures: review and update. *Epilepsy Behav* 2003; 4:205–16.
24. Charcot JM, Richer P. *Les Demoniaques Dans l'Art 1887*. Reprint by Kessinger Publishing Company USA. 2008; 96.

Section 2 Chapter 13

Nonepileptic seizures: culture, cognition, and personality clusters

Use of neuropsychological and personality testing to identify adults with psychogenic nonepileptic seizures

Carl B. Dodrill

The identification of adults with psychogenic nonepileptic seizures (PNES) in contradistinction to epileptic seizures (ES) is a continuing challenge. The possible roles that neuropsychological and personality testing might have in making this differentiation are explored in this chapter.

Evaluation of neuropsychological functioning

Neuropsychological testing

The evaluation of mental abilities by tests sensitive to the condition of the brain would seem to immediately have potential to differentiate between patients with ES and those with PNES. In our current understanding, ES is, after all, a neuronally related condition, and PNES is primarily behavioral and psychiatric. Thus, patients with ES should as a whole do more poorly on neuropsychological tests than patients with PNES. Some preliminary studies addressing this question were summarized by Hermann [1] in the first edition of this book, while a series of chapters in the second edition [2–5] addressed the same question. By 2002, there were actually 23 such studies in print [6], and perhaps because the results of these studies were sufficiently uniform, few general investigations of this type have appeared since that time.

The results of all papers published to date do not confirm the previously stated hypothesis and can be summarized fairly succinctly: (1) no significant differences beyond those expected by chance were typically found between patients with PNES and patients with ES on tests of mental abilities; (2) when differences were found between the groups, they favored PNES over ES; (3) all differences found were limited in magnitude and they were never clearly able to reliably predict group placement for individual patients; (4) where differences between the groups were found, there was no consistency in cognitive domains; (5) both PNES and ES groups typically performed outside normal limits on tests of mental abilities; and (6) when a normal control group was studied along with ES and PNES groups, both the ES and PNES groups routinely performed more poorly than the controls.

The consistency in findings across all the published studies in the area makes it unnecessary to go through the investigations in a detailed manner. However, the fact that PNES patients generally do not do better than patients with ES has been puzzling, and this question is provocative enough that it requires specific attention.

Possible reasons for a similarity in neuropsychological test results of patients with ES or PNES

A review of the literature reveals that two general hypotheses have been advanced to account for the remarkably similar neuropsychological performances of patients with ES or PNES.

The first hypothesis is that there are actually diminished mental abilities in PNES which reflect a compromised condition of the brain. If this is the case, positive neurological histories should be found frequently in cases with PNES as well as cases with ES, and this in fact has been demonstrated repeatedly [7–10]. The same studies demonstrated equivalency of family histories of epilepsy. Focal findings on the neurological examination tend to be more frequent in ES, but not significantly so [9–10]. None of these findings provide hard evidence for brain impairment in PNES, but the findings do provide hints of compromised brain functions in PNES. Diminished adaptive abilities may be

Gates and Rowan's Nonepileptic Seizures, 3rd edn. ed. Steven C. Schachter and W. Curt LaFrance, Jr. Published by Cambridge University Press. © S. Schachter and W. C. LaFrance, Jr. 2010.

best picked up by neuropsychological tests, and this lessened ability to cope with the stressors of life may in fact predispose people to PNES, especially when these diminished adaptive abilities are found in combination with other critical factors such as female gender and early sexual molestation.

A second explanation for diminished scores on neuropsychological tests by patients with PNES is that the test results are not valid. This could be due to ongoing depression and anxiety, but solid evidence for this is lacking and most investigators seem to have put aside this explanation as an important factor. Instead, in recent times some researchers have suggested that the primary reason for diminished test scores relates to diminished test-taking motivation. This possibility requires specific attention.

The first investigator to seriously raise the possibility of diminished effort or test-taking motivation in PNES was Binder [11–13]. On the Portland Digit Recognition Test (an easy test but one which requires consistent attention to the task), people with PNES performed more poorly than patients with ES, with the suggestion that those with PNES had less consistent motivation to do well. Less convincing but somewhat similar findings were reported for the California Verbal Learning Test [14] and the Test of Memory Malingering [15].

In more recent times, the Word Memory Test (WMT) has been used as a test of effort with patients with ES and PNES. In one study reported on two occasions [9, 16], it was found that 51% of the patients with PNES "failed" the WMT (had scores in a range suggestive of poor effort) while only 8% of the patients with ES performed in the same range. When the patients with PNES who had "failed" the WMT were dropped, the remaining patients with PNES performed much better on the neuropsychological tests than the patients with ES. The authors concluded that the lack of differences between PNES and ES groups on neuropsychological tests in most studies is due to poor effort by patients with PNES.

The conclusions drawn in the prior two paragraphs have been challenged. Cragar et al. [8] studied four tests of motivation or effort (Portland Digit Recognition Test, Digit Memory Test, Letter Memory Test, Test of Memory Malingering), and found that none of these tests could differentiate between patients with ES or PNES. Even when the tests were considered in an additive manner to maximize discrimination between the groups, patients with ES or PNES demonstrated equivalent effort. The study utilizing the WMT was also followed up by an investigation at the same institution where the original work was done [10]. It was noted that the prior study had numerous restrictions on subject selection and that when most of the restrictions were eliminated the differences between the PNES and ES groups on the WMT completely disappeared. Thus, there was no evidence whatever for diminished effort by patients with PNES when a broader and more representative sample was employed.

Comment is required on these conflicting results. First, in every study concluding that patients with PNES have lowered scores due to diminished effort, patients with ES had been eliminated who likely would have scored poorly on measures of effort. Patients who had any evidence for any type of brain injury, previous surgery, diminished intelligence, fixed neurological deficits, etc. were routinely excluded. While this practice is generally common in studies of effort, it is self-fulfilling in nature since it tends to eliminate patients with ES that may not have done well on effort testing with the result that the effort hypothesis is artificially strengthened. In the first WMT study [9], for example, 47% of all patients with ES had been eliminated for a series of reasons, and each reason likely resulted in omitted patients who may not have done well on effort testing [10].

The second comment is that ES and PNES groups are very different than the compensation-seeking and litigating groups upon which effort tests were developed. Therefore, an uncritical transfer of the information on effort testing to these groups may not be warranted. For example, in the two compendiums of literature on effort testing which are now available [17, 18], it is repeatedly *assumed* that tests labeled as tests of "effort" do in fact measure that construct for groups to which they are applied. Further, axiomatic to the entire effort testing movement is the belief that these tests are unrelated to general intelligence and insensitive to impairment in brain functions. However, the WMT is strongly related to intelligence in both patients with ES and PNES as can be illustrated with data from one of the studies using the WMT [10]. These data, presented for the 93 subjects with ES or PNES who completed the Wechsler Adult Intelligence Scale III (WAIS-III), are presented in Table 13.1. Within each IQ range, there was never a difference in frequency of passing and failing the WMT across the ES and PNES groups (Fisher's exact probabilities always greater than 0.14). However, the rate of

Table 13.1 Probability of passing and failing on the WMT in relationship to range of intelligence considering patients with ES and PNES separately and together

WAIS-III FSIQ range	ES (n = 63) WMT Pass	ES (n = 63) WMT Fail	PNES (n = 30) WMT Pass	PNES (n = 30) WMT Fail	All patients WMT Pass	All patients WMT Fail
58–79	10 (56%)	8 (44%)	3 (60%)	2 (40%)	13 (57%)	10 (43%)
80–89	15 (79%)	4 (21%)	3 (43%)	4 (57%)	18 (69%)	8 (31%)
90–100	13 (87%)	2 (13%)	7 (78%)	2 (22%)	20 (83%)	4 (17%)
101–135	11 (100%)	0 (0%)	9 (100%)	0 (0%)	20 (100%)	0 (0%)

Note: Within each IQ range, there was never a difference in frequency of passing and failing the WMT across the ES and PNES groups (Fisher's Exact probabilities always greater than 0.14). However, the rate of failing the WMT decreased systematically as level of intelligence increased (χ^2 12.58, p = 0.006). ES, epileptic seizures; PNES, psychogenic nonepileptic seizures; FSIQ, Full Scale Intelligence Quotient. Dodrill [10]

failing the WMT dramatically decreased as level of intelligence increased (χ^2 12.58, p = 0.006). This is directly contrary to the axioms of effort testing. In fact, the WMT may merely be another test of mental abilities in these groups rather than a test of "effort." If one were to maintain that it is a test of effort, obviously erroneous conclusions could be drawn based upon Table 13.1 such as, "The duller you are the less you will try to do your best," and "All patients with IQs of 101 and higher have good test-taking motivation."

Conclusions for neuropsychological evaluation

In conclusion, it is evident that patients with either ES or PNES perform approximately the same on neuropsychological tests. The performances of both groups often fall in a mildly impaired range, and both groups perform more poorly than normal controls. The reason(s) why patients with PNES perform as poorly as those with ES has not been definitely established, but these patients do have positive neurological histories as frequently as do patients with ES, and they may in fact be neurologically impaired in ways appreciated by neuropsychological tests. It does not seem likely that a simple explanation that patients with PNES are not trying hard enough while taking tests will ultimately be held responsible for the similarity of neuropsychological performances of the two groups. By its nature, PNES is complex and multifaceted, and it is suggested that unraveling this disorder will require explanations equal to its complexity. Regardless of the ultimate answer(s) to the question at hand, the fact remains that neuropsychological tests as currently applied do not differentiate these groups to a clinically useful degree.

Evaluation of personality and emotional adjustment

Minnesota Multiphasic Personality Inventory (MMPI/MMPI-2)

Major reviews of the MMPI and MMPI-2 and their use in PNES were published in 2000 and 2002 [5–6]. These reviews covered 26 investigations with 22 using the MMPI and 4 using the MMPI-2. Every research report but one evaluated patients with PNES in comparison with patients with ES. At least six more papers have been published since the reviews on the ability of the MMPI or MMPI-2 to differentiate between ES and PNES [19–24]. The results on all 32 papers can be summarized as follows.

First, the MMPI and MMPI-2 were routinely found to be useful in differentiating between ES and PNES, and the authors of at least 80% of the papers drew this conclusion. In a small number of reports, the MMPI was not found to be especially helpful, but the reasons for these atypical findings have been examined, and these reasons focus upon unusual characteristics of the samples studied [5]. The Hypochondriasis (Hs) and Hysteria (Hy) scales are the most useful scales in making the discrimination between the groups. The approach of using rules based upon profile configurations (e.g., "conversion V" rules of Wilkus *et al.* [7])

produce results typically in the 70% to 75% range of correct classification for both ES and PNES groups, and factor scores also appear useful.

Second, the results on the MMPI and the MMPI-2 (thus far) are essentially equivalent in their ability to discriminate between the groups. Note is made that there are a series of supplemental scales on the MMPI-2 which were not on the original form of the MMPI. An example of this is the Fake Bad Scale, but other supplemental scales and subscales have been developed as well. As only four studies have utilized the MMPI-2 thus far, and as these studies have not utilized the additional scales in any systematic way, it is too early to determine if these additional scales might be of value in distinguishing between ES and PNES groups.

Third, the highest discrimination rates between the groups have been obtained when MMPI/MMPI-2 variables have been combined with EEG and seizure history data. There are just two papers supporting this, but in both cases it was found that combining the MMPI with video-EEG data and the historical variable of length of time since diagnosis resulted in correct classification rates which were about 10 points higher than when any one set of variables was used alone [23, 24]. This approach deserves definite attention in the future.

Tests other than the MMPI/MMPI-2

While the MMPI/MMPI-2 unquestionably dominated the scene until recently, other inventories and approaches are now being used. A few papers have appeared with regard to health-related quality of life, for example. In the first of these [25], it was determined that patients with PNES saw themselves as having poorer physical health than patients with ES on the Quality of Life in Epilepsy Inventory-89 (QOLIE-89), but differences in all other areas were less evident. In contrast, another study using the same quality-of-life inventory found broadly decreased quality of life in PNES [26]. Finally, in a third paper using the QOLIE-89, only the overall scale was reported with poorer scores for PNES than ES but without the indication of how well this scale or other scales separated the groups [27]. In all three of these studies, while there were statistical differences in mean scores across ES and PNES groups, it was not possible to discover the degree to which various quality-of-life scales could differentiate the groups on a case-by-case basis.

Other inventories have also occasionally been used in the comparison of patients with ES and PNES, but reports on them are often in abstract form only. Possibly most promising is the Personality Assessment Inventory (PAI), although there is only one study using the PAI which is published in two places [28, 29]. These investigators found that by subtracting the Health Concerns scale score from the Conversion scale score, the resulting index would provide 84% sensitivity and 73% specificity for the diagnosis of PNES versus ES. This result needs to be cross-validated with new samples of patients before being accepted at face value. The one study using the PAI which is available in abstract form only at this time is of merit since it used larger groups of patients (58 ES, 41 PNES) than all other studies and since it also provided a comparison with the MMPI-2 [29]. Using standard PAI scales, it found results slightly better than with the MMPI-2.

In summary, for tests other than the MMPI/MMPI-2, there is simply insufficient information to show how well these inventories can differentiate patients with ES from those with PNES. The available information suggests that they are roughly comparable to the MMPI/MMPI-2, but it is possible that they are easier to administer than the MMPI/MMPI-2, and they may have other advantages. Hopefully, more research on these other tests will be forthcoming.

Conclusions and recommendations for personality and emotional adjustment

Inventories such as the MMPI, MMPI-2, and possibly others continue to be useful clinically, and used in combination with EEG and seizure history variables, they may make a greater contribution than has been the case thus far. Another way of maximizing their potential is to take advantage of subgroupings of patients with PNES. For example, a division by gender might improve prediction of group placement since there is now evidence that men with PNES have much poorer adjustment than women with PNES [19].

It is further evident that division of patients by their behavior (both motor and affective) during their events is also directly related to their emotional status [30, 31]. Also, it has been shown that likely relief from PNES is directly related to behavior during the events [32], and it is not a big jump to suggest that the inventories discussed here might be of considerable assistance in identifying likely effective therapies for subgroups of cases with PNES. All of these areas have had limited attention to date, but they are truly promising areas for future research.

References

1. Hermann BP. Neuropsychological assessment in the diagnosis of non-epileptic seizures. In: Rowan AJ, Gates JR, eds. *Non-Epileptic Seizures*. Boston, MA: Butterworth-Heinemann. 1993; 221–32.
2. Walker JA. Use of neuropsychological testing to differentiate neurologic from non-neurologic disorders. In: Gates JR, Rowan AJ, eds. *Non-Epileptic Seizures*, 2nd ed. Boston, MA: Butterworth-Heinemann. 2000; 113–22.
3. Swanson SJ, Springer JA, Benbadis SR, Morris III GL. Cognitive and psychological functioning in patients with non-epileptic seizures. In: Gates JR, Rowan AJ, eds. *Non-Epileptic Seizures*, 2nd edn. Boston, MA: Butterworth-Heinemann. 2000; 123–37.
4. Risse GL, Mason SL, Mercer DK. Neuropsychological performance and cognitive complaints in epileptic and non-epileptic seizure patients. In: Gates JR, Rowan AJ, eds. *Non-Epileptic Seizures*, 2nd edn. Boston, MA: Butterworth-Heinemann. 2000; 139–50.
5. Dodrill CB, Holmes MD. Psychological and neuropsychological evaluation of the patient with non-epileptic seizures. In Gates JR, Rowan AJ, eds. *Non-Epileptic Seizures*, 2nd edn. Boston, MA: Butterworth-Heinemann. 2000; 169–81.
6. Cragar DE, Berry DTR, Fakhoury TA, Cibula JE, Schmitt FA. A review of diagnostic techniques in the differential diagnosis of epileptic and nonepileptic seizures. *Neuropsychol Rev* 2002;12:31–63.
7. Wilkus RJ, Dodrill CB, Thompson PM. Intensive EEG monitoring and psychological studies of patients with pseudoepileptic seizures. *Epilepsia* 1984;25:100–7.
8. Cragar DE, Berry DTR, Fakhoury TA, Cibula JE, Schmitt FA. Performance of patients with epilepsy or psychogenic non-epileptic seizures on four measures of effort. *Clin Neuropsychol* 2006;20:552–66.
9. Drane DL, Williamson DJ, Stroup ES, *et al.* Cognitive impairment is not equal in patients with epileptic and psychogenic nonepileptic seizures. *Epilepsia* 2006;47:1879–86.
10. Dodrill CB. Do patients with psychogenic non-epileptic seizures produce trustworthy findings on neuropsychological tests? *Epilepsia* 2008;49:691–95.
11. Binder LM, Salinsky MC, Smith SP. Psychological correlates of nonepileptic seizures. *J Clin Exp Neuropsychol* 1994;16:524–30.
12. Binder LM, Kindermann SS, Heaton RK, Salinsky MC. Neuropsychologic impairment in patients with nonepileptic seizures. *Arch Clin Neuropsychol* 1998;13:513–22.
13. Binder LM, Salinsky MC. Psychogenic nonepileptic seizures. *Neuropsychol Rev* 2007;17:405–12.
14. Bortz JJ, Prigatano GP, Blum D, Fisher RS. Differential response characteristics in nonepileptic and epileptic seizure patients on a test of verbal learning and memory. *Neurology* 1995;45:2029–34.
15. Hill SK, Ryan LM, Kennedy CH, Malamut BL. The relationship between measures of declarative memory and the Test of Memory Malingering. *J Forensic Neuropsychol* 2003;3:1–18.
16. Williamson DJ, Drane DL, Stroup ES. Symptom validity tests in the epilepsy clinic. In: KB Boone, ed. *Assessment of Feigned Cognitive Impairment: A Neuropsychological Perspective*. New York: Guilford Press. 2007; 346–65.
17. Boone KB, ed. *Assessment of Feigned Cognitive Impairment: A Neuropsychological Perspective*. New York: Guilford Press, 2007.
18. Larrabee GJ, ed. *Assessment of Malingered Neuropsychological Deficits*. Oxford: Oxford University Press, 2007.
19. Holmes MD, Dodrill CB, Bachtler S, *et al.* Evidence that emotional maladjustment is worse in men than in women with psychogenic nonepileptic seizures. *Epilepsy Behav* 2001;2:568–73.
20. Owczarek K. Anxiety as a differential factor in epileptic versus psychogenic pseudoepileptic seizures. *Epilepsy Res* 2003;52:227–32.
21. Owczarek K. Somatisation indexes as differential factors in psychogenic pseudoepileptic and epileptic seizures. *Seizure* 2003;12:178–81.
22. Owczarek K, Jedrzejczak J. Patients with coexistent psychogenic pseudoepileptic and epileptic seizures: a psychological profile. *Seizure* 2001;10:566–9.
23. Storzbach D, Binder LM, Salinsky MC, Campbell BR, Mueller RM. Improved prediction of nonepileptic seizures with combined MMPI and EEG measures. *Epilepsia* 2000;41:332–7.
24. Schramke CJ, Valeri A, Valeriano JP, Kelly KM. Using the Minnesota Multiphasic Personality Inventory-2, EEGs, and clinical data to predict nonepileptic events. *Epilepsy Behav* 2007;11:343–6.
25. Breier JI, Fuchs KL, Brookshire BL, *et al.* Quality of life perception in patients with intractable epilepsy or pseudoseizures. *Arch Neurol* 1998;55:660–5.
26. Szaflarski JP, Hughes C, Szaflarski M, *et al.* Quality of life in psychogenic nonepileptic seizures. *Epilepsia* 2003;44:236–42.
27. Testa SM, Schefft BK, Szaflarski JP, Yeh H-S, Privitera MD. Mood, personality, and health-related quality of

life in epileptic and psychogenic seizure disorders. *Epilepsia* 2007;**48**:973–82.

28. Wagner MT, Wymer JH, Topping KB, Pritchard PB. Use of the Personality Assessment Inventory as an efficacious and cost-effective diagnostic tool for nonepileptic seizures. *Epilepsy Behav* 2005; **7**:301–4.

29. Stroup E, Chaytor N, Drane D, Coady E, Holsman M. PAI vs. MMPI in the classification of patients with epileptic and psychogenic nonepileptic seizures: overall accuracy and advantages. *J Int Neuropsychol Soc* 2006;**12**:92.

30. Griffith NM, Szaflarski JP, Schefft BK, *et al*. Relationship between semiology of psychogenic nonepileptic seizures and Minnesota Multiphasic Personality Inventory profile. *Epilepsy Behav* 2007;**11**:105–11.

31. Wilkus RJ, Dodrill CB. Factors affecting the outcome of MMPI and neuropsychological assessments of psychogenic and epileptic seizure patients. *Epilepsia* 1989;**30**:339–47.

32. Selwa LM, Geyer J, Nikakhtar N, *et al*. Nonepileptic seizure outcome varies by type of spell and duration of illness. *Epilepsia* 2000;**41**:1330–4.

Section 2 Chapter 14

Nonepileptic seizures: culture, cognition, and personality clusters

Cognitive complaints and their relationship to neuropsychological function in adults with psychogenic nonepileptic seizures

George P. Prigatano and Kristin A. Kirlin

In this chapter, we will review the studied cognitive complaints of persons with psychogenic nonepileptic seizures (PNES) and the relationship of these complaints to their actual neuropsychological test performance. We also will consider the relationship of anxiety and depression to their cognitive complaints and neuropsychological test performance. Our guiding hypothesis, based on clinical observation, is that patients with PNES may overestimate their cognitive limitations. Poor neuropsychological test performance in these patients is often associated with elevated signs of anxiety and depression. This pattern is generally not observed in patients with epileptic seizures (ES).

Whether patients' self-perceived cognitive (and possibly affective) difficulties contribute to a diagnosis of PNES is not well understood; however, patients with PNES often describe cognitive symptoms that appear disparate with their day-to-day functioning and neuropsychological test performance. Therefore, a careful assessment of subjective cognitive and affective symptoms, in conjunction with their neuropsychological test performance, may further help identify this complex group of individuals. In this chapter we focus on cognitive and affective aspects of neuropsychological testing. Effort testing, which is frequently done in neuropsychological batteries, is covered in Chapter 13.

Cognitive complaints of patients with PNES

The cognitive complaints of patients with PNES are as variable as the underlying psychiatric disorders that have been identified for this patient group (see Table 21.1 in current edition and Figure 3.3 in [1]). However, some authors contend that many (but not all) patients with PNES appear to present with some form of an underlying dissociative condition [2]. As a group, they tend to focus on physical complaints, but also report significant memory impairment [3]. When further questioned, some of these patients report language difficulties, especially problems with word-finding in free speech. This is often not observed consistently when interviewing them. Moreover, on formal neuropsychological testing they frequently perform within normal limits on measures of language functioning [4, 5].

Depending on the underlying psychiatric diagnosis, a wide range of cognitive and affective disturbances might be elicited in persons with presumed PNES. We have observed patients with PNES who report no cognitive complaints, but who emphasize their severe distress with their uncontrollable "seizures," while other patients may report severe memory impairment associated with disorientation. For example, one patient reported no memories whatsoever of several days' events and an inability to recognize her husband. She also would report episodes of confusion in which she could not find her way home or even form questions to get help. The patient's spouse reported that these episodes seemed to be associated with his wife's extreme distress. When hearing this, the patient reported that stress had nothing to do with her symptoms. Other patients with PNES report difficulties remembering why they have entered a room and associated difficulties completing their thoughts when talking with others.

Patients with PNES and a history of borderline personality disorder may not spontaneously report cognitive difficulties, but do note significant problems maintaining relationships and holding down a job. Likewise, patients with PNES and borderline intellectual functioning or mild mental retardation may not spontaneously describe any cognitive limitation, but

Gates and Rowan's Nonepileptic Seizures, 3rd edn. ed. Steven C. Schachter and W. Curt LaFrance, Jr. Published by Cambridge University Press. © S. Schachter and W. C. LaFrance, Jr. 2010.

will admit to having difficulties with new learning and getting "confused" when confronted with different life situations.

Unfortunately, the literature on cognitive complaints of patients with PNES often has not studied the specific subgroups of PNES identified by Gates and Erdahl [1] and compared and contrasted their subjective appraisal of their cognitive functioning to other patient groups. Rather, there has been a strong preference to administer standardized questionnaires to sample areas of cognitive functioning that might separate patients with many different types of PNES from patients with ES. To date, most studies addressing this issue have utilized the cognitive functioning domain of the Quality of Life in Epilepsy Inventory-89 (QOLIE-89) [6] to quantify subjective cognitive difficulties in patients with PNES. The items comprising this domain ask respondents to rate their degree of difficulty with memory, attention/concentration, and language abilities. Among the QOLIE-89 normative sample of 304 individuals with epilepsy, the mean ratings for the cognitive items suggested mild-to-moderate difficulties with memory, and more mild language and attentional problems. Difficulties with emotional functioning were also rated as mild among the normative epilepsy sample.

Several studies have compared the responses of patients with NES and PNES on this measure, with mixed results. Breier *et al.* [5] examined the relationship between self-reported and objective measures of cognitive functioning among 43 patients with intractable epilepsy versus 25 with PNES. Comparison of the two groups' QOLIE-89 profiles yielded no significant differences in their levels of self-reported cognitive dysfunction, despite the fact that their sample with PNES performed better than the ES group on objective cognitive measures. The PNES group rated themselves as more fatigued and in worse health overall. Their results suggested the relationship between patients' subjective and objective cognitive abilities was independent of their degree of depression among those with ES, but not among those with PNES. Loring *et al.* [7] also found no significant difference between patients with ES and PNES in scores on the QOLIE-89 cognitive domains. In contrast, Szaflarski *et al.*'s [8] comparison of the QOLIE-89 ratings of patients with ES or PNES yielded significantly lower (worse) ratings in the group with PNES on all three of the cognitive subscales. The patients with PNES reported memory to be their weakest cognitive domain. The higher levels of depression and medication side effects in the patients with PNES were found to negatively influence their QOLIE-89 overall scores.

Fargo *et al.* [4] examined the accuracy (rather than concordance) of patients with ES or PNES in rating their own memory, language abilities, and concentration (via the QOLIE-89) relative to their performance on neuropsychological tests. Patients with PNES rated memory as their greatest area of cognitive difficulty (almost 1.5 SD below the mean of the QOLIE-89 normative sample); their ratings for language and attentional problems were both within a half of a standard deviation of the mean. The results suggested patients with ES accurately rated their memory, but overestimated their language and attentional abilities. In contrast, the participants with PNES accurately rated their attention, but underestimated their memory and overestimated their language abilities. The participants' mood state was found to be the strongest predictor of their subjective ratings of their cognition for both ES and PNES groups, but not their psychometric test scores.

The use of a measure such as the QOLIE-89 to assess patients' subjective cognitive complaints has its benefits in that it is a standardized instrument and yields normative scores relative to a sample of adults with mild-to-moderate epilepsy. However in clinical practice, subjective cognitive complaints are typically elicited via clinical interview of the patient rather than by a self-report questionnaire. The use of an interview also has several potential benefits, including allowing the examiner to assess the patients' ratings of any perceived change in their cognition relative to "normal" or their individual baseline (rather than relative to other patients with epilepsy), as well as asking for examples of the patients' cognitive difficulties. How patients describe their cognitive difficulties may provide qualitative information suggestive of either a neurological or psychiatric etiology.

As an example of the use of the clinical interview in this area of research, Risse *et al.* [9] asked their samples of 43 patients with ES and 43 with PNES an open-ended question regarding their cognitive function (i.e., "Have you been having any difficulty with your thinking?"). Memory dysfunction was the most common complaint among both patient groups. Patients with PNES had more frequent complaints in the other cognitive domains assessed (attention, confusion, language) than the ES group. In contrast to their subjective description of their cognition, the PNES group's

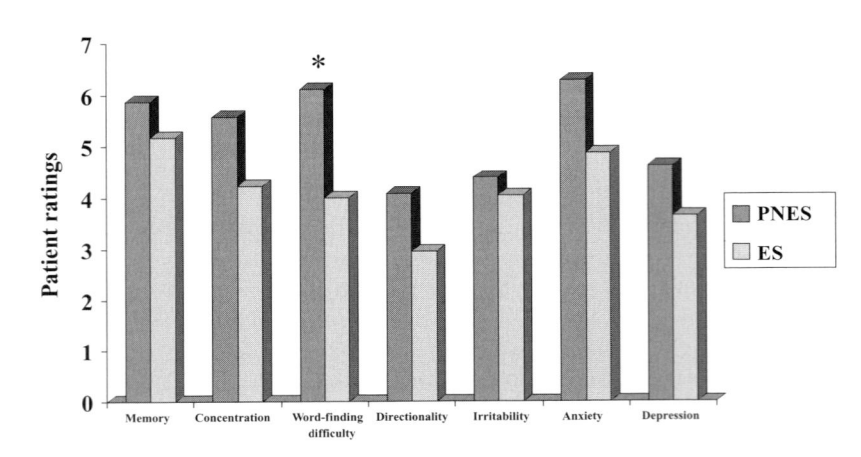

Figure 14.1. Mean ratings of subjective complaints in patients with epileptic seizures (ES) and patients with psychogenic nonepileptic seizures (PNES). (PNES = 23; ES = 22)
Note: *F(1, 43) = 5.70, p = 0.02. From Prigatano and Kirlin [10], with permission from Elsevier.

mean neuropsychological test scores were within normal limits.

Subjective appraisal and objective neuropsychological findings of cognitive and affective functioning in persons with presumed PNES

Recently, Prigatano and Kirlin [10] had patients rate their level of cognitive and affective difficulties as a part of their clinical interview on an epilepsy monitoring unit (EMU). These patients were then administered neuropsychological tests of both cognitive and affective functioning. Data were obtained *before* the attending neurologists arrived at a final diagnosis of PNES versus ES.

Figure 14.1 compares the subjective ratings of 23 patients with PNES versus 22 patients with ES on a variety of cognitive and affective domains. Patients were asked to rate on a scale from 0 to 10 (with 0 meaning no difficulty and 10 a severe problem) their level of difficulty with memory, concentration, word-finding, irritability, anxiety, depression, and problems "getting lost in space" or directionality.

On all domains, the mean ratings of patients with PNES were higher than those of patients with ES. The only statistically significant difference, however, was in word-finding difficulties. The correlation of one's subjective ratings of word-finding difficulties and actual performance on the Boston Naming Test, however, differed between the patients with PNES and ES. For the patients with ES, there was a statistically significant correlation ($r = -0.47$, $p = 0.03$). For those with PNES, the correlation was nonsignificant ($r = -0.29$, $p = 0.18$). That is, higher ratings of word-finding difficulties were clearly related to lower scores on a confrontation naming task for the patients with ES. The relationship appeared weaker for patients with PNES.

Another finding of the Prigatano and Kirlin [10] study was that the performance on tasks of affect expression and perception significantly correlated with the ratings by patients with PNES of word-finding difficulty, but this was not observed in the patients with ES. In their study, Prigatano and Kirlin [10] used the affect subtest of the BNI Screen for Higher Cerebral Functions (BNIS), which includes items that ask patients to read a sentence in both a happy and angry tone of voice, perceive facial affect, and produce spontaneous affect in response to humorous or incongruent stimuli [11]. Patients with PNES performed worse on this affect subtest compared to those with ES ($p = 0.02$). Those with PNES who had the worst performance in affect expression and perception rated their word-finding difficulties at a higher level of impairment ($r = -0.40$, $p = 0.01$), whereas patients with ES did not show this statistically significant finding ($r = -0.19$, $p = 0.40$). The findings suggest that sampling the patients' affective responses (rather than just having them self-report their affective functioning) may help identify patients with PNES.

One final observation of the Prigatano and Kirlin [10] study is relevant to the present discussion. While patients with PNES did not differ from those with ES on two of the three memory measures employed, the correlation of the patients' self-reported level of anxiety and depression and their memory performance was strikingly different. As Table 14.1

Table 14.1 Correlation coefficients between self-ratings of anxiety and depression and actual memory performance for patients with epileptic seizures (ES) and patients with psychogenic nonepileptic seizures (PNES)

	Patients with ES (n = 22)	
	RAVLT-D[a] (T)	BVMT-R-D[b] (T)
Self-ratings of anxiety	r = −0.15 (p = 0.50)	r = −0.05 (p = 0.81)
Self-ratings of depression	r = −0.20 (p = 0.39)	r = 0.02 (p = 0.93)
	Patients with PNES (n = 23)	
	RAVLT-D[a] (T)	BVMT-R-D[b] (T)
Self-ratings of anxiety	r = −0.56 (p = 0.01)	r = −0.57 (p = 0.01)
Self-ratings of depression	r = −0.42 (p = 0.05)	r = −0.25 (p = 0.26)

[a] Rey Auditory Verbal Learning Test 20-minute delayed recall (T score value).
[b] Brief Visuospatial Memory Test-Revised 25-minute delayed recall (T score value).

illustrates, there was no indication of a relationship between self-rated level of anxiety and depression and the performance of patients with ES on the delayed recall of the Rey Auditory Verbal Learning Test and the Brief Visuospatial Memory Test-Revised. In contrast, there was a strong relationship between the anxiety ratings of patients with PNES (and to some degree depression) and their performance on memory measures. Compatible with other study findings [4, 5], the patients' level of emotional distress was significantly correlated with their memory performance in those with PNES, but not patients with ES.

Why do self-perceived levels of anxiety particularly relate to cognitive complaints in patients with PNES but not those with ES?

There is a large literature that implicates hippocampal dysfunction with memory impairment in both animals and humans [12]. Small or atrophic hippocampal volume has been repeatedly related to verbal and nonverbal learning and memory deficits in patients with temporal lobe epilepsy who have complex partial seizures [13]. We could not locate any study that compared hippocampal volume with memory performance in patients with PNES. There are case reports of MRI evidence of mesial temporal sclerosis (MTS) in four patients with PNES [14]; however, MTS is the exception, not the rule, in patients with PNES.

A few studies have appeared on the relationship of hippocampal volume to memory performance in persons with posttraumatic stress disorder (PTSD). Bremner et al. [15] found slightly smaller left hippocampal volume (an average of 12% smaller than controls) in persons with PTSD. There was, however, no statistically significant correlation of hippocampal volume and recall on the Logical Memory subtest of the Wechsler Memory Scale. Patients with PTSD, however, did perform worse on this test compared to normal controls.

In a later, more comprehensive study, Bremner et al. [16] demonstrated smaller hippocampal volumes in women with a history of abuse with and without PTSD. This study is more relevant to the study of patients with PNES because, as Bremner et al. [16] noted, dissociative reactions are common in cases of abuse. The same is true for patients with PNES [2, 3].

In the Bremner et al. study [16], a significant relationship was found between a smaller left hippocampal volume and the severity of the patients' dissociative symptoms ($R^2 = 0.30$, $p < 0.05$). Positron emission tomography findings on the same subjects revealed less activation of hippocampal structures during a verbal encoding task in abused women with PTSD versus abused women without PTSD. However, and most important for the study of patients with PNES who have a high incidence of dissociative features, no relationship was reported between the severity of dissociative features, level of memory functioning, and hippocampal volumes.

While a history of PTSD and severity of dissociative features statistically are associated with hippocampal abnormalities, they do not seem to account for the level of memory dysfunction in patients with non-neurological disorders. This is not to say that patients with psychiatric disorders do not have "real" memory difficulties; only that the mechanism and expression of their memory difficulties may be different.

In dissociative states, the defense mechanisms of denial and repression have traditionally been thought to play an important role in symptom formation. In an experimental study on intentional forgetting of unwanted memories (an analogue to repression), Anderson et al. [17] reported that in 24 healthy subjects, motivated forgetting or suppression of memories for paired associate words was associated with increased activation of the dorsal lateral prefrontal cortex and decreased hippocampal activation. Thus, the process of not thinking about something you do not want to remember requires "effort" associated with a sustained shift of attention. Hippocampal areas become less activated during these times.

Vuilleumier *et al.* [18] studied the neuroimaging correlates of sensorimotor loss associated with a conversion disorder in a sample of seven patients and observed decreased activation (using SPECT) in the thalamus, the caudate, and the putamen. Equally important, after the patients improved in their functioning, activation patterns increased in these subcortical regions. The implication of these two studies is that deep brain structures (versus cortical structures) become less activated during the time a symptom associated with denial or repression occurs.

A study by Mailis-Gagnon *et al.* [19] suggests that the cingulate-thalamic connections may be important in keeping unwanted sensory experiences from reaching consciousness. They studied patients with chronic pain and "hysterical" anesthesias. A general suppression of brain activation was observed in the patients when the "affected" limb was exposed to noxious mechanical stimuli. A shift from posterior cingulate activation to more anterior activation was noted.

In our previous work, we reported two phenomena in patients with PNES. First, a negative response bias was observed in some patients when asked to perform a verbal recognition test [20]. Despite repeatedly hearing words that were read on five previous learning trials, some of these patients reported not hearing those words when they were presented on a recognition task. This may be a behavioral marker of the defense mechanism of denial.

Second, when attempting group psychotherapy with patients with PNES, many reported that during the times in which they were sexually abused, they shifted their attention to some other thoughts or activities so they did not have to experience the emotions associated with the episodes of abuse [3]. This activity might well implicate changes in cingulate-thalamic activation as well as suppression of hippocampal activation.

In dissociative states, memories may be suppressed by means of shifting attention and concentration away from an anxiety-producing stimulus. The process of suppression requires effort. Oftentimes the suppression is incomplete and the patient remains distressed and/or anxious. During these times, they may experience some anxiety, but not know why. McAdams [21] notes that the role of any defense mechanism is to keep anxiety at a minimum for purposes of adaptability. The defense mechanism of denial is often used for this purpose. When the defense is only partially effective, the person will experience anxiety in daily activities.

We propose that this process accounts for the relationship between level of self-perceived anxiety (and to some degree depression) and memory performance in patients with PNES, but not those with ES. In the latter group, memory performance is indirectly related to the patients' emotional state, but directly related to the intactness of brain structures involved in new learning and memory. The opposite pattern is seen in many (but not all) patients with PNES. Memory performance is directly related to their affective state (mainly anxiety) and indirectly related to possible subtle disturbances in hippocampal function that might impede new learning and later retrieval of memories.

Implications for clinical practice and research

The findings reviewed suggest that careful assessment of patients' cognitive complaints may help identify patients with PNES. As a group, they often report higher memory and word-finding difficulties than what is observed on examination and when compared to patients with ES. In at least three studies, the mood state of patients with PNES appeared to strongly correlate with their subjective cognitive complaints [4–5, 10]. This pattern has been less often observed in patients with ES [10, 22].

In addition to having patients rate both cognitive and affective states, it may be helpful to directly assess their ability to generate positive and negative affect in their tone of voice upon command, as well as identify facial emotions. Just as the literature demonstrating a discrepancy between patients' self-reported cognitive difficulties and their neuropsychological test performance supports the need for formal psychometric testing of patients' cognitive abilities, the present findings suggest that patients' self-report (via interview or questionnaire) regarding their emotional functioning should not be taken at face value. This may be particularly the case in patients with PNES who may have dissociative tendencies or a somatoform disorder, which by its nature limits their ability to accurately appraise their own affective functioning. Further research is needed addressing the performance of patients with PNES on non-self-report measures of affective processes such as identification of facial expression, modulation of affect expression, and generation/recognition of prosody. Prigatano and Kirlin [10] reported that patients with PNES performed less well than those with ES on these types of tasks. Moreover, difficulties carrying out the tasks significantly correlated with word-finding difficulties in patients with PNES, but not those with ES.

When word-finding difficulties are emphasized by a patient with potential PNES, we suggest that the clinical assessment focus on answering the following questions. Can the patients generate anger and happiness in their tone of voice upon command? Are the patients' subjective ratings of memory impairment and word-finding difficulties greater than what is observed in the clinical interview and on objective neuropsychological tests? Does the patient appear highly anxious and/or depressed, irrespective of their subjective reports and answers on questionnaires? A positive answer to each of these three questions may help identify patients with PNES evaluated on EMUs who present with an underlying dissociative condition associated with somatic and cognitive complaints.

Finally, we encourage researchers to study the cognitive complaints of patients with PNES as a function of their specific psychiatric diagnosis. We believe this is preferable to studying cognitive complaints of these patients as a large but heterogeneous group. Such an approach may also help explain the variability of findings that are reported in the literature.

References

1. Gates JR, Erdahl P. Classification of non-epileptic events. In: Rowan AJ, Gates JR, eds. *Non-Epileptic Seizures*. Boston, MA: Butterworth-Heinemann. 1993; 21–30.
2. Bowman ES, Markand ON. Psychodynamics and psychiatric diagnosis of pseudoseizure subjects. *Am J Psychiatry* 1996;**153**:57–63.
3. Prigatano GP, Stonnington C, Fisher RS. Psychological factors in the genesis and management of nonepileptic seizures: clinical observations. *Epilepsy Behav* 2002;**3**:43–9.
4. Fargo JD, Schefft BK, Szaflarski JP, *et al*. Accuracy of self-reported neuropsychological functioning in individuals with epileptic or psychogenic nonepileptic seizures. *Epilepsy Behav* 2003;**5**:143–50.
5. Breier JI, Fuchs KL, Brookshire BL, *et al*. Quality of life perceptions in patients with intractable epilepsy or pseudoseizures. *Arch Neurol* 1998;**55**:660–5.
6. Vickery BG, Perrine KR, Hays RD, *et al. Quality of Life in Epilepsy. QOLIE-89 Scoring Manual and Patient Inventory*. Santa Monica: Rand, 1993.
7. Loring DW, Meador KJ, King DW, Hermann BP. Relationship between quality of life variables and personality factors in patients with epileptic and non-epileptic seizures. In: Rowan AJ, Gates JR, eds. *Non-Epileptic Seizures*, 2nd edn. Boston, MA: Butterworth-Heinemann. 2000; 159–68.
8. Szaflarski JP, Szaflarski M, Hughes C, *et al*. Psychopathology and quality of life: psychogenic non-epileptic seizures versus epilepsy. *Med Sci Monit* 2003;**9**(2):113–18.
9. Risse GL, Mason SL, Mercer DK. Neuropsychological performance and cognitive complaints in epileptic and non-epileptic seizure patients. In: Rowan AJ, Gates JR, eds. *Non-Epileptic Seizures*, 2nd edn. Boston, MA: Butterworth-Heinemann. 2000, 139–50.
10. Prigatano GP, Kirlin KA. Self-appraisal and objective assessment of cognitive and affective functioning in persons with epileptic and nonepileptic seizures. *Epilepsy Behav* 2009;**14**(2):387–92.
11. Prigatano GP, Amin K, Rosenstein LD. *Administration and Scoring Manual for the BNI Screen for Higher Cerebral Functions*. Phoenix AZ: Barrow Neurological Institute, 1995.
12. Squire LR. *Memory and Brain*. New York: Oxford University Press, 1987.
13. Smith ML. Memory disorders associated with temporal-lobe lesions. In: Boller F, Grafman J, eds. *Handbook of Neuropsychology*. Amsterdam: Elsevier. 1989; 91–106.
14. Benbadis SR, Tatum IV, WO, Murtagh FR, Vale FL. MRI evidence of mesial temporal sclerosis in patients with psychogenic nonepileptic seizures. *Neurology* 2000;**55**:1061–5.
15. Bremner JD, Randall P, Vermetten E, *et al*. Magnetic resonance imaging-based measurement of hippocampal volume in posttraumatic stress disorder related to childhood physical and sexual abuse–a preliminary report. *Biol Psychiatry* 1997;**41**:23–32.
16. Bremner JD, Vythilingam M, Vermetten E, *et al*. MRI and PET study of deficits in hippocampal structure and function in women with childhood sexual abuse and posttraumatic stress disorder. *Am J Psychiatry* 2003;**160**:924–32.
17. Anderson MC, Ochsner KN, Kuhl B, *et al*. Neural systems underlying the suppression of unwanted memories. *Science* 2004;**303**:232–5.

18. Vuilleumier P, Chicherio C, Assal F, *et al.* Functional neuroanatomical correlates of hysterical sensorimotor loss. *Brain* 2001;**124**:1077–90.
19. Mailis-Gagnon A, Giannoylis I, Downar J, *et al.* Altered central somatosensory processing in chronic pain patients with "hysterical" anesthesia. *Neurology* 2003;**60**:1501–7.
20. Bortz JJ, Prigatano GP, Blum D, Fisher RS. Differential response characteristics in nonepileptic and epileptic seizure patients on a test of verbal learning and memory. *Neurology* 1995;**45**:2029–34.
21. McAdams DP. The role of defense in the life story. *J Pers* 1998;**66**:1125–46.
22. Elixhauser A, Leidy NK, Meader K, Means E, Willian MK. The relationship between memory performance, perceived cognitive functioning, and mood in patients with epilepsy. *Epilepsy Res* 1999;**37**:13–24.

Section 2 Chapter 15

Nonepileptic seizures: culture, cognition, and personality clusters

Health Related Quality of Life: utility and limitation in patients with psychogenic nonepileptic seizures

Gemma Mercer, Roy C. Martin, and Markus Reuber

Over the last decade, increasing prominence has been placed on patient reported outcome measures, especially on Health Related Quality of Life (HRQoL). These measures are now used routinely in the evaluation of intervention effects and the allocation of healthcare resources. This chapter will focus on HRQoL research in patients with psychogenic nonepileptic seizures (PNES). After describing the concept and measures of HRQoL, we will summarize the results of studies which have observed HRQoL in patients with PNES. Next, we will put the findings in patients with PNES in context by comparing them with those in two other patient groups – patients with epilepsy and patients with anxiety disorders and depression. Finally we discuss the current state of knowledge, the scope, and limitation of using HRQoL measures in patients with PNES.

The concept of HRQoL

Health Related Quality of Life (HRQoL) is the most commonly used framework to assess the impact of illness [1]. According to the World Health Organization, HRQoL is

[…] an individual's perception of their position in life in the context of the culture and value systems in which they live, in relation to their goals, expectations, standards and concerns. It is a broad ranging concept affected in a complex way by the person's physical health, psychological state, level of independence, social relationships and their relationships to salient features of the environment [2].

Typically, HRQoL is operationalized as a multidimensional concept, encompassing items describing physical, functional, psychological, social, and sexual aspects of life. It involves both "objective" and "subjective" domains. Whereas the objective domains concern aspects of physical functioning or limitations, the subjective domains are concerned with the patient's perception of how their life matches with some internal standard [3]. Health status, functional status, and quality of life are three concepts often used interchangeably to refer to the same domain of "health" [4].

Health Related Quality of Life is important for measuring the impact of chronic disease [5]. One reason for the success of HRQoL measures is that physical disease markers often correlate poorly with functional capacity and well-being, or aspects of life most important for patients' everyday lives. For example, in patients with chronic heart and lung disease, exercise capacity in the laboratory is only weakly related to exercise capacity in daily life [6].

Measures of HRQoL

Typically, HRQoL instruments are self-report questionnaires. The questionnaire items can be summed to produce scores across a number of different domains. Domains might include mobility and self-care (which could be subsumed into physical function), or depression, anxiety, and well-being (which together would form an emotional-function domain). Health Related Quality of Life measures broadly fall into two categories; generic and disease-specific instruments.

Generic instruments

Generic health status measures are designed to be valid across disease types and severity of illness. These measures are designed to capture information about a range of the domains of quality of life. Generic measures can take the form of health profiles or utility measures. Health profiles are instruments that attempt to measure all important aspects of HRQoL while utility measures are an indirect measure of quality of life based on the patient's preference for a particular health

Table 15.1 Domains included in SF-36 and QOLIE measures

	SF-36	QOLIE-89	QOLIE-31	QOLIE-10
No. of items	36	89	31	10
No. of scales or subscales	8 (2 component scores)	17	2	10
Overall quality of life/life satisfaction		✓	✓	✓
General health perception	✓	✓	✓	
Global change in health	✓			
Physical functioning	✓	✓		
Limitation due to physical health	✓		✓	
Energy, fatigue, tiredness, vitality	✓	✓	✓	✓
Social activity, adjustment, relationships, leisure	✓	✓	✓	✓
Social support, social isolation, social behavior		✓		
Emotional well-being, mental health, psychological disturbances	✓	✓	✓	✓
Limitation due to emotional health	✓	✓		
Sexual relationship		✓		
Pain	✓	✓		
Driving		✓	✓	
Cognitive functions		✓	✓	
Medicine, medical management, physicians, medical costs		✓	✓	✓
Adverse events profile, medication side effects		✓	✓	✓
Fear of attacks, attitude towards, worry, agitation, distress, relative reactions		✓		✓

Adapted from Leone *et al.* [11]

state. Utility measures incorporate preference measurements and relate health states to death; HRQoL is summarized as a single number along a continuum that usually extends from death (zero) to full health (one). Scores less than zero, representing states worse than death, are possible. Utility measures can be used in cost-utility analyses that combine duration and quality of life [7]. The results of such analysis can be expressed as "cost per Quality Adjusted Life Year (QALY)" and are used by healthcare purchasers to help them decide whether interventions represent acceptable value for money [8]. Some health profiles (such as the SF [Short Form]-36 [9]) can be statistically transformed into utility measures.

Disease-specific instruments

Disease-specific measures are developed for specific diagnostic groups or patient populations, and seek to sample clinically important changes. These are changes that clinicians and patients think are important for that particular disease. The major advantage of this approach lies in the potential for increased responsiveness that may result from including only those aspects of HRQoL that are relevant to the patient group of interest. The Quality of Life in Epilepsy Inventory-89 (QOLIE-89) is a disease-specific measure that has been validated in patients with epilepsy (although it actually incorporates the "generic" questions of the SF-36) [10]. Shorter versions (QOLIE-31 and -10) have also been developed. The SF-36 and the QOLIE family of questionnaires are some of the most commonly used measures in patients with epilepsy and PNES [11]. Table 15.1 illustrates the range of domains covered in these measures.

HRQoL and PNES

Several studies have investigated HRQoL in PNES; the majority of these are comparison studies with patients with epileptic seizures (ES) as the control group. Although there are no studies in which patients with PNES were compared with any other control group directly, the profile of HRQoL scores reported by the PNES groups in these studies can also be compared to general population norms (see below for further discussion).

At first glance, all studies show that patients with PNES experience a reduced HRQoL when compared to the general population or patients with ES. However, closer inspection of the data suggests that the relationship between PNES and HRQoL may not be direct.

For instance, Testa et al. [12, 13] found that current mood state moderated the relationship between diagnosis (ES versus PNES); that is, when patients demonstrate lower levels of mood disturbance (as measured by the Profile of Mood State scale), patients with PNES reported lower HRQoL than did patients with ES. However, where mood disturbance is high, this difference in HRQoL disappears. In addition, when more chronic aspects of psychological distress and somatization (as measured by the Minnesota Multiphasic Personality Inventory [MMPI-2]) were introduced into their model, this moderating effect of mood was no longer significant, suggesting that it may actually be these factors which account for the interaction between seizure diagnosis and HRQoL. These authors also identified a subset of individuals with PNES who rated their HRQoL as lower than those with ES despite nonclinical levels of mood state. They concluded that some patients with PNES may have a tendency to overreport difficulties related to health and physical functioning while neglecting symptoms related to emotional states and mood.

Szaflarski et al. [14] demonstrated that the difference in self-reported HRQoL of patients with PNES and ES was explained by higher levels of depression and adverse events in those with PNES. However, they also found that HRQoL was reduced by psychopathology independent of the diagnosis: patients with PNES and depression reported a lower quality of life than patients with PNES alone. This finding was replicated in the patients with ES in their study [15].

Quigg et al. [16] found that in their retrospective sample of 30 patients with PNES, complete seizure cessation was required to demonstrate a significantly higher HRQoL. Lawton et al. [17] argued that the examination of correlations between PNES frequency and HRQoL, psychological distress, and the number of somatic symptoms could distinguish between the effects of the seizures themselves on HRQoL and the consequences of less specific psychological distress or somatization tendencies. They found a significant relationship between PNES frequency and HRQoL, although this relationship failed to achieve significance when the degree of psychological distress or the number of other physical symptoms was taken into account.

All of these findings suggest that HRQoL in patients with PNES is closely linked to underlying psychopathology, and that the seizures themselves make a relatively insignificant contribution to HRQoL overall. In terms of treatment this could mean that it may not be sufficient to focus on the reduction or control of seizures without addressing the psychosocial factors which underpin the disorder. Having said that, it has been shown that HRQoL can be a sensitive measure of treatment associated change in patients with PNES. One study, in which 63 patients with functional neurological symptoms (of whom 68.3% had PNES) self-reported HRQoL immediately before and after a brief psychodynamically oriented therapeutic intervention, showed that 36% of patients improved by at least one standard deviation on the SF-36. These improvements were maintained at six months follow-up and were achieved at modest cost ($5159 to $10 317/QALY) [18].

HRQoL in other disorders: epilepsy

In a recent review, Schachter [19] described a number of psychosocial factors that have been shown to influence HRQoL in patients with ES. He concluded that in addition to seizure control and side effects of antiepileptic drugs, quality of life is determined by depression, anxiety (including seizure worry, social anxiety, and parental anxiety), stigma, and self-mastery. However, unlike in patients with PNES [17], the significant relationship between HRQoL and epilepsy severity markers is not lost when psychopathology is introduced as covariate [20]. Many studies have examined HRQoL of patients with PNES in comparison to patients with ES. Table 15.2 presents the differences in HRQoL between these two patient groups.

Overall, patients with PNES report significantly lower HRQoL than patients with epilepsy, although there are some discrepancies between studies in terms of differences at the level of the subscales. Figure 15.1 presents the profiles of HRQoL subscores. All studies

Table 15.2 HRQoL and PNES study summary table

Study	Control group	Sample	Sample recruitment	Demographics Age (years)	Gender (% Female)	Relevant measures	Significant difference in HRQoL
Breier et al. [35]	Temporal lobe epilepsy	68 epilepsy; 25 PNES	Inpatients	35.7 epilepsy; 35.1 PNES	50 epilepsy; 88 PNES	QOLIE-89	PNES significantly more limited on domains of physical and mental health
Szaflarski et al. [36]	Intractable epilepsy	45 epilepsy; 40 PNES	Inpatients	36 epilepsy; 37.6 PNES	60 epilepsy; 85 PNES	QOLIE-89	PNES significantly lower on all subscales except; Role Limitations: Emotional, Emotional Well-being, Medical Effects and Social Isolation
Szaflarski et al. [14]	Intractable epilepsy	53 epilepsy; 53 PNES	Inpatients	36 epilepsy; 36 PNES	62.3 epilepsy; 77.4 PNES	QOLIE-89	PNES significantly lower on overall HRQoL score
Al Marzooqi et al. [37]	Epilepsy (age and sex matched)	97 epilepsy; 97 PNES	Outpatients	34	69	SF-36	PNES significantly lower on all subscales except Physical or Social Functioning
Szaflarski & Szaflarski [15]	Intractable epilepsy	99 epilepsy; 95 PNES	Inpatients	36.5 epilepsy; 36.3 PNES	64.6 epilepsy; 81.1 PNES	SF-36	PNES with depression have significantly lower scores on all subscales than PNES without depression and epilepsy with and without depression
Testa et al. [12]	Epilepsy	69 epilepsy; 45 PNES	Inpatients	35.9 epilepsy; 37.42 PNES	55.1 epilepsy; 68.9 PNES	QOLIE-89	PNES significantly lower on overall HRQoL score

PNES, psychogenic nonepileptic seizures.

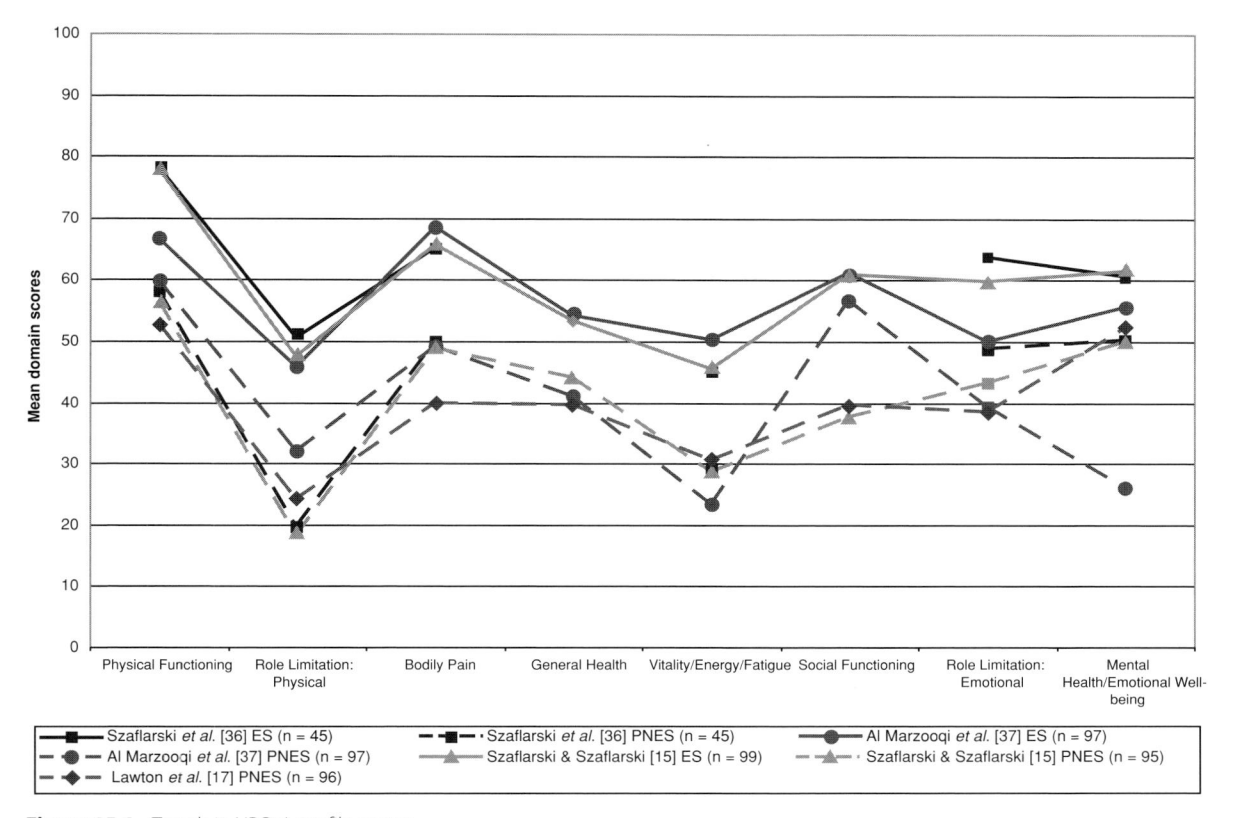

Figure 15.1. Trends in HRQoL profile scores.

utilized the SF-36, except Szaflarski et al. [14] who utilized the QOLIE-89. Only those subscales contained in both the SF-36 and the QOLIE-89 are presented. The findings in the PNES groups are represented by the scored lines. Lower values represent poorer self-reported HRQoL.

The graph illustrates the general pattern for patients to report lower HRQoL across all domains. Although patients with both ES and PNES tend to report greater role limitations in relation to their physical functioning relative to the reported physical functioning, this difference appears to be pronounced in patients with PNES.

HRQoL in other disorders: anxiety and depression

As there is a high level of psychopathology in the population of patients with PNES [21–23], and PNES are considered as a manifestation of psychiatric disorder in the current nosologies [21, 22], it makes sense to compare the HRQoL of patients with PNES with that of patients with other psychiatric disorders. Here, we focus on anxiety disorders and depression because they are particularly common. Table 15.3 provides the profile of scores on the SF-36 for patients with depression, anxiety, or PNES, as well as normative scores for the UK population. As the data have been assembled from four different studies, the comparison in Table 15.3 between the different disorders should be seen as a guide rather than a direct comparison. Given that the patients described are likely to have disorders of different severity, the profiles of the different domain scores are more relevant than the absolute values.

The main difference in the profiles of patients with PNES and patients with depression, social anxiety disorder, or panic disorder is that the patients with PNES report less impairment in the domains mental health and role limitation emotional. This is not unexpected; patients with PNES have been found to have high levels of alexithymia [23], and they have a tendency to attribute their illness as being of a more physical than emotional or psychiatric nature [24].

Table 15.3 Means and standard deviations on the SF-36 for general population, patients with depression, anxiety, or psychogenic nonepileptic seizures

SF-36 domains	General population[a]	Depression[b] (n = 250)	Anxiety — Social anxiety disorder[c] (n = 33)	Anxiety — Panic disorder[c] (n = 33)	PNES[d] (n = 96)
Physical function	88.4 (18.0)	80.2 (22.2)	92.9 (14.4)	79.6 (20.9)	52.78 (33.99)
Role limitation physical	85.8 (29.9)	44.9 (39.4)	86.4 (23.5)	54.9 (42.4)	24.26 (33.84)
Bodily pain	81.5 (21.7)	60.5 (27.1)	80.0 (20.3)	68.1 (24.4)	39.86 (27.07)
General health perception	73.5 (19.9)	53.9 (21.6)	80.1 (19.6)	71.1 (23.0)	39.63 (19.72)
Energy/vitality	61.1 (19.7)	23.6 (18.4)	59.4 (18.5)	51.1 (21.6)	30.57 (18.55)
Social functioning	88.0 (19.9)	49.5 (22.9)	65.9 (28.5)	61.0 (25.2)	39.56 (20.26)
Role limitation emotional	82.9 (31.8)	19.8 (30.1)	67.9 (42.1)	55.5 (43.8)	38.61 (43.22)
Mental health	73.8 (17.2)	33.9 (16.3)	58.5 (19.4)	47.7 (18.6)	52.13 (23.20)

[a] Oxford Health and Life Survey [38]
[b] The Counseling versus Antidepressants in Primary Care Study Group [28]
[c] Simon et al. [29]
[d] Lawton et al. [17]

Conclusion

There is currently only a small body of literature examining the HRQoL in patients with PNES. There is a clear need for more and larger scale, prospective longitudinal studies. Most importantly, we need to know much more about the relationship between HRQoL and other outcomes, including disability status, healthcare utilization, and family function.

The majority of studies currently published in this area involve a comparison to patients with epilepsy. The validity of such a comparison is questionable, particularly given the involvement of other psychological factors. Use of an epilepsy comparison group may have some face validity, but it is likely that the choice of this particular disease control group is usually based on opportunity rather than scientific justification. It may be more appropriate to compare PNES with other emotional or psychiatric disorders. In relation to this, the use of epilepsy-specific measures may be called into question. To our knowledge, there are no published studies demonstrating the validity of using such measures in this population. The assumption that the concerns relating to quality of life are the same between these two groups needs to be tested, particularly in light of the results of the studies that have been carried out which suggest that the profiles of domain scores differ between the two disorders. For example, the Liverpool group developed a model of quality of life in epilepsy [25] based on a model described by Spitzer [26]. However, to date, the development of such a model has not been attempted in PNES.

There seems to be a trend for patients with PNES to report only average levels of limitations on the activities described due to actual physical disabilities, yet to report high levels of impairment in their role functioning related to their physical health. One explanation for this is that the questions contributing to the Physical Functioning score of the SF-36 are quite strongly based on patients' mobility and they do not reflect other aspects of physical dysfunction associated with PNES sufficiently well. It is also possible that for many patients with PNES, impairment of role functioning is related to avoidance and self-imposed restrictions on activity due to fear of having a seizure rather than actual physical disability. Avoidance has certainly been reported as a prominent coping strategy in this patient group [27–29]. On the other hand it may be characteristic of patients with PNES to overstate disability despite relatively well-preserved functioning. This interpretation would be supported by studies which suggest that patients with PNES are more likely to receive benefits than patients with epilepsy despite comparable severity of their seizure disorders [30, 31].

There are a number of concerns about the measurement of HRQoL in general. Although the concept of HRQoL was introduced in part to resolve some of the issues of ambiguity in measures of quality of life, these measures still ignore the context of the patient's illness. Hunt [32] argues that it is not possible to separate the effects due to health and the consequences of changes in finance, friendships, family life, responsibilities, expectations, occupation, ageing, etc. In patients with PNES who are known to have difficult interpersonal relationships and be dependent on benefits this may be particularly pertinent.

Despite these concerns, measures of HRQoL fill an important gap in the assessment of therapeutic interventions. They give patients or service users a voice and are likely to be used more, rather than less, in the future. However, the research summarized above raises some critical questions about the validity of these measures, and a greater understanding of the relationship between these self-report scales and objectively observable outcome measures is urgently required, especially in patients with PNES. Until we have a better understanding of how patients with PNES rate their HRQoL, it may be prudent to use these self-report measures in combination with other observations, such as caregiver reports and objective behavioral measures (for instance healthcare utilization) [33, 34].

References

1. Ashing-Giwa KT. The contextual model of HRQoL: a paradigm for expanding the HRQoL framework. *Qual Life Res* 2005;**14**(2):297–307.
2. World Health Organization Quality of Life Group. *What Quality of Life?* World Health Organization Quality of Life Assessment: World Health Forum. 1996; 354–6.
3. Romney DM, Evans DR. Toward a general model of health-related quality of life. *Qual Life Res* 1996;**5**(2):235–41.
4. Patrick DL, Bergner M. Measurement of health status in the 1990s. *Annu Rev Public Health* 1990;**11**:165–83.
5. Patrick DL, Erickson P. *Health Status and Health Policy: Quality of Life in Health Care Evaluation and Resource Allocation*. New York: Oxford University Press, 1993.
6. Guyatt GH, Thompson PJ, Berman LB, *et al.* How should we measure function in patients with chronic heart and lung disease? *J Chronic Dis* 1985;**38**(6):517–24.
7. Brazier J, Roberts J, Deverill M. The estimation of a preference-based measure of health from the SF-36. *J Health Econ* 2002;**21**(2):271–92.
8. Green C, Brazier J, Deverill M. Valuing Health-Related Quality of Life: a review of health state valuation techniques. *PharmacoEconomics* 2000;**17**:151–65.
9. Ware J, Sherbourne C. The MOS 36-Item Short Form Health Survey (SF-36). I. Conceptual framework and item selection. *Med Care* 1992;**30**: 473–82.
10. Devinsky O, Vickrey BG, Cramer J, *et al.* Development of the Quality of Life in Epilepsy Inventory. *Epilepsia* 1995;**36**(11):1089–104.
11. Leone MA, Beghi E, Righini C, Apolone G, Mosconi P. Epilepsy and quality of life in adults: a review of instruments. *Epilepsy Res* 2005;**66**(1–3):23–44.
12. Testa SM, Schefft BK, Szaflarski JP, Yeh H-S, Privitera MD. Mood, personality, and health-related quality of life in epileptic and psychogenic seizure disorders. *Epilepsia* 2007;**48**(5):973–82.
13. Testa SM, Schefft BK, Getzoff EA, Fargo JD. Tripartite model of depression and anxiety in epileptic and psychogenic seizures [abstract]. *J Int Neuropsychol Soc* 2003;**9**(02):277.
14. Szaflarski J, Szaflarski M, Hughes C, *et al.* Psychopathology and quality of life: psychogenic non-epileptic seizures versus epilepsy. *Med Sci Monit* 2003;**9**(4):CR165–70.
15. Szaflarski JP, Szaflarski M. Seizure disorders, depression, and health-related quality of life. *Epilepsy Behav* 2004;**5**(1):50–7.
16. Quigg M, Armstrong RF, Farace E, Fountain NB. Quality of life outcome is associated with cessation rather than reduction of psychogenic nonepileptic seizures. *Epilepsy Behav* 2002;**3**(5):455–9.
17. Lawton G, Mayor RJ, Howlett S, Reuber M. Psychogenic nonepileptic seizures and health-related quality of life: the relationship with psychological distress and other physical symptoms. *Epilepsy Behav* 2009;**14**(1):167–71.
18. Reuber M, Burness C, Howlett S, Brazier J, Grunewald R. Tailored psychotherapy for patients with functional neurological symptoms: a pilot study. *J Psychosom Res* 2007;**63**(6):625–32.
19. Schachter SC. Quality of life for patients with epilepsy is determined by more than seizure control: the role of psychosocial factors. *Exp Rev Neurother* 2006;**6**(1):111–18.
20. Suurmeijer TPBM, Reuvekamp MF, Aldenkamp BP. Social functioning, psychological functioning, and quality of life in epilepsy. *Epilepsia* 2001;**42**(9): 1160–8.
21. Benbadis SR. A spell in the epilepsy clinic and a history of "chronic pain" or "fibromyalgia" independently predict a diagnosis of psychogenic seizures. *Epilepsy Behav* 2005;**6**(2):264–5.
22. Bowman ES, Markand ON. Psychodynamics and psychiatric diagnoses of pseudoseizure subjects. *Am J Psychiatry* 1996;**153**(1):57–63.

23. Reuber M. Psychogenic nonepileptic seizures: Diagnosis, aetiology, treatment and prognosis. *Schweizer Archiv fur Neurologie und Psychiatrie* 2005;**156**(2):47–57.

24. Binzer M, Stone JON, Sharpe M. Recent onset pseudoseizures–clues to aetiology. *Seizure* 2004;**13**(3):146–55.

25. Baker GA, Smith DF, Dewey M, Jacoby A, Chadwick DW. The initial development of a health-related quality of life model as an outcome measure in epilepsy. *Epilepsy Res* 1993;**16**(1):65–81.

26. Spitzer WO. State of science 1986: Quality of life and functional status as target variables for research. *J. Chronic Dis* 1987;**40**(6):465–71.

27. Frances PL, Baker GA, Appleton PL. Stress and avoidance in pseudoseizures: Testing the assumptions. *Epilepsy Res* 1999;**34**(2–3):241–9.

28. Goldstein LH, Drew C, Mellers J, Mitchell-O'Malley S, Oakley DA. Dissociation, hypnotizability, coping styles and health locus of control: Characteristics of pseudoseizure patients. *Seizure* 2000;**9**(5):314–22.

29. Goldstein LH, Mellers JDC. Ictal symptoms of anxiety, avoidance behaviour, and dissociation in patients with dissociative seizures. *J Neuro, Neurosurg Psychiatry* 2006;**77**(5):616–21.

30. Binder LM, Salinsky MC, Smith SP. Psychological correlates of psychogenic seizures. *J Clin Exp Neuropsychol* 1994;**16**(4):524–30.

31. Kristensen O, Alving J. Pseudoseizures–risk factors and prognosis. A case-control study. *Acta Neurol Scand* 1992;**85**:177–80.

32. Hunt SM. The problem of quality of life. *Qual Life Res* 1997;**6**(3):205–12.

33. Martin RC, Gilliam FC, Kilgore M, Faught E, Kuzniecky R. Improved health care resource utilization following video-EEG-confirmed diagnosis of nonepileptic psychogenic seizures. *Seizure* 1998;**7**(5):385–90.

34. Reuber M, Mitchell AJ, Howlett S, Elger CE. Measuring outcome in psychogenic nonepileptic seizures: how relevant is seizure remission? *Epilepsia* 2005;**46**(11):1788–95.

35. Breier JI, Fuchs KL, Brookshire BL *et al*. Quality of life perception in patients with intractable epilepsy or pseudoseizures. *Arch Neurol* 1998;**55**:660–5.

36. Szaflarski JP, Hughes C, Szaflarski M *et al*. Quality of life in psychogenic nonepileptic seizures. *Epilepsia* 2003;**44**(2):236–42.

37. Al Marzooqi SM, Baker GA, Reilly J, Salmon P. The perceived health status of people with psychologically derived non-epileptic attack disorder and epilepsy: a comparative study. *Seizure* 2004;**13**(2):71–5.

38. Wright L, Harwood D, Couldter A. *Health and Life Styles in the Oxford Region*. Oxford: Health Services Research Unit, University of Oxford, 1992.

Section 2 Chapter 16

Nonepileptic seizures: culture, cognition, and personality clusters

Legal medicine considerations related to nonepileptic seizures

Roy G. Beran, John A. Devereux, and W. Curt LaFrance, Jr.

Epilepsy is a medical condition that evokes many legal issues impacting on the patient and his/her quality of life as well as the therapeutic relationship [1]. As many people who have nonepileptic seizures (NES) manifest their disorder with alterations of consciousness, similar to some epileptic seizures (ES), it follows that the legal ramifications that impact on epilepsy, and those who have it, are just as relevant to many people with NES. The fact that these patients have NES, whether alone or with comorbid epilepsy, does not diminish the legal ramifications that already exist because of the seizures.

The majority of people with NES do not have epilepsy [2] and thus there is need to consider those additional legal issues that are directly referrable to the NES. Psychogenic NES (PNES) represent a form of psychosomatic illness, where an underlying psychological stressor manifests as a neurological event [3, 4]. It is therefore imperative to differentiate between physiological nonepileptic events (NEE) that also have no relationship to epilepsy, such as dyskinetic movements associated with movement disorders like Parkinson's disease [5], from PNES, which have a psychological etiology.

Psychogenic nonepileptic seizures represent a form of conversion reaction [2, 6]. Some patients with PNES are presumed to have a model upon which their behavior is based [2] and a secondary gain that "rewards" such behavior [7]. Once these have been identified, then it is possible to offer appropriate remedies that address the underlying issues [8]. This does not negate any legal implications that such PNES evoke.

What follows is consideration of some of the specific legal implications of PNES, as compared to NEE, which may, or may not, affect the patient's life.

Driving

Many people with PNES have episodes in which, for all appearances, they lose contact with their environment. The fact that these are not epileptic in nature does not mean that it is safe for the person to drive.

Some people have placed driving and PNES in the "too hard to decide" basket. The alternate argument is that because PNES are not ES, the person should be safe to drive. Such an argument ignores the possible triggers that evoke PNES. Should stress be a provocateur for PNES, then it seems reasonable to assume that drivers with PNES will be exposed to stress, possibly while driving, and hence may experience PNES at this time. If this is the case, it also seems reasonable to assume that these patients are at increased risk of accidents due to their PNES.

Unlike ES, for which one can prescribe appropriate medications and hence fully control seizures in up to 80% of patients [9], PNES are much less predictably controlled. The assessment of risk for a person with epilepsy who drives relies on a level of predictability which indicates that if a person is seizure-free for a predetermined period of time then the risk of further seizures while driving is sufficiently low to be acceptable to the wider community [10]. Some patients with PNES do not experience such a level of predictability, and hence it could be argued that they present a greater safety risk than ES with respect to driving.

The management of PNES is such that it is occasionally difficult to determine either the model upon which the behavior is based or the secondary gain and hence success of treatment is less positive than is the case with ES. Mixed ES/PNES presents unique challenges. In those who have both epilepsy and PNES it is often possible to stop the ES without stopping the PNES [11].

Gates and Rowan's Nonepileptic Seizures, 3rd edn. ed. Steven C. Schachter and W. Curt LaFrance, Jr. Published by Cambridge University Press. © S. Schachter and W. C. LaFrance, Jr. 2010.

One study addresses driving in patients with PNES [12]. In a survey of physician members of the American Epilepsy Society on whether patients with PNES should be able to drive, of the 82 physicians questioned, 37 (45%) responded. The distribution among respondents was as follows: 49% applied the same restrictions as for patients with epilepsy; 32% did not place patients under any restrictions; and 19% decided on a case-by-case basis. In the same study, crash records were reviewed in patients with PNES and compared with state records from the same year. Patients with PNES reported eight crashes, all of which were nonfatal. What is not available consequent to these data is the consideration of possible accidents caused by, but not involving, people with PNES as a result of potentially erratic driving that may have ensued as a result of PNES.

It could well be argued that the person with PNES still needs to satisfy the community that he/she is safe to drive. To do that also dictates the need to demonstrate a seizure-free period for the PNES before being allowed to drive. Sometimes it is very difficult to differentiate between ES and PNES without video-EEG, which may confirm an absence of epileptic activity at the time of the PNES [13]. If this be the case, in a given patient, then it follows that a reasonably safe procedure is to impose those restrictions referrable to epilepsy, as it is unclear which are ES and which are PNES.

Privacy

Patients with PNES have a psychiatric disorder typically classified within the category of conversion disorders [3, 6]. Therefore it is instructive to briefly review legal aspects of psychiatric disorders.

A medical practitioner who divulges details of psychiatric illnesses to other people may be liable in tort law for negligence if doing so causes further psychiatric illness. The New Zealand case of *Furniss v Fitchett* [14] is instructive in this regard. That case dealt with a husband and wife who were patients of the same doctor. The doctor advised the husband of the wife's mental state without her consent. This later came to light during legal proceedings for separation, causing her stress, for which she sued the doctor for "nervous shock." The doctor was found negligent in breaching expected professional standards and to have knowingly caused her foreseeable harm by the disclosure.

Of course, a patient with PNES is, in any event, owed a duty of confidentiality in equity and at common law (with respect to tort law and consideration of negligence). McMahon [15] identified the three elements referable to the healthcare relationship, namely a confidential relationship, the information becoming available because of that confidential relationship, and that the confidential information was misused to the detriment of the patient.

The duty of confidentiality is not absolute. The duty of confidentiality is a public good, which may be outweighed by competing and more compelling public interests. In the English case of *Egdell* [16], a psychiatrist disclosed information concerning a patient, in a secured psychiatric facility, to the Assistant Medical Director of that facility and the Home Office to prevent transfer to a less secure facility, which resulted in an action for breach of confidence. Both the trial court and the subsequent appeal found in favor of the doctor as the duty of care to the wider community outweighed that owed to the patient concerning confidentiality. The duty of confidentiality is only outweighed by public safety concerns in circumstances where the need to disclose is urgent, is made in response to a real threat, and where disclosure is made to people only no wider than is necessary to avoid the threat. So, for example, disclosure made only to a media outlet, such as a reporter or the producer of a show, may result in dissemination of the material well beyond that which is acceptable within this framework and may not fall within this category.

Different states, even within the same country, have different requirements regarding reporting patients with epilepsy to the division of motor vehicles. Doctors reporting patients to the driving authority are generally indemnified, so long as the reporting is done in good faith [1]. This would be true for PNES but the response from the licensing authority is less easy to predict, as is suggested above. The reporting of those with epilepsy is mandated in some jurisdictions [1] but the position concerning PNES is less well defined because the impact of PNES on driving is less certain, making reporting less clear.

The duty to warn is another legal medicine aspect to be considered by clinicians. *Tarasoff* [17], a US case, dealt with a psychologist who failed to warn an identifiable victim about a person diagnosed with paranoid schizophrenia, resulting in Tarasoff's death. The Supreme Court of California found that the psychologist's duty to protect Tarasoff overrode the duty of confidentiality to the patient. This raises the potential for an injured third party to sue the doctor should a person with PNES cause injury because the doctor allowed activity without disclosure where there existed a predictable, foreseeable risk that the injury would occur.

Having said that, doctors and healthcare professionals have a duty not to disclose information gleaned consequent to the professional relationship. Such duty is enforceable in equity, breach of confidence, at common law (intentional infliction of psychiatric injury), in negligence, and subject to professional disciplinary standards according to relevant ethical codes of conduct [18]. Obvious exceptions to such duty are when the patient consents to disclosure or when this is authorized by statute [13, 17].

Discrimination

Discrimination against people with epilepsy is well recognized [1] but discrimination against people with PNES is less clear. Once it is acknowledged that the episodes are PNES there is a tendency to categorize the patient as a malingerer [19]. (Malingering accounts for only a small number of patients presenting with seizures, and is addressed below in a discussion of establishing medico-legal causation. Likewise, factitious disorder is covered in Chapter 20 on Munchausen syndrome.) The patient may feel stigmatized by the diagnosis of PNES [20] and feel the doctor does not take him/her seriously. This may result in the patient either changing doctors inappropriately or alternatively making vexatious claims against the doctor [20]. The patient's impression that the complaint "is not real" (according to the doctor) has the potential to make the patient feel rejected and angry and it is possible that this hostility becomes directed towards the therapist [20]. Such an attitude may cause the patient to malign the doctor and, depending on the sphere of influence the patient controls, may have detrimental impact on the doctor's clinical practice.

Again, recognizing that PNES are due to a psychiatric disorder, patients with PNES may thus suffer the discrimination relevant to epilepsy per se to which may be added the discrimination referrable to psychiatry, should the diagnosis become disclosed [21]. If this is the case then all the legal avenues to protect against discrimination become relevant. These include statutory protection [22, 23], but to invoke the rights that such laws are designed to protect requires the patient to initiate litigation against the perceived offender. Such litigation is time consuming, expensive, and itself may exacerbate any deep-seated psychological problem [24].

Disability

Patients with epilepsy have access to advocacy organizations, such as the Epilepsy Foundation in the US or Epilepsy Australia, which will mediate on their behalf should perceived discrimination occur [25]. Disability laws also protect against discrimination in the workplace, including recent legislation in the US incorporating epilepsy in the Americans with Disabilities Act and its recent Amendment. Patients with PNES may be less fortunate. Litigation for workers' compensation or long-term disability may not receive the same review as does epilepsy. Further complications may result because people with PNES sometimes deny the psychogenic nature of their disorder and rely on a diagnosis of epilepsy to access the same services as are available to those with epilepsy. This may reinforce the wrong messages, validating the wrong diagnosis and instigation of the wrong therapeutic intervention, and thus represent a reversed form of discrimination, which may help to entrench "sickness" behavior that could be counterproductive to the patient's long-term well-being.

Causation

Litigation sometimes arises after injuries or traumas where subsequent PNES or other psychogenic disorders develop. LaFrance and Self [26] examined the difficult issue of addressing insult-injury from an immediate proximate cause perspective. Legal causation and medical causation use separate metrics in evaluating causation. Neuropsychiatric aspects of an individual's developmental history and exposures add a further level of complexity to determining causation, especially in the population with somatoform disorders. Determining whether symptoms are intentionally produced or are the result of an unconscious process remains a significant challenge in the courtroom.

As noted above, conversion seizures are produced unconsciously. Malingering is not a psychiatric diagnosis, rather it is the intentionally feigned production of a symptom. Malingering accounts for a small number of those with seizures. These individuals may use a symptom to extricate themselves from military service, incarceration, or to obtain compensation or prescription medications. Neuropsychological tests may be useful in individuals with a question of feigned symptoms related to memory.

Conclusion

The legal implications of PNES encompass all those considerations that apply to epilepsy. In addition to those legal considerations referable to the person with epilepsy, there may be additional legal ramifications that impact upon the person with PNES.

To emphasize this point, five such areas have been further explored – driving, privacy, discrimination, disability, and causation. This chapter is in no way intended to be an exhaustive review, but topics were chosen to describe potential areas where PNES may involve specific legal consequences and have implications separate from, or complementary to, those relevant to epilepsy.

References

1. Beran RG. Epilepsy and the law. *Epilepsy Behav* 2008;**12**(4):644–51.
2. Gates JR. Non-epileptic seizures: classification co-existence with epilepsy: diagnosis, therapeutic approaches and consensus. *Epilepsy Behav* 2002;**3**:28–33.
3. LaFrance Jr WC, Blum AS, Miller IW, Ryan CE, Keitner GI. Methodological issues in conducting treatment trials for psychological nonepileptic seizures. *J Neuropsychiatry Clin Neurosci* 2007;**19**(4):391–8.
4. Gates JR. Nonepileptic seizures: time for progress. *Epilepsy Behav* 2000;**1**:2–6.
5. Kehdi EE, Huynh W, Kim SD, Beran RG. Non-epileptic seizures in Parkinson's Disease. ESA 22nd Annual Scientific Meeting, Adelaide, Australia, 2007.
6. Stonnington CM, Barry JJ, Fisher RS. Conversion disorder. *Am J Psychiatry* 2006;**163**:1510–17.
7. Lambert MV, Schmitz EB, Ring HA, Trimble M. Neuropsychiatric aspects of epilepsy. In: Schiffer RB, Rao SM, Fogel BS, eds. *Neuropsychiatry: Drug and Disease Management*. Philadelphia: Lippincott Williams & Wilkins. 2003; 1071–131.
8. Reuber M. Psychogenic nonepileptic seizures: answers and questions. *Epilepsy Behav* 2008;**12**:622–35.
9. Herkes GK. Antiepileptics – clinical applications. *Aust Prescr* 1994;**17**:9–12.
10. Assessing Fitness To Drive – Commercial & Private Vehicle Drivers: Medical Standards for Licensing and Clinical Management Guidelines. AUSTROADS & National Road Transport Commission, Sydney. Sept. 2003; 55–60.
11. DiMario FJ. Paroxysmal nonepileptic events of childhood. *Semin Pediatr Neurol* 2006;**13**:208–21.
12. Benbadis SR, Blustein JN, Sunstad L. Should patients with psychogenic nonepileptic seizures be allowed to drive? *Epilepsia* 2000;**41**(7):895–7.
13. Devinsky O, Sanchez-Villasenor F, Vazquez B, et al. Clinical profile of patients with epileptic and nonepileptic seizures. *Neurology* 1996;**46**: 1530–3.
14. *Furniss v Fitchett* [1958] NZLR 396.
15. McMahon M. Rethinking confidentiality. In: Freckelton I, Petersen K, eds. *Disputes and Dilemmas in Health Law*. Sydney: Federation Press. 2006; 563–603.
16. *Wyes v Egdell* [1990] 1 All ER 835.
17. *Tarasoff v Regents of the University of California; Tarasoff v Regents of the University of California* 17 Cal 3d 425; 131 Cal Rptr 14; 551 P2d 334 (1976).
18. Iacovino L, Mendelson D, Paterson M. Privacy issues, health connect and beyond. In: Freckelton I, Petersen K, eds. *Disputes and Dilemmas in Health Law*. Sydney: Federation Press. 2006; 604–21 at 607.
19. Binder LM, Kindermann SS, Heaton RK, Salinsky MC. Neuropsychologic impairment in patients with nonepileptic seizures. *Arch Clin Neuropsychol* 1998;**13**(16):513–22.
20. Thompson NC, Osorio I, Hunter EE. Nonepileptic seizures: reframing the diagnosis. *Perspect Psychiatr Care* 2005;**41**(2):71–8.
21. Byrne P. Psychiatric stigma: past, passing and to come. *J R Soc Med* 1997;**90**(11):618–21.
22. *Disability Discrimination Act* 1992 (Cth), Australia.
23. *Americans with Disability Act* 42 U.S.C. 12101 et seq 1990 USA.
24. Douglas KS, Koch WJ. Psychological injuries and tort litigation: sexual victimisation and motor vehicle accidents. In: Ogloff JRP, Schuller RA, eds. *Introduction to Psychology and Law*. Toronto, ON: University of Toronto Press. 2001; 407–26.
25. Beran RG, Devereux JA, McLin WM, et al. Legal concerns and effective advocacy strategies. In: Engel J, Jr., Pedley TA, eds. *Epilepsy – A Comprehensive Textbook*, Vol. 3 (221), 2nd edn. Philadelphia: Lippincott-Raven. 2008; 2277–82.
26. LaFrance Jr WC, Self JA. Do bus accidents cause nonepileptic seizures?: Complex issues of medicolegal causation. *J Am Acad Psychiatry Law* 2008;**36**(2):227–33.

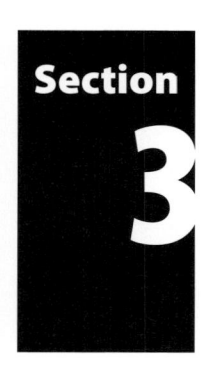

Section 3: Psychiatric and neuropsychological considerations in children and adolescents with psychogenic nonepileptic seizures

Section 3 Chapter 17

Psychiatric and neuropsychological considerations in children and adolescents with psychogenic nonepileptic seizures

Psychiatric features and management of children with psychogenic nonepileptic seizures

Rochelle Caplan and Sigita Plioplys

Risk factors that play unique roles in determining children's mental functioning include genetic predisposition to mental illness; reactivity to stress; cognitive, linguistic, and social skills deficits; medical history; as well as environmental variables including socioeconomic status, family functioning, and social milieu [1–4]. A disruptive change in the balanced and dynamic interaction between these child- and environment-related risk factors can cause mental health problems in childhood. In some cases this imbalance results in pediatric psychogenic nonepileptic seizures (PPNES), a conversion disorder with seizure-like manifestations.

Despite the marked morbidity of PPNES (see review in [5]), there is limited information available on the psychiatric manifestations and risk factors of this disorder, and what is known is based on a few small case series [6–11] and retrospective studies [12–20]. Consequently, there is a dearth of knowledge about the etiology and pathogenesis of PPNES. Adding to this, difficulties making this diagnosis and lack of pragmatic clinical information on how to evaluate these children and adolescents contribute to the challenges of advancing research on the psychiatric aspects of PPNES [21].

This chapter describes models of PPNES followed by the spectrum of its psychiatric manifestations (i.e., primary and associated psychiatric diagnoses), and range of treatment options. It then provides clinical guidelines, such as when, how, and with whom to make this diagnosis and give diagnostic feedback (i.e., the "do's"), as well as what not to do (i.e., the "don'ts"). Three clinical vignettes illustrate successful and unsuccessful approaches to PPNES diagnosis and feedback.

Models of PPNES

Overview

The following models of PPNES integrate information from developmental models of pediatric psychopathology, specifically somatization [1, 4, 21–24], extant studies of psychopathology [6, 7, 9–14, 17, 25–27], and the authors' clinical experience with PPNES. Based on conventional psychodynamic formulation [28, 29], PPNES result from the displacement of an unresolved intrapsychic conflict, the primary pathology, and its conversion to behavioral manifestations that are similar to epileptic seizures (ES). The sources of the primary conflict might be interpersonal (e.g., having one's feelings hurt; being ignored, mocked, rejected, or in a competitive situation; arousing a parent's anger; feeling angry towards others) or intrapersonal (e.g., poor self-esteem; emotional maladjustment; learning, language, or social deficits; difficulties with sport). The severity of associated stress ranges from mild (e.g., social slights or hurt feelings) to severe (e.g., physical, sexual, and emotional abuse as well as other types of trauma). Due to inadequate problem solving of the underlying conflict, the associated negative affect (e.g., tension, anxiety, anger, helplessness, hopelessness) is channeled through the body and expressed as neurological symptoms.

The expression of negative affect through neurological symptoms might reflect the social acceptance of medical rather than psychiatric symptoms in some cultures [30], rural regions, and among low-income individuals and those with limited medical knowledge [31]. Significantly higher rates of physical symptoms and medical illness in the parents of children with

PPNES compared to the parents of children with ES without PPNES also imply the importance of modeling of parental somatisizing behaviors [32]. Future studies are needed to distinguish the child- and environment-related risk factors that predispose children to somatisizing disorders, such as PPNES, rather than psychiatric disorders.

Pediatric PNES symptoms obviate fulfilling duties, such as going to school, doing homework, or participating in sports, and temporarily relieve the patient from dealing with the underlying conflict. Despite this respite, the secondary gain, recurrent seizures, behavioral and cognitive adverse effects of antiepileptic drug (AED) treatment, and the cumulative effects of inadequate problem solving (e.g., increased workload due to missing school in an already overburdened child with undiagnosed learning difficulties) make it even more difficult for the child to problem solve and deal with the primary pathology. The resulting increased tension further exacerbates "seizures," while increasing the secondary gain, thus creating a vicious cycle that perpetuates and increases the clinical morbidity. Left untreated, habitual maladaptive problem solving and coping through physical symptoms can impair psychosocial and academic development and lead to lifelong unsuccessful functioning and disability in terms of continued seizures and economic independence [33].

Models

Studies of children with somatization disorders reveal low thresholds for developing conversion symptoms from stress associated with behavioral inhibition, fear of uncertainty, and generalized sensitivity to stimuli they perceive as threatening [34]. Several researchers have suggested that conversion symptoms develop when youngsters with inhibited or difficult temperament and high reactivity to stress perceive emotional experiences as threatening [22, 34–36].

Based on the dynamic-maturational model [37] and attachment theory [38], Kozlowska [24] considers conversion symptoms in children as rudimentary and primal unconscious self-protective behavioral strategies with phylogenetic roots in innate animal defense behaviors, such as the "freeze" and "appeasement defense" responses. In some parent–child relationships, youngsters learn to inhibit negative affect and unacceptable behaviors to "secure" attachment, decrease parental withdrawal or hostility, and elicit adult attention and approval [31]. Kozlowska [24] posits that these youngsters perceive distressful emotional experiences as physiological threats due to their immature or ineffective cognitive processing of emotional information. In this context, children with PPNES are viewed as unable and ill-equipped to resolve distress, and unconsciously displace distressful affect into more acceptable and less cognitively distorted behavioral "markers" – the neurological conversion symptoms. When psychologically distressed, these children are thus thought to experience an automatically activated and innate "freeze response" (e.g., staring spell, "loss of consciousness") coupled with learned inhibition of negative affect and unacceptable behaviors.

This theory further suggests that youngsters who cannot completely inhibit motor behaviors associated with their negative affect will clinically present with disorganized motor activity, the seizure-like behaviors, in addition to the inhibited subjective awareness (i.e., "loss of consciousness") associated with the "freeze response." Kozlowska elegantly depicts the phenomenon of *la belle indifference* as the ultimate "freezing" of cognitive and emotional recognition of distress [39].

Children who "freeze" without recognizing their distress and its causes are unable to verbalize and inform their parents or others about the source of their stress. As a result, the parents of these children are unaware of their children's emotional difficulties. In other cases in which neurological symptoms have not yet developed, children may know the reasons for their stress and try to communicate this to their parents. However, their parents might not understand or acknowledge their difficulties. For example, parents might accuse a child with learning difficulties of being lazy and not applying his/herself or might turn a deaf ear when told of familial incest. Unable to successfully problem solve, the child gives up trying to inform the parents of the problem. The "unsolved" underlying distress subsequently worsens, and the child experiences what Taylor [40] calls the "predicament." In this situation, the child sees no way out, and becomes "physically ill."

Summary

Pediatric PNES, like other conversion symptoms, are conceptualized to represent the displacement of negative affect associated with the primary psychopathology (underlying conflict) and its conversion to seizure-like symptoms. Increased emotional reactivity coupled with phylogenetically immature problem solving and poor family communication might underlie the development of PPNES. In this context, secondary gain together with ineffective coping and maladaptive problem solving exacerbate and perpetuate PPNES.

Primary and comorbid psychiatric diagnoses

Primary diagnosis

Although PPNES is not a recognized Diagnostic and Statistical Manual of Mental Disorders, Fourth Edition (Text Revision) (DSM-IV-TR) [41] diagnostic category, these patients meet criteria for one of the following DSM-IV-TR primary diagnoses: conversion disorder with seizures, dissociative disorder, and factitious disorder. Since factitious disorder is rarely identified in PPNES in contrast to adult PNES (see review in [5]), this chapter focuses on conversion disorders, found in 52% to 100% of the cases [6, 17, 42], and on dissociative disorders [6, 10, 17, 43].

A necessary but not sufficient criterion for the diagnosis of a primary conversion disorder in a child or adolescent is that their characteristic seizure-like episode is not associated with epileptiform activity during a simultaneous video-(VEEG) recording. Psychiatric symptoms suggesting displaced distress (i.e., the primary psychopathology), as well as the secondary gain should be apparent in the history and examination. As previously described and further detailed in the "Diagnosis: how to, do's and don'ts" section of this chapter, the psychiatric symptoms might only suggest the presence of "significant psychological problems and stressors" as these patients are generally unaware of their distress and/or unable to verbalize their problem. Alternatively, their parents do not acknowledge or understand when their children tell them about their stressors.

Similar to children with other pediatric conversion disorders [39], youngsters with PPNES often experience transformation of their initial symptoms and develop secondary somatic complaints, such as headaches, abdominal or chest pain, gait disturbance, abnormal movements, motor weakness, and loss of sensation or vision. These secondary somatic symptoms reflect a more severe conversion disorder and inappropriate treatment of the underlying conflict or source of distress. Thus, Pakalnis and Paolicchi [15] noted that more medical investigations, treatment, and a higher risk for iatrogenic complications contribute to making children with secondary somatic symptoms more functionally impaired than patients with PPNES without symptomatic transformation.

Dissociative disorder, characterized by medically unexplained loss of consciousness, stupor, or coma [41], is most commonly found following physical and sexual abuse [43–45]. However, other than a single report of dissociative disorders in 3 of 21 (14%) Brazilian children with PPNES [10], dissociative disorders are rare in PPNES. By contrast, dissociative symptoms, such as staring and daydreaming, are primary human responses to stress that are frequently found in youth with posttraumatic stress disorder (PTSD), some of whom also have PPNES [6, 10, 17, 43].

Comorbid psychiatric diagnoses

Similar to other pediatric conversion disorders, PPNES is a "low-incidence" but "high-impact" disorder [39] with psychiatric problems in 16% to 100% of the cases [10, 16, 17]. The rate and severity of psychopathology is higher in adolescents (48.6%) than in children younger than 13 years (16%) [16]. Whereas females predominate in adolescents with PPNES [16], boys either outnumber girls [13] or have PPNES at the same frequency as girls in 5- to 13-year-old children [6, 16].

Youth with PPNES have a wide range of comorbid psychopathology with mood disorders (e.g., depression, anxiety) in 32% to 67% and disruptive behavioral disorders (e.g., ADHD, oppositional defiant, and conduct disorders) in 10% to 25% of cases [6, 10, 16, 17, 26]. However, at the time of the initial diagnosis of PPNES, 72% to 90% of the cases have previously diagnosed comorbid psychopathology [16] and 71% have undergone psychiatric treatment [46]. Moreover, the association of depression and history of abuse with secondary somatic symptoms in some children with PPNES is thought to reflect more dysfunctional and ineffective coping [15].

The wide range of comorbid psychopathology and the relationship with secondary somatic symptoms might reflect the difficulties clinicians have diagnosing PPNES. These comorbidities also imply that some vulnerable children with mental health problems, whose primary psychopathology is poorly understood and unsuccessfully managed, subsequently develop conversion disorders.

In terms of informants, although adolescents with PPNES and their parents report symptoms suggestive of different types of comorbid psychiatric diagnoses with different frequencies, both groups describe symptoms of anxiety and depression as the most common problems [46]. In one study, whereas parents reported symptoms that met criteria for PTSD, panic, and obsessive compulsive disorder, those reported by the youths support dysthymia, specific phobia, and social phobia diagnoses [46]. Interestingly, in this study 22% of youth with PPNES also confirmed symptoms commensurate with somatization and 22% with eating disorder diagnoses. Their parents, however, did not corroborate these symptoms.

Furthermore, self-report scores of social anxiety related to fear of performance and physical symptoms (i.e., somatic autonomic) suggest that youth with PPNES may perceive their high levels of social anxiety as somatic symptoms [46]. Supporting this finding, children with PPNES had significantly higher parent-based Child Behavior Checklist [47] scores of somatic and internalizing problems, as well as more functional disability compared to children with epilepsy [48].

These findings emphasize the importance of interviewing both parents and children as informants to obtain a comprehensive picture of the primary and comorbid psychopathology in individual patients with PPNES. They also suggest that the somatic symptoms and disability of youth with PPNES might reflect social and performance-related anxiety.

Evidence of cognitive deficits in 5% to 14.8% [14, 17–20] and learning problems in 14% to 45.7% of patients with PPNES [16, 18] corroborate the possible role of performance anxiety in PPNES. In fact, academic difficulties can limit a child's effectiveness with problem solving and coping with their academic and social demands. Associated poor self-esteem, sad or angry mood, and worries and fears, together with parents' misunderstanding of their children's cognitive or learning difficulties might all interact in the development of PPNES. However, studies of stressors, such as linguistic and social deficits, are lacking in youngsters with PPNES.

Summary

The most frequent primary diagnosis in PPNES is conversion disorder and the wide range of comorbid psychiatric diagnoses spans mood and disruptive disorders which often antedate the diagnosis of PPNES. Recent findings imply that youth with PPNES might channel social, academic, and/or performance anxiety through somatic symptoms.

Diagnosis: how to, do's and don'ts

The problem of diagnosing PPNES

As previously emphasized, PPNES is not simply a default diagnosis made following a negative VEEG in a child or adolescent with poorly controlled seizures. To make this diagnosis, it is necessary to demonstrate the psychiatric hallmarks of this syndrome – denial of any ongoing stressors, negative affect (e.g., anxiety, anger, sadness), or distress together with secondary gain and seizure-like behaviors. However, it is often difficult to identify the primary pathology, stressors, emotional problems, or the "predicament" [40] since most youth with PPNES and their parents acknowledge the seizures, but often deny the presence of non-physical problems, such as emotional, behavioral, social, or learning difficulties. Unable to penetrate the "everything is fine other than seizures" barrier, physicians may focus only on the seizures.

There are two main reasons for this barrier. The first and previously described reason involves impaired emotional insight, coping, and communication. The second reason is the co-occurrence of PPNES with ES [13]. In terms of insight, coping, and communication, the child with PNES might be unable to recognize or verbalize difficulties other than "seizures" and physical symptoms. Alternatively, the youth recognizes the stressors, is unable to deal with them, and has communicated or attempted to communicate these difficulties to the parents to get their help. The parents, however, either fail to understand the child's distress or are unable to acknowledge it due to their own emotional difficulties. In some cases, the child has difficulty identifying and/or verbalizing his/her problems and the parents are emotionally unable to "hear" or "accept" the presence of these problems. In PPNES with comorbid psychiatric diagnoses, these children acknowledge and talk about the symptoms of their comorbid disorders but not about the primary emotional difficulties underlying their conversion disorder.

Regarding the high rate of PPNES of 35% to 44% in children who also have ES [13, 16, 19, 20], the physicians and parents of these children and adolescents may focus only on the epilepsy and assume that all the seizure-like manifestations including those that are actually due to PPNES are epileptic in origin. This often leads to unnecessary emergency room visits and frequent changes in AED dosage, type of AED, and AED polytherapy. By increasing the child's secondary gain (e.g., absence from school, not participating in competitive sports or other events, not dealing with social difficulties), this medical approach can make the neurological symptoms more persistent. Similarly, adverse behavioral and cognitive effects of high AED doses and AED polytherapy (see review in [49]) exacerbate the PPNES by further compromising the child's coping and problem-solving skills, particularly the ability to deal with ongoing emotional, behavioral, social, or learning problems.

Five "diagnostic clues" should alert clinicians to the possibility of PPNES in children: (1) movements and behaviors not typical of ES that present in an inconsistent and changing pattern, (2) a change in the typical clinical manifestations of the seizures of a child with well established ES, (3) the occurrence of episodes only in the presence of others, (4) prolonged "seizures" (i.e., hours, days), and (5) *la belle indifférence*. A detailed history provides information on the first four diagnostic clues, and the clinical interview of the child reveals *la belle indifférence*. Unlike the classical indifference to conversion symptoms in adults with *la belle indifférence*, in children it presents as indifference to problems and stressors in their lives but intense emotional investment with and concern about their "seizures."

Summary

Youth with PPNES and their parents focus on the neurological manifestations of the disorder and often deny possible underlying emotional problems. Physicians, therefore, who do not explore the possibility of PPNES conclude the child has either developed epilepsy *de novo* or breakthrough seizures in a child with confirmed epilepsy. A history suggesting a changing and inconsistent pattern of "prolonged seizures" only in the presence of other people and associated with secondary gain as well as minimal concern about life problems should alert physicians to the possibility of PPNES.

Timing and techniques used in the diagnosis of PPNES

When?

A timely diagnosis of PPNES is important because the treatment outcome is better the shorter the lag time from the onset of symptoms to diagnosis and treatment [12]. In addition, early diagnosis decreases the morbidity and high costs associated with repeated emergency room visits and medical care. However, establishing rapport with these children and their parents, determining how invested the parents are in the child having a medical rather than a psychiatric diagnosis, and penetrating the "everything is fine" barrier take time. Therefore, the psychiatric diagnostic process should start as soon as the neurologist begins to suspect PPNES and parallel the neurological workup including inpatient telemetry and outpatient evaluation.

How to

The first step in the diagnostic process is a detailed neurological history taken from the parents without the youth present to determine the pattern and consistency of seizures, conditions and situations that preceded the development of the illness and those related to recurrent episodes, when and where episodes occur and who is present, duration of the episodes, as well as AED changes and associated frequency of episodes. It is essential to ascertain information on the child's emotional/behavioral functioning by asking the parents about the child's prevalent mood and mood changes, how the child deals with and expresses anger, stress, and fears, as well as changes in sleep patterns. It is also crucial to inquire about the child's academic functioning in terms of strengths and weaknesses, ability to pay attention, grades, homework patterns, and nervousness prior to tests or projects as well as changes in functioning prior to onset of the illness. Clarification of the child's social functioning, such as whether he/she has friends, interacts with them at and/or after school, or participates in organized social activities, as well as recent changes in how the child feels with peers is also imperative.

During this process, it is important for the clinician to establish the parents' trust, give them a sense that the clinician understands how difficult the illness has been for them, appreciates their level of investment in a medical diagnosis, comprehends how the PPNES symptoms might prevent the child from meeting their parents' expectations and aspirations for the child, and sympathizes with pertinent ongoing life stresses for the parents and family. If the parents deny that the child has emotional, behavioral, academic, or social difficulties including how to handle stress and anger, the clinician should clarify that she/he is interested in this information because stress can impact seizure control.

To establish rapport with the child, the clinician should see the child alone and be cognizant of the child's potential difficulty acknowledging and verbalizing emotional difficulties. Asking the child a few questions about the episodes helps to develop rapport and trust. After explaining to the child that stress might make "seizures" worse, the clinician should explain that he/she will be asking questions about different aspects of the child's life including mood, sources of anger and its management, school, social life, relationships with parents and siblings, ambitions, self-esteem, issues that cause stress, and how the child deals with them. The clinician should also find out what problem solving techniques the patient uses, how well they work, and parent involvement in this process. In addition, the clinician should gently ask the child about possible abuse.

It is not unusual for the child to deny problems other than seizures at the first meeting. When the clinician describes to the child what other children with seizures have said about stress and their seizures, the difficulties they experience due to their seizures, how seizures might make school work, social activities, and life at home more problematic, this normalizes things for the child and improves the rapport and trust for the clinician. As a result, the patient gradually begins to reveal some of the difficulties he/she faces. If the clinician is empathetic and indicates an understanding for what the child is trying to communicate, the child realizes that this is a person who can be trusted and who might be able to help with the "predicament." Sometimes, this might not occur until the second or third meeting with the child.

If there is evidence for unresolved stressors and/or negative affect and feelings (i.e., the conflict) that have been channeled into physical symptoms, it is necessary to determine if the obstacles are child-based, parent-based, or both. The clinician should also ascertain the extent of the child's secondary gain and its effect on the parents' functioning (e.g., missed work days; expectations from child regarding homework and tests; participation in competitive sports, dancing, or academic events; enforcement of disciplinary measures; coming together of separated/divorced parents to manage the child). Finally, detailed questions on mood including suicidal ideation, plans, and acts; fears, apprehensions and worries; type of learning and attentional difficulties; prior physical, sexual, or other trauma; social problems; and psychotic symptoms will help rule out or support the presence of comorbid psychiatric diagnoses.

Once the clinician has obtained good rapport with the parents and with the child, a joint interview with the child and the parents provides additional important information on family interaction. This includes how the child communicates with the parents, as well as their sensitivity and response to the child's communications.

Don'ts

In terms of interview techniques, when first meeting the parents, clinicians should not rely on the seizure history obtained in the past by the epileptologist (neurologist), but rather obtain a seizure history that includes questions on the previously described diagnostic clues for PPNES. In addition, the child should not be interviewed together with the parents to ensure that the clinician establishes firm rapport with the child. The child's permission should be obtained before information is shared with the parents, and only if this is relevant to the diagnosis and treatment plan. Rather than accepting denial of any psychological problems and distress as evidence for the absence of psychopathology in a child with PPNES, clinicians should recognize that this is, in fact, a diagnostic clue and the hallmark of an underlying conversion disorder. Knowing that all parents and children with and without medical disorders will acknowledge some ongoing problems will help the clinician in this process.

Summary

To overcome the obstacle of denial of problems other than seizures, both parents and child should be separately interviewed using the seizure history to obtain relevant information (i.e., diagnostic clues) as well as to establish rapport and trust. By discussing difficulties involved in having seizures, clinicians should establish rapport and use empathy to elicit information on what the child perceives as stressors and how the child and family deal with and respond to the child's stressors. In this way, obstacles to healthy problem solving for the child and the parents can be identified.

Feedback

Feedback provides the parents and the child with a PPNES diagnosis and a treatment plan. It is problematic because the parents frequently want a neurological diagnosis as they have difficulty accepting that the child might have learning, social or other emotional difficulties. As a result, the parents might become enraged with the medical team "that does not know what it is doing" and/or with their child if they interpret a PPNES diagnosis as meaning that the child has been "faking" neurological symptoms.

When?

Feedback should be given only after enough information is collected to confirm or rule out a PPNES diagnosis and the team (pediatric neurologist, epileptologist, mental health clinician, EEG technician, epilepsy nurse) has had a chance to discuss and fully understand the case. If the child is undergoing VEEG monitoring, this typically occurs at the end of the telemetry admission. For outpatients, the diagnostic process might involve several sessions depending on how difficult it is to establish rapport and trust both with the parents and child and to penetrate the "everything is fine" barrier. Pediatric PNES feedback can take a long time due to the difficulty the parents and the child have understanding this diagnosis, what it means to them, how it is treated, and the long-term implications if not treated. Therefore, both the neurologist and the mental health clinician need to schedule a block of time of adequate length for the feedback between the clinicians, child, and parents.

How to

Team. Since parents differ in their level of investment in the child having epilepsy or a neurological or medical diagnosis, feedback stating that the child has a psychiatric rather than a neurological diagnosis that involves psychological and/or psychopharmacological treatment rather than treatment specific for epilepsy may be problematic. In our experience, this feedback works best if the pediatric neurologist (epileptologist) acts as team leader and the mental health clinician as team member. The team gives feedback separately to the parents and to the child. Having a clear presentation of PNES in mind and familiarity with delivery of the diagnosis of PNES facilitates communication among the team members, the parents, and the child.

Parent feedback. The pediatric neurologist (epileptologist) typically begins the feedback process to the parents with the VEEG findings for inpatients and with the EEG and neurological findings for outpatients using a positive approach indicating that there is "good and informative news." The "good news" is that the child's EEG indicates no evidence for epilepsy or a severe illness of the brain in those with PNES alone. For children who have both ES and PNES, the "good news" is that the monitoring revealed a better picture of the child's different types of seizures.

However, it is important that the team leader clearly states that the child does have an illness (alluding to the "informative news"). For parents not wholly invested in a neurological diagnosis, the pediatric neurologist (epileptologist) should then explain that the child's seizures are probably due to emotional causes and stressors, supported with examples obtained from the history and detailed evaluation. The pediatric neurologist (epileptologist) should spell out for the parents of children who also have epilepsy the manifestations of the child's ES and differentiate them from the PNES symptoms.

It is essential to clarify for parents that in the presence of the stressors, the child's tension is channeled into the body and expressed though physical symptoms. Further, it should be explained that this is not a volitional process, and that the child is not "faking" seizures. To underscore this, say "The seizures are real, they are just not caused by epilepsy." In addition, the physician should underscore that the intervention will focus on helping the child identify and verbalize his/her problems as well as learning to problem solve in socially accepted and functional ways rather than through physical symptoms. From this point on, the pediatric neurologist (epileptologist) refers to the conversion symptoms as "episodes" rather than "seizures." So as to not convey the impression that the seizures are "faked," we also discourage the use of the term "pseudoseizures."

The pediatric neurologist (epileptologist) should use a different approach for parents who have difficulty accepting a psychological basis for the child's symptoms. In these cases, the "good and bad news" approach can be used. However, the focus should be that whereas there is no evidence for a serious disease of the brain (the "good news"), stress plays a role in aggravating seizures and the child's difficult-to-control condition (the "bad news"). This approach can be used whether the child has both epilepsy and PPNES or only PPNES.

With the child's permission, it is also possible to let the parents know that the child is quite aware of several stressors (e.g., emotional, academic, social, and familial). If, until now, parents have resisted talking about the possible role of stress, they often begin to open up and discuss potential stress factors, particularly when they hear the child has spoken about them. The clinician should clarify that intervention is needed to recognize and identify the stressors so as to help the child cope better and decrease seizure frequency. With these parents, we only use the term "episodes" when they have accepted that the child has PNES.

It is important to emphasize that the feedback frequently leads to marked emotional responses as the parents experience relief that the child does not have something very wrong with their brain and begin to understand what the child has and what they are dealing with. As mentioned earlier, in some cases they experience varying degrees of anger towards the child because they think a diagnosis of PNES means the child is "faking" symptoms. The team should carefully process these emotional responses with the parents.

This challenging process is crucial because it determines if the parents will accept the diagnosis and treatment plan or simply decide to go to another professional who will provide them with the medical diagnosis and treatment they want for their child. If the parents continue to "doctor shop," the child's underlying problems go untreated, and maladaptive problem solving through medical symptoms becomes the child's way of dealing with life's problems. Without treatment, these "psychological and emotional handicaps" can result in dysfunctional outcomes [12]. An additional untoward effect of feedback on parenting could be that the parents feel they are guilty, "incompetent," or "bad" parents for not recognizing the child's emotional problems. They then overcompensate by being overprotective and reward the child unnecessarily and excessively. This parenting style increases the child's secondary gain.

Child feedback. When giving feedback to the child, clinicians should first present the "good news" and then follow with the "other news." More specifically, assure that the child knows that his/her brain is "okay" and that, as discussed with him/her, stress and some of the things the child has spoken about as stressful might be making seizures worse. It is most important to explain to the child that this does not mean the child is "faking" seizures. These "episodes" are real (the "bad news") and have caused the child a lot of distress and trouble but their cause seems to be related to stress or emotional causes that are difficult for most physicians to understand and identify. From this point on, the clinician should replace the word "seizures" with "episodes" or some other term with which the child feels comfortable.

Discussing the frequency of PPNES and the difficulty doctors have making this diagnosis, with the parents and child separately, helps "normalize" the illness so that the parents and child feel that the child is not unique, unusual, or very impaired. It also serves to assuage parent anger and guilt feelings and relieve the child about how long it took to get the correct diagnosis and how no one understood that psychological factors might be involved in the child's uncontrolled "seizures." In addition, the complex medical nature of the case and time involved in obtaining the diagnosis also provide the child with a "face-saving device" for return to school and providing an explanation to the school, friends, peers, and extended family.

Recommendations and treatment plan. In addition to recommending educational testing to complete the evaluation, the team should outline the medical and psychological treatment plan separately for both the parents and the child with appropriate modifications based on the child's mental and emotional age. Assuming the child does not also have epilepsy, the pediatric neurologist (epileptologist) should provide a schedule for AED tapering/discontinuation (if applicable or unless continuation is warranted for the AED's psychotropic effects), and the mental health clinician should present the aims of the psychological treatment. These aims typically involve a short-term approach to stop the "episodes" so the child can resume regular daily functioning, including school attendance, and a long-term approach to first help the child recognize and verbalize difficulties and then use appropriate and functional problem-solving techniques.

Concurrent work with the parents to help them understand how the child communicates with them about his/her problems and stressors and how they can best encourage and support the child's efforts to problem solve is essential to attain these goals. Treatment of the comorbidities of PPNES should also be discussed and outlined. For children who have psychiatric diagnoses in addition to conversion disorder, the mental health clinician should also describe the relevant treatment approaches (e.g., psychopharmacological treatment and/or cognitive behavioral therapy for depression and anxiety).

Don'ts

None of the team members (e.g., interns, residents, and nurses) should provide any interim diagnostic feedback to the parents or child until both the neurological/VEEG and psychiatric evaluations are completed. In particular, they must refrain from suggesting a possible psychiatric basis to the disorder with parents who are wholly vested in a medical diagnosis before all the results are known and discussed by the team. It is important not to rush the feedback and to allow the parents and child time for questions. Feedback should be given to both parents in a two-parent family. Similarly, a post-feedback processing session will clarify what the parents and child heard, understood, and took away from the feedback. This is imperative to prevent misconceptions and to diffuse parental anger towards the child and/or prior treating physicians, and guilt. Finally, clinicians should not insist on focusing on the psychological basis of the disorder for parents who are wholly invested in a neurological diagnosis.

Summary

The pediatric neurology or epileptology treatment team leader should use a sensitive approach to provide separate feedback to the parents and to the child that highlights the potential of emotional, academic, or social stressors to trigger the seizures, which represent the child's maladaptive attempt to problem solve and/or cry for help. The neurologist and mental health clinician should outline a treatment plan that involves changes in AEDs, a short-term behavioral approach to decrease the frequency of PNES, and a long-term psychological intervention focused on the child's ability to identify difficulties and problem solve as well as the family's role in this process. The team should give the feedback allowing enough time for questions and a post-feedback processing session.

Clinical vignettes

Case 1: parent focus on neurological symptoms and multiple diagnoses

Two years prior to her initial psychiatric assessment, this 17-year-old adolescent female was involved in a car accident in which she was the driver and her younger brother was thrown out of the car. The patient was uninjured and her brother sustained mild injuries. She had previously experienced two "grand mal seizures," one at age 11 years while in a discussion with her father in a restaurant and another at age 14 years while on a school trip for a sports event. Her routine EEG was normal and she received carbamazepine for about two years after the first seizure.

About six months after the car accident, she presented with a variety of neurological impairments that included altered superficial sensations in the limbs, impaired mobility, stiffness, and pain in her back and limbs. She was treated with physical therapy and analgesics and her symptoms underwent remission after about one and a half years. Several months later and shortly after starting twelfth grade, she began to experience memory loss and her neurologist was concerned that this might reflect uncontrolled ES. In contrast to the patient, the mother provided no information on the accident and denied that the patient had current or past mood or other emotional or behavioral symptoms, learning, social or family problems. Her main concern was that the patient was having uncontrolled seizures.

The patient described her memory difficulties in detail, thought she was having seizures, and was very concerned about her memory loss and its impact on her schoolwork and daily activities. For example, she would forget why she was walking down the street or what she needed to buy when in a store. She would also forget what she was talking about in the middle of a sentence. She nevertheless got A's on her final examinations in her Advanced Placement physics and calculus classes.

The patient described estrangement from both her parents, a restrictive and unpleasant home environment in which she, as the female and oldest child, had to do most of the chores, including driving her brothers around because her mother was working. On two occasions when she could no longer tolerate the restrictive environment, she left home for the night but returned because she felt guilty. She also acknowledged frequent crying, losing her temper with her mother, and two suicide attempts in which she swallowed a large number of tablets. When she awoke after these attempts, she told her parents that she had wanted to die. They were angry with her for attempting suicide but sought no professional help for their daughter. The patient denied any posttraumatic symptoms after the car accident and appeared quite unconcerned about what could have happened to her brother when he was thrown from the car. However, she cried frequently when discussing her relationship with her parents, and was hopeless about any change in her relationship with them. She had no social interest, poor appetite, and confirmed occasional suicidal thoughts.

This patient had a neurological evaluation that was normal and routine EEGs that were negative for epileptiform activity. She was given a diagnosis of PNES with dissociative episodes (mimicking memory loss following absence seizures) associated with PTSD, as well as both past and current diagnosis of major depression.

Comments: this case demonstrates the importance of diagnosing conversion disorder even when a patient has additional psychiatric diagnoses. Identification of her primary and comorbid diagnoses was essential to design appropriate short- and long-term combined psychopharmacological and individual therapy to stop the episodes and resolve both the depression and PTSD. In fact, medical treatment of the patient's multiple physical symptoms rather than treatment focused on the underlying conversion disorder was associated with the progression of her disorder to dissociative states.

In terms of the history, the mother's focus on the neurological aspects of the disorder, without mentioning her daughter's past depression, suicide attempts, and difficult relationship with her parents, is striking. Furthermore, the patient's past history of two "grand mal" seizures in socially challenging situations (arguing with her father in a restaurant, being away from home in a socially challenging environment with peers on a sports trip) suggest onset of the PNES even prior to the dissociative episodes of "memory loss."

Case 2: resistance to psychiatric involvement and "seizures = the problem"

This 11-year-old boy had a confirmed diagnosis of epilepsy based on clinical history and right posterior epileptic activity on routine EEG recordings. His pediatric epileptologist first referred him for a psychiatric evaluation to rule out the role of psychological factors for "breakthrough" seizures despite treatment with carbamazepine and that began shortly after the beginning of the school year (six months prior to the psychiatric referral). The father accompanied the patient, but knew little about the child's medical, neurological, and emotional history. He claimed that other than seizures and some mild learning problems, maybe ADHD, the child had no emotional or behavioral problems.

In some detail, the child described his seizures as staring, clonus of the jaw, and subsequent sleep. He voiced his hatred for carbamazepine because it made him sleepy at school and prevented him from doing his work. He, too, denied any problems other than his seizures. Due to increasing frequency of episodes both at school and at home while doing homework, he missed a lot of school and was unable to do his homework. A quick assessment of his basic reading and math skills during the interview suggested that he had learning difficulties. However, the child denied learning problems. His only acknowledged problem was tiredness in class and when he had to do homework, and this was "all because of my medicine." Prior outside neuropsychological testing revealed evidence for a wide range of learning difficulties, confirming the presence of a learning disorder.

Preliminary feedback to the father emphasized that to complete the psychiatric evaluation and determine if psychological factors might play a role in the child's uncontrolled seizures, it was necessary to obtain information from the mother and meet again with the child. The child insisted that his only problem was the medication and that he did not need to "talk any more." The mother and child did not show up for the appointment.

Several months later, the pediatric epileptologist made an emergency referral of the patient to rule out PPNES because the child had experienced repeated seizures and emergency room visits night after night despite changes in AEDs and their dosages, and VEEG had showed no epileptic activity during the captured seizures. Once again the father accompanied the child and described the mother's resistance to psychiatric involvement in the case. However, he maintained that she would come later that day after she picked up their other children from school.

The second interview with the child was similar to the first interview with the exception that he felt he was less tired since replacement of his carbamazepine with lamotrigine and levetiracetam. He now attended a school for children with learning disabilities, claimed that it was a good move and that he was doing well at school. But he added that he missed a lot of school because of his seizures. He repeatedly denied any problem other than his seizures.

When the psychiatrist mentioned that stress could make children's seizures worse, he stared into space for a few seconds. As he "regained consciousness," the psychiatrist rephrased the question, and the child fell asleep. The psychiatrist gently aroused the child who said, "I have had a few seizures." The psychiatrist mentioned that it looks like the patient does not like the word stress and the patient said, "People say all kind of things about stress and faking seizures." When the psychiatrist asked him who had said that he was faking seizures, he lapsed into a deep sleep, and could not be roused.

In the meantime, his mother arrived, and the child awoke and was happy for the psychiatrist to see his parents without him. Aware that the parents appeared divided regarding a possible psychological basis for the child's poor seizure control, the psychiatrist focused on establishing rapport with the mother and determining if, in fact, she was resistant to "a psychological" approach to the case. To help decrease her resistance, the psychiatrist discussed the difficulties parents experience when a child has seizures, particularly when the seizures are not controlled, emphasized the impact on the rest of the family, and highlighted how parents can frequently experience increased tension between them on how to manage and divide their attention equally among their children. The mother reported that the patient's younger brother had asthma with repeated emergency room visits and that she did not have the emotional energy for psychiatric involvement with her child with epilepsy.

Discussing the guilt and torn feelings the parents felt due to the father's involvement with the child with PNES and the mother with the asthmatic child helped foster rapport with the parents. They realized that the physician understood them, did not judge them, and could be trusted to help with their child with PNES. Not surprisingly, once the parents were part of the team, it became easier to establish rapport with the child at the next diagnostic meeting. In response to questions about his learning problems, he again denied any type of difficulty, but was able to acknowledge that he really did not like the school. He then appeared to space out and fell asleep.

Comments: this child had well controlled ES until the development of PNES. From the neurological perspective, this case, therefore, underscores that the PNES of children with epilepsy can go undiagnosed for extensive periods because the parents and physician assume the child has experienced breakthrough seizures. It also highlights the importance of ruling out the possibility of PNES in a child with epilepsy who has breakthrough seizures. To do this, the epileptologist (pediatric neurologist) needs to reassess the diagnosis of epilepsy in terms of re-obtaining a careful history of the pattern of seizures, where and when they occur (their occurrence at school and when mother sat him down to do homework were important diagnostic clues), and possible emotional triggers.

From the psychiatric perspective, this case demonstrates the difficulties involved in penetrating the child's "everything is fine except my seizures" and the mother's resistance to psychiatric involvement. It also describes the approaches used to overcome these obstacles. If the epileptologist had handled the "psychological" aspects of the case, the mother probably would have had less difficulty accepting the psychiatric basis for the child's disorder. Of note, this case also alerts clinicians to the fact that sleep, after what might appear to be a postictal event, can be a conversion symptom.

Case 3: unsuccessful feedback

This 15-year-old ninth grade girl was referred for a psychiatric evaluation following negative VEEG findings and a diagnosis of PPNES given by the epileptologist to the mother and daughter together. The patient, who experienced one "grand mal" seizure at age 11 years treated by a community neurologist with topiramate, had chosen to be the main caretaker of her younger developmentally delayed brother who had poorly controlled generalized tonic-clonic seizures since infancy. Her "breakthrough seizures," which involved sudden screaming and walking around, occurred with increasing frequency and duration at school.

The mother's history revealed no problems other than the girl's seizures, and the mother found it hard to believe that her daughter had PPNES. She also described the patient as an excellent reader even though she was reading fifth grade-level "girlie" fiction books. The patient did not understand the neurologist's feedback about PNES and was very concerned about her seizures. She described herself as a good student who had many friends even though her closest friends were her older sister, who recently began spending most of her time with her boyfriend and peers, and her younger developmentally delayed brother.

The psychiatric evaluation revealed awkward social skills, poor reading comprehension, and difficulties with math, as well as the "everything-is-fine barrier" and significant secondary gain due to being repeatedly sent home from school. The academic and social demands of high school for this girl with learning and social difficulties and the lack of support from her older sister triggered the PNES.

The father was unable to participate in the evaluation due to his busy work schedule, and both he and the community neurologist did not attend the feedback session. The psychiatrist gave separate feedback to the mother and the daughter, and recommended educational testing and treatment. Nevertheless, the mother was concerned about the girl's seizures and did not think she had learning or social difficulties. In contrast, the daughter was "relieved" to hear that someone else understood how much difficulty she was having academically and socially at school, and was highly motivated to get help with these aspects of her life.

Subsequent to the feedback, the community neurologist made no change in the patient's AED treatment even though the psychiatric evaluation confirmed the PPNES diagnosis. The parents also did not pursue the recommendations for educational testing and treatment. The "untreated" patient began to have dissociative episodes in which she wandered off from school and was found on a bus, not knowing who or where she was. The community neurologist who believed the patient had underlying epilepsy as well as PPNES then prescribed multiple AEDs due to repeated "seizures" at school, and the patient became psychotic when given high doses of lamotrigine and levetiracetam.

Comments: this case highlights how lack of teamwork, failure to include both parents in the diagnostic evaluation and feedback, absence of post-feedback processing, and unnecessary treatment with high doses of multiple AEDs can lead to increased PPNES and the development of psychosis. In terms of teamwork, the psychiatrist was not involved in the case during the VEEG, and the epileptologist made a "default" PPNES diagnosis based on lack of positive EEG findings but without considering whether psychiatric symptoms confirmed PPNES. By giving feedback about this diagnosis alone rather than involving the psychiatrist, the epileptologist minimized the importance of the mental health component of the girl's illness for her and her mother. After the patient's discharge, the neurologist increased the dose and number of AEDs but did not redirect the mother's repeated calls about continued "episodes" to the psychiatrist. For both the mother and patient this further confirmed the presence of epilepsy, not PPNES, and increased their resistance to the psychiatrist's treatment and educational recommendations. Not surprisingly, the frequency of PPNES and school absences then increased.

Regarding parental involvement, clarification of the reasons the father did not participate in the diagnostic evaluation and feedback and his role in the family's functioning were essential both for the comprehensive diagnostic evaluation and the treatment planning. Since neither the epileptologist nor the psychiatrist was able to conduct post-feedback processing, the psychiatrist could not adequately understand nor address the level of the mother's resistance to the diagnosis and recommendations. Similarly, post-feedback processing would have been important to clarify the lack of understanding the patient had regarding PPNES, particularly given the resistance the mother (and perhaps the father) had to this diagnosis.

Treatment

In a textbook chapter [50], Aldenkamp and colleagues described a controlled trial comparing adolescent patients with PNES who underwent inpatient behavioral therapy (n = 15), inpatient wait and see or milieu treatment (n = 15), and outpatient treatment by a neurologist (n = 15). Other than a significantly lower seizure frequency in the behavioral therapy group in the first week of treatment, there was no significant difference in seizure frequency in the three treatment arms. There have been no other treatment studies of PPNES.

From the clinical perspective, there are short-term, intermediate, and long-term goals to the treatment of

Table 17.1 Summary of the psychiatric features of PPNES

Diagnosis/Procedure	Features
Primary Psychopathology	High emotional reactivity, poor problem solving
	Displacement and somatic conversion of negative affect (anger, anxiety, sadness) triggered by an underlying conflict or predicament
	Poor family communication
Primary DSM-IV diagnoses	
Conversion Disorder with Seizures	Changing, inconsistent, prolonged "seizures" in the presence of others with no epileptic activity on VEEG
	Denial of emotional distress and negative mood (anger, anxiety, sadness)
	Seizure-related respite from responsibilities (secondary gain) temporarily relieves need to deal with the underlying conflict and perpetuates seizures
	Minimal concern about problems other than seizures
	Secondary somatic complaints and symptoms reflect more severe disorder
Dissociative Disorder	Rare
Factitious Disorder	Rare
Malingering Disorder	Rare
Comorbid psychopathology	
Current	
Anxiety Disorders	Social, academic, and performance anxiety may be perceived through "seizure" symptoms
Depression	With secondary somatic complaints, more severe
Disruptive Behavioral Disorders	ADHD, Oppositional Defiant Disorder
Cognitive and Learning Disorders	
Past	
Preexisting psychopathology	Poorly understood and managed mental health and learning problems may evolve into PPNES
Psychiatric treatment	
Rule out PPNES diagnosis	In the differential diagnosis of all youth with seizures
Diagnostic interview	Separate detailed history from child and parents on the development, pattern, and course of seizure-like events, pattern of controlled seizures prior to onset of PPNES in a child with confirmed epilepsy, medical, emotional, cognitive, linguistic, and social stressors, prior or ongoing abuse, the child's coping and problem solving skills, family functioning, parenting, parents, medical and psychiatric history
Feedback	Joint feedback by team given separately to parents and child on PPNES diagnosis, the psychological elements involved in the development of PPNES, where indicated need for educational testing, and treatment goal to promote the child's healthy adaptive coping with life's stressors
Treatment	Short-term goals include reducing PPNES, tapering AEDs when appropriate, and, if needed, psychopharmacological treatment of comorbidities
	Improved school attendance is an intermediate goal
	Long-term goals focus on helping the child identify and verbalize difficulties and negative feelings and to successfully problem solve. Parallel family therapy goals include acknowledging the child's communications about difficulties and supporting his/her healthy efforts to problem solve

PPNES. The main short-term goal, reduction of the frequency of PNES, is accomplished by integrating a behavioral approach, decrease in AEDs, and efforts to alleviate triggers, with a focus on learning problems, social difficulties, or family stressors. If indicated, psychopharmacological treatment is also initiated for comorbid psychiatric diagnoses. As the frequency of PNES decreases, the intermediate goal, school attendance, is achieved through assessment of the child's educational needs and close work with the teachers.

The Appendix includes a clinician's template letter for communicating with school departments regarding PPNES.

The long-term individual psychotherapy goals are for the child to recognize, identify, and verbalize his/her difficulties or negative feelings and learn to successfully problem solve. Parallel family therapy is essential to help the parents "hear" and acknowledge the child's difficulties and provide the support needed to ensure that the child problem solves successfully and no longer "communicates" about ongoing difficulties through physical symptoms, such as PNES.

Cooperation and communication between the child's epilepsy and mental health professionals is essential during the short-term treatment phase of PPNES. The need for continued long-term work with the epilepsy team varies in individual cases but is essential in children who also have ES.

Conclusions

Given the clinical morbidity and poor long-term psychosocial outcome of untreated PPNES, this diagnosis should be part of the differential diagnosis of every child or adolescent with seizures. As summarized in Table 17.1, the most common psychiatric features of PPNES include conversion disorder as the primary diagnosis with or without comorbid psychiatric diagnoses such as depression, anxiety, and disruptive disorders.

To diagnose conversion disorder in PPNES, it is necessary to document seizure-like behaviors but no epileptic activity on VEEG and identify the psychiatric hallmark of this syndrome, the denial of any ongoing stressors or intrapsychic distress, such as anger, anxiety, and sadness (i.e., negative affect). Key elements supporting this diagnosis include a history of a changing and inconsistent pattern of "prolonged seizures" that occur only in the presence of other people, as well as minimal concern about ongoing problems and temporary respite from responsibilities (i.e., secondary gain) including school attendance, homework, chores, participation in competitive activities, and others.

The main clinical challenge to diagnosing PPNES and clarifying the nature of the primary pathology (underlying conflict) is the "everything is fine other than seizures" barrier put up by the child and frequently also by the parents. However, a detailed history of the child's seizures, sensitive assessment of possible emotional, cognitive, linguistic, social, abuse, familial, and other stressors in the child's life, the child's coping patterns, and family functioning obtained separately from the child and parents provide the information needed to make this diagnosis.

Joint feedback by the epileptologist (pediatric neurologist) and mental health clinician given separately to the parents and child informs them of the PPNES diagnosis, explains the nature of the disorder, clarifies how it has developed in the patient, and outlines the treatment recommendations. During this process, the team underscores that the psychological basis for this disorder should not be confused with "faking" and that psychological/psychiatric treatment is essential to resolve the seizures and promote the child's healthy adaptive coping and problem solving with life's stressors. Treatment consists of short-term goals for reducing PNES, tapering AEDs when appropriate, and addressing comorbidities. Return to school or improvement of school attendance is an intermediate goal. The long-term psychotherapy goals are for the child to recognize, identify, and verbalize his/her difficulties or negative feelings and successfully problem solve. Parallel family therapy helps the parents "hear" and acknowledge the child's difficulties and, if indicated, provide the support needed to ensure adaptive rather than maladaptive problem solving through physical symptoms, such as PNES. Cooperation and communication between the child's epilepsy and mental health professionals is essential for successful diagnosis, feedback, and treatment of youth with PNES.

References

1. Cadoret R, Winokur G, Langbehn D, et al. Depression spectrum disease, I: The role of gene-environment interaction. *Am J Psychiatry* 1996;**153**:892–9.
2. Carmant L, Kramer U, Holmes GL, et al. Differential diagnosis of staring spells in children: a video-EEG study. *Pediatr Neurol* 1996;**14**:199–202.
3. Kraemer H, Stice E, Kazdin A, Offord D, Kupfer D. How do risk factors work together? Mediators, moderators, and independent, overlapping, and proxy risk factors. *Am J Psychiatry* 2001;**158**:848–56.
4. Rutter M. Categories, dimensions, and the mental health of children and adolescents. *Ann NY Acad Sci* 2003;**1008**:11–21.
5. LaFrance Jr WC, Alper K, Babcock D, et al. Nonepileptic seizures treatment workshop summary. *Epilepsy Behav* 2006;**8**:451–61.
6. Bhatia MS, Sapra S. Pseudoseizures in children: a profile of 50 cases. *Clin Pediatr (Phila)* 2005;**44**: 617–21.
7. Lancman ME, Asconape JJ, Graves S, Gibson PA. Psychogenic seizures in children: long-term analysis of 43 cases. *J Child Neurol* 1994;**9**:404–7.
8. Pakalnis A, Paolicchi J, Gilles E. Psychogenic status epilepticus in children: psychiatric and other risk factors. *Neurology* 2000;**54**:969–70.

9. Papavasiliou A, Vassilaki N, Paraskevoulakos E, et al. Psychogenic status epilepticus in children. *Epilepsy Behav* 2004;**5**:539–46.

10. Vincentiis S, Valente KD, Thomé-Souza S, et al. Risk factors for psychogenic nonepileptic seizures in children and adolescents with epilepsy. *Epilepsy Behav* 2006;**8**:294–8.

11. Wyllie E, Friedman D, Luders H, et al. Outcome of psychogenic seizures in children and adolescents compared with adults. *Neurology* 1991;**41**:742–4.

12. Gudmundsson O, Prendergast M, Foreman D, Cowley S. Outcome of pseudoseizures in children and adolescents: a 6-year symptom survival analysis. *Dev Med Child Neurol* 2001;**43**:547–51.

13. Kotagal P, Costa M, Wyllie E, Wolgamuth B. Paroxysmal nonepileptic events in children and adolescents. *Pediatrics* 2002;**110**:e46.

14. Kramer U, Carmant L, Riviello JJ, et al. Psychogenic seizures: video telemetry observations in 27 patients *Pediatr Neurol* 1995;**12**:39–41.

15. Pakalnis A, Paolicchi J. Frequency of secondary conversion symptoms in children with psychogenic nonepileptic seizures. *Epilepsy Behav* 2003;**4**:753–6.

16. Patel H, Scott E, Dunn D, Garg B. Nonepileptic seizures in children. *Epilepsia* 2007;**48**:2086–92.

17. Wyllie E, Glazer JP, Benbadis S, Kotagal P, Wolgamuth B. Psychiatric features of children and adolescents with pseudoseizures. *Arch Pediatr Adolesc Med* 1999;**153**:244–8.

18. Plioplys S. Epidemiological, clinical, and developmental characteristics of pediatric psychogenic nonepileptic seizures. *Sci Proc: Am Acad Child Adolesc Psychiatry* 2006;**33**:115.

19. Bye A, Kok DJ, Ferenschild FT, Vles JS. Paroxysmal nonepileptic events in children: a retrospective study over a period of 10 years. *J Paediatr Child Health* 2000;**36**:244–8.

20. Montenegro MA, Sproule D, Mandel A, et al. The frequency of nonepileptic spells in children: results of video-EEG monitoring in a tertiary care center. *Seizure* 2008;**17**:583–7.

21. Plioplys S, Asato MR, Bursch B, et al. Multidisciplinary management of pediatric nonepileptic seizures *J Am Acad Child Adolesc Psychiatry* 2007;**46**:1491–5.

22. Boyce W, Ellis BJ. Biological sensitivity to context: I. An evolutionary-developmental theory of the origins and functions of stress reactivity. *Dev Psychopathol* 2005;**17**:271–301.

23. Essex M, Kraemer HC, Armstrong JM, et al. Exploring risk factors for the emergence of children's mental health problems. *Arch Gen Psychiatry* 2006;**63**:1246–55.

24. Kozlowska K. The developmental origins of conversion disorders. *Clin Child Psychol Psychiatry* 2007;**12**:487–510.

25. Irwin K, Edwards M, Robinson R. Psychogenic nonepileptic seizures: management and prognosis. *Arch Dis Child* 2000;**82**:474–8.

26. Pakalnis A, Paolicchi J. Psychogenic seizures after head injury in children. *J Child Neurol* 2000;**15**:78–80.

27. Wyllie E, Friedman D, Rothner AD, et al. Psychogenic seizures in children and adolescents: outcome after diagnosis by ictal video and electroencephalographic recording. *Pediatrics* 1990;**85**:480–4.

28. Goodyer I, Taylor DC. Hysteria. *Arch Dis Child* **60**:680–1.

29. Stuart S, Noyes R. Attachment and interpersonal communication in somatization. *Pychosomatics* 1999;**40**:34–43.

30. Srinath S, Bharat S, Girimaji S, Seshadri S. Characteristics of a child inpatient population with hysteria in India. *J Am Acad Child Adolesc Psychiatry* 1993;**32**:822–5.

31. American Psychiatric Association. *Diagnostic and Statistical Manual of Mental Disorders*, 4th edn. (DSM-IV). Washington, DC: American Psychiatric Association, 1994.

32. Plioplys S, Siddarth P, Asato M, et al. Psychological and medical features of parents of children with nonepileptic events (NEE) versus epilepsy. *Sci Proc: Am Acad Child Adolesc Psychiatry* 2008;**35**:227.

33. Reuber M, Pukrop R, Bauer J, et al. Outcome in psychogenic nonepileptic seizures: 1 to 10-year follow-up in 164 patients. *Ann Neurol* 2003;**53**:305–11.

34. Campo J, Bridge J, Ehmann M, et al. Recurrent abdominal pain, anxiety, and depression in primary care. *Pediatrics* 2004;**113**:817–24.

35. Millikan E, Wamboldt MZ, Bihun JT. Perceptions of the family, personality characteristics, and adolescent internalizing symptoms. *J Am Acad Child Adolesc Psychiatry* 2002;**41**:1486–94.

36. Neiderhiser J, Pike A, Hetherington EM, Reiss D. Adolescent perceptions as mediators of parenting: genetic and environmental contributions. *Dev Psychol* 1998;**34**:1459–69.

37. Crittenden P. A dynamic-maturational model of attachment. *Aust NZ J Fam Therapy* 2006;**27**:105–15.

38. Crittenden P. Attachment and risk for psychopathology: the early years. *J Dev Behav Pediatr* 1995;**16**:12–16.

39. Kozlowska K, Nunn KP, et al. Conversion disorder in Australian pediatric practice. *J Am Acad Child Adolesc Psychiatry* 2007;**46**:68–75.

40. Taylor D. The sick child's predicament. *Aust N Z J Psychiatry* 1985;**19**:130–7.
41. American Psychiatric Association. *Diagnostic and Statistical Manual of Mental Disorders*, 4th edn., Text Revision (DSM-IV-TR). Washington, DC: American Psychiatric Association, 2000.
42. Plioplys S, Szwed S, Varn M. Psychiatric problems in children with psychogenic nonepileptic seizures (NES). *Epilepsia* 2005;**46** Suppl 8:159.
43. Perry B, Pollard R. Homeostasis, stress, trauma and adaptation – a neurodevelopmental view of childhood trauma. *Child Adolesc Psychiatr Clin N Am* 1998;**7**:33–51.
44. Kisiel C, Lyons JS. Dissociation as a mediator of psychopathology among sexually abused children and adolescents. *Am J Psychiatry* 2001;**58**:1034–9.
45. Yeager C, Lewis DO. Mental illness, neuropsychologic deficits, child abuse, and violence. *Child Adolesc Psychiatr Clin N Am* 2000;**9**:793–813.
46. Plioplys S. Children with psychogenic nonepileptic seizures – high incidence of comorbid medical illnesses. *Sci Proc: Am Acad Child Adolesc Psychiatry* 2006;**33**:235.
47. Achenbach T. *Manual for the Child Behavior Checklist and Revised Child Behavior Profile*. Vermont: Department of Psychiatry, University of Vermont, 1991.
48. Salpekar J, Siddarth P, Plioplys S, et al. Behavioral profiles of children with nonepileptic events versus epilepsy. *Epilepsia* 2008;**49** Suppl 7:269.
49. Loring DW, Meador KJ. Cognitive side effects of antiepileptic drugs in children. *Neurology* 2004;**62**:872–7.
50. Aldenkamp AP, Mulder OG. Pseudoepileptic seizures in adolescents. In: Manelis J, Bental E, Loeber JN, Dreifuss FE, eds. *Advances in Epileptology: XVIIth Epilepsy International Symposium*. New York: Raven Press. 1989; 445–9.

Section 3 Chapter 18

Psychiatric and neuropsychological considerations in children and adolescents with psychogenic nonepileptic seizures

Neuropsychological and psychological aspects of children presenting with psychogenic nonepileptic seizures

Ann Hempel, Julia Doss, and Elizabeth Adams

Children presenting with psychogenic nonepileptic seizures (PNES) pose a challenge to healthcare professionals, largely given the complexity and multitude of physical and psychological variables that need to be clarified in order to establish the correct diagnosis and guide appropriate treatment planning. Video-EEG (VEEG) recording remains the main physiological assessment tool for ruling out epileptiform discharges or other electrographic abnormalities as possible etiologies for the patient's symptoms [1]. Cognitive evaluations [2] and psychological assessments are an invaluable supplement to the diagnostic process, because they provide the opportunity to clarify nonphysiological factors that may underlie and/or contribute to the manifestation of physical symptoms that do not have a clear physiological basis. A combination of VEEG recording, cognitive evaluation, and psychological assessment therefore provide the optimal standard of care for differentiating PNES from epileptic seizures (ES).

Nonepileptic seizures are but one type of symptom with which a psychogenic disorder, a presumptive conversion disorder, can present. Patients with PNES often present with a history of acute and/or chronic stressors that have challenged their coping capabilities. Though not diagnostic in itself, a history of multiple stressors may be one discriminating factor, in addition to normal EEG findings, that differentiates the PNES group, as a whole, from pediatric patients with ES [3]. While it is widely accepted that adult patients with PNES present with histories of both family difficulties and psychopathology [4, 5], this has been less frequently examined in the pediatric population.

Academic difficulties were among the most frequently reported stressors for conversion disorders in pediatric patients in several previous studies [6, 7]. Bowman [8] reported on early research on PNES, and indicated that the early studies, which were often in the form of case reports, suggested that whether PNES were of childhood or adult onset, they were often preceded by a traumatic event, such as child abuse. In a review of the literature from the 1980s and early 1990s, it was found that, across studies, 38% of pediatric patients with conversion disorders displayed a comorbid psychological condition, 36% experienced school problems, and 64% had a background of psychopathology in family members [3]. This review also demonstrated that while a history of sexual abuse was not uncommon in this group, when studies were aggregated, only 17% were found to experience a sexual stressor, which was not higher than the general population base rate at that time [9]. Several recent studies demonstrated that some patients with PNES do have a history of childhood physical and sexual trauma, though this does not characterize all or even most of the persons who develop PNES [10, 11]. More recent research suggests that psychological stress can be subtle, persistent, and chronic [12, 13, 14].

Consideration of both the individual and his/her family system is essential in the assessment and treatment of pediatric patients with PNES. Family conflict was the most frequently reported psychosocial stressor in a study of pediatric patients with conversion disorder at a Chinese hospital [14]. Results of our own patient sample [3] documented a higher proportion of patients with PNES experiencing family conflict (45%) relative to a sample of children with ES (11%), whereas similar rates of school problems (70% and 67%), peer relationship problems (45% and 37%) and below-average IQ (40% and 44%) were

Gates and Rowan's Nonepileptic Seizures, 3rd edn. ed. Steven C. Schachter and W. Curt LaFrance, Jr. Published by Cambridge University Press. © S. Schachter and W. C. LaFrance, Jr. 2010.

observed in patients with PNES and ES. This finding was confirmed by a subsequent study that found family psychopathology to be more prevalent among patients with PNES than in those with ES alone [15].

Since the printing of the second edition of this book, subsequent studies on conversion disorder or PNES have been largely consistent with previous findings. Anxiety regarding school or academic testing was relatively common (30%) among one sample of patients with PNES [16]. Both family and school problems were common in a Japanese sample [17]. Acute stressors remain possible contributing factors in many children/adolescents, however. For example, in a recent study, trauma, family problems, and bereavement were identified as some of the most salient characteristics in the histories of patients with PNES [5].

While current literature examining treatment outcome in pediatric patients with PNES is sparse, one study showed that severity of comorbid psychopathology is one of the strongest predictors of prognosis in children who present with PNES [18]. Thus, consideration of psychiatric problems, often identified prior to onset of PNES symptoms [19], is essential for both initial evaluation and ongoing treatment planning. However, it is important to note that, in our previous study [3], the most common comorbid psychiatric or behavioral diagnosis among children in both the ES and PNES groups was a disruptive behavior disorder such as ADHD. Nearly half of those in each patient group evidenced a disruptive behavior disorder. These data suggest that, contrary to clinical lore, "internalizing" psychological disorders (e.g., depression or anxiety) does not necessarily precede psychogenic physical symptoms.

Taken together, currently available data suggest that patients with PNES may be distinct from the sample with ES by virtue of increased psychopathology within the family, increased incidence of comorbid psychological conditions within the child, and recent experience of emotionally taxing events. However, previous findings also indicate a high incidence of cognitive/learning and peer relationship difficulties among both patients with PNES and patients with ES. It may be helpful to know that patients with PNES and those with ES often experience learning and peer relationship problems, and that this may be an important source of psychological stress that needs to be mitigated in these groups. The presence of a learning disability in itself, however, is unhelpful in clarifying the PNES diagnosis, as the base rate of learning disabilities in the general population is high. For example, the prevalence of dyslexia has been estimated at 17.5% in the general population [20].

To re-examine the nature of the cognitive and academic difficulties commonly experienced by pediatric patients with PNES, we describe a sample of our patients. We will also describe psychosocial stressors and comorbid psychiatric diagnoses commonly observed in our sample, particularly when there is an absence of significant learning or cognitive problems.

Study methods

The records of 15 child and adolescent patients with PNES were reviewed retrospectively. These patients were admitted to the epilepsy unit for long-term VEEG monitoring to clarify whether their possible seizure episodes were epileptic or nonepileptic. Patients were included in the sample if they were intellectually normal (IQ $\geq$ 70), evidenced a normal interictal EEG, and did not have a history of neurological insult. Magnetic resonance imaging was normal in all patients who had this procedure as part of their workup, with the exception of one patient whose study revealed an otherwise asymptomatic Chiari I malformation. In all patients the typical seizure-like event was recorded on EEG, and was not found to be associated with epileptiform activity.

Patients were also included in the sample if they underwent some form of cognitive testing. When possible, all patients suspected of PNES were referred for neuropsychological testing unless logistical factors (patient seen on a weekend when psychology staff members were unavailable) precluded a cognitive assessment. In addition, all patients received a psychological evaluation consisting of a diagnostic interview and behavior rating scales and/or self-report psychological measures, either as part of a separate psychological assessment or as a component of the neuropsychological evaluation. Because the patients did not have a history of a neurological condition, an abbreviated battery of cognitive measures was administered to assess intellectual functioning, academic skills and sustained attention.

Patients were administered either a short form or a full Wechsler Intelligence Scale for Children – Third or Fourth Edition [21] to assess intellectual development. They were also administered selected subtests of the Woodcock-Johnson Tests of Achievement – Third

Table 18.1 Patient characteristics

Number of females	13
Number of males	2
Mean age (range)	14 years (11–16)
Mean age at onset of PNES (range)	13.6 years (11–16)
Number of patients with duration of PNES ≤ 12 months	13
Number of patients with duration of PNES > 12 months	2

Table 18.2 Percentage of patients with PNES evidencing each diagnosis

Diagnosis	N	% of sample
ADHD/ADD	4	27
Reading disability	2	13
Mathematics disorder	5	33
Disorder of written language	2	13
ADHD and/or learning disability	7	47
Any cognitive[a]	10	67

[a] Any cognitive = Confirmed or suspected attention deficit or learning disability.

Table 18.3 Cognitive performance of patients with PNES

Scale/Subject	N	mean	SD	range
VIQ	15	99	10	83–123
PIQ	15	99	12	75–119
FSIQ	14	99	9.9	83–114
Letter-word identification	11	97	10.1	78–116
Calculation	15	99	14.3	79–124
Math fluency	13	89	15.3	64–122
Spelling	11	98	11.4	77–114

V, Verbal; P, Performance; FS, Full Scale.

Table 18.4 Number of patients performing at least one grade level below grade placement

Subject	N	% of sample
Letter-word	5	33
Calculation	6	40
Math fluency	9	60
Spelling	5	33

Edition [22] to assess basic academic skills. Additional measures of reading and written language skills and the Gordon Diagnostic System [23] were administered as needed to clarify a learning disability or attention deficit diagnosis, respectively.

Results

Table 18.1 presents data on the background characteristics of the patient sample. Most patients were female (87%), and all but one patient were between the ages of 12 and 16 at the time of the neuropsychological evaluation (93%). The majority of the patients had experienced symptoms for less than 12 months. Twelve patients presented with some shaking or twitching of extremities, usually accompanied by unresponsiveness, although those who displayed movements of extremities as one aspect of their symptoms often experienced other physical symptoms, such as headache, hyperventilation, nausea, dizziness, eye-fluttering, and light-headedness. The three remaining patients displayed unresponsiveness, which was accompanied by staring in one patient, by falling and "blacking out" in one patient, and by head rolling in one patient.

Only three patients were of low normal intellectual development (IQ = 80 to 89). The remaining 12 patients were of average or better IQ. Seven patients (47%) experienced at least one formally diagnosed learning disability or had ADHD. However, an additional five patients displayed sufficiently prominent learning or attention problems to suggest at least a provisional diagnosis of a learning disability or attention deficit; in these patients there was insufficient information available at the time of neuropsychological evaluation to confirm a formal diagnosis. In total, ten patients (67%) evidenced prominent attention or learning problems in some form (Table 18.2).

It should be noted that the mean standard scores on tests of academic skills were often in the normal range (Table 18.3), whereas number of grade levels below grade placement were often significant, and appeared to more fully convey the extent of the patients' skill weaknesses. Table 18.4 indicates that a high proportion of the sample experienced underachievement of at least one grade level in each basic academic skill area.

Not surprisingly, a large proportion of patients experienced at least one psychological stressor, independent of the expected school problems in those with learning or attention problems (Table 18.5). Peer relationship problems (e.g., peer rejection, bullying, exclusion from activities) was the most common stressor experienced by the group as a whole (73%). One

Table 18.5 Percentage of patients with PNES experiencing each stressor

Stressor	N	% of sample
Parent/child conflict	3	20
Parental psychopathology	6	40
Parental alcohol dependence	0	0
Parental marital discord	2	13
School problems	10	67
Peer relationship problems	11	73
Sexual stressor[a]	2	13
History of parental divorce/separation	2	13
High parental or child expectations	2	13
Parent emotionally unavailable	3	20
Recent loss (e.g., death of grandparent, pet)	4	27
Low-average FSIQ (80–89)	3	20

Average number of stressors per patient = 3.2, SD = 2.0

[a] Any inappropriate or unwanted sexual contact with a peer or relative.
FSIQ, Full Scale Intelligence Quotient.

Table 18.6 Percentage of patients with PNES evidencing psychiatric diagnosis

Diagnosis	N	% of sample
Anxiety disorder	8	53
Depressive disorder	5	33
Anxiety or depressive disorder	9	60
Any cognitive[a] **and** Anx/Dep[b]	6	40
Any cognitive[a] **or** Anx/Dep[b]	14	93

[a] Any cognitive = Confirmed or suspected attention deficit or learning disability.
[b] Anx/Dep = Either anxiety or depressive disorder.

patient experienced relational aggression to the extent that the school environment no longer felt safe. Due to this patient excelling academically and wanting to attend college, there seemed little other choice but to remain in this environment or jeopardize the chances of attending the college of choice. Other patients described pervasive peer rejection, resulting in little to no daily interaction with peers that was considered positive. There were only two patients whose stressors appeared to be limited to attention or learning problems.

The second most common type of stressor was parental psychopathology, with 40% of all patients experiencing this. In those children whose parents experienced psychopathology, history of anxiety disorder was most prevalent, with four patients' mothers or fathers experiencing panic attacks. History of parental depression was also common. It was common for the patients with PNES to experience some form of stressor relating to their parents (47%), either in the form of parent/child conflict, parental psychopathology, or parental unavailability. For example, one patient felt pressure to be the one "normal" child in a family whose members experienced considerable psychological distress. Another patient had an otherwise supportive parent whose time was inordinately consumed by having to care for the patient's chronically ill sibling.

Seven patients experienced two or more stressors apart from school issues. Some of these issues included loss of contact with one biological parent, history of sexual assault, parent emotional unavailability, or excessive parental expectations for behavior and achievement. Of those patients who experienced multiple stressors, recent loss, including death of a grandparent or pet, was described as being quite distressing. One patient, who suffered from significant peer rejection, described the death of the family dog as completely overwhelming, resulting in inability to function for some time afterward. Emotional unavailability by a parent was also significant. Reasons for this unavailability ranged from the parent caring for other siblings to the parent not recognizing the impact of certain stressors the patient was identifying.

Table 18.6 indicates the number of patients in our sample with an anxiety or depressive disorder of some kind. Both were found to be common conditions, and most patients (60%) evidenced either an anxiety or depressive disorder. Forty percent of the patients displayed both a cognitive condition and an anxiety or depressive disorder. Of the five patients who displayed an absence of learning or attentional issues, all but one had either an anxiety or depressive disorder. Prominent in this subgroup of patients was the relative lack of awareness or acknowledgment by the patient of significant social stressors, such as peer rejection. While social relationships seemed a particular struggle in this subgroup, they were frequently functioning at an average or above average level academically. Also, each of the patients who did not demonstrate learning or attentional issues had at least one first-degree relative with a history of an anxiety disorder.

Discussion

Results from our most recent sample of pediatric patients with PNES are compatible with our previous findings [3]. We once again found a surprisingly large proportion of patients with PNES who, on careful assessment, were found to have a developmental cognitive condition, such as a specific learning disability or a form of ADHD. Somewhat fewer patients in our present sample (20%) than in the previous study (40%) had a below-normal IQ, suggesting that generally limited cognitive aptitude can accompany PNES, but is not the norm. As in our previous study, we found that most patients with PNES and ADHD or learning disability also experienced prominent psychosocial stressors outside of the academic/school domain. Peer relationship and parent factors were the most common psychological stressors independent of learning or attention problems, which is not surprising given that peer and family life constitute most children's major life domains. In some children the stressors were often subtle, and not readily acknowledged by parents or patients, whereas in other children there was such a plethora of stressors as to challenge even the most sanguine individual's ability to cope.

Nearly half of those patients with a developmental learning or attention problem also experienced an anxiety or depressive disorder. The majority of the sample as a whole displayed either a depressive or anxiety disorder, whether or not there were also learning or attentional difficulties, although it is unclear to what extent these internalizing psychological disorders may have been secondary to, or coincident with, persistent stressors or could be considered primary conditions. In the majority of these cases, the stressors occurred prior to the reported onset of the psychological symptoms. This implies that the stressors were a factor in the later development of the internalizing disorders.

Current findings suggesting that learning disabilities and attentional difficulties are common in the pediatric PNES population, and that these patients often experience multiple chronic psychosocial stressors, are hardly novel revelations. Academic difficulties are common among pediatric patients with conversion disorders in general [6, 24]. Previous studies have also indicated that the presence of multiple psychosocial stressors are typical of PNES more so than in pediatric patients with ES [3, 13]. Our findings once again demonstrate that, although PNES are sometimes preceded by a traumatic event, children with PNES are more likely to experience mundane and chronic psychological stressors, such as school and peer difficulties and family discord. A history of sexual abuse is present in some patients with PNES [13], but our results again suggest that the incidence of sexual abuse in these patients does not appear to exceed the population base rate. Even with the presence of chronic stressors in our sample, there was often a recent history of a particularly poignant stressor, such as death of a grandparent, or departure for college of an emotionally supportive older sibling, that, although not highly traumatic in the usual sense, may have made the difference between the patient coping or failing to cope with other stressors.

It remains unclear to what extent patients with PNES might be unaware of their psychological distress, and either consciously or subconsciously express this unacknowledged distress in the form of physical symptoms. It is equally unclear to what extent they may be fully aware of psychological stress, and capable of expressing their feelings, but do not have a receptive and empathic audience among family members or friends, or perceive their support systems as lacking in this regard. Among the minority who did not have ADHD or specific learning disabilities, there appeared to be a lack of acknowledgment or awareness of psychosocial stressors, or the stressors, when acknowledged by the adolescent, were either unknown to the parents or perceived to be benign.

Implications for diagnosis and treatment

As in previous studies on PNES and conversion disorder [12], the majority of our sample was female and adolescent age. Nonepileptic seizures were of recent onset, typically less than one year in duration at the time of evaluation. Hence, in addition to symptom presentation that is atypical of ES, older age of onset than is usually seen in pediatric patients with ES and recent age of onset should heighten the treating pediatric neurologist's attention to the possibility that a patient's events could be psychogenic in nature [3, 24].

Current results support our previous recommendation that, because learning and attention problems are so common in the PNES population, patients should routinely be referred for a neuropsychological assessment to evaluate for these conditions, even when patients' or parents' first instinct is to assure the clinician that there are no problems in these regards. Careful enumeration of other possible psychosocial stressors, including the role of family dynamics, and assessment for an anxiety or depressive disorder should also be considered the standard of care for evaluation of possible PNES. Ideally, this should occur over multiple interview sessions, to allow sufficient time to develop rapport with patients and family members who may be reticent to disclose uncomfortable feelings or stressors that may directly or indirectly contribute to the current symptom presentation [25]. Merely diagnosing the events as nonepileptic on the basis of EEG recording and sending the patient home without an appropriate plan does a disservice to the patient and the family.

The family system sometimes inadvertently maintains stress or internal conflict underlying a child's PNES. For example, other urgent or acute issues (e.g., divorce, a relative's passing, a sibling's illness, a parent's psychological distress) may obscure parents' awareness of a child's seemingly mild or chronic stress, thus limiting parents' capacity to attend to the relatively less pressing needs of the child. Families with one or more medically ill children are particularly vulnerable to overlooking the needs of the sibling whose suffering is emotional rather than physiological. Children in these situations often perceive that, in comparison to the problems of family members, their concerns are minimal and might be discounted or overlooked if brought to parents' attention. Therefore, the clinician should maintain awareness of the family system, as seemingly unrelated systemic issues could directly or indirectly influence the child's ability to cope.

Children who adapt to potentially distressing situations and appear unscathed to the outside observer can still have a very real subjective experience of stress. Common reactions to stress include insomnia/hypersomnia, headaches, and gastrointestinal problems. PNES can also be conceptualized as a somatic response to overwhelming and sometimes unrecognized stress. Therefore, physicians and other clinicians should approach each patient with PNES with careful consideration of issues that are particularly salient for the individual, bearing in mind that some or all of the presenting concerns may appear relatively mild and/or irrelevant to the current symptom cluster. As with many other psychogenic disorders, it may be the patient's perception and subjective experience of the stressor, not necessarily the nature of the stressor itself, that underlies the maladaptive coping reaction. This may require multiple or extended interview sessions with the child, to allow opportunity for him/her to express thoughts or feelings that he/she may assume would be perceived as unimportant.

There are a host of issues on which to provide the family assistance. Accepting the diagnosis can be difficult, particularly when extended family and community members have rallied about the patient in support of a presumed physical disorder [25]. Parents may have concern about how to inform others of the diagnosis in a face-saving manner and what family, friends, and community members might think about a PNES diagnosis. Parents may have a persisting concern that the events might still have a physiological basis, or may feel they are inadequate as parents for overlooking or minimizing the extent of the child's psychological distress. A PNES diagnosis may contradict the child's and/or family's perception of the child's identity as an "epileptic [26]," and pose the perhaps greater challenge of helping the child to cope with difficult emotions and stressors that heretofore may have been discussed minimally in the context of routine family conversations. As such, therapeutic intervention with the family is usually an integral part of the evaluation and treatment process. Family therapy could provide a framework for developing appropriate communication between family members, empathic and nonjudgmental acceptance of emotional distress, and adaptive management of family conflict [15]. Therapy may provide resources for the parents to better understand and manage their child's symptoms. It is also necessary to provide strategies for coping with those family issues that contribute to maintenance of the symptoms.

Comorbid depressive and anxiety disorders, if present and not treated, could impact the effective management of the PNES symptoms [19]. A thorough psychological evaluation is an integral part of the initial PNES evaluation, as uncovering comorbid disorders aids in understanding the patient's symptoms and planning for treatment. Therapeutic interventions must address both family dynamics and psychological symptoms associated with comorbid psychopathologies. Strategies may include developing appropriate anxiety reduction techniques aimed both at addressing the PNES symptoms while also managing the underlying stressors. A trial of psychotropic medications may prove helpful in managing mood symptoms as well.

Although providing the family and child with psychotherapeutic strategies to enhance more adaptive coping is a primary treatment aim, meaningful changes to the child's academic environment are equally important. Realistic and truly helpful accommodations for learning disabilities and attention problems should be considered. These might include such provisions as decreased length or quantity of assignments without sacrificing mastery of content, extended time on some tests, note-taking assistance, and resource room support or individualized assistance for particularly challenging subject areas. In addition, school-based support systems should be implemented to provide the student with guidance in managing peer interactions, especially when he/she is at risk for bullying or being bullied. Extracurricular activities such as sports, musical groups, and student government are often helpful in encouraging development of positive peer relationships.

Summary

Empirical findings demonstrate that pediatric patients with PNES, as a group, share certain clinical characteristics, such as comorbid psychological conditions, academic or attentional difficulties, relationship conflicts, and family history of psychopathology. One or a combination of several characteristics could precede and maintain the symptoms of PNES.

Because pediatric patients with PNES often do not demonstrate severe academic problems, it is important to consider the psychological impact of even the mildest or well circumscribed learning difficulties. This is particularly salient for children whose academic performances produce satisfactory grades but require excessive effort, and for children with normal to low normal academic aptitude whose immediate family members have demonstrated above normal achievements. Children often feel ashamed about their school struggles, and subsequently work harder to avoid being recognized by parents or teachers.

Taken together, evaluation of the pediatric patient with PNES requires thorough understanding of the individual's experience of stress. Though the child's academic, emotional, social, or family challenges may seem mild or irrelevant to the outside observer, it is the child's perception, not necessarily the objective situation, that remains the crux of successful assessment and treatment planning. Careful listening without expectation or judgment may facilitate accurate diagnosis and effective treatment of the child with PNES.

References

1. Krebs PP. Psychogenic seizures. *Am J Electroneurodiagnostic Technol* 2007;**47**(1):20–8.
2. Drane DL, Williamson DJ, Stroup ES, *et al.* Cognitive impairment is not equal in patients with epileptic and psychogenic nonepileptic seizures. *Epilepsia* 2006; **47**:1879–86.
3. Hempel, A. Cognitive features and predisposing factors in children with psychogenic seizures. In: Gates JR, Rowan AJ, eds. *Non-Epileptic Seizures*. Boston, MA: Butterworth-Heinemann. 2000; 185–95.
4. Binzer M, Stone J, Sharpe M. Recent onset pseudoseizures: clues to aetiology. *Seizure* 2003;**13**: 146–55.
5. Reuber M, Howlett S, Khan A, Grunwald P. Non-Epileptic seizures and other functional neurological symptoms: predisposing, precipitating, and perpetuating factors. *Psychosomatics* 2007; **48**:230–8.
6. Silver LB. Conversion disorder with pseudoseizures in adolescence: a stress reaction to unrecognized and untreated learning disabilities. *J Am Acad Child Psychiatry* 1982;**21**:508–12.
7. Wynick S, Hobson RP, Jones RB. Psychogenic disorders of vision in childhood ("visual conversion reactions"): perspectives from adolescence: a research note. *J Child Psychol Psychiatry* 1997;**38**:375–9.
8. Bowman ES. Relationship of remote and recent life events to the onset and course of non-epileptic seizures. In Gates JR, Rowan AJ, eds. *Non-Epileptic Seizures*. Boston, MA: Butterworth-Heinemann. 2000; 269–84.
9. Finkelhor D, Hotaling G, Lewis IA, Smith C. Sexual abuse in a national survey of adult men and women: prevalence, characteristics, and risk factors. *Child Abuse Negl* 1990;**14**:9–28.
10. Reuber M, Pukrop R, Bauer J, Derfuss C, Elger C. Multidimensional assessment of personality in patients with psychogenic non-epileptic seizures. *J Neurol Neurosurg Psychiatry* 2004;**75**:743–8.
11. Sharpe D, Faye C. Non-epileptic seizures and child sexual abuse: a critical review of the literature. *Clin Psychol Rev* 2005;**26**:1020–40.
12. Leary PM. Conversion disorder in childhood – diagnosed too late, investigated too much? *J R Soc Med* 2003;**96**:436–8.
13. Williams J, Grant ML. Characteristics of pediatric non-epileptic seizure patients: a retrospective study. In: Gates JR, Rowan AJ, eds. *Non-Epileptic Seizures*. Boston, MA: Butterworth-Heinemann. 2000; 197–206.
14. Yang CH, Lee YC, Lin CH, Chang K. Conversion disorders in childhood and adolescence: a psychiatric

consultation study in a general hospital. *Acta Paed Sin* 1996;**37**:405–9.

15. Krawetz P, Fleisher W, Pillay N, *et al*. Family functioning in subjects with pseudoseizures and epilepsy. *J Nerv Ment Dis* 2001;**189**:38–43.

16. Bhatia MS, Sapra MA. Pseudoseizures in children: a profile of fifty cases. *Clin Pediatr (Phila)* 2005;**44**: 617–21.

17. Murase S, Sugiyama T, Ishii T, Wakako R. Polysymptomatic conversion disorder in childhood and adolescence in Japan. Early manifestation or incomplete form of somatization disorder? *Psychother Psychosom* 2000;**69**:132–6.

18. Wyllie E, Glazer J, Benbadis S, Kotagal P, Wolgumuth B. Psychiatric features of children and adolescents with pseudoseizures. *Arch Pediatr Adolesc Med* 1999;**153**: 244–8.

19. van Merode T, Twellaar M, Kotsopoulos IA, *et al*. Psychological characteristics of patients with newly developed psychogenic seizures. *J Neurol Neurosurg Psychiatry* 2004;**75**:1175–7.

20. Swanson HL, Harris KR, Graham S. *Handbook of Learning Disabilities*. New York: Guilford Press, 2003.

21. Wechsler D. *Wechsler Intelligence Scale for Children – Fourth Edition*. Texas: The Psychological Corporation, 2003.

22. Woodcock RW, McGrew KS, Mather N. *Woodcock-Johnson III Tests of Achievement*. Illinois: Riverside Publishing Company, 2001.

23. Gordon M. *Gordon Diagnostic System*. New York: Gordon Systems, 1983.

24. Ritter FJ, Kotagal P. Non-epileptic seizures in children. In: Gates JR, Rowan AJ, eds. *Non-Epileptic Seizures*. Boston, MA: Butterworth-Heinemann. 2000; 185–95.

25. Plioplys S, Asato MR, Bursch B. Multidisciplinary management of pediatric nonepileptic seizures. *J Am Acad Child Adolesc Psychiatry* 2007;**46**:1491–5.

26. Lach LM, Peltz L. Adolescents' and parents' perception of non-epileptic seizures and related symptoms in children and adolescents. In: Gates JR, Rowan AJ, eds. *Non-Epileptic Seizures*. Boston, MA: Butterworth-Heinemann. 2000; 227–36.

Section 3 Chapter 19

Psychiatric and neuropsychological considerations in children and adolescents with psychogenic nonepileptic seizures

Adolescents' and parents' perceptions of psychogenic nonepileptic seizures

Manjeet S. Bhatia and Ravi Gupta

A plethora of literature is available regarding adult conversion disorder; however, controlled data are less extensively available in children and adolescents. Common presentations of the conversion disorder symptoms in children and adolescents are similar to presentations in adults, and include neurological features: anesthesia/paresthesia, headache, loss of muscle power, ataxia, movement disorders, etc. However, the most frequent presentation is epilepsy-like symptoms, hereafter referred to as psychogenic nonepileptic seizures (PNES).

We can gain some knowledge of PNES by drawing from the child and adolescent conversion literature, where similarities between PNES and other conversion disorders may exist. In the adolescent conversion disorder, PNES is the most common presentation, especially in girls. A sizable number of patients with PNES have other comorbid psychiatric ailments such as depression and anxiety disorders [1–3]. However, the prevalence of PNES as a manifestation of conversion disorder varies in the different age groups. Kotagal *et al.* reported that conversion disorder is seen in children after five years of age and its frequency increases with age to 83% of all patients brought to the epilepsy unit during adolescence [2].

There are multiple theories regarding the origin of PNES. Because of the different prognoses and psychiatric comorbidities in patients with PNES, some authors propose different etiologies of PNES in adults and children. Freud based his psychoanalytic theories on psychosexual stages of development during childhood. According to psychological theory proposed by Freud [4], during what was then referred to as hysteria, emotional conflicts are converted and expressed as physical symptoms. This theory underlines the emotional origin of somatic symptoms in circumstances where the emotions are hurting the patient to such an extent that the patient is not able to tolerate them. The second important part of the theory is the origin of somatic symptoms at an unconscious level, thus differentiating them from malingering. Behavioral theory views conversion as a learned response by children to use their somatic symptoms in anxiety provoking situations [5]. Leybourne and Churchill [5] insisted that the children are aware of their actions, thus overlapping with the definition of malingering. Some patients with PNES have dysfunctional coping skills and mainly use escape-avoiding strategies [6]. They also feel more external control compared to healthy persons [6]. Ercan *et al.* emphasized the role of the family in the development of PNES [3], while other researchers reported that continued stress, e.g., broken family, separated parents, communication problems in the family, and highly expressed emotions, are important factors in the development of PNES among children [7–10]. In addition, a predisposition to psychiatric disorder also increases the chances of conversion disorder among adolescents. While sexual abuse is considered to increase the chances of developing a conversion disorder, a review of 34 studies examined this relationship and was followed by a meta-analysis of 19 effect sizes. Statistical results supported the professed link between child sexual abuse and PNES, however, the authors suggested that because of research design limitations, it is premature to draw definitive conclusions regarding a relationship [11].

Adolescents' and parents' perceptions about PNES

Although there is a paucity of literature addressing PNES in adolescents, the available literature concerning adults may provide clues to the understanding of PNES. Many patients feel offended when their symptoms are given labels that suggest a psychological origin for their symptoms [12]. The more "unscientific" labels like "symptoms in the mind" are most offensive followed by "hysterical seizures" and "pseudoseizures" [13]. This suggests that patients do not like their symptoms to be ascribed to a mental origin and prefer a diagnosis that suggests a neurological nature to the illness. A clear diagnosis is important while educating the patient regarding PNES and explaining the potential therapeutic options.

From the adult literature, Carton *et al.* reported that most patients with PNES do not adequately understand the nature of the diagnosis and were unaware that their symptoms were nonepileptic [12]. Still, a sizable number of patients endorsed that their symptoms were triggered by their emotions and confirmed the precipitation of PNES during stressful periods. Since these patients had all received the diagnosis of PNES after a revision of their diagnosis from epilepsy, which was diagnosed earlier and consequently had been treated with antiepileptic drugs (AEDs), most were confused regarding the contradictory nature of the earlier diagnosis of epilepsy and revised diagnosis of PNES. About one-fifth reported relief from not having epilepsy. However, most of the patients did not follow through with adequate psychological interventions. In addition, this study showed that those patients who did not accept the diagnosis continued to suffer from recurrent PNES [12].

Subjects with PNES perceive their health to be poorer as compared to patients with epilepsy, which contributes to the chronicity of their symptoms [8]. They focus more upon their physical symptoms than their psychological symptoms as an explanation to the stress, which in turn may also be related to the mood and anxiety disorders in these patients [9]. Patients with PNES are not able to express their needs and emotions in an effective verbal manner [13]. This manifests with their tendency for somatisizing their stress rather than gain an understanding of the underlying problems. This process also reveals that these patients are less psychologically minded and lack insight, which make them poor candidates for psychodynamic psychotherapy. Poor verbal communication may also be the "effect" rather than the cause of PNES. Poor verbal communication may be due to the presence of constant stress or perpetrator with the patient [14] (Table 19.1).

Patients with PNES perceive and report more traumatic events in their life as compared to patients with epilepsy [10], and perceive their cognitive functioning to be poorer than their actual functioning, as measured by objective tests, an effect that is mediated by mood [9].

When compared to patients with motor conversion disorder, patients with PNES feel that less warmth was provided by their parents during childhood and they feel that they were often rejected by their father [15]. They contend that their family members do not communicate with them, frequently engage in conflict, and are unable to provide the affection that they require. They also feel that overall functioning of their family system is poor and that their family members do not allow them to communicate effectively [14].

Family members show emotional over-involvement in the initial phase of the PNES as compared to the parents of children with epilepsy but develop more negative views about the patients with protracted symptoms [7]. Most family members, like PNES patients, lack the understanding of the nature of symptoms and remain puzzled regarding the consequences. In due course, they start criticizing

Table 19.1 Adolescents' and parents' perception of psychogenic nonepileptic seizures (PNES)

Adolescents' emotional responses
Positive: Feeling relieved for not having epilepsy
Hopeful for future
Negative: Confusion, frustration, uncertainty, anger
Denial of life stress

Adolescents' behavioral responses
Acceptance and coping with diagnosis
Staying calm
Seeking parental support
Keeping up with schoolwork in spite of the intrusiveness of episodes

Adolescents' cognitive responses
More likely to have external locus of control
Accepting that NES related to stress and thus using coping devices to contain it
Term "pseudo" upsetting, reflecting false or unreal

Parents' emotional responses
Positive: Feeling relieved for not having epilepsy
Hopeful for future
Negative: Shame, frustration, chances of being misunderstood
Inability to discuss the diagnosis
Emotional problems
Guilt for not being able to recognize child's emotional distress
Fear of response of friends and community

Parents' behavioral responses
Difficulty in managing anxiety
Difficulty in telling adolescent Do's and Don'ts

Parents' cognitive responses
Matching their experiences with information
Understanding that physical symptoms are due to emotional stress and critical events

the patient and hold the patient responsible for their illness [7].

Indian experience

The majority of parents of children and adolescents with PNES in India are unable to differentiate PNES from epileptic seizures and thus take their children to an outpatient pediatric department for evaluation. If need be, they are referred to a psychiatrist to rule out a comorbid psychiatric disorder [16, 17]. School phobia, fear of examination, and parental pressure for performance are the common precipitating factors for PNES [16]. Overprotection and rigidity are important parental attitudes that tend to perpetuate conflict. Physical and sexual abuse are important family-related etiological factors, which can be addressed in family therapy [18].

Summary

Psychogenic nonepileptic seizures is a fairly prevalent disorder among adolescents and most of them suffer from other comorbid psychiatric disorders, commonly anxiety disorders and depression. These disorders negatively affect the perception of adolescents about their symptoms and their functioning capabilities. Similarly, recurrent symptoms and a protracted course, for which often no obvious neurological cause can be found, are problems for their parents, who gradually start rejecting the child's symptoms as genuine illness. This in turn augments the number of episodes and a vicious cycle starts. Looking at the role of family and other environmental factors in development and perpetuation of PNES, these factors must be addressed early in the course. However, the available literature is scarce and more research is required in this overlooked area.

References

1. Pehlivanturk B, Unal F. Conversion disorder in children and adolescents: clinical features and comorbidity with depressive and anxiety disorders. *Turk J Pediatr* 2000;**42**:132–7.
2. Kotagal P, Costa M, Wyllie E, Wolgamuth B. Paroxysmal nonepileptic events in children and adolescents. *Pediatrics* 2002;**110**:e46, 1–5.
3. Ercan ES, Varan A, VeznedaroGlu B. Associated features of conversion disorder in Turkish adolescents. *Pediatr Int* 2003;**45**:150–5.
4. Freud S. *Collected Papers*. New York: Churchill Livingstone, 1954.
5. Leybourne P, Churchill S. Symptom discouragement in treating hysterical reactions of childhood. *Int J Child Psychother* 1972;**1**:111–14.
6. Goldstein LH, Drew C, Mellers J, Mitchell-O'Malley S, Oakley DA. Dissociation, hypnotizability, coping styles and health locus of control: characteristics of pseudoseizure patients. *Seizure* 2000;**9**:314–22.
7. Stanhope N, Goldstein LH, Kuipers E. Expressed emotions in relatives of people with epileptic and non-epileptic seizures. *Epilepsia* 2003;**44**:1094–102.
8. Mazooqi SMA, Baker GA, Reilly J, Salmon P. The perceived health status of people with psychologically derived non-epileptic attack disorder and epilepsy: a comparative study. *Seizure* 2004;**13**:71–5.
9. Breier J, Fuchs KL, Brookshire BL, *et al.* Quality of life perception in patients with intractable epilepsy or pseudoseizures. *Arch Neurol* 1998;**55**:660–5.
10. Fleisher W, Staley D, Krawetz P, *et al.* Comparative study of trauma-related phenomena in subjects with pseudoseizures and subjects with epilepsy. *Am J Psychiatry* 2002;**159**:660–3.
11. Sharpe D, Faye C. Non-epileptic seizures and child sexual abuse: a critical review of the literature. *Clin Psychol Rev* 2006;**26**:1020–40.
12. Carton S, Thompson PJ, Duncan JS. Non epileptic seizures: patient's understanding and reaction to the diagnosis and impact on outcome. *Seizure* 2003;**12**:287–94.
13. Stone J. What should we call pseudoseizure? A patient's perspective. *Seizure* 2003;**12**:568–72.
14. Krawetz P, Fleisher W, Pillay N, *et al.* Family functioning in patients with pseudoseizure and epilepsy. *J Nerv Ment Dis* 2001;**189**:38–43.
15. Stone J, Sharpe M, Binzer M. Motor conversion symptoms and pseudoseizures: a comparison of clinical characteristics. *Psychosomatics* 2004;**45**:492–9.
16. Bhatia MS, Dhar NK, Nigam VR, Bohra N, Malik SC. Hysteria in childhood and adolescence. *Indian Pract* 1990;**4**:307–13.
17. Bhatia MS, Sapra S. Pseudoseizures in children: a profile of 50 cases. *Clin Pediatr* 2005;**44**:617–21.
18. Bhatia MS. Pseudoseizures. *Indian Pediatr* 2004;**41**:673–9.

Section 3 Chapter 20

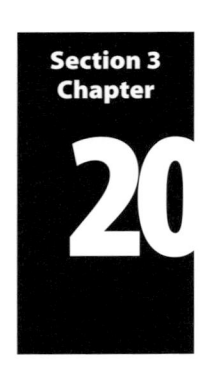

Psychiatric and neuropsychological considerations in children and adolescents with psychogenic nonepileptic seizures

Munchausen syndrome

Ghislaine Savard, Frederick Andermann, and Renée Fugère

Munchausen syndrome is a severe variant of chronic factitious disorder. The eponym "Munchausen Syndrome" refers to Karl Friedrich Hieronymus von Münchhausen, born in 1720 in the small town of Bodenwerder near Hannover, Germany. The Baron Münchhausen, returning in 1750 to his hometown after military campaigns against Russia, acquired quite some fame as a brilliant storyteller at aristocratic parties. In his audience was a geologist, Rudolph Eric Raspe.

In 1775, Raspe sailed to London in an effort to escape accusations of fraud. His criminal reputation followed him and his fellow scientists at the Royal Society rejected him. He found himself penniless. To survive, Raspe published anonymously those thrilling tales of travels and exploits, both real and imagined, that he had heard from the Baron. His writing of tall tales proved very popular and his book was translated into French, Spanish, and German. It circulated widely and reached back to Bodenwerder, where it disgraced the Baron's name, ruining the social life of Münchhausen the Lügenbaron or "Baron of lies" [1–3].

This story, some 150 years after the Baron's death, inspired Richard Asher when he described a medical syndrome in which patients travel widely from hospital to hospital, intentionally produce episodes that appear like seizures or injuries, and lie, telling physicians fantastic stories about how their sickness happened [4]. Asher named it Munchausen syndrome, modifying somewhat the spelling of the Baron's name [4].

It is interesting to know that, to this day, touristic Bodenwerder and the Baron's manor are visited by readers of the *Singular Travels, Campaigns and Adventures of Baron Munchausen* [1]. As well, physicians from all specialties continue to witness cases of Munchausen syndrome.

Definitions

In Diagnostic and Statistical Manual of Mental Disorders, Fourth Edition (DSM-IV), factitious disorder is categorized as an Axis 1 diagnosis, in contrast to malingering, which is not a psychiatric disorder but a "condition that may be a focus of attention" [5]. In both, there is intentional lying or deceit, however, with factitious disorder, there is prominent psychopathology. The diagnostic construct of factitious disorder as a legitimate illness is not accepted by all [6, 7].

In factitious disorder, the willful fabrication of symptoms takes place; first, in the absence of a clear or preponderant "external reality" incentive and second, in the presence of an "internal psychological" need to assume the sick role. In this clinical situation, the doctor must not be deterred by the false symptoms and signs; rather, he/she must attend to the "genuine" need to act sick. Factitious disorder sufferers not only lie about their medical history, they often self-inflict injuries or illnesses, presenting with real symptoms as well as with false ones, vexing even more the distinction between ill and not ill. In DSM-IV, the exact nature of the psychological motive for seeking the relationship with the doctor remains elusive, as does the degree of control the patient has on self-harming and acting.

In contrast, in malingering, the willful fabrication of symptoms takes place in the presence of a clear external incentive or motive. Malingering is not a medical condition. Once the deceit is uncovered, doctors protect themselves and quickly find ways to end being duped.

In factitious disorder, the patients' efforts, sometimes heroic, to deceive doctors as well as their staunch silence about motive, severely challenge the patient–doctor dyad. Once deceit is uncovered, doctors find it difficult to protect themselves as there is no quick way

Gates and Rowan's Nonepileptic Seizures, 3rd edn. ed. Steven C. Schachter and W. Curt LaFrance, Jr. Published by Cambridge University Press. © S. Schachter and W. C. LaFrance, Jr. 2010.

to end being duped. Protecting the patients is difficult as well [8]. It is said that treatment is rarely successful [9]. Our experience is that few physicians have the training to manage the dangers of self-harming and the potential for severe boundary transgressions as is the case with factitious disorder, and especially with Munchausen syndrome. Referral to general psychiatry is met with ambivalence by both patients and doctors, with the result that patients are lost to follow-up or do not progress well. We have long advocated joint follow-up by neurology and neuropsychiatry in the neurology clinic, but this outpatient medical setting has obvious limitations when in-depth psychiatric care is embarked on. In our opinion, collaboration with units specializing in the treatment of patients with severe personality disorders who also present with self-harming and severe boundary violations appears essential for developing clinical guidelines and corridors of care for factitious disorder sufferers. Well-researched therapeutic interventions for self-abusing personality disorders and for medical patients with severe health risk behaviors, from motivational interviewing [10] to comprehensive dialectical behavior therapy that successfully address self-defeating behaviors, interpersonal and quality-of-life choices, might improve prognosis in factitious disorder in the consenting patient [11].

Review of literature

A MEDLINE bibliographic search with the keywords factitious disorder and Munchausen syndrome reveals many case histories and short case series reported by members of various medical specialties including neurology, neurosurgery, dermatology, psychiatry, otorhinolaryngology, plastic surgery, hematology, and others. These are an invaluable source of information since the secretive behavior in factitious disorder thwarts traditional epidemiological research [12–22]. The incidence of factitious disorder in neurology is hard to assess. The Munchausen variant is felt to be rare, but in any given case the number of hospital visits where the diagnosis was missed is typically very high. The dire consequences for the patient with factitious disorder, the high cost to society, and the strong emotions raised in healthcare providers are typically emphasized.

Internet health support groups have struggled with cases of Munchausen syndrome and their deceptive postings [23]. Pediatricians and even veterinarians have reported on Munchausen syndrome occurring by proxy with illnesses inflicted on children by parents or on house pets by their owners [24, 25].

We have published a case of epileptic Munchausen syndrome who presented to our neurological intensive care unit three consecutive times under three aliases, with pseudostatus epilepticus and iatrogenic complications. She also had a history of faked suicidal attempts. Despite her self-injurious behavior and active seeking of invasive procedures, she was assessed by us as competent to consent to care and offered joint psychiatric and neurological follow-up. Upon her defiant refusal and self-discharge against medical advice, she was thus left to continue her hospital peregrinations. She later died from hanging while in confined psychiatric treatment [19]. To this day, we do not know whether she died from a faked suicide attempt that accidentally turned fatal or whether she meant to end her life by hanging that day. Other cases of pseudostatus epilepticus have since been published [14, 15, 21, 22].

There are clinical and theoretical similarities in the challenges that psychogenic nonepileptic seizures and movement disorders present. Prior international meetings on either topics have led to relevant publications as well [26–29].

The neurological history and examination

Usually, the neurologist first suspects deceit from inconsistencies or contradictions in history and examination, from presentations incompatible with anatomy or physiology, from worsening on attention and disappearance on distraction, from responsiveness to neutral provocative measures like a tuning fork applied on the middle forehead and lack of response to usual treatments, or from refusal of access to past charts. A host of maneuvers during examination are available to show healthy function despite the patient's report of a deficit in true Charcot tradition [30]. Due attention is given to the exclusion of medical disease with proper investigations. If malingering is not clearly the issue, and if psychological distress is deemed present, some neurologists reveal to the patient that symptoms are "functional" early on and some even apply self-taught cognitive behavioral therapy techniques in therapeutic interventions. If patients do not get better, they cordially end the therapeutic encounters and transfer the patient to the primary care physician for long-term chronic care or refer to psychiatry [31, 32]. This approach has its merit, in our view, in that it sets practical limits in the context of the neurological setting, but it cannot help sicker patients reach remission or even improve significantly.

The psychiatric consultation

While a standard and thorough psychiatric assessment must be completed, the "funnel" question format has advantages in the presence of suspected deceit. Open questions are preferred at first ("What happened? When were you last well?"), suggestive questions are best avoided ("Did you know that this medication can cause this or that?"), and more specific questions are kept for the end ("Have you been told of a possible link with your psychological state? Do you endorse that formulation?").

With a neutral attitude, it is helpful to explore the core beliefs about health and disease, about perceived causes of current pseudoneurological symptoms and signs, and about the nature of hoped for treatments. It is informative to review past encounters with the medical system and with authoritative bodies such as litigation lawyers, employers, or compensating agencies when applicable. We have seen patients prolong psychiatric interviews asking for more tests on the basis of paramedical opinions that they value but that invalidate the medical opinion, or patients who write down every word spoken by the psychiatrist only to quote them back with an unsuspected bias to other doctors. Patients may challenge the credibility of the psychiatrist, interrupt the psychiatric inquiry repeatedly by their focus on somatic issues, and ignore, sidetrack, or dismiss psychological reality. Resistance to psychiatric interviewing takes many forms. It may be necessary to articulate agendas: "Since you have been referred and are here, is there any way that, as a psychiatrist, I can be of help to you?"

The patient may have denied the signs and symptoms of affective, anxiety, and psychotic disorders, so that psychopharmacological interventions are not an option. Temperament, character, and personality would seem key areas to explore in depth. The opportunity to assess these formally may not be forthcoming given the context of assessing patients who present first and foremost with somatic complaints [33]. At a minimum, the clinician will aim to get an impression with regard to the degree of self-efficacy or belief that one can get better, degree of readiness to improve, and degree of willingness to reevaluate the pros and cons of past attempts to get better [10].

The risk of suicide is present in factitious disorders, especially in the presence of serious self-harming [9, 16, 19, 20]. While predicting which patient will commit suicide remains difficult, the systematic assessment, documentation, and management of suicidal risk is essential in the individual patient [34]. As well, the thorough assessment of the patient's competency to consent or to refuse care is crucial, given the likelihood of discharge against medical care for inpatients, or, importantly in the outpatient setting, the possibility of refusing to engage in psychological treatment. How well the diagnosis was formulated, and how well it was communicated and explained to the patient matter in this regard. Does the patient understand the condition for which the treatment is proposed? Does the patient understand the nature and the purpose of treatment? Does the patient understand the risks involved in undergoing the treatment? Does the patient understand the risks involved in refusing the treatment? Is the patient's ability to consent affected by the factitious disorder [35]?

It is our opinion that the sharpness of distinction between malingering, conversion and factitious disorder is often blurred. It is very difficult for the clinician and the patient alike to weigh internal or external incentives, conscious and unconscious motivation, and true rather than tampered evidence, especially since all these often coexist. Insistence on precise DSM-IV diagnostic labeling may not be as pertinent as insistence on the pros and the cons, from the patient's perspective, of leaving the self-defeating, high-risk health behavior untreated by psychotherapy. Qualifying degree of diagnostic certainty as either possible, probable, clinically definite, or documented, as Fahn *et al.* have proposed for psychogenic movement disorders, is another consideration since as in all psychogenic disorders, a fair degree of skepticism is in order [36].

Issues of special concern

It is helpful to remember that detecting lies during a clinical encounter is very difficult, with an efficacy at chance level for most interviewers. An interesting self-administered test from Paul Ekman's Facial

Action Coding System on the World Wide Web will likely amuse and convince clinicians of this [37]. More robust electrophysiological lie detection techniques such as those used in the forensic laboratory do not have their place in the neurological or psychiatric clinic [38]. Of note, there is no rigorous published study on the use of hypnosis or of sodium amytal interview in factitious disorder. As a result, clinicians tend to disregard early on the lies to avoid futile confrontations, and to focus on elements of truth such as the high-risk health behaviors.

The psychiatric interview from the first encounter or during any follow-up may be interrupted by episodes of nonepileptic seizures with risk of self-injury. We have encountered patients who threw themselves on the floor in the psychiatric office, at times banging their heads or limbs on furniture, screaming or, on the contrary, conspicuously mute, eyes shut or looking away. What is the psychiatrist to do when feigned alteration of consciousness, wild screams, or feigned muteness prevent informed dialogue from taking place? Whether the psychiatrist offers to resume talk, move furniture away for safety, give a hand to get up, or call security or a neurologist, the factitious disorder sufferer may distort any well-meaning intervention on the part of the therapist as rejection, intrusion, or limitless love nurturing only further dependency. A cautious case-by-case approach is warranted. The trans-theoretical model of intentional human behavior change appears most helpful here to understand and manage such resistance, and maybe even prevent it [39]. Psychiatrists working in this field will benefit from familiarity with this model.

Patients diagnosed with factitious disorder ask whether they can drive cars, engaging the physicians' responsibility and raising the issue of safety on the roads (see also Chapter 16). This question can be answered according to regional jurisdiction and following clinical guidelines to the medical assessment of driving ability [40]. This question goes to the core of the degree of control that the patient has in factitious disorder. Since there is an element of fabrication in factitious disorder, these patients are generally felt to be responsible to decide when they can drive safely and when they are to abstain, and thus are liable to prosecution if their driving is reckless, whether they have nonepileptic seizures or not. Of course, the clinician needs to assess whether there is a suicidal risk at the wheel and manage it accordingly [34].

Psychiatric treatment

There is only one systematic review of the literature on the management of factitious disorders [9]. It concludes that there is an absence of any reported rigorous evidence of efficacy of any treatment modality, confrontational or not. There is a lack of controlled trials. Many factitious disorder sufferers never engage in treatment or are lost early to follow-up. Pharmacological therapy is felt to be helpful mainly for the treatment of comorbid affective or anxiety disorders, when present. The authors suggest that a network of interested clinicians be established and that a central registry of standardized patient data be developed. The issue of obtaining consents for the registry is not raised by the authors and seems problematic to us.

There is one case report of a woman who recovered from Munchausen syndrome, who wished to be available to support other sufferers, and who clearly consented to the publication of her story [17].

We believe that joint care from neurologists and psychiatrists remains essential to address the clinical presentation with both physical and behavioral symptoms and signs, to prevent division between caregivers, to safely watch for evidence of iatrogenic complications, and to share the burden of care.

With time, the relevance of a psychological model of care becomes paramount. Motivational interviewing [10] can be a prelude to other forms of psychotherapy. If patients give informed refusal to psychiatric treatment, end of care should be accepted.

Conclusions

The following professional vignette is interesting historically and from an ethical point of view [41–43]. Doctor Pallis and Doctor Bamji, a rheumatologist and a neurologist respectively, lost track of a patient with Munchausen syndrome whose peregrinations they had followed for years. In 1979, the doctors coauthored the patient's obituary and published it, "hoping it was premature." In truth, soliciting information about the patient's whereabouts was their aim, and one year later, a reply publication reported that patient McIlroy was alive and still an active Munchausen case. This vignette got great coverage in the lay press thereafter, involving even prestigious journals such as the *Times of London* and others. The use of deception by a physician to fight deception of a patient is indicative of a personal obsession with a case by the physician and is a sign of professional boundary violation and can lead to exploitative management of factitious disorder [7].

By fooling the doctor, the impostor could come to control the doctor. He may dictate the length of the interview or hospitalization, the number of tests, the prescription of medications or of mobility aids that are not indicated. The peculiar and demanding interpersonal style of factitious disorder patients, and especially of Munchausen syndrome sufferers, may provoke physicians into violating therapeutic boundaries themselves. Ethically, the physician has a professional code to honor and is responsible for maintaining professional boundaries. The doctor must be vigilant of any personal risk increasing his likelihood of boundary problems such as narcissistic needs that are unmet [44, 45].

References

1. Raspe RE. *Singular Travels, Campaigns and Adventures of Baron Munchausen*. London: Cresset Press, 1948.
2. Duranano L. Raspe the rascal. *Mineral Digest*, 1976.
3. Fisher JA. Investigating the Barons: narrative and nomenclature in Munchausen syndrome. *Perspect Biol Med* 2006;**2**:250–62.
4. Asher R. Munchausen's syndrome. *Lancet* 1951;**1**: 339–41.
5. American Psychiatric Association. *Diagnostic and Statistical Manual of Mental Disorders*, 4th edn., Text Revision (DSM-IV-TR). Washington DC: American Psychiatric Association, 2000.
6. Bass C, Halligan PW. Illness related deception: social or psychiatric problem? *J R Soc Med* 2007;**100**:81–4.
7. Fisher JA. Playing patient, playing doctor: Munchausen Syndrome, clinical S/M, and ruptures of medical power. *J Med Humanit* 2006;**27**:135–49.
8. Case records of the Massachusetts General Hospital. Weekly clinicopathological exercises. Case 28–1984. A 39-year-old man with gas in the soft tissues of the left forearm. *N Engl J Med* 1984;**311**:108–15.
9. Eastwood S, Bisson JI. Management of factitious disorders: a systematic review. *Psychother Psychosom* 2008;**77**:209–18.
10. DiClemente CC, Velasquez MM. Motivational interviewing and the stages of changes. In: Miller WR, Rollnick S, eds. *Motivational Interviewing, Preparing People for Change*, 2nd edn. New York: Guilford Press. 2002; 201–16.
11. Lynch ER, Trost WT, Salsman N, Linehan MM. Dialectical behavior therapy for borderline personality disorder. *Annu Rev Clin Psychol* 2007;**3**:181–205.
12. Krahn LE, Li H, O'Connor MK. Patients who strive to be ill: factitious disorder with physical symptoms. *Am J Psychiatry* 2003;**160**:1163–8.
13. Huffman JC, Stern TA. The diagnosis and treatment of Munchausen's syndrome. *Gen Hosp Psychiatry* 2003;**25**:358–63.
14. Pakalnis A, Drake ME, Jr, Phillips B. Neuropsychiatric aspects of psychogenic status epilepticus. *Neurology* 1991;**41**:1104–6.
15. Christensen RC, Szlabowicz JW. Factitious status epilepticus as a particular form of Munchausen's syndrome. *Neurology* 1991;**41**:2009–10.
16. Eisendrath SJ, McNiel DE. Factitious physical disorders, litigation, and mortality. *Psychosomatics* 2004;**45**:350–3.
17. Feldman MD. Recovery from Munchausen syndrome. *South Med J* 2006;**99**:1398–9.
18. Diefenbacher A, Heim G. Neuropsychiatric aspects in Munchausen's syndrome. *Gen Hosp Psychiatry* 1997;**19**:281–5.
19. Savard G, Andermann F, Teitelbaum J, et al. Epileptic Munchausen's syndrome: a form of pseudoseizures distinct from hysteria and malingering. *Neurology* 1988;**38**:1628–9.
20. Hirayama Y, Sakamaki S, Tsuji Y, et al. Fatality caused by self-bloodletting in a patient with factitious anemia. *Int J Hematol* 2003;**78**:146–8.
21. Peters G, Leach JP, Larner AJ. Pseudostatus epilepticus in pregnancy. *Int J Gynaecol Obstet* 2007;**97**:47.
22. Howell SJL, Owen L, Chadwick DW. Pseudostatus epilepticus. *Q J Med* 1989;**71**:507–19.
23. Feldman MD. Legal issues surrounding the exposure of "Munchausen by internet". *Psychosomatics* 2007;**48**:451–2.
24. Stirling J Jr. American Academy of Pediatrics Committee on Child Abuse and Neglect. Beyond Munchausen syndrome by proxy: identification and treatment of child abuse in a medical setting. *Pediatrics* 2007;**119**:1026–30.
25. Milani M. Problematic client-animal relationships: Munchausen by proxy. *C Vet J* 2006;**47**:1161–4.
26. Rowan AJ, Gates JR, eds. *Non-Epileptic Seizures*. Boston, MA: Butterworth-Heinemann, 1993.
27. Hallet M, Fahn S, Jankovic J, et al. *Psychogenic Movement Disorders*. Philadelphia: Lippincott Williams & Wilkins, 2006.
28. Kapfhammer H-P, Rothenhausler H-B. Malingering/Munchausen: factitious and somatoform

disorders in neurology and clinical medicine. In: Hallet M, Fahn S, Jankovic J, *et al.*, eds. *Psychogenic Movement Disorders*. Philadelphia: Lippincott Williams & Wilkins. 2006; 163–79.

29. Lesser RP. Treatment and outcome of psychogenic nonepileptic seizures. In: Hallett M, Fahn S, Jankovic J, *et al.*, eds. *Psychogenic Movement Disorders*. Philadelphia: Lippincott Williams & Wilkins. 2006; 82–7.

30. Goetz CG. J-M Charcot and simulated neurologic disease. Attitudes and diagnostic strategies. *Neurology* 2007;**69**:103–9.

31. Stone J, Carson A, Sharpe M. Functional symptoms and signs in neurology: assessment and diagnosis. *J Neurol Neurosurg Psychiatry* 2005;**76**(Suppl I): i2–12.

32. Stone J, Carson A, Sharpe M. Functional symptoms in neurology: management. *J Neurol Neurosurg Psychiatry* 2005;**76**(Suppl I): i13–21.

33. Cloninger CR, Przybeck TR, Svrakic DM, *et al. The Temperament and Character Inventory: A Guide to its Development and Use*. St Louis, MO: Washington University Center for Psychobiology of Personality, 1994. www.psychobiology.wustl.edu.

34. Simon RI. *Assessing and Managing Suicide Risk. Guidelines for Clinically Based Risk Management*. Washington, DC: American Psychiatric Publishing Inc., 2004.

35. Evans KG. *Consent. A Guide for Canadian Physicians*, 4th edn. Ottawa: Canadian Medical Protective Association, 2006.

36. Fahn S, Williams DT. Psychogenic dystonia. *Adv Neurol* 1988;**50**:431–55.

37. Ekman P, Friesen MV. Facial Action Coding System. www.bbc.co.uk/science/humanbody/mind/surveys/smiles.

38. Vrij A. *Detecting Lies and Deceit. The Psychology of Lying and the Implications for Professional Practice*. Chichester: John Wiley and Sons, 2000.

39. Miller WR, Rollnick S. *Motivational Interviewing: Preparing People for Change*, 2nd edn. New York: Guilford Press, 2002.

40. Bouchard C. L'évaluation du conducteur au cabinet, clé en main. *Médecin du Québec* 2006;**41**:27–71.

41. Pallis CA, Bamji AN. McIlroy was here. Or was he? *Br Med J* 1979;**1**:973–5.

42. Bamji AN, Pallis CA. McIlroy, the media, and the macabre. *Br Med J* 1980;**280**:641–2.

43. Manning GC. Munchausen's Syndrome. *Med Press* 1960;**243**:232–5.

44. Gutheil TG. Boundary issues and personality disorders. *J Psychiatr Pract* 2005;**11**:88–96.

45. Gutheil TG, Simon RI. Non-sexual boundary crossings and boundary violations: the ethical dimension. *Psychiatr Clin North Am* 2002;**25**:585–92.

Section 4: Psychiatric considerations in adults with psychogenic nonepileptic seizures

Section 4 Chapter 21

Psychiatric considerations in adults with psychogenic nonepileptic seizures

Classification of nonepileptic seizures

W. Curt LaFrance, Jr. and Mark Zimmerman

In the chapter on nosology in the second edition of this book, published in 2000, Ronald L. Martin and John Gates discussed the purposes and principles of classification of nonepileptic seizures (NES), identified problems with inconsistent application of terminology, and proposed an algorithm for classification of NES [1].

These same issues remain relevant today and are discussed in this chapter on classification of NES. At the time of the last edition, the *Diagnostic and Statistical Manual of Mental Disorders*, Fourth Edition (DSM-IV), was the official diagnostic manual for psychiatric disorders [2]. The hope for the DSM was for: (1) widespread use, thereby facilitating communication among professionals; (2) clear definition and delineation of the disorders; (3) compatibility with the International Classification of Diseases (ICD) diagnostic system; (4) clear guidelines for compilation and reporting of patient diagnostic data; (5) comprehensive collection of diagnostic terms in one source; and (6) ease of use [3]. The DSM is now undergoing its fifth revision, and varied opinions exist on the most appropriate means of classifying psychosomatic syndromes in the somatoform disorders section [4].

As Martin and Gates noted, a great deal of time and effort can be spent debating definitions and terminology [1]. Productive study of a medical condition demands a clear, precise, logically coherent, universally applicable, consistently interpreted descriptive nosology. Such a nosology allows unambiguous communication and fosters meaningful classification, which in turn facilitates differential diagnosis. In years past, the study of "seizure-like events," unfortunately, has been marred by the lack of such a nosology and classification.

Terminology

Prior terms used for seizure-like events that do not have associated epileptiform activity and have psychological process underpinnings have ranged from hystero-epilepsy, pseudoseizures, hysterical pseudoseizures, spells, nonepileptic attack disorder (used in the UK), as well as hysterical, nonphysiological, functional, dissociative, and psychogenic seizures. Parenthetically, the term "psychogenic seizures" is a misnomer, as psychogenic seizures actually are epileptic seizures that are triggered by cognitive, emotional, or environmental stimuli [5–7]. The histories, rationales, and disadvantages of such terms have been well described many times [8–10]. One study in the UK examined the meanings of these labels for patients, and which have the least potential to offend [11]. Some labels were deemed highly offensive by patients, e.g., "symptoms all in the mind" and "hysterical seizures." The authors found that "stress-related seizures" and "functional seizures" were significantly less offensive than other terms; however, the term "nonepileptic seizures" was not included among the patient choices.

In a survey of treatment providers for patients with NES, neurologists, psychiatrists, and psychologists reported that "nonepileptic seizures" was the term they used most frequently to communicate to patients regarding their seizures [12]. Over the past two decades, the term nonepileptic seizures emerged as the most appropriate term and has been endorsed by patients, neurologists, and psychiatrists because of its nonpejorative description of the events [13, 14]. This term was adopted after a long process of considering traditional terms, including those listed previously. Of

Table 21.1 DSM-IV compatible nosology and classification of seizure-like events

I. Explained by a general (nonpsychiatric) medical condition or the direct effect of a substance (intoxication or withdrawal)
   A. Paroxysmal physiological nonseizure signs or symptoms of a general medical condition (e.g., syncope, transient ischemic attacks, tremors, dystonias, tics, migraine auras)
   B. Seizures (associated with abnormal paroxysmal discharge of cortical neurons)
      1. Symptomatic nonepileptic seizures (i.e., usually isolated seizures provoked by an identified precipitant [e.g., metabolic disturbances, high fever, blow to the head, electric shock, the direct effects of a substance])
      2. Epileptic seizures (chronic recurrent and unprovoked seizures, further differentiated according to the International League Against Epilepsy classification of epileptic seizures)

II. Not explained by a general medical condition or the direct effects of a substance
   A. Feigned seizures (i.e., intentionally produced)
      1. Malingered seizures (motivated by external incentives, such as avoiding military duty or work, obtaining financial compensation or drugs, evading criminal prosecution)
      2. Factitious seizures (apparent goal is to assume the patient role but is not otherwise motivated by objective external incentives or environmental advantages as in malingering)
   B. Paroxysmal signs or symptoms explained by anxiety, mood, psychotic, or other mental disorder (e.g., panic attacks, profound psychomotor agitation or retardation, catatonia, hallucinations)
   C. Psychogenic nonepileptic seizures
   1. Somatoform seizures (not intentionally produced)
      a. Conversion seizures (presence of voluntary motor and/or sensory dysfunction or deficits)
         i. In conversion disorder (conversion symptoms only)
         ii. In somatization disorder (multiple somatic symptoms: pseudoneurological somatoform symptoms and also at least four pain, two nonpain gastrointestinal, and one nonpain sexual or reproductive symptoms; for several years, begins before age 30 years)
         iii. In undifferentiated somatoform disorder (at least 6 months' duration; also other somatoform symptoms but criteria for somatization disorder not met)
         iv. In somatoform disorder not otherwise specified (less than 6 months' duration; also other somatoform symptoms)
      b. Dissociative seizures (dysfunction in consciousness, identity, or memory; in the absence of motor sensory components)
         i. In depersonalization disorder
         ii. In dissociative disorder not otherwise specified

Modified from Martin and Gates [1] with permission.

particular concern was the pejorative connotation of terms with the prefixes *hystero-*, *psycho-*, and *pseudo-*. *Hystero-* and *psycho-* may impart "it's all in your head," and *pseudo-* might indicate that something is not "real" and perhaps is even deliberately falsified, faked, or feigned [15].

Given the importance of the presentation of the diagnosis of psychogenic NES (PNES) with its potential downstream effects on treatment, building an alliance with patients and families is paramount. In today's medical practices, clear clinician communication with patients and families for informed diagnosis is needed. Patients and families have reacted to some of the pejorative terminology used. One of the authors knows a mother who described a medical encounter in frustration noting, "When the doctor in the emergency room saw my daughter, he said, 'It's a pseudoseizure; just step away from the gurney.' I was hurt. Why would my daughter fake these seizures?" In working towards treatments, healthcare providers should build rapport with patients and their families. Ultimately, *pseudo-* implies false or fake, and the use of such terms may compromise the establishment of an alliance with the patient.

The resistance of some clinicians to adopt the term NES is based on a misinformed defense that seizures are, by nature, epileptic. As noted by the International League Against Epilepsy consensus, the word *seizure* derives from the Greek, meaning *to take hold*. A seizure, by definition, is a sudden onset of symptoms [16]. The seizure may be descriptively modified by the preceding, "epileptic," but that it is attributed to epileptiform activity is not inherently invested in the word "seizure." An analogy that illustrates the irrationality of the idea that seizure is only associated with epilepsy is found in the term headache. Clinicians use descriptors for various headaches to differentiate the type of headache, such as migraine headache, rebound headache, posttraumatic headache, and tension headache, without giving it a second thought. This thinking easily applies to seizure, also. In paroxysmal, time-limited, ictal presentations, there are epileptic seizures, physiological nonepileptic seizures, and psychogenic nonepileptic seizures.

Chapter 21: Classification of nonepileptic seizures

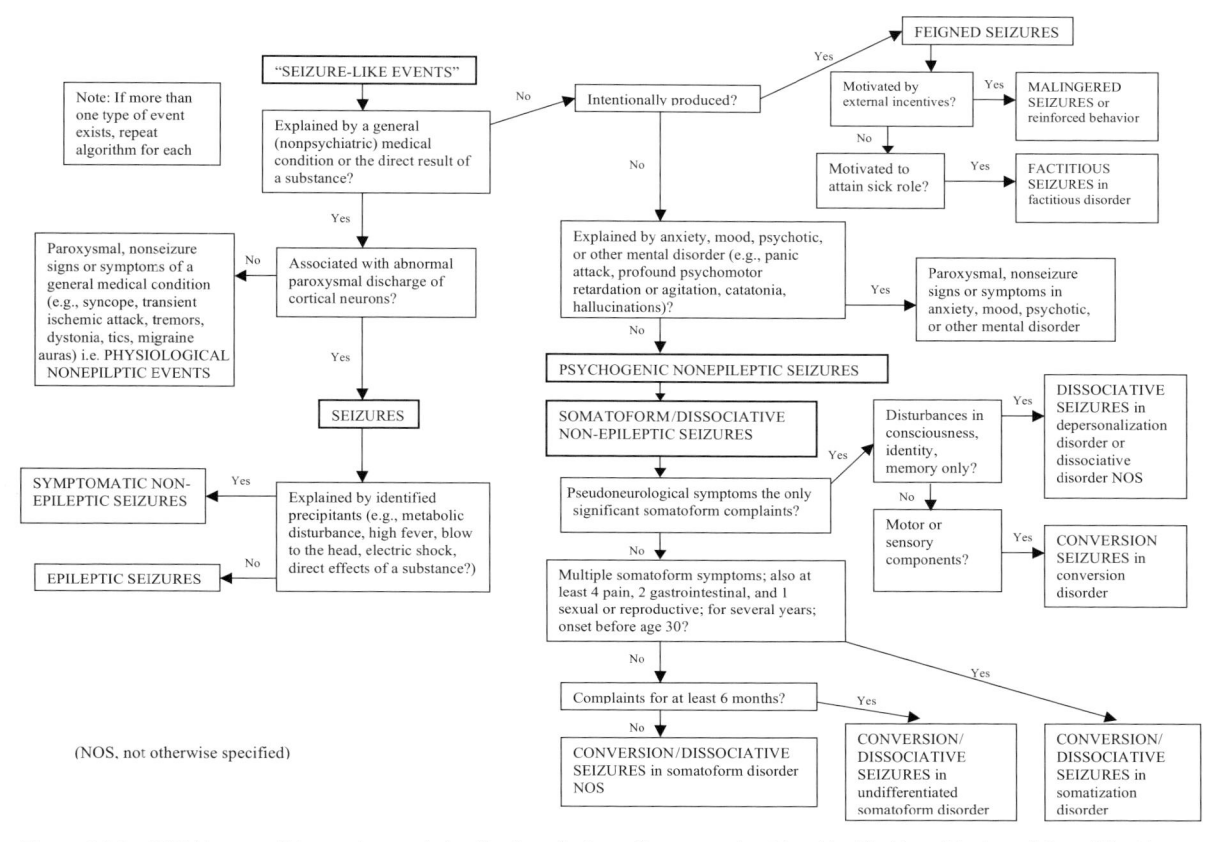

Figure 21.1. DSM-IV compatible nosology and classification of seizure-like events algorithm. Modified from Martin and Gates [1] with permission.

Classification of nonepileptic seizures

As in the prior edition's chapter [1], it is the purpose of this chapter to describe a nosology and classification system that is (1) descriptively accurate, (2) logically consistent throughout, (3) compatible with the classification systems accepted in neurology and epileptology (International League Against Epilepsy classification) [17], and psychiatry (DSM-IV) [2], (4) able to facilitate differential diagnosis, and (5) appropriate for communication with patients and families. The proposed system is shown in outline form in Table 21.1 and algorithmically in the decision tree in Figure 21.1.

Nonepileptic seizures have been traditionally classified by etiology, semiology, and nosology. Each of these classifications has their strengths and weaknesses, and we briefly review these three approaches.

Etiology

Etiology is discussed elsewhere in this book, but a review here is important because etiological distinction may have different treatment implications (see Chapter 28). A few authors have proposed etiological categories for PNES. According to Kalogjera-Sackellares, there are two major etiological categories that account for the majority of cases of PNES, posttraumatic PNES and developmental PNES [18]. From a psychodynamic perspective, it is important to recognize these two patterns because they represent different sets of psychological difficulties. Understanding these difficulties and the psychodynamic processes that underlie them is essential for formulating an effective psychodynamic therapeutic approach. Posttraumatic PNES are thought to develop in response to acute or chronic exposure to traumatic experience, such as physical or psychological trauma, sexual or physical abuse. Developmental PNES refers to coping difficulties with tasks and milestones along the individual's continuum of psychosocial development.

Bowman approaches etiology from a perspective of psychodynamic *pathways* to PNES, which include a history of childhood physical or sexual abuse, recent sexual assault, multiple life stresses that overwhelm the individual's coping abilities, and panic attacks mistaken for PNES [19, 20]. In a variation of the above noted conceptualizations, Porter describes pathways in three categories of causes for PNES [13]: psychopathological processes, such as conversion or dissociative disorder; acute response to stress without evidence of psychopathology (or "situational"), and malingering. Conversion PNES are seen as nonverbal communications facilitated by nonspecific factors that inhibit more articulate verbal expression of ideas or emotions [21]. Ford and Folks [21] describe the utility of the conversion symptom as a solution to an unconscious conflict, a means to express forbidden feelings or ideas, an acceptable means to enact a sick role, or a conditioned response learned in childhood that is a maladaptive coping mechanism in adulthood. Somatization is a process where bodily symptoms are used when factors such as amplification, alexithymia, systems issues (such as family problems), avoiding stigmatizing psychiatric disorders, or impaired verbal expression are present [22].

It is notable that in a series of patients with PNES, no psychiatric diagnosis or psychosocial stressor or precipitant was found in only 5% of cases [23]. Also note that only a small minority of individuals malinger seizures, and they would not fall into the psychologically based etiological categories named above. Etiology in the form of mechanisms for PNES has been listed as: (1) inadequate coping mechanisms, (2) misinterpretation of physical sensations, (3) psychosis, (4) "highlighting" (embellishment of an aura in those with a true partial or absence seizure followed by a psychogenic event), and (5) emotional conflict expression as somatic symptoms [24].

Semiology

Psychogenic nonepileptic seizures can present in the same manner as epileptic seizures; i.e., as a simple partial, complex partial or a generalized absence, myoclonic or tonic-clonic seizure, with or without changes in level of consciousness during events [25]. Semiological descriptions have been used to differentiate PNES by some authors [26] who have emphasized the importance of classifying the kind of nonepileptic event from which the patient suffers. The authors described the events as: swoons (unconscious collapse), tantrums (thrashing with vocalizations), and abreactive attacks (convulsive attack with hypersexual movements). The significance of the ictal characteristics is thought to have a relationship to the presence of traumatic exposure, with higher prevalences of abuse in the swoon and abreactive presentations. The swoon was seen as a "cut-off phenomenon" in which the patient has an automatic reaction to intrusion into consciousness of unpleasant memories or flashbacks. The abreactive attack was viewed as acting out of the memory of the abuse, part of a posttraumatic stress disorder (PTSD) [27].

van Merode *et al.* [28] examined the relationship between gender and semiological presentation of PNES. Males tended to suffer especially from tonic-clonic type seizures (80% of cases), while in women tonic-clonic type events were observed in equal numbers with complex partial type attacks. The authors explained the gender differences by proposing that the clinically more impressive tonic-clonic attack would more readily be suspected to be real, making these types of seizures a more "male" form of acting out. Special types of attacks (swoons, tantrums, abreactive attacks, and forthright simulation) were observed at the same proportion in both sexes. Eighteen women endorsed a history of sexual abuse, though there were no differences between women with and without such a history. Other researchers have likewise found a lack of association between semiological classification and trauma [29].

Nosology

The nosological approach classifies PNES according to the symptomatology found in the DSM, and the ICD. One study classified PNES based on the psychiatric symptomatology, which was reported to inform the type of psychotherapy given [29]. The six patient groupings were conceptualized as: Anxious; Ambivalent (abused [Borderline]); Somatic; Dysthymic; Avoidant (abused [PTSD]); and Mentally Retarded [30]. For nosological clarification we provide definitions of various paroxysmal disorders and their relationship to PNES.

Dissociative states. Dissociation is both a mechanism and a disorder. It is defined in DSM-IV as "a disruption in the usual integrated functions of consciousness, memory, identity, or perception of environment" [2]. Dissociation occurs in a variety of neurological and psychiatric disorders, ranging from temporal lobe epilepsy (TLE), to PTSD, to dissociative disorders, to PNES [31, 32]. Some dissociative episodes are thus due to ictal manifestations of abnormal neuronal firing, and others due to anxiety-based defense responses to physical and psychological trauma [33]. The World Health Organization (WHO) diagnostic categorization of dissociation suggests a mechanistic relationship to psychological etiology, related to "trauma, insoluble or intolerable problems or disturbed relationships" [34]. Along with acute and chronic posttraumatic disorders, dissociation occurs in affective disorders and in certain personality disorders. Dissociation in PNES may lead to the misdiagnosis of epilepsy, with the reporting of amnesia and with EEG abnormalities found in some patients having dissociative episodes [35]. While the patient may report being "unconscious" during an ictus, the term "loss of consciousness" means different things to doctors and to patients [36]. Many patients with PNES actually present with a dissociative alteration in consciousness, rather than loss of consciousness, and this amnestic report must not be equated with an epileptic event.

Other dissociative symptoms include depersonalization and derealization, referring to a disturbance of feeling about the self or the surrounding world, respectively. Autoscopy refers to the "out of body experience" where an individual reports standing outside his/her body and looks down on it. Déjà vu and jamais vu represent amnestic dislocations, with déjà vu most commonly occurring in anxiety disorder. The dissociative symptoms of the TLE aura are more vivid and often more repetitive than those of the psychologically associated symptoms [37].

Catatonia. As is the case with dissociation, alterations in motoric behavior and consciousness are found in catatonic states and may be associated with cerebral dysfunction, toxic metabolic states, or psychogenic causes. Among the psychiatric diagnoses, catatonia is often associated with schizophrenia; however, catatonia occurs in severe affective disorders also. Catatonia is a disturbance of motor behavior with psychological or neurological etiologies, which manifests as rigid immobility for extended periods of time, or as agitated purposeless motor activity [2]. Medically emergent forms of catatonia can be found in neuroleptic malignant syndrome, associated with antipsychotic use, stiff-person syndrome, or epilepsy. Primavera *et al.* emphasized the necessity of using EEG in the diagnostic evaluation of the acute catatonic patient. They found seizures in 4 patients and nonconvulsive status epilepticus in another in their series of 29 patients [38].

Panic. Panic attacks present as paroxysmal episodes with autonomic symptomatology, including a combination of tachycardia, palpitations, hyperventilation, dyspnea, diaphoresis, angina, tremulousness, presyncope, visual changes, and "an impending sense of doom." They may occur in stressful situations or sporadically, once they have been entrained apart from the feared stimulus. Differentiating epileptic seizures from PNES when the primary symptom is anxiety, with the overlap between ictal fear and panic symptoms, can be difficult. Indeed, some patients who meet DSM criteria for panic attacks have actually been found to have evidence of partial seizure activity when monitored [39, 40]. Clinically, however, the diffuse symptoms of anxiety differ from the "dreamy state" and automatisms described by Hughlings Jackson [41] and the epigastric rising sensation reported in TLE prior to loss of consciousness, and personality measures of anxiety are higher in patients with PNES than in patients with epilepsy [42].

Conversion disorders. Symptoms in conversion disorders are defined as "a loss of, or alteration in, voluntary motor or sensory functioning suggesting a neurological or general medical condition. Psychological factors are judged to be associated with the development of the symptom, and the symptom is not fully explained by a neurological or general medical condition or the direct effects of a substance." Conversion disorders may occur in the presence of neurological disease, and the two are not mutually exclusive. Briquet's syndrome (somatization disorder) is a more chronic, stable form of "hysteria" that may present with numerous somatic complaints, various neurological symptoms, and a history of abnormal illness behaviors [43, 44]. The PNES that are described as types of conversion disorders or as dissociative phenomena are usually considered as unconscious processes.

Malingering. In contrast to unconscious processes in conversion disorder, malingering, which makes up a small subset of NES patients and is not considered as a psychiatric illness, is thought of as a conscious process of deception. Malingering using epileptic-like symptoms has been documented in the medical literature for over a century [45, 46]. The DSM-IV categorizes malingering in "additional conditions that may be a focus of clinical attention," defining it as "the intentional production of false or exaggerated symptoms, motivated by external incentives" [2]. Examples of the goals of malingering include avoiding military service, jail, work, or a difficult social situation, though malingering is most often discovered in settings of obtaining drugs or compensation.

Episodic dyscontrol. Episodic dyscontrol is a condition of repeated paroxysmal episodes of rage and violence, which often occur sporadically without precipitant, and are relatively short lived [47]. Similarly, individuals diagnosed with "intermittent explosive disorder" (IED) may be amnestic of the events that result in serious assaults towards people or property destruction [2]. Episodic dyscontrol and IED are found in boys, in urban areas, often with a family history of violence [47]. IED may be confused with epilepsy, with the transient change in consciousness, the response to antiepileptic/mood stabilizing drugs, some association with a history of head injury, and an abnormal EEG with nonspecific slowing [48, 49].

One of the controversies surrounding PNES is whether the disorder should be classified as a dissociative disorder or a somatoform conversion disorder [50–52]. The question of dimensional versus categorical approaches toward classification may be less controversial than for other psychiatric disorders – a patient either has events or does not. The categorical-dimensional debate in PNES has been addressed somewhat using dissociative scales and personality profiles in patients with PNES, epilepsy, and dissociative disorders [32, 53–60]. As it stands now, in the DSM-IV, under the heading of somatoform disorders, conversion disorder with seizures (code 300.11) exists, and in the ICD-10, dissociative (conversion) disorders with seizures (code F44) is the equivalent. With only a limited understanding of the neuropathophysiology in somatoform and dissociative disorders (discussed in the next section), the classification debate continues and will not be resolved in this edition.

Classification considerations and consciousness

Because the issue of conversion disorder historically hinged on the presence of an unconscious psychological conflict, we briefly discuss neuroanatomical and neurophysiological aspects of consciousness, and conscious and unconscious processes. Consciousness has been described as "the subjective awareness of something," having "limited awareness of [its] processes; it perceives the products of cognition" [61]. Proponents of a hippocampal/medial temporal lobe based, modular memory theory argue that awareness is always present with declarative memory (episodic or semantic memory) [62]. In contrast, certain precepts and nonconscious behaviors, as in procedural memory, are fully unconscious (or inaccessible to consciousness). The interaction between procedural and declarative knowledge is seen in hypnosis and implicit memory, which are posited as examples of the individual's operational cognitive unconscious, where innate and over-learned behaviors may use declarative memory while being inaccessible to consciousness [63].

From a neurophysiological perspective, consciousness is state-dependent, requiring the forebrain to be in an operational state that is conducive to the representation of images, thoughts, and emotions, and is characterized by general neuronal depolarizations and readiness of cortical and thalamic networks [64, 65]. A disruption of consciousness in epilepsy is associated with abnormal synchronized oscillations of activity that disrupt normal neurological function [66].

Consciousness in epilepsy has been conceptualized as bidimensional with axes of level of consciousness and content of consciousness [67]. In a study that compared the semiology of PNES to TLE, patients with TLE had disordered levels of consciousness, while patients with PNES showed self-directed consciousness disturbances [68]. Awareness and arousal were not disordered during the ictus in the patients with PNES. Conversion disorders frequently present as alterations of sensory, motor or behavioral functions and may result from nonconscious elements of mind associated with restriction of conscious awareness.

While the underlying neuroanatomy in pathophysiological alterations of consciousness is documented, the role of neurobiological factors in PNES and consciousness itself is less well understood. Along with mediation of nonverbal, visuospatial, and topographic perception, the right hemisphere has functional correlates of corporeal awareness or the bodily sense of self [69]. The prefrontal cortex has been proposed as a substrate for inhibitory mechanisms altering attention and awareness in conversion reactions [70]. Right hemispheric dysfunction may impair recognition of the body's sense of self (e.g., anosognosia), and conversion disorders have been associated with right hemispheric laterality [71]. Brain abnormalities, such as stroke, vascular malformations, infections, and traumatic brain injury, are found in almost one-quarter of patients with lone PNES and in over 90% of patients with mixed epilepsy and PNES [72]. In one study, right hemispheric structural lesions or electrophysiological abnormalities were found in 71% of patients with PNES [73].

These findings bring together functional neuroanatomical connections between consciousness, an individual's awareness of self, and conversion symptoms, manifesting as PNES. Theories on the etiology of conversion symptoms range historically from psychodynamic to neuroanatomical. A unified theory acknowledges that environmental influences, in the presence of macro-anatomic or distributed network brain abnormalities, in the vulnerable individual may contribute to the development of PNES and other conversion disorders.

Decision tree for the differential diagnosis of seizure-like events

Following the algorithm of Figure 21.1, modified from Martin and Gates [1], the process of differential diagnosis using the proposed nosology and classification can be determined by a series of "yes-no" questions in a decision-tree model. The following narrative describes the decision-making process in using the algorithm.

Explained by a general (nonpsychiatric) medical condition or the direct effects of a substance?

By design, seizure-like events represent a broad inclusive category of events intended to encompass a wide variety of paroxysmal events that are or could be misinterpreted as epileptic seizures. Whether the seizure-like events are explained by a general medical condition or are the direct effects of a substance is perhaps the most important question and should first be applied to any paroxysmal event. This delineation is a basic dichotomization in psychiatry. Stated here in DSM-IV terminology, it corresponds to separating what was termed "organic" from "functional" conditions in previous classifications. The "organic" designation was abandoned as anachronistic, given progress in implicating "biological" (in many ways akin to organic) factors in traditionally designated functional disorders, such as depressive or bipolar mood disorders, schizophrenia and other psychotic disorders, panic disorder, and obsessive compulsive disorder, to name a few [74]. In DSM-IV, the term *general medical condition* refers to all medical conditions that are not "psychiatric" or "mental." This is to emphasize that psychiatric conditions are still medical conditions. Thus, general medical conditions would include cardiovascular conditions that result in episodes of syncope, neurological disorders with movements resembling seizures, and metabolic disturbances or epilepsy itself as an explanation for seizures. Various substances also fully explain seizures, some during intoxication (e.g., cocaine), others during withdrawal (e.g., alcohol and other sedative-hypnotics).

Yes

A yes answer signifies that the seizure-like event is fully explained as an effect of either an identified or presumed general medical condition or the direct effects of a substance as described previously.

No

A no answer signifies that the event is not fully explained on one of the previously mentioned bases and would lead to determination on the psychiatric arm of the algorithm. Intentionality is then addressed (see below).

Before addressing the psychiatric arm, in this discussion, the "medically explained" arm is reviewed first.

Associated with abnormal paroxysmal discharge of cortical neurons?

No

Not all medically explained events that are paroxysmal, and thereby may resemble seizures, meet the previously given definition of an epileptic seizure [75]. Such events would be classified as "paroxysmal, nonseizure signs or symptoms of a general medical condition." Included here would be manifestations of a general medical condition such as vascular conditions that cause syncope or transient ischemic attacks. In convulsive syncope, brief loss of clear consciousness, sometimes accompanied by some spasmodic jerks, may resemble a seizure [76, 77]. In transient ischemic attacks, transient neurological deficits may appear suddenly and then promptly resolve, resembling a seizure [78]. Neurological conditions, such as tremors, dystonias, and tics, may all be associated with sudden involuntary movements that may resemble seizures [79]. Migraine auras may manifest with the sudden onset of sensory experiences (e.g., scintillating scotomas) or deficits that may be misinterpreted as seizures. However, none of these events, although paroxysmal, are temporally associated with the abnormal discharges of cortical neurons as in an epileptic seizure. These events are termed "Physiological nonepileptic events."

Yes

A yes answer to the presence of abnormal paroxysmal cortical neuron discharges designates that events are seizures. This leads to the question of cause, particularly as to whether they are symptomatic nonepileptic or epileptic seizures.

Explained by identified precipitants?

Yes

A yes answer designates that the seizures are provoked by identified factors, such as metabolic disturbances (e.g., hypoxia or an electrolyte disturbance), high fever, or external causes such as a blow to the head, an electric shock, or the direct effects of a substance, whether it be intoxication or withdrawal [10]. With this definition, the occurrence of such seizures would parallel the precipitants and in most instances would be isolated events, limited to times during which the provoking precipitants were operative. These seizures, it can be argued, are symptomatic, whereby the events meet the definition of a seizure yet are not considered a result of epilepsy. This question is of major clinical importance because such symptomatic seizures generally are not chronically treated with antiepileptic drugs.

No

Exclusion of such factors leads to a determination of epileptic seizures. Epileptic seizures can be differentiated extensively according to current neurological concepts [80], but this is not the focus of this chapter, which is intended to expand on seizure-like events that do not have such physiological explanations. Readers are directed to the International League Against Epilepsy classification for differentiation of epileptic seizures [17].

Having determined that the event is not medically associated or epilepsy, the next task is to decide whether the event is produced intentionally, as alluded to above.

Intentionally produced (feigned)?

Yes

As used in DSM-IV, the term *intentionally* means conscious intent. Something can be unconsciously intentional but not fulfill the DSM-IV definition of intentional production. Determining whether conscious intent is present is difficult and not always clear-cut, if not impossible. Some would argue that it should be abandoned. Yet, it remains a task intrinsic to Western legal systems, in which ascertaining intent is instrumental in determining the level of criminal responsibility (consider the differentiations of manslaughter versus second-degree murder). Even manslaughter is further subdivided as voluntary or involuntary.

Although imperfect, methods used in determining whether a seizure-like event is intentionally produced involve a "contextual analysis" [2]. The presence of obvious objective goals or external incentives, such as avoiding military duty or work, obtaining financial compensation or drugs, or evading criminal prosecution, should make one especially suspicious of intentionality. The setting is also important to consider. In court or legal referrals, the military, or prison settings, intentionality is much more common.

If it is decided that a seizure is intentionally produced, it is designated a *feigned seizure*. The next question pertains to the motivation for its conscious production.

Motivated by external incentives?
This question involves whether the production of the seizure is motivated by obvious external incentives as were listed previously.

Yes
If the answer is yes, the events are considered malingered seizures.

No
A no answer leads to the next question.

Motivation to attain the sick role?
Yes
In the case of a yes answer, a diagnosis of factitious disorder would be considered, whereby the motivation is less obvious and involves the goal of assuming the "sick role." This is described elsewhere in DSM-IV as the "patient role," which is more accurate descriptively. In factitious disorders, there is some aspect about being a patient that is motivating for such individuals, perhaps in terms of the personal attention or perhaps in the procedures performed (which would be noxious to most people). In the case of a factitious seizure, the motivation could be the process of being evaluated and perhaps hospitalized, with the resultant care, concern, and attention that would be involved, as well as obtaining sometimes dramatic diagnostic procedures, such as EEG, MRI, and CT. In the past, the motivation may have been to receive earlier versions of brain scans, angiography, and even pneumoencephalography. These motivations must be differentiated from others such as gaining admission to a hospital as a place to sleep and be given food and shelter, which would be considered malingering.

Another interesting although rare presentation is "factitious disorder by proxy" [81], whereby a person, often a parent or caretaker, contrives to make it appear that another person, generally under his/her control or influence, such as a child, has some medical condition. In the case of seizures, the perpetrator might report symptoms that suggest a seizure, thereby obligating healthcare professionals to evaluate the victim, perform diagnostic procedures, and so forth.

Intentionally produced?
No
In the absence of intentional production, PNES are designated as somatoform or dissociative seizures either as symptoms of a dissociative or a conversion disorder itself or, depending on whether other somatoform symptoms are present, as components of another somatoform disorder. It is unfortunate that DSM-IV requires that a categorical distinction between dissociative and somatoform disorders must be made. As is explained below, perhaps a varietal differentiation would be more appropriate. In DSM-IV, dissociative disorders are not included as somatoform disorders in that, although they are medically unexplained symptoms that suggest a general medical condition, they do not involve *physical* symptoms. This distinction is arbitrary, however, because it appears that dissociative and conversion symptoms are closely related etiologically as well as phenomenologically [34, 50]. They often coexist in the same patient. Even in DSM-IV, dissociative symptoms are included as examples of pseudoneurological symptoms in the criteria for somatization disorder.

Explained by an anxiety, mood, psychotic, or other mental disorder?
Backtracking to those events that are not explained by a general medical condition or the direct effects of a substance and having excluded intentional production of events, the question of whether the event can be explained by an anxiety, mood, psychotic, or other mental disorder can be asked.

Yes
A yes designation signifies that the events are paroxysmal signs or symptoms of a mental disorder but that any resemblance to a seizure is incidental, that is, not consciously intended or motivated by factors out of awareness (i.e., "unconscious") to simulate a seizure. Examples of such events would include panic attacks, which may come on suddenly and be associated with some change in the level of awareness, resembling changes that occur with seizures. More rarely, profound psychomotor retardation or agitation also comes on suddenly and may be associated with apparent change in the level of awareness. Likewise, hallucinatory phenomena can come on suddenly and also may affect the level of awareness, thereby

resembling a seizure. Paroxysms of false perceptions may resemble complex partial seizures, and disturbances in level of awareness may suggest absence seizures. As described above, given that some atypical epileptic seizure presentations may have surface-negative EEGs, the greatest perspicacity needs to be exercised in labeling seizure-like activity associated with anxiety or stressors as nonepileptic.

No

Having excluded intentional production of events earlier in the algorithm, and in the absence of such explanations, one is left with the probability that an event is psychogenic. That is, resemblance of the events to seizures is not incidental, as in the previously described events associated with anxiety, mood, or psychotic disorders. Rather, they actually simulate seizures unintentionally – that is, without conscious intent (unconsciously) – as in conversion or dissociative seizures. In each of these, there are some assumptions about psychological motivation or explanation, as are discussed later.

Pseudoneurological symptoms the only significant somatoform complaints?

Yes

If the somatoform symptoms are limited to pseudoneurological complaints, the somatoform seizure would be considered a part of either a dissociative or conversion disorder.
(See below for "No".)

Disturbances in consciousness, identity, or memory only?

Yes

If the answer is yes, the event would be considered a dissociative seizure. Dissociative seizures may resemble complex partial seizures or even absence attacks. It has been argued by some that such events were actually associated with seizure activity, but this is not necessarily the case [82, 83].

No

If, on the other hand, only voluntary motor or sensory components are involved, the event would represent a conversion seizure. In some instances, of course, both voluntary motor or sensory and dissociative components may be involved. In such cases, a mixed conversion/dissociative seizure would be diagnosed. DSM-IV subtypes conversion disorder as "with motor symptom or deficit," "with sensory symptom or deficit," "with seizures or convulsions," or "with mixed presentation." If seizures are the only conversion symptoms, "conversion disorder with seizures or convulsions" would be diagnosed; if other conversion symptoms were seen as well, "with mixed presentation" would be the subtype.

Pseudoneurological symptoms the only significant somatoform complaints?

Returning to the question of whether pseudoneurological somatoform symptoms are present, the question of whether these symptoms are the only significant somatoform complaints should be asked.

No

According to DSM-IV definitions, if multiple nonpseudoneurologic somatoform symptoms are present, the next questions involve the following: Of which of the somatoform disorders are the somatoform seizures (whether dissociative or conversion) a component?

Multiple somatoform symptoms: in addition to pseudoneurological symptoms, also at least four pain, two nonpain gastrointestinal, and one nonpain sexual or reproductive symptoms, with an onset before age 30 years and a duration of at least several years?

Yes

If the criteria of multiple somatoform symptoms are met, somatization disorder is diagnosed. In such cases the conversion or dissociative seizures would be subsumed under this diagnosis because, as pseudoneurological symptoms, they are a subset of the symptomatology of this disorder. Conversion or dissociative disorder would not be diagnosed in addition.

No

If criteria for somatization disorder are not met but the symptoms have been present for at least six months, the conversion or dissociative seizures would be considered part of an undifferentiated somatoform disorder. If symptoms have been present for less than six months, somatoform disorder not otherwise specified would be diagnosed.

A tool to classify NES

Based on the classification algorithm described above, we generated a semi-structured clinical interview for diagnosis (SCID) module to categorize patients with confirmed PNES. Modifications occurred as listed in Figure 21.1. There were two main modifications to the decision tree from the original Martin and Gates version. The first was incorporation of a branch that allows for the subset of patients who have more than one type of event. Roughly 10% of patients with PNES have comorbid epilepsy, and the NES SCID module allows for questions to be asked for classification of the various types of events. The second modification was to move the intentionality question up the decision tree to exclude malingering, which is not a psychiatric disorder, and therefore should not be classified under "psychogenic" questions. While factitious disorder has the component of the motivation to assume the sick role, it is included under the feigned seizure groups apart from the "psychogenic" NES category because of the intentional element. The unconscious aspect of the conversion/dissociative seizures potentially makes this patient group vastly different from those intentionally producing their symptoms. A study comparing conversion to factitious to malingering would be of great benefit.

When applying the NES SCID module to our sample of 43 patients with confirmed PNES who enrolled in PNES treatment trials over the past 5 years, only 3 were classified as Dissociative Seizures in Depersonalization Disorder. The other 40 patients were diagnosed with Conversion Seizures in Conversion Disorder. This was not an epidemiological assessment, rather an attempt to classify those persons with confirmed PNES by the Martin and Gates algorithm. Future studies could apply the PNES SCID module across seizure types for an epidemiological assessment of nosology (LaFrance, submitted for publication).

Conclusion

As is the case in discerning the nature of any medical disorder, classification schemes in NES are just as important. Nosology can be one of the first steps in understanding etiology, and with that, potentially informs appropriate treatment. We have found an approach as being beneficial, one which separates out epileptic seizures, from physiological nonepileptic events, from feigned seizures, from PNES. The outlined nosology initially proposed by Martin and Gates has the advantage over previously proposed systems of significantly aiding in differential diagnosis of seizure-like events. The algorithm begins with a fundamental dichotomization of seizure-like events as fully explained on the basis of a general medical condition or the direct effects of substances versus those not explained as such. On the "medical" side of the algorithm, physiological nonepileptic events are then differentiated as due to a medical condition or to an identified precipitant. Symptomatic seizures are then differentiated from epileptic seizures. The events associated with a psychiatric correlate or that are intentionally produced are designated as malingering or factitious. The rest of the algorithm differentiates somatoform/dissociative seizures. Martin and Gates argued that this nosology and classification could virtually cover any seizure-like event, placing the event unambiguously in the classification. Conversion or somatoform seizures were thought to be neutral, nonpejorative terms in the classification scheme. Clinical experience and the literature confirm that confronting the individual who is malingering may be problematic. This individual typically withdraws from treatment, and sometimes seeks treatment elsewhere.

In the late twentieth century and early twenty-first century, we increasingly have had at our disposal powerful tools to help better understand and visualize neuroanatomy coupled with neurophysiology. Functional neuroimaging and electrophysiological assessments provide enhanced neurobiological examination, with better spatial and temporal resolution in brain processes. Along with the neurological and mental status examination, neurologists, psychiatrists, psychologists, and neuroscientists may employ these tools to evaluate patients with NES. The technologies used to assess neurophysiology, however, still do not have the power to distinguish conscious vs. unconscious, or volitional vs. involuntary, or feigned vs. unfeigned behaviors in individual patients. Ultimately, to better classify NES, we potentially will require a better understanding of the conscious and unconscious mind and the brain processes that correlate with behavior.

References

1. Martin RL, Gates JR. Nosology, classification, and differential diagnosis of non-epileptic seizures: an alternative proposal. In: Gates JR, Rowan AJ, eds. *Non-Epileptic Seizures*, 2nd edn. Boston, MA: Butterworth-Heinemann. 2000; 253–67.
2. American Psychiatric Association. *Diagnostic and Statistical Manual of Mental Disorders*, 4th edn. (DSM-IV). Washington, DC: American Psychiatric Association; 1994.
3. Zimmerman M, Spitzer RL. Psychiatric classification. In: Sadock BJ, Sadock VA, Kaplan HI, eds. *Kaplan & Sadock's Comprehensive Textbook of Psychiatry*, 8th edn. Philadelphia: Lippincott Williams & Wilkins. 2004; 1003–34.
4. Mayou R, Kirmayer LJ, Simon G, Kroenke K, Sharpe M. Somatoform disorders: time for a new approach in DSM-V. *Am J Psychiatry* 2005;**162**(5): 847–55.
5. Ingvar DH, Nyman GE. A new psychological trigger mechanism in a case of epilepsy. *Neurology* 1962;**12**:282–7.
6. Fenwick P. Precipitation and inhibition of seizures. In: Reynolds EH, Trimble MR, eds. *Epilepsy and Psychiatry*. Edinburgh; New York: Churchill Livingstone. 1981; 306–21.
7. Mattson RH, Heninger GR, Gallagher BB, Glaser GH. Psychophysiologic precipitants of seizures in epileptics. *Neurology* 1970;**20**(4):407.
8. Fenton GW. Epilepsy and hysteria. *Br J Psychiatry* 1986;**149**:28–37.
9. Trimble MR. Pseudoseizures. *Neurol Clin* 1986;**4**(3): 531–48.
10. Gates JR, Mercer K. Nonepileptic events. *Semin Neurol* 1995;**15**(2):167–74.
11. Stone J, Campbell K, Sharma N, *et al.* What should we call pseudoseizures? The patient's perspective. *Seizure* 2003;**12**(8):568–72.
12. LaFrance Jr WC, Rusch MD, Machan JT. What is "treatment as usual" for nonepileptic seizures? *Epilepsy Behav* 2008;**12**(3):388–94.
13. Porter RJ. Diagnosis of psychogenic and other nonepileptic seizures in adults. In: Devinsky O, Theodore WH, eds. *Epilepsy and Behavior*. New York: Wiley-Liss. 1991; 237–49.
14. Scull DA. Letter to the Editor: Pseudoseizures or non-epileptic seizures (NES); 15 synonyms. *J Neurol Neurosurg Psychiatry* 1997;**62**(2):200.
15. Chabolla DR, Krahn LE, So EL, Rummans TA. Psychogenic nonepileptic seizures. *Mayo Clin Proc* 1996;**71**(5):493–500.
16. Fisher RS, van Emde Boas W, Blume W, *et al.* Epileptic seizures and epilepsy: definitions proposed by the International League Against Epilepsy (ILAE) and the International Bureau for Epilepsy (IBE). *Epilepsia* 2005;**46**(4):470–2.
17. Commission on Classification and Terminology of the ILAE. Proposal for revised classification of epilepsies and epileptic syndromes. *Epilepsia* 1989;**30**(4): 389–99.
18. Kalogjera-Sackellares D. Psychological disturbances in patients with pseudoseizures. In: Sackellares JC, Berent S, eds. *Psychological Disturbances in Epilepsy*. Oxford, England: Butterworth-Heinemann. 1996; 191–217.
19. Bowman ES. Etiology and clinical course of pseudoseizures. Relationship to trauma, depression, and dissociation. *Psychosomatics* 1993;**34**(4):333–42.
20. Bowman ES, Markand ON. The contribution of life events to pseudoseizure occurrence in adults. *Bull Menninger Clin* 1999;**63**(1):70–88.
21. Ford CV, Folks DG. Conversion disorders: an overview. *Psychosomatics* 1985;**26**(5):371–4, 380–3.
22. Ford CV. The somatizing disorders. *Psychosomatics* 1986;**27**(5):327–31, 335–7.
23. Moore PM, Baker GA. Non-epileptic attack disorder: a psychological perspective. *Seizure* 1997;**6**(6):429–34.
24. Gumnit RJ, Gates JR. Psychogenic seizures. *Epilepsia* 1986;**27** Suppl 2:S124–9.
25. Gates JR, Ramani V, Whalen S, Loewenson R. Ictal characteristics of pseudoseizures. *Arch Neurol* 1985;**42**(12):1183–7.
26. Betts T, Boden S. Diagnosis, management and prognosis of a group of 128 patients with non-epileptic attack disorder. Part I. *Seizure* 1992;**1**(1):19–26.
27. Betts T, Boden S. Diagnosis, management and prognosis of a group of 128 patients with non-epileptic attack disorder. Part II. Previous childhood sexual abuse in the aetiology of these disorders. *Seizure* 1992;**1**(1):27–32.
28. van Merode T, de Krom MC, Knottnerus JA. Gender-related differences in non-epileptic attacks: a study of patients' cases in the literature. *Seizure* 1997;**6**(4):311–16.
29. Rusch MD, Morris GL, Allen L, Lathrop L. Psychological treatment of nonepileptic events. *Epilepsy Behav* 2001;**2**:277–83.
30. LaFrance Jr WC, Devinsky O. Treatment of nonepileptic seizures. *Epilepsy Behav* 2002;**3**(5 Suppl 1):S19–23.
31. Dietl T, Bien C, Urbach H, Elger C, Kurthen M. Episodic depersonalization in focal epilepsy. *Epilepsy Behav* 2005;7(2):311–15.

32. Dikel TN, Fennell EB, Gilmore RL. Posttraumatic stress disorder, dissociation, and sexual abuse history in epileptic and nonepileptic seizure patients. *Epilepsy Behav* 2003;**4**(6):644–50.
33. Sivec HJ, Lynn SJ. Dissociative and neuropsychological symptoms: the question of differential diagnosis. *Clin Psychol Rev* 1995;**15**(4):297–316.
34. World Health Organization, ed. *The ICD-10 Classification of Mental and Behavioural Disorders: Clinical Descriptions and Diagnostic Guidelines.* Geneva, Switzerland: World Health Organization, 1992.
35. Jawad SS, Jamil N, Clarke EJ, *et al.* Psychiatric morbidity and psychodynamics of patients with convulsive pseudoseizures. *Seizure* 1995;**4**(3):201–6.
36. Gloor P. Consciousness as a neurological concept in epileptology: a critical review. *Epilepsia* 1986;**27** Suppl 2:S14–26.
37. Trimble MR. Non-epileptic seizures. In: Marshall JC, ed. *Contemporary Approaches to the Study of Hysteria: Clinical and Theoretical Perspectives.* Oxford, New York: Oxford University Press. 2001; 143–54.
38. Primavera A, Fonti A, Novello P, Roccatagliata G, Cocito L. Epileptic seizures in patients with acute catatonic syndrome. *J Neurol Neurosurg Psychiatry* 1994;**57**(11):1419–22.
39. Weilburg JB, Schachter S, Worth J, *et al.* EEG abnormalities in patients with atypical panic attacks. *J Clin Psychiatry* 1995;**56**(8):358–62.
40. Weilburg JB, Schachter S, Sachs GS, *et al.* Focal paroxysmal EEG changes during atypical panic attacks. *J Neuropsychiatry Clin Neurosci* 1993;**5**(1):50–5.
41. Hogan RE, Kaiboriboon K. The "dreamy state": John Hughlings-Jackson's ideas of epilepsy and consciousness. *Am J Psychiatry* 2003;**160**(10):1740–7.
42. Owczarek K. Anxiety as a differential factor in epileptic versus psychogenic pseudoepileptic seizures. *Epilepsy Res* 2003;**52**(3):227–32.
43. Guze SB. The validity and significance of the clinical diagnosis of hysteria (Briquet's syndrome). *Am J Psychiatry* 1975;**132**(2):138–41.
44. Wetzel RD, Guze SB, Cloninger CR, Martin RL, Clayton PJ. Briquet's syndrome (hysteria) is both a somatoform and a "psychoform" illness: a Minnesota Multiphasic Personality Inventory study. *Psychosom Med* 1994;**56**(6):564–9.
45. MacDonald CF. Feigned epilepsy. Case of James Clegg, alias James Lee, the "Dummy Chucker." *Am J Insanity* 1880;**37**:1–22.
46. Hammond RD. Simulated epilepsy: report of a case. *Arch Neurol Psychiatry* 1948;**60**:327–8.

47. Gordon N. Episodic dyscontrol syndrome. *Dev Med Child Neurol* 1999;**41**(11):786–8.
48. Drake ME, Jr. Saline activation of pseudoepileptic seizures: clinical EEG and neuropsychiatric observations. *Clin Electroencephalogr* 1985;**16**(3):171–6.
49. Olvera RL. Intermittent explosive disorder: epidemiology, diagnosis and management. *CNS Drugs* 2002;**16**(8):517–26.
50. Brown RJ, Trimble MR. Dissociative psychopathology, non-epileptic seizures, and neurology. *J Neurol Neurosurg Psychiatry* 2000;**69**(3):285–8.
51. Kuyk J, Van Dyck R, Spinhoven P. The case for a dissociative interpretation of pseudoepileptic seizures. *J Nerv Ment Dis* 1996;**184**(8):468–74.
52. Bowman ES. Why conversion seizures should be classified as a dissociative disorder. *Psychiatr Clin North Am* 2006;**29**(1):185–211, x.
53. Marchetti RL, Kurcgant D, Neto JG, *et al.* Psychiatric diagnoses of patients with psychogenic non-epileptic seizures. *Seizure* 2008;**17**(3):247–53.
54. Tabassum K, Farooq S. Sociodemographic features, affective symptoms and family functioning in hospitalized patients with dissociative disorder (convulsion type). *J Pak Med Assoc* 2007;**57**(1):23–6.
55. Goldstein LH, Mellers JD. Ictal symptoms of anxiety, avoidance behaviour, and dissociation in patients with dissociative seizures. *J Neurol Neurosurg Psychiatry* 2006;**77**(5):616–21.
56. Sar V, Akyuz G, Kundakci T, Kiziltan E, Dogan O. Childhood trauma, dissociation, and psychiatric comorbidity in patients with conversion disorder. *Am J Psychiatry* 2004;**161**(12):2271–6.
57. Fiszman A, Alves-Leon SV, Nunes RG, D'Andrea I, Figueira I. Traumatic events and posttraumatic stress disorder in patients with psychogenic nonepileptic seizures: a critical review. *Epilepsy Behav* 2004;**5**(6):818–25.
58. Akyuz G, Kugu N, Akyuz A, Dogan O. Dissociation and childhood abuse history in epileptic and pseudoseizure patients. *Epileptic Disord* 2004;**6**(3):187–92.
59. Reuber M, House AO, Pukrop R, Bauer J, Elger CE. Somatization, dissociation and general psychopathology in patients with psychogenic non-epileptic seizures. *Epilepsy Res* 2003;**57**(2–3):159–67.
60. Prueter C, Schultz-Venrath U, Rimpau W. Dissociative and associated psychopathological symptoms in patients with epilepsy, pseudoseizures, and both seizure forms. *Epilepsia* 2002;**43**(2):188–92.

61. Devinsky O. Neurological aspects of the conscious and unconscious mind. *Ann N Y Acad Sci* 1997;**835**:321–9.
62. Moscovitch M. Recovered consciousness: a hypothesis concerning modularity and episodic memory. *J Clin Exp Neuropsychol* 1995;**17**(2):276–90.
63. Kihlstrom JF. The cognitive unconscious. *Science* 1987;**237**(4821):1445–52.
64. McCormick DA. Cortical and subcortical generators of normal and abnormal rhythmicity. *Int Rev Neurobiol* 2002;**49**:99–114.
65. Hasenstaub A, Sachdev RN, McCormick DA. State changes rapidly modulate cortical neuronal responsiveness. *J Neurosci* 2007;**27**(36):9607–22.
66. McCormick DA, Contreras D. On the cellular and network bases of epileptic seizures. *Annu Rev Physiol* 2001;**63**:815–46.
67. Monaco F, Mula M, Cavanna AE. Consciousness, epilepsy, and emotional qualia. *Epilepsy Behav* 2005;**7**(2):150–60.
68. Oana Y. Epileptic seizures and pseudoseizures from the viewpoint of the hierarchy of consciousness. *Epilepsia* 1998;**39** Suppl 5:21–5.
69. Devinsky O, D'Esposito M. Neuroanatomy and assessment of cognitive-behavioral function. In: Devinsky O, D'Esposito M, eds. *Neurology of Cognitive and Behavioral Disorders*. Oxford; New York: Oxford University Press. 2004; 1–51.
70. Sierra M, Berrios GE. Towards a neuropsychiatry of conversive hysteria. *Cogn Neuropsychiatry* 1999;**4**(3):267–87.
71. Devinsky O, D'Esposito M. The right hemisphere, interhemispheric communication, and consciousness. In: Devinsky O, D'Esposito M, eds. *Neurology of Cognitive and Behavioral Disorders*. Oxford; New York: Oxford University Press. 2004; 68–95.
72. Reuber M, Fernandez G, Helmstaedter C, Quirishi A, Elger CE. Evidence of brain abnormality in patients with psychogenic nonepileptic seizures. *Epilepsy Behav* 2002;**3**:249–54.
73. Devinsky O, Mesad S, Alper K. Nondominant hemisphere lesions and conversion nonepileptic seizures. *J Neuropsychiatry Clin Neurosci* 2001;**13**(3):367–73.
74. Tucker G, Popkin M, Caine E, Folstein M, Grant I. Reorganizing the "organic" disorders. *Hosp Community Psychiatry* 1990;**41**(7):722–4.
75. Rothner AD. 'Not everything that shakes is epilepsy'. The differential diagnosis of paroxysmal nonepileptiform disorders. *Cleve Clin J Med* 1989;**56** Suppl Pt 2:S206–13.
76. Grubb BP, Gerard G, Wolfe DA, *et al*. Syncope and seizures of psychogenic origin: identification with head-upright tilt table testing. *Clin Cardiol* 1992;**15**(11):839–42.
77. Grubb BP, Gerard G, Roush K, *et al*. Differentiation of convulsive syncope and epilepsy with head-up tilt testing. *Ann Intern Med* 1991;**115**(11):871–6.
78. Gerstner E, Liberato B, Wright CB. Bi-hemispheric anterior cerebral artery with drop attacks and limb shaking TIAs. *Neurology* 2005;**65**(1):174.
79. Fisher RS. Imitators of epilepsy. *CNS Spectr* 1997;**2**(6):39–55.
80. Martin RL. Diagnostic issues for conversion disorder. *Hosp Community Psychiatry* 1992;**43**(8):771–3.
81. O'Shea B. Factitious disorders: the Baron's legacy. *Int J Psychiatr Clin Prac* 2003;**7**:33–9.
82. Devinsky O, Putnam F, Grafman J, Bromfield E, Theodore WH. Dissociative states and epilepsy. *Neurology* 1989;**39**(6):835–40.
83. Ross CA, Heber S, Anderson G, *et al*. Differentiating multiple personality disorder and complex partial seizures. *Gen Hosp Psychiatry* 1989;**11**(1):54–8.

Section 4 Chapter 22

Psychiatric considerations in adults with psychogenic nonepileptic seizures

Posttraumatic stress disorder, abuse, and trauma: relationships to psychogenic nonepileptic seizures

Elizabeth S. Bowman

Psychogenic nonepileptic seizures (PNES) are part of the ancient disease of hysteria, attributed for 3800 years to uterine wandering by Egyptians and early Greeks [1]. PNES are linked to trauma via hysteria's association with sexuality and trauma. American psychiatry abandoned the diagnosis of hysteria when the Diagnostic and Statistical Manual of Mental Disorders, Third Edition (DSM-III) [2] split hysteria into somatoform and dissociative disorders, posttraumatic stress disorder (PTSD), and other diagnoses. PNES are classified in DSM-IV [3] within the somatoform disorders as "conversion disorder, with seizures or convulsions." The International Classification of Diseases, Tenth Edition (ICD-10 [4]) classifies PNES as "dissociative seizures."

The connection of hysteria and PNES with sexual traumas was popularized in the nineteenth century by Pierre Janet and Charcot [5]. Briquet, Charcot, and Janet [5–9] described seizures and other conversion symptoms in response to traumas such as marital stress, divorce, injuries, and unwanted pregnancies. Janet's hysteria/conversion case histories connected PNES onset with frights, and abusive relationships, accidents, and bereavement traumas [5, 6–8]. Janet posited that conversion symptoms were symbolic reenactments of traumas split off (dissociated) from consciousness and associated with fixed unconscious ideas [8]. His theories of PNES from dissociated trauma remain valid today. Reports of childhood sexual abuse in late-nineteenth-century PNES literature created controversies. After Freud discarded the sexual seduction (trauma) theory of hysteria and proposed his infantile sexuality theory [5], interest in a connection between trauma and PNES waned until the late twentieth century.

Modern data on the interrelationships of trauma/abuse, PTSD, and PNES

Studies of PNES have burgeoned since the advent of video-EEG (VEEG) recording in the 1970s. Video-EEG studies enabled neurologists to be certain of PNES diagnoses and created awareness of their unsuspected high prevalence. Sufficient studies of trauma and PTSD in PNES exist to justify a literature review [10]. Two categories of data exist on the relationship of PNES to trauma/abuse and PTSD: direct evidence from assessment of abuse/trauma and PTSD in patients with PNES, and indirect evidence from studies of comorbid abuse-related psychiatric conditions in persons with PNES. This chapter considers direct and indirect evidence, and theoretical explanations for the association of PNES with abuse/trauma and PTSD.

Direct evidence associating PNES with abuse/trauma

"Abuse" usually designates interpersonal trauma, while "trauma" encompasses a wide range of phenomena. We consider both abuse and trauma in PNES.

Physical, sexual, and emotional abuse

Numerous reports exist on the association of abuse/trauma with PNES. Initially, the focus was on childhood sexual abuse in persons with PNES [11–15]. The focus of research widened to physical and psychological childhood abuse, and now includes studies of nonabuse traumas/stresses and adult trauma [16–22]. PNES studies have become more sophisticated, but

Gates and Rowan's Nonepileptic Seizures, 3rd edn. ed. Steven C. Schachter and W. Curt LaFrance, Jr. Published by Cambridge University Press. © S. Schachter and W. C. LaFrance, Jr. 2010.

are still retrospective, cross sectional, and reflect association rather than causality [10].

Not all of the modern studies of abuse and trauma in PNES have utilized comparison subjects, VEEG diagnosis, or validated assessment methods. Fiszman *et al.*'s [10] review of studies (1950–2004) of traumatic events and PTSD in patients with PNES cites 17 studies before April 2004 that utilized VEEG and explicit diagnostic criteria. They reviewed how research methodology complicates comparison of studies of abuse and trauma in PNES, including failure to account for the proportion of females in patients with PNES and comparison subjects. Women report more physical and sexual trauma than men. Thus, higher proportions of women in PNES samples than in controls may falsely elevate reported abuse in PNES. However, one study that controlled gender proportions in PNES and epilepsy subjects found significantly more reported childhood sexual abuse (70% vs. 32%, $p<0.05$) and general traumatic events (100% vs. 68%, $p<0.05$) in patients with PNES [21].

Fiszman *et al.* [10] reported rates of traumatic events of 76% to 100% in subjects with PNES, with a lower rate (44%) in a study of minors [23] that considered only "severe family stressors" such as parental divorce, discord, or death of a family member. Fiszman *et al.* reported on a meta-analysis of other studies of trauma, abuse and PTSD in PNES subjects [10]. They did not define traumatic events. Reported lifetime rates of physical and/or sexual abuse in subjects with PNES were 50% to 77%, far higher than in general populations. Lower overall abuse rates (27% to 38%) were found in three studies of patients with PNES whose abuse occurred before age 18 [17, 24, 25]. Higher rates of general trauma in subjects with PNES have been found in some [26, 27], but not all, controlled studies. Rates of childhood abuse, usually defined as interpersonal physical, sexual, or emotional abuse occurring before age 18, were significantly higher in patients with PNES (9% to 70%) compared to comparison subjects in three [27–29] of five controlled studies.

Since 2004, some controlled studies of subjects with PNES have found more sexual (30%), nonsexual (73% to 86%), and overall (44% to 90%) trauma in these patients [22, 28] compared to controls. Studies differ on which types of trauma occur at significantly higher rates in patients with PNES than in controls, but adult physical abuse [22] and childhood psychological abuse [21, 28] significantly distinguish PNES groups from controls. Studies [20, 22, 28] employing systematic inquiry by a psychotherapist interviewer in an individual confidential setting study found overall lifetime trauma in 84% [20] to 90% [28] of patients with PNES. Studies using self-report or unsystematic assessment report lower rates of trauma in those with PNES.

Childhood neglect

Child neglect is rarely mentioned in the PNES literature but could contribute to PNES by creating a disorganized attachment style in infants that has been empirically linked with dissociation at age 20 [30–32]. Internationally, PNES experts posit that dissociation is the likely mechanism that produces PNES [33–40]. This theoretical link between neglect and PNES does not yet have the support from data compared to the link between PNES and child abuse. Child abuse generally occurs in the context of neglectful, disorganized family settings, creating the possibility that abused children are neglected [19, 21, 26], but researchers infrequently assess neglect in subjects with PNES. Persons with PNES report significantly less parental warmth and more parental rejection in childhood than do comparison subjects with epileptic seizures (ES) [17, 21].

Other traumas

Increasingly, studies now assess other traumas in subjects with PNES, and have reported higher rates of nonabuse stressful life events [16, 21, 22, 26] in those with PNES compared to controls with functional neurological symptoms [26]. Bereavement commonly precipitates PNES [16, 26]. Family dysfunction is highly associated with perpetuating PNES [19, 26], especially in women [26], and was found as the factor mediating the association of PNES with abuse and with somatization [21]. Health anxiety commonly precipitates PNES in men [26]. Compared to patients with epilepsy, those with PNES have significantly more negative life events, perceive events as significantly more stressful, have higher stress scores and significantly more dysfunctional cognitions and ruminations about stress, more stress-related disease, more social pressures, more health anxiety (in males), and report poorer childhood relationships with fathers and less perceived parental care [22, 26, 31]. Recent work [18, 21, 27, 30] highlights the role of family dysfunction in creating insecure attachment that predisposes to somatization in creating PNES.

Summary of trauma/abuse

Most, but not all, studies of patients with PNES in comparison to patients with ES have found higher prevalence of abuse, trauma, and life stresses in those with PNES, despite rates of abuse in patients with ES that exceed general population rates. Diverse methodology limits generalization from these studies. Clear trends include the association of PNES with nonsexual abuse, adult trauma/abuse, multiple traumas and the role of family dysfunction and insecure attachment [11, 16, 18, 19, 21, 22, 26, 27, 30–32]. Childhood sexual abuse is no longer held to be a unique or even necessary precipitant for PNES. The most significant association between PNES and trauma appears to be a family environment that fosters attachment trauma and produces tendencies toward somatization.

Direct evidence associating PNES with PTSD

Experience of a significant trauma is a criterion for diagnosis of DSM-IV PTSD. Persons who report enough symptoms for a DSM-IV PTSD diagnosis also report trauma, but evaluators do not always have confirmation of those trauma reports. Many studies have evaluated patients with PNES for PTSD. Symptoms of PTSD abound in the hysteria/conversion seizure case studies of Janet [6–8] and in war trauma survivors for millennia [33]. Since DSM-III in 1980 [2], the term Posttraumatic Stress Disorder and specific criteria have enabled study of PTSD. Not all traumatized persons develop PTSD. Is there evidence that rates of PTSD in patients with PNES exceed those of patients with ES or general population groups? Eleven studies provide us these data.

Fiszman et al.'s review of these 11 studies [10] noted current PTSD in 14% to 100% of subjects with PNES [26, 27, 34, 35] (median 33%). Patients with PNES had a higher prevalence of PTSD than comparison subjects in four studies, but this reached statistical significance in only one study [34]. The prevalence of PTSD in populations with ES is also high (11% to 37%) [28, 34, 35,]. Two literature reviews [10, 35] and other studies report current PTSD in 4% to 49% of adults [17, 20, 36–40] and 8.8% of children and adolescents [41] with PNES. The lifetime prevalence of PTSD in patients with PNES is reported as 36% to 100% (median 60% to 61%) [20, 29, 35, 41], and nearly all studies have cited rates that exceed the prevalence in the general population (9%) [42] and in combat veterans (15% to 25%) [43]. These rates of PTSD are understandable in the highly traumatized population of patients with PNES.

In summary, there is evidence that persons with PNES have a higher prevalence of current (14% to 100%) and lifetime (36% to 100%) PTSD than the general population or comparison samples with ES. The wide range of PTSD prevalence in patients with PNES in research reports reflects diverse subject populations and methodology. Studies that systematically assessed PTSD or used multiple assessment tools reported higher rates of PTSD. Giving a PTSD checklist or self-report form to a patient with PNES is unlikely to ascertain all persons with this illness, since not all subjects are aware that their PTSD symptoms are traumatic in origin. It is likely that elevated PTSD rates in patients with PNES are related to reported adulthood and childhood physical and sexual abuse, but insufficient data exist to draw firm conclusions about whether the high rates of PTSD in these subjects reflect a traumatic etiology [27]. Confirmation of abuse or trauma reports cannot easily be obtained during most research studies.

Two types of PTSD have been proposed [44–47], based on distinct types of neurophysiological responses to trauma [47, 48]: a primarily intrusive hyperaroused PTSD and a dissociative type. In persons with PTSD, these persistent distinct neurophysiological responses to reminders of trauma suggest different underlying neuronal mechanisms for PTSD [47, 49]. Peri-traumatic dissociation predicts development of PTSD [50–52]. Patients with PNES report considerable trauma, PTSD, and dissociative symptoms. Thus, Fiszman et al. [10] propose that PNES may be a clinical expression of the dissociative type of PTSD, but acknowledge that this categorization will not apply to all patients with PNES. This author agrees that patients with PNES are not all characterized by PTSD but observes that some exhibit both dissociative and intrusive forms of PTSD. Evidence that PNES are a dissociative form of PTSD awaits further studies.

Indirect evidence associating PNES with trauma: comorbid disorders

Indirect evidence for a relationship between PNES and trauma comes from the association of PNES with other disorders that are linked to trauma by association. Due to space limitations, this chapter discusses only two of these associations: dissociative disorders and nonconversion somatoform disorders. Their association with PNES does not imply causality; each could be causally related to mutual intervening third factors such as disordered attachment or family environment (summarized in [27] and [32]).

Dissociative disorders

The dissociative nature of PNES symptoms, as part of hysteria, has been noted from Janet [1, 6–8] through the present time [33–42]. After DSM-III, conversion disorder (PNES) was classified with the somatoform disorders in the DSMs and dissociative disorders in the ICDs [4]. Nemiah [53] and others [33–35, 37, 54] advocated for returning PNES to the DSM dissociative disorders for a better diagnostic fit with some cultures [54]. Not all events diagnosed (accurately or inaccurately) as PNES have psychological dissociation, such as simple partial PNES without change in level of consciousness, and reclassification would require a redefining of "dissociation" to be included in this category. PNES have been called somatoform dissociation [39]. Somatoform and psychoform dissociation (e.g., amnesia, depersonalization, identity alteration) correlate [55], so the association of PNES with psychoform dissociative disorders could imply a somatoform dissociative mechanism for PNES.

Dissociative disorders have been robustly associated with trauma [53–63]. Current and lifetime prevalence of nonconversion dissociative disorders in patients with PNES is 11% to 100% [64], with median prevalence of 33% [14, 20, 65–69]. DSM-IV Dissociative Identity Disorder (DID) in patients with PNES has been reported in 15% and 16% [20, 38] but a study of ICD-10 dissociative disorder patients (mixed DSM-IV dissociative and conversion) found no DID [54]. DSM-IV Dissociative Disorder Not Otherwise Specified (DDNOS) has been found in 27% to 62% [20, 66] of patients with PNES and in 55% of those patients with both PNES and ICD-10 dissociative disorders [54]. The symptom of dissociative amnesia occurs in up to 98% in patients with PNES [20], but the diagnosis of DSM-IV Dissociative Amnesia is made less often (13%, 53%) [20, 64, 68] because its criteria exclude amnesia occurring only in the course of DID, PTSD, or Somatization Disorder [3]. Patients with PNES have rates of DSM-III-R dissociative disorders above those of populations of psychiatric patients [57].

The reverse – high rates of conversion in patients with dissociative disorder – also occurs. Six studies of all conversion types in patients with DID or its predecessor, multiple personality disorder (MPD) (summarized in [33]) found some type of conversion in 10% to 57%. Conversion in patients with DDNOS and Dissociative Amnesia is reported in 14% and 24% respectively [66, 67]. The occurrence of PNES in MPD/DID is unknown, but "seizures" (cause unknown, possibly epilepsy) are reported in 11% to 67% [38, 63, 69–70]. These rates of conversion far exceed the 0.022% prevalence in the US general population and 4.5% in psychiatric outpatients [71].

The relationship of dissociation to conversion seizures is complex. Despite very high prevalences of conversion seizures in patients with DID [38, 63], and of dissociative disorders in patients with PNES [20, 35, 38], levels of dissociation do not differentiate ES from PNES [70]. PNES cannot only be solely due to dissociation, despite their proposed dissociative mechanism [34, 35, 37–39]. Likewise, other conversion disorder manifestations, such as in patients with psychogenic movement disorders or conversion paralysis, do not always demonstrate dissociative states with their symptoms. This confusing situation is likely related to imprecision in DSM-IV diagnostic criteria for conversion disorder and to differences between diagnosis of conversion in DSM-IV [3] and the ICD-10 [4].

Other somatoform disorders

Psychogenic nonepileptic seizures are highly comorbid with adulthood and childhood abuse and with other DSM-IV somatoform disorders (reviewed in [72]).

Somatoform pain disorder has been reported in 14% to 77% of patients with PNES [35]. Chronic unexplained headaches are especially common (61% to 73%) [20, 63, 64, 72] in subjects with PNES, in patients with DSM dissociative disorders, and in survivors of childhood abuse [63, 69, 71–78] compared to controls. In patients with somatoform pain, especially those with chronic pelvic pain (CPP), the prevalence of childhood sexual abuse has been reported as 36% to 70% [79, 80]. Chronic pelvic pain has been proposed as a somatoform disorder [80] but has not been studied in patients with PNES. With rare exception [77], women with nonsomatic CPP have significantly more childhood [80–83] and adulthood [81] sexual abuse than women with somatically based pelvic pain.

The prevalence of physical or sexual abuse in patients with general pain is over 50% [84] and correlates with number of body areas and severity of pain symptoms, and higher levels of medical care utilization [84, 85]. Patients with irritable bowel syndrome (IBS) or functional abdominal pain have a high prevalence of PTSD (36%) [86] and more childhood sexual abuse than comparison groups with medical (i.e., nonfunctional) disease [87, 88].

Childhood maltreatment (physical, sexual, and emotional) has been found to be a general risk factor for fibromyalgia [89–94]. Generally, particular forms of childhood maltreatment (e.g., sexual abuse) have not been found to be specific fibromyalgia risk factors [90], but rape was significantly associated with fibromyalgia in one study [95]. The reported lifetime prevalence of physical and sexual abuse in fibromyalgia patients is 53% to 64% [91, 92, 94–96]. In persons with refractory seizures, a fibromyalgia diagnosis predicts PNES on VEEG in 75% of patients [97]. Patients with fibromyalgia report more adulthood physical and sexual abuse than do controls with physically explained pain [90]. Psychogenic nonepileptic seizures are linked to fibromyalgia and both diagnoses are significantly associated with abuse, often with childhood abuse, and poor relationships with parents [89, 90].

One study [93] found a strong and specific relationship between adult physical assault and unexplained pain. Patients with PNES, a group that reports a significant lifetime prevalence of physical assault [10, 20], exhibit high rates of unexplained pain, as mentioned above [20, 62–64, 72]. Given the link between fibromyalgia and abuse, an association between fibromyalgia and PTSD might be expected. Comorbidity between PTSD and fibromyalgia significantly exceeds chance expectations [98]. Men with PTSD have a significantly higher point prevalence of fibromyalgia (49%) compared to normal controls (0%) [98]. Community women with fibromyalgia have been found to be significantly ($p < 0.01$) more likely to have PTSD symptoms or a PTSD diagnosis compared to women without fibromyalgia [96]. Among female outpatients, a diagnosis of PTSD nearly doubles the odds of having a fibromyalgia diagnosis [99, 100]. PTSD is strongly linked to chronic widespread pain (as occurs in fibromyalgia), but the link does not appear related to genetic vulnerability to both pain and PTSD [101]. Overall, PNES is associated with fibromyalgia and PTSD, and all three conditions are significantly associated with trauma.

Somatization disorder (Briquet's syndrome) has been associated with reports of psychological, sexual, and physical trauma precipitants since Briquet's original report [9]. DSM-IV somatization disorder requires eight symptoms, including one conversion symptom. Consistently, higher levels of somatization, with and without formal somatization disorder, are found in clinical and nonclinical samples of sexual abuse survivors than in comparison groups without sexual abuse [102–107].

In 11 studies of patients with PNES, the prevalence of any DSM somatoform diagnosis ranged from 2% to 100% (median prevalence 33%) [63]. With systematic assessment, DSM-III-R [108] or DSM-IV somatization disorder has been found in 13% of subjects with PNES [20] compared to 0.38% in the US [105, 107] and 1.6% in the German general population [109]. Patients with PNES have a strikingly high (42% to 93%) prevalence of other conversion symptoms [64] and have a lifetime mean of 5.9 different conversion symptoms [68]. DSM-IV undifferentiated somatoform disorder (less than eight somatoform symptoms) in those with PNES has been found in 18% to 25% [22, 110]. PNES appear to be only one manifestation of widespread somatic defenses in these persons. Somatoform symptoms, dissociation, PTSD, and trauma are highly associated in many studies, with levels of pain predicting higher levels of dissociation [82, 111, 112] but these associations may imply a shared causal pathway of neurobehavioral development rather than trauma as the causal factor for PNES.

Theories of the etiology of PNES, in relation to trauma and PTSD

Theories abound regarding the etiology of PNES, indicating its etiology remains uncertain. For 120 years, the major etiological theory for PNES has been trauma/abuse with dissociation, but other theories are supportable [1, 6–9, 113]. The specific symptom production mechanism of PNES remains unknown. Below are major theories of PNES etiology and discussion of their possible relationship to trauma or PTSD.

PNES as dissociation

Dissociation is a common theory for the etiology of PNES [34–39, 53, 111–115], but actually explains the mechanism rather than etiology of PNES. Dissociation in PNES is posited as a somatic coping response to trauma [34, 35, 39, 56], a symptom of PTSD [10], or as somatic dissociation itself [39, 55, 115, 116]. Nijenhuis et al. [55] proposed that dissociative and conversion disorders are psychological and somatoform types of dissociation that can be reliably measured by the Somatoform Dissociation Questionnaire (SDQ-5 and SDQ-20) [39, 116]. The SDQ-20 screens for psychoform dissociation (DSM-IV dissociative disorders) and includes an item on "pseudo-epileptic attacks" [39]. Somatoform dissociation is linked to reported trauma, emotional numbing, and neurobiological animal defensive reactions of freezing and analgesia [39]. The somatoform dissociation theory is supported by somatoform dissociation (SDQ-20), but not psychoform dissociation, discriminating patients with PNES from those with ES [70]. Physical and sexual trauma, occurring in emotionally neglectful contexts, predict somatoform dissociation [39]. The traumatic somatoform dissociation theory of the etiology of PNES is well supported empirically.

PNES as a manifestation of PTSD

From PTSD neuroimaging studies, Fiszman et al. [10] propose a mechanism by which trauma and dissociation may produce PNES and suggest that PNES may be an expression of the dissociative type of PTSD. When people with PTSD recall trauma, perfusion of the left hemisphere Broca's area (expressive speech) decreases [117]. Persons with PTSD lateralize trauma memory function to the usually nonverbal right hemisphere [118]. Patients with PNES lack adequate verbal expression [19, 21], often have PTSD, and have considerable dissociation. Peri-traumatic dissociation generally predicts development of PTSD [50–52]. Neurophysiological and neuroimaging responses to trauma scripts in patients with PTSD fall into two distinct categories: dissociative and hyperaroused [51, 118, 119]. Fiszman et al. [10] do not explain why PNES would fall into the dissociative rather than the hyperaroused category of PTSD. Their intriguing theory of PNES as a type of PTSD awaits further confirmation by functional neuroimaging of subjects with PNES. This author hypothesizes that subjects with PNES may fall into both categories of PTSD, with some PNES representing flashbacks of trauma [114, 120–122] and others unresponsive dissociative states. This theory predicts cessation of PNES when PTSD is treated in patients with PNES [10].

Quinn et al. [27] rearranged Bowman's [114] proposed four etiological pathways to PNES by proposing three groups of patients with PNES. Three of Bowman's and all of Quinn et al.'s groups are related to trauma, but not specifically to PTSD. Quinn et al.'s theory includes attachment trauma.

PNES as attachment trauma and family dysfunction

This theory proposes that attachment trauma from disturbed family relationships predisposes patients with PNES to abuse, dissociation, PTSD, and somatization [10, 27, 43], explaining the dissociative and posttraumatic mechanism of PTSD. Disorganized attachment predicts the development of dissociation after trauma [31, 32, 72]. Trauma and insecure attachment style in adults make independent contributions to levels of somatization [26, 32]. Childhood familial abuse in patients with PNES occurs in emotionally abusive and dysfunctional families [19, 21, 26, 122, 123]. Dysfunctional families produce disorganized attachment and offspring predisposed to somatization [21, 32, 72, 122, 123]. In patients with PNES, abuse appears to be a marker for family dysfunction that produces somatization [21].

How might disrupted attachment predict PNES? From neuroimaging data, Quinn et al. [27] propose that attachment disruption and ongoing trauma are associated with underdevelopment of left hemisphere neural connections (limbic system to cingulate gyrus and frontal cortex) related to verbal expression, right hemisphere dominance, and reduced right hemisphere regulation of affect and impulsivity. Overwhelmed by poorly regulated affect, patients with PNES dissociate and utilize somatic flashbacks rather than verbal coping, i.e., express both types of PTSD. Quinn et al.'s theory may explain how early trauma predisposes to adult somatization [120, 123]. Supportive evidence for this theory awaits controlled studies of adult attachment styles in patients with PNES.

PNES as panic attacks

Some PNES are theorized to be related to unrecognized panic disorder [124–127]. Panic is common (14% to 90%) in patients with PNES [64, 68, 69, 110,

127] and has been proposed as one cause of PNES [110]. Quinn *et al.* [27] proposes that one group of patients with PNES has underdeveloped emotional regulation skills, experiences trauma, and develops panic attacks. Agreement exists that some persons with supposed PNES actually are exhibiting misdiagnosed panic attacks [27, 69, 110, 127]. Panic attacks should not be diagnosed as PNES; panic is not strictly a cause of PNES but should be in the differential diagnosis of evaluations for possible PNES.

PNES as brain trauma

This theory posits that repetitive brain trauma from head injuries (accidental and abusive) [16, 20] or poorly controlled epilepsy [124] may cause PNES by impairing affect regulation and disrupting a coherent sense of self, leading to somatic expressions of affect via PNES [27]. This theory may explain coexisting epilepsy and PNES, but needs more research for support.

Conclusions

The association of PNES with trauma and dissociation is robust [128]. PTSD is frequently associated with PNES, but the significance of this association is unclear. PNES is related to trauma and PTSD by association, which does not imply causality by trauma. Indeed, a minority of patients with PNES does not report a trauma history. The field of PNES has moved from assuming that childhood sexual abuse caused PNES [123] to demonstrating that multiple abuses and non-abuse traumas are associated with PNES. The focus has moved toward assessing data on brain laterality in patients with PTSD, attachment trauma, and dysfunctional families to more comprehensive theories linking PNES to trauma and PTSD via mediating causes of disrupted attachment creating dissociation.

Clinical observations and research data provide evidence that no single cause exists for all patients with PNES. Some events resemble the dissociative flashbacks seen in patients with PTSD; others are simple dissociative trance states suspected as absence epilepsy without a DSM-IV diagnosis, and fall outside dissociative seizures in the ICD-10 [4], and some appear to have no change in level of consciousness. It is not clear whether those patients without changes in level of consciousness truly have PNES or have motor type conversion misdiagnosed as seizure type conversion. Nearly all patients with PNES have dissociative symptoms; this author argues for a dissociative pathway for most patients with PNES. In some patients, panic attacks may be misdiagnosed as PNES.

In many patients with PNES, a mélange of stresses and traumas have overwhelmed affect regulation systems already impaired by invalidating family environments that suppressed emotional and verbal expression. Trauma and PTSD are intimately related to PNES, but PNES has no single cause, as elegantly stated by Pierre Janet [8]: "The hysterical fit of convulsions, far from being a simple phenomenon, is, on the contrary, a very variable and complex symptom. The convulsions have all sorts of meanings..."

References

1. Veith I. *Hysteria. The History of a Disease*. Chicago: University of Chicago, 1965.
2. American Psychiatric Association. *Diagnostic and Statistical Manual of Mental Disorders*, 3rd edn. (DSM-III). Washington, DC: American Psychiatric Association, 1980.
3. American Psychiatric Association. *Diagnostic and Statistical Manual of Mental Disorders*, 4th edn. Washington, DC: American Psychiatric Association, 1994.
4. World Health Organization. *The ICD-10 Classification of Mental and Behavioural Disorders. Clinical Descriptions and Diagnostic Guidelines*. Geneva, Switzerland: World Psychiatric Association. 1992; 151, 737–9.
5. Ellenberger, HF. *The Discovery of the Unconscious. The History and Evolution of Dynamic Psychiatry*. New York: Harper Basic Books, 1970.
6. Janet P. *L'Automatisme Psychologique*. Paris: Alcan, 1889.
7. Janet P. *Contribution a l'études accidents mentaux chez les hystériques*. Paris: Rueff et Cie, 1893.
8. Janet P. *The Major Symptoms of Hysteria*. London: MacMillan Co., 1907.
9. Briquet P. *Traité d'hysterie*. Paris: Ballière et Fils, 1859.
10. Fiszman A, Alves-Leon SV, Nunes RG, D'Andea I, Figueira I. Traumatic events and posttraumatic stress disorder in patients with psychogenic nonepileptic seizures: a critical review. *Epilepsy Behav* 2004;**5**:818–25.
11. Goodwin J, Simms M, Bergman R. Hysterical seizures: a sequel to incest. *Am J Orthopsychiatry* 1979;**49**:698–703.

12. Goodwin J. Pseudoseizures and incest. *Am J Psychiatry* 1979;**136**:1231.

13. LaBarbera JK, Dozier JE. Psychologic responses of incestuous daughters: emerging patterns. *South Med J* 1981;**74**:1478–80.

14. Gross M. Incestuous rape: a cause for hysterical seizures in our adolescent girls. *Am J Orthopsychiatry* 1979;**49**:704–8.

15. Betts T, Boden S. Diagnosis, management and prognosis of a group of 128 patients in non-epileptic attack disorder. Part II. Previous childhood sexual abuse in the etiology of these disorders. *Seizure* 1992;**1**:27–32.

16. Bowman ES, Markand ON. The contribution of life events to pseudoseizure occurrence in adults. *Bull Menninger Clin* 1999;**63**(1):70–88.

17. Binzer M, Stone J, Sharpe M. Recent onset pseudoseizures – clues to aetiology. *Seizure* 2004;**13**:146–55.

18. Krawetz P, Fleisher W, Pillay N, *et al.* Family functioning in subjects with pseudoseizures and epilepsy. *J Nerv Ment Dis* 2001;**189**:38–43.

19. Griffith JJ, Polles A, Griffith ME. Pseudoseizures, families and unspeakable dilemmas. *Psychosomatics* 1998;**39**:144–53.

20. Bowman ES, Markand ON. Psychodynamics and psychiatric diagnoses of pseudoseizure subjects. *Am J Psychiatry* 1996;**153**:57–63.

21. Salmon P, Al-Marzooqi SM, Baker G, Reilly J. Childhood family dysfunction and associated abuse in patients with nonepileptic seizures: toward a causal model. *Psychosom Med* 2003;**65**:695–700.

22. Tojek TM, Lumley M, Barkley G, Mahr G, Thomas A. Stress and other psychosocial characteristics of patients with psychogenic nonepileptic seizures. *Psychosomatics* 2000;**41**:221–6.

23. Wyllie E, Glazer JP, Benbadis S, *et al.* Psychiatric features of children and adolescents with pseudoseizures. *Arch Pediatr Adolesc Med* 1999;**153**:244–8.

24. Alper K, Devinsky O, Perrine K, Vazquez B, Luciano D. Nonepileptic seizures and childhood sexual and physical abuse. *Neurology* 1993;**43**:1950–3.

25. Alper K, Devinsky O, Perrine K, *et al.* Dissociation in epilepsy and conversion nonepileptic seizures. *Epilepsia* 1997;**38**:991–7.

26. Reuber M, Howlett S, Khan A, Grünewald RA. Non-epileptic seizures and other functional neurological symptoms: predisposing, precipitating, and perpetuating factors. *Psychosomatics* 2007;**48**(3):230–8.

27. Quinn M, Schofield M, Middleton W. Conceptualization and treatment of psychogenic non-epileptic seizures. *J Trauma Dissociation* 2008;**9**(1):63–84.

28. Dikel TN, Fennell EB, Gilmore RL. Posttraumatic stress disorder, dissociation, and sexual abuse history in epileptic and nonepileptic seizure patients. *Epilepsy Behav* 2003;**4**:644–50.

29. Arnold LM, Privitera MD. Psychopathology and trauma in epileptic and psychogenic seizure patients. *Psychosomatics* 1996;**37**:438–43.

30. van Ijzendoorn M, Schuengel C, Bakermans-Kranenburg MJ. Disorganized attachment in early childhood: meta-analysis of precursors, concomitants, and sequelae. *Dev Psychopathol* 1999;**11**:225–49.

31. Ogawa JR, Sroufe LA, Weinfield NS, *et al.* Development and the fragmented self: longitudinal study of dissociative symptomatology in a nonclinical sample. *Dev Psychopathol* 1997;**9**:855–79.

32. Harari D, Bakersman-Kranenburg MJ, van Ijzendoorn MJ. Attachment, disorganization, and dissociation. In: Vermetten E, Dorahy MJ, Spiegel D, eds. *Traumatic Dissociation: Neurobiology and Treatment.* Washington: American Psychiatric Press. 2007;31–54.

33. van der Kolk BA, Weisaeth L, van der Hart O. History of trauma in psychiatry. In: van der Kolk BA, McFarlane AC, Weisaeth L, eds. *Traumatic Stress.* New York: Guilford Press. 1996; 47–74.

34. Bowman ES. Why conversion seizures should be classified as a dissociative disorder. *Psychiatr Clin North Am* 2006;**29**:185–211.

35. Harden CL. Pseudoseizures and dissociative disorder: a common mechanism involving traumatic experiences. *Seizure* 1997;**6**:151–5.

36. Spitzer C, Spelsberg B, Grabe H-J, Mundt B, Freyberger HJ. Dissociative experiences and psychopathology in conversion disorders. *J Psychosom Res* 1999;**46**(3):291–4.

37. Kuyk J, Van Dyck RV, Spinhoven P. The case for a dissociative interpretation of pseudoepileptic seizures. *J Nerv Ment Dis* 1996;**184**:408–74.

38. Tezcan E, Atmaca M, Kuloglu M, *et al.* Dissociative disorders in Turkish inpatients with conversion disorder. *Compr Psychiatry* 2003;**44**(4):324–30.

39. Nijenhuis ERS. *Somatoform Dissociation.* Assen, Netherlands: Van Gorcum, 1999.

40. Tomb DA. Psychogenic seizures. *Neurology* 1992;**42**:1848–9.

41. Wyllie E, Glazer JP, Benbadis S, Kotagal P, Wolgamuth B. Psychiatric features of children and adolescents with

pseudoseizures. *Arch Pediatr Adolesc Med* 1999;**153**:244–8.

42. Breslau N, Davis GC, Andreski P, Peterson E. Traumatic events and posttraumatic stress disorder in an urban population of young adults. *Arch Gen Psychiatry* 1991;**48**:216–22.

43. Kulka RA, Schlenger WE, Fairbank JA, *et al*. *Trauma and the Vietnam War Generation: Report of Findings from the National Vietnam Veterans' Readjustment Study*. New York: Brunner Mazel, 1990.

44. Bremner JD, Narayan M, Staib LH, *et al*. Neural correlates of childhood sexual abuse in women with and without posttraumatic stress disorder. *Am J Psychiatry* 1999;**156**:1787–95.

45. Bremner JD, Staib L, Kaloupek D, *et al*. Neural correlates of exposure to traumatic pictures and sound in Vietnam combat veterans with and without posttraumatic stress disorder: a positron emission tomography study. *Biol Psychiatry* 1999;**45**:806–16.

46. Lanius RA, Williamson PC, Boksman K, *et al*. Brain activation during script-driven imagery induced dissociative responses in PTSD: a functional magnetic resonance imaging investigation. *Biol Psychiatry* 2002;**52**:305–11.

47. Lanius RA, Williamson PC, Densmore M, *et al*. Neural correlates of traumatic memories in posttraumatic stress disorder: a functional MRI investigation. *Am J Psychiatry* 2001;**158**:1920–2.

48. Lanius RA, Bluhm R, Lanius U. Posttraumatic stress disorder symptom provocation and neuroimaging. In: Vermetten E, Dorahy MJ, Spiegel D, eds. *Traumatic Dissociation. Neurobiology and Treatment*. Washington, DC: American Psychiatric Press. 2007; 191–217.

49. Alper K. Nonepileptic seizures. *Neurol Clin* 1994;**12**:153–73.

50. Koopman C, Classen C, Spiegel D. Predictors of posttraumatic stress symptoms among survivors of the Oakland-Berkeley, California firestorm. *Am J Psychiatry* 1994;**151**:888–94.

51. Brewin CR, Andrews B, Rose S, Kirk M. Acute stress disorder and posttraumatic stress disorder in victims of violent crime. *Am J Psychiatry* 1999;**156**:360–6.

52. Classen C, Koopman C, Hales R, Spiegel D. Acute stress disorder as a predictor of posttraumatic stress symptoms. *Am J Psychiatry* 1998;**155**:620–4.

53. Nemiah JC. Dissociation, conversion, and somatization. In: Tasman A, Goldfinger SM, eds. *Review of Psychiatry*, Vol. 10. Washington, DC: American Psychiatric Press. 1991; 249–60.

54. Alexander PJ, Joseph S, Das A. Limited utility of ICD-10 and DSM-IV classification of dissociative and conversion disorders in India. *Acta Psychiatr Scand* 1997;**95**:177–92.

55. Nijenhuis ERS, Spinhoven P, van Dyck R, van der Hart O, Vanderlinden J. Degree of somatoform and psychological dissociation in dissociative disorder is correlated with reported trauma. *J Trauma Stress* 1998;**11**:711–30.

56. van der Hart O, Horst R. The dissociation theory of Pierre Janet. *J Trauma Stress* 1989;**2**(4): 397–412.

57. Ross CA, Anderson G, Fleisher WP, Norton GR. The frequency of multiple personality disorder among psychiatric inpatients. *Am J Psychiatry* 1991;**148**:1717–20.

58. Coons PM. Dissociative disorders not otherwise specified: a clinical investigation of 50 cases with suggestions for treatment. *Dissociation* 1992;**5**: 187–95.

59. Coons PM, Milstein V. Psychogenic amnesia: a clinical investigation of 25 cases. *Dissociation* 1992;**5**: 73–9.

60. Coons PM, Bowman ES, Milstein V. Multiple personality disorder: a clinical investigation of 50 cases. *J Nerv Ment Dis* 1988;**176**:519–27.

61. Ross CA, Miller SD, Reagor P, *et al*. Structured interview data on 102 cases of multiple personality disorder from four centers. *Am J Psychiatry* 1990;**147**:596–601.

62. Dell PF, Eisenhower JW. Adolescent multiple personality disorder: a preliminary study of eleven cases. *J Am Acad Child Adolesc Psychiatry* 1990;**29**:359–66.

63. Putnam FW, Guroff JJ, Silberman EK, *et al*. The clinical phenomenology of multiple personality disorder: review of 100 recent cases. *J Clin Psychiatry* 1986;**47**:285–93.

64. Bowman ES, Kanner AM. Psychopathology and outcome in psychogenic nonepileptic seizures. In: Ettinger AB, Kanner AM, eds. *Psychiatric Issues in Epilepsy: A Practical Guide to Diagnosis and Treatment*. Philadelphia: Lippincott Williams & Wilkins. 2007; 432–60.

65. Jawad SSM, Jamil N, Clarke EJ, *et al*. Psychiatric morbidity and psychodynamics of patients with convulsive pseudoseizures. *Seizure* 1995;**11**: 458–63.

66. Kanner AM, Parra J, Frey M, *et al*. Psychiatric and neurologic predictors of psychogenic pseudoseizure outcome. *Neurology* 1999;**53**:933–8.

67. Ramchandani D, Schindler B. Evaluation of pseudoseizures. A psychiatric perspective. *Psychosomatics* 1993;**34**:70–9.

68. Martínez-Taboas, A. Multiple personality in Puerto Rico: analysis of fifteen cases. *Dissociation* 1991;**4**:189–92

69. Vein AM, Djukova GM, Vorobieva OV. Is panic attack a mask of psychogenic seizures? A comparative analysis of phenomenology of psychogenic seizures and panic attacks. *Funct Neurol* 1994;**9**:153–9.

70. Litwin R, Cardeña E. Demographic and seizure variables, but not hypnotizability or dissociation differentiated psychogenic from organic seizures. *J Trauma Dissociation* 2000;**1**(4):99–122.

71. Stefánsson JG, Messina JA, Meyerowitz S. Hysterical neurosis, conversion type: clinical and epidemiological considerations. *Acta Psychiatr Scand* 1976;**53**:119–38.

72. Loewenstein RJ. Somatoform disorders in victims of incest and child abuse. In: Kluft RP, ed. *Incest-Related Syndromes of Adult Psychopathology*. Washington: American Psychiatric Press. 1990; 75–107.

73. Tietjen GE, Brandes JL, Digre KB, *et al*. History of childhood maltreatment is associated with comorbid depression in women with migraine. *Neurology* 2007;**69**:959–68.

74. Felitti VJ. Long-term medical consequences of incest, rape, and molestation. *South Med J* 1991;**84**:328–31.

75. Glod CA. Long-term consequences of childhood physical and sexual abuse. *Arch Psychiatr Nurs* 1993;**7**:163–73.

76. Arnow BA, Hart S, Hayward C, *et al*. Severity of child maltreatment, pain complaints, and medical utilization among women. *J Psychiatr Res* 2000;**34**:413–21.

77. Sack M, Lahmann C, Jaeger B, Henningsen P. Trauma prevalence and somatoform symptoms. Are there specific somatoform symptoms related to traumatic experiences? *J Nerv Ment Dis* 2007;**195**:928–33.

78. Blumer D. The paroxysmal somatoform disorder: a series of patients with non-epileptic seizures. In: Rowan AJ, Gates JR, eds. *Non-Epileptic Seizures*. Boston, MA: Butterworth-Heinemann. 1993; 165–72.

79. Ettinger AB, Devinsky O, Weisbrot DM, *et al*. Headaches and other pain symptoms among patients with psychogenic non-epileptic seizures. *Seizure* 1999;**8**:424–6.

80. Heim C, Ehlert U, Hanker JP, Hellhammer DH. Abuse-related posttraumatic stress disorder and alterations of the hypothalamic-pituitary-adrenal axis in women with chronic pelvic pain. *Psychosom Med* 1998;**6**:309–18.

81. Ehlert U, Heim C, Hellhammer DH. Chronic pelvic pain as a somatoform disorder. *Psychother Psychosom* 1999;**68**:87–94.

82. Walker E, Katon W, Harrop-Griffiths J, *et al*. Relationship of chronic pelvic pain to psychiatric diagnoses and childhood sexual abuse. *Am J Psychiatry* 1988;**145**:75–80.

83. Walker E, Katon W, Hansom J, *et al*. Medical and psychiatric symptoms in women with childhood sexual abuse. *Psychosom Med* 1992;**54**:658–64.

84. Reiter RC, Shakerin LR, Gambone JC, Milburn AK. Correlation between sexual abuse and somatization in women with somatic and nonsomatic chronic pelvic pain. *Am J Obstet Gynecol* 1991;**165**:104–9.

85. Draijer N. Long-term psychosomatic consequences of child sexual abuse. In: van Hall EV, Everaerd W, eds. *The Free Woman: Women's Health in the 1990s*. Cornforth, UK: Parthenon Publishing Group. 1989; 969–709.

86. Finestone HM, Stenn P, Davies F, *et al*. Chronic pain and health care utilization in women with a history of childhood sexual abuse. *Child Abuse Negl* 2000;**24**:547–56.

87. Irwin, C, Falsetti SA, Lydiard RB, *et al*. Comorbidity of posttraumatic stress disorder and irritable bowel syndrome. *J Clin Psychiatry* 1996;**57**:576–78.

88. Drossman DA, Leserman J, Nachman G, *et al*. Sexual and physical abuse in women with functional or organic gastrointestinal disorders. *Ann Intern Med* 1990;**113**:828–33.

89. Bass C, Bond A, Gill D, Sharpe M. Frequent attenders without organic disease in a gastroenterology clinic. *Gen Hosp Psychiatry* 1999;**21**:30–8.

90. Imbierowicz K, Egle UT. Childhood adversities in patients with fibromyalgia and somatoform pain disorder. *Eur J Pain* 2003;**7**(2):113–19.

91. McBeth J, Macfarlane GJ, Benjamin S, Morris S, Silman AJ. The association between tender points, psychological distress, and adverse childhood experiences: a community-based study. *Arthritis Rheum* 1999;**42**:1397–404.

92. Goldberg RT, Pachas WN, Keith D. Relationship between traumatic events in childhood and chronic pain. *Disabil Rehabil* 1999;**21**(1):23–30.

93. Alexander RW, Bradley LA, Alarcon GS, *et al*. Sexual and physical abuse in women with fibromyalgia: association with outpatient health care utilization and pain medication usage. *Arthritis Care Res* 1998;**11**(2):102–15.

94. Walker EA, Keegan D, Gardner G, *et al*. Psychosocial factors in fibromyalgia compared with rheumatoid arthritis: II. Sexual, physical, and emotional abuse and neglect. *Psychosom Med* 1997;**59**:572–7.

95. Boisset-Pioro MH, Esdaile JM, Fitzcharles MA. Sexual and physical abuse in women with fibromyalgia syndrome. *Arthritis Rheum* 1995;**38**:235–41.

96. Ciccone DS, Elliott DK, Chandler HK, Nayak S, Raphael KG. Sexual and physical abuse in women with fibromyalgia syndrome: a test of the trauma hypothesis. *Clin J Pain* 2005;**21**:378–86.

97. Benbadis SR. A spell in the epilepsy clinic and a history of "chronic pain" or "fibromyalgia" independently predict a diagnosis of psychogenic seizures. *Epilepsy Behav* 2005;**6**(2):264–5.

98. Schur EA, Afari N, Furberg H, *et al*. Feeling bad in more ways than one: comorbidity patterns of medically unexplained and psychiatric conditions. *J Gen Intern Med* 2007;**22**:818–21.

99. Amital D, Fostick L, Polliack ML, *et al*. Posttraumatic stress disorder, tenderness, and fibromyalgia syndrome: are they different entities? *J Psychosom Res* 2006;**61**:663–9.

100. Seng JS, Clark MK, McCarthy AM, Ronis DL. PTSD and physical comorbidity among women receiving Medicaid: results from service-use data. *J Trauma Stress* 2006;**19**(1):45–56.

101. Arguelles LM, Afari N, Buchwald DS, *et al*. A twin study of posttraumatic stress disorder symptoms and chronic widespread pain. *Pain* 2006;**124**(1–2):150–7.

102. Briere J, Runtz M. Symptomatology associated with childhood sexual victimization in a nonclinical adult sample. *Child Abuse Negl* 1988;**12**:51–9.

103. Springs FE, Friedrich WN. Health risk behavior and medical sequelae of childhood sexual abuse. *Mayo Clin Proc* 1992;**67**:527–32.

104. Polusny MA, Follette VM. Long-term correlates of child sexual abuse: theory and review of the empirical literature. *Appl Prev Psychol* 1995;**4**:143–66.

105. Morrison J. Childhood sexual histories in women with somatization disorder. *Am J Psychiatry* 1989;**146**:239–41.

106. Swartz M, Blazer D, George L, Landerman R. Somatization disorder in a community population. *Am J Psychiatry* 1986;**143**:1403–8.

107. Escobar JI, Burnam MA, Karno M, Forsythe A, Golding JM. Somatization in the community. *Arch Gen Psychiatry* 1987;**44**:713–18.

108. American Psychiatric Association. *Diagnostic and Statistical Manual of Mental Disorders*, 3rd edn., Revised (DSM-III-R). Washington, DC: American Psychiatric Association, 1987.

109. Wittchen HU, Essau CA, von Zerssen D, Krieg JC, Zaudig M. Lifetime and six-month prevalence of mental disorders in the Munich follow-up study. *Eur Arch Psychiatry Clin Neurosci* 1992;**241**:247–58.

110. Snyder SL, Rosenbaum DH, Rowan AJ, *et al*. SCID diagnosis of panic disorder in psychogenic seizure patients. *J Neuropsychiatry Clin Neurosci* 1994;**6**:261–6.

111. Badura AS, Reiter RC, Altmaier EM, Rhomberg A, Elas D. Dissociation, somatization, substance abuse and coping in women with chronic pelvic pain. *Obstet Gynecol* 1997;**90**:405–10.

112. Watson CG, Tilleskjor C. Interrelationships of conversion, psychogenic pain, and dissociative disorder symptoms. *J Consult Clin Psychol* 1982;**51**:788–9.

113. Kihlstrom JF. One hundred years of hysteria. In: Lynn SJ, Rhue JW, eds. *Dissociation: Clinical and Theoretical Perspectives*. New York: Guilford Press. 1994; 365–94.

114. Bowman ES. Etiology and clinical course of pseudoseizures: relationship to trauma, depression and dissociation. *Psychosomatics* 1993;**34**:333–42.

115. Kuyk J, Spinhoven P, van Emde Boas MD, van Dyck R. Dissociation in temporal lobe epilepsy and pseudo-epileptic seizure patients. *J Nerv Ment Dis* 1999;**187**:713–20.

116. Nijenhuis ERS, Spinhoven P, van Dyck R, van der Hart O, Vanderlinden J. The development of the somatoform dissociation questionnaire (SDQ-5) as a screening instrument for dissociative disorders. *Acta Psychiatr Scand* 1997;**96**:311–18.

117. Rauch, van der Kolk BA, Fisler RE, *et al*. A symptom provocation study of posttraumatic stress disorder using positron emission tomography and script-driven imagery. *Arch Gen Psychiatry* 1996;**53**:380–7.

118. Schiffer F, Teicher MH, Papanicolou AC. Evoked potential evidence for right brain activity during the recall of traumatic memories. *J Neuropsychiatry Clin Neurosci* 1995;**7**:169–75.

119. Marshall RD, Spitzer R, Liebowitz MR. Review and critique of the new DSM-IV diagnosis of acute stress disorder. *Am J Psychiatry* 1999;**156**:1677–85.

120. Bryant RA, Harvey AG. New DSM-IV diagnosis of acute stress disorder. *Am J Psychiatry* 2000;**157**: 1889–91.

121. Cartmill A, Betts T. Seizure behavior in a patient with a post-traumatic stress disorder following rape. *Seizure* 1992;**1**:33–6.

122. Betts T, Duffy N. Non-epileptic attack disorder (pseudoseizures) and sexual abuse: a review. In: Gram L, Johannessen SI, Osterman PO, Sillanpää M, eds. *Pseudo-Epileptic Seizures*. Petersfield, UK: Wrightson Biomedical Publishing. 1993; 55–65.

123. Waldinger RJ, Schulz MS, Barsky AJ, Ahern AK. Mapping the road from childhood trauma to adult somatization: the role of attachment. *Psychosom Med* 2006;**68**:129–35.

124. Cunningham J, Pearce T, Pearce P. Childhood sexual abuse and medical complaints in adult women. *J Interpers Violence* 1988;**3**(2):131–44.

125. Trimble MR. Pseudoseizures. *Neurol Clin* 1986;**4**: 531–48.
126. Gates JR, Erdahl P. Classification of non-epileptic events. In: Rowan AJ, Gates JR, eds. *Non-Epileptic Seizures*. Boston, MA: Butterworth-Heinemann. 1993; 21–30.
127. Russell JL, Kushner MG, Beitman BD, *et al*. Nonfearful panic disorder in neurology patients validated by lactate challenge. *Am J Psychiatry* 1991;**148**:361–4.
128. Sar V. The scope of dissociative disorders: an international perspective. *Psychiatr Clin North Am* 2006;**29**:227–45.

Section 4 Chapter 23

Psychiatric considerations in adults with psychogenic nonepileptic seizures

Comorbidities in psychogenic nonepileptic seizures: depressive, anxiety, and personality disorders

Adriana Fiszman and Andres M. Kanner

Psychogenic nonepileptic seizures (PNES) are recurrent paroxysmal episodes of presumed psychogenic origin that are identified in 20% to 30% of patients referred to epilepsy centers, often with a diagnosis of pharmacoresistant epilepsy. The availability of video-EEG (VEEG) monitoring in the last four decades has been instrumental in the establishment of this diagnosis. From the psychiatric standpoint, PNES are the expression of heterogeneous psychopathology presenting as psychiatric disorders coded on Axis I in the Diagnostic and Statistical Manual of Mental Disorders, Fourth Edition (DSM-IV) [1–4]. Yet, in a small minority of patients, no significant psychopathology may be identified at the time of diagnosis [5]; in these few cases, PNES sometimes remit immediately following the establishment of the diagnosis even without any therapeutic interventions [6]. The aim of this chapter is to review the most frequent psychiatric disorders associated with PNES, with particular attention to depressive, anxiety, and personality disorders.

Primary psychiatric disorders in PNES

In general terms, PNES can be classified as a conversion disorder, which is classified within the somatoform disorders according to the DSM-IV. Other somatoform disorders can be present such as somatization disorder and undifferentiated somatoform disorder [7]. PNES alternatively occur as a dissociative process in dissociative disorders – dissociative amnesia, dissociative fugue, dissociative identity disorder, depersonalization – and posttraumatic stress disorder (PTSD). In fact, conversion and dissociation have been classically considered manifestations of a sole underlying condition, "hysteria." For this reason, the International Classification of Diseases, Tenth Edition (ICD-10) has included both conversion and dissociation under the rubric of dissociative disorders and classified dissociative and conversion PNES as "dissociative convulsions (seizures)" [8]. In addition, symptoms similar to PNES may also be the expression of panic disorder, impulse control disorders (episodic dyscontrol), psychotic disorders, factitious disorder, and malingering [9–11]. The reader is referred to the DSM-IV classification for a review of the specific diagnostic criteria of each condition [1].

Comorbid psychiatric disorders in PNES

The psychiatric disorders outlined above occur together with other psychiatric conditions in patients with PNES, the most frequent being depressive, anxiety, and personality disorders. Unfortunately, the reported prevalence of the comorbidities varies among the various studies, likely because of methodological differences. Some studies relied on self-rating screening instruments and others on structured or semi-structured interviews based on DSM-III-revised (DSM-III-R) or DSM-IV criteria, while others were carried out with interviews that did not follow the diagnostic criteria suggested by a DSM classification.

In the DSM-IV classification, depressive and anxiety disorders are coded as Axis I and personality disorders as Axis II disorders. The DSM-IV multi-axial classification allows the coding of diagnoses from both Axis I and Axis II.

Table 23.1 Prevalence of *current* depressive and anxiety disorders in patients with psychogenic nonepileptic seizures (PNES)

Authors, date Diagnostic criteria	N PNES N control group	Depressive disorders % PNES	Depressive disorders % control group	Anxiety disorders % PNES	Anxiety disorders % control group
Snyder et al., 1994 [9] DSM-III-R SCID	20 PNES	45 major depression 10 dysthymia		70 panic 20 phobia	
Bowman and Markand, 1996 [10] DSM-III-R SCID	45 PNES	60 depressive disorders 47 major depression 13 dysthymia		47 PTSD 20 panic 33 phobia 9 GAD 4 OCD 2 anxiety NOS	
Arnold and Privitera, 1996 [28] DSM-III-R SCID	14 PNES 27 ES	21 major depression	18 major depression 7 dysthymia	14 PTSD 14 panic 7 phobia	3 PTSD 13 panic 14 phobia
Kanner et al., 1999 [5] DSM-III-R SCID	45 PNES	60 major depression 7 dysthymia		2 panic 9 GAD	
Mökleby et al., 2002 [48] DSM-IV MINI	23 PNES 23 somatoform disorder sex-age matched	57 depressive disorders	52 depressive disorders	35 PTSD 13 phobia 39 GAD 9 OCD	13 PTSD 26 phobia 30 GAD 4 OCD
Kuyk et al., 2003 [12] DSM-III-R Past year CIDI	60 PNES 25 mixed group	28 depressive disorders	32 depressive disorders	38 anxiety disorders	48 anxiety disorders
Galimberti et al., 2003 [4] DSM-III-R SCID Patient version	31 PNES 38 mixed group 31 ES sex-age matched	13 depressive disorders	Mixed group 16 depressive disorders ES 45 depressive disorders	16 anxiety disorders	Mixed group 30 anxiety disorders ES 9 anxiety disorders
Baillés et al., 2004 [30] DSM-IV SCID	30 PNES	30 depressive disorders 13 major depression 17 dysthymia		10 panic 3 GAD 3 anxiety NOS	
D'Alessio et al., 2006 [27] DSM-IV SCID	24 PNES 19 mixed group	54 depressive disorders	74 depressive disorders	29 PTSD 25 other anxiety disorders	5 PTSD 11 other anxiety disorders

ES, patients with epileptic seizures; Mixed group, patients with PNES and epileptic seizures; PTSD, posttraumatic stress disorder; GAD, generalized anxiety disorder; OCD, obsessive compulsive disorder; NOS, not otherwise specified; DSM-III-R, Diagnostic and Statistical Manual of Mental Disorders – third edition, revised; DSM-IV, Diagnostic and Statistical Manual of Mental Disorders – fourth edition; SCID, Structured Clinical Interview for DSM-III-R/DSM-IV Disorders; CIDI, Composite International Diagnostic Interview; MINI, Mini-International Neuropsychiatric Interview for DSM-IV Disorders.

Comorbid depressive and anxiety disorders in PNES

Table 23.1 summarizes the prevalence of current depressive and anxiety disorders in patients with PNES assessed with structured or semi-structured interviews based on DSM-III-R or DSM-IV diagnostic criteria. The depressive disorders evaluated in patients with PNES were mostly major depression and/or dysthymic disorder; only two studies included bipolar disorder [12]. A review of Table 23.1 clearly shows high prevalence rates of depressive disorders (21%, 28%, 30%,

45%, 54%, 57%, and 60%), which are significantly higher than the rates reported in the general population [13, 14]. Of note, the prevalence of current depressive disorders in patients with PNES did not differ from those observed in control groups composed of patients with refractory epileptic seizures (ES) and mixed ES/PNES. Only one study reported significantly higher rates of depressive disorders in the epilepsy group (45%) than in the PNES group (14%) and in patients with mixed ES/PNES (16%). In that study [4], the low prevalence of depressive disorders may have resulted from assessing depression as one of the primary diagnoses of PNES and not as comorbid, which is how this condition commonly appears in PNES populations.

The reported prevalence of anxiety disorders in PNES varied significantly among the studies included in Table 23.1. The possible cause of such variable rates may reflect the lack of an agreement about which disorders are "primary causes" of PNES and which are comorbid. For example, Snyder et al. [9] reported a prevalence of 70% for panic disorder, when classified as one of the primary conditions underlying PNES, while Kanner et al. [5] only found a prevalence of 2%, classifying it as an accompanying comorbidity. The prevalence of generalized anxiety disorder (GAD), obsessive compulsive disorder (OCD), and phobias also varied among the different studies; yet, as in the case of depressive disorders, prevalences were in general much higher in patients with PNES than those found in general populations [15]. In addition, patients with PNES were not found to experience anxiety disorders with greater frequency than the control groups composed of patients with refractory epilepsy, mixed ES/PNES, or somatoform disorder. The presence of PTSD was an exception since it was significantly more prevalent in patients with PNES than in control groups. This is explained by the fact that PTSD is highly associated with dissociative disorders, which are one of the most prevalent primary diagnoses underlying PNES [7, 16].

In conclusion, despite differences in definition and assessment of comorbid disorders, our review found high rates of current depressive and anxiety disorders in patients with PNES. However, with the exception of PTSD, depressive and anxiety disorders were reported with comparable frequencies in control groups composed of patients with refractory ES, mixed ES/PNES or somatoform disorder. The lack of differences with patients with ES stems from the relatively high prevalence of comorbid psychiatric disorders in patients with refractory epilepsy referred to specialized centers, where PNES samples are studied. In particular, depressive disorders are the most common comorbid psychiatric disorders in patients with pharmacoresistant epilepsy, ranging from 20% to 50% [17, 18]. Yet, one would expect significantly higher prevalence of psychiatric disorders in patients with PNES, when compared to seizure-free patients with epilepsy. Unfortunately, no data are available to support this speculation.

While depressive and anxiety disorders – other than PTSD and panic disorder – may be comorbid psychiatric conditions, their identification and treatment are as important as those of the primary psychiatric diagnoses in order to achieve a successful outcome from treatment of the PNES. In fact, chronic depressive and anxiety disorders that have failed to respond to treatment or were never treated were more often associated with persistent PNES after diagnosis than in patients with a psychiatric history of mild severity [5, 6].

Comorbid personality disorders in PNES

Personality disorders are defined as an enduring pattern of inner experiences and behaviors that deviates markedly from the expectations of the culture of the individual who exhibits it [1]. Personality disorders are postulated to have their origins in childhood or adolescence, with deficits in the development of affect regulation, self-consciousness, impulse control, and identity consolidation, all of which have adverse and persistent effects on the person's adaptation to occupational and social demands. Some authors have suggested that personality disorders may result from early onset, chronic, untreated Axis I disorders in the form of depressive, anxiety, attention-deficit hyperactivity disorders, or a combination of some or all of these conditions, often in the setting of chaotic family environments. Family psychiatric history is frequent in patients with personality disorders [19, 20]. Personality disorders lead to serious interpersonal disturbances and a negative impact on the course and response to treatment of comorbid Axis I disorders [21], which in turn worsen the severity of personality disorders.

Unfortunately, systematic screenings of personality disorders using validated instruments and well-defined criteria are lacking in patients with PNES, in spite of their negative impact on outcome [5, 22, 23]. Indeed, a majority of studies have relied on self-rating screening instruments such as the Minnesota Multiphasic Personality Inventory (MMPI)[24, 25]. Some investigators [23] have questioned the MMPI's usefulness as a diagnostic tool in PNES, since it does not measure personality deviations equivalent to diagnostic categories coded on Axis II of the DSM-IV or the ICD-10. These authorities highlighted that the MMPI identifies symptoms of a broad range of Axis I disorders, such as hypochondriasis, conversion disorder, depression, schizophrenia, fear, and others. The use of the MMPI in PNES is discussed in Chapter 13.

Our review of the literature found only eight studies examining personality disorders in PNES samples using SCID II (Structured Clinical Interview for DSM Personality Disorders) [26] or other reliable instruments based on DSM-III-R or DSM-IV diagnostic criteria (Table 23.2). Out of these eight studies, five compared the prevalence of personality disorders between patients with PNES and control groups, composed of patients with mixed ES/PNES [4, 12, 27] or patients with only ES [4, 28, 29]. Personality disorders were grouped into three clusters according to the DSM-IV classification: cluster A disorders (paranoid, schizoid, schizotypical), cluster B disorders (antisocial, borderline, histrionic, narcissistic), and cluster C disorders (avoidant, dependent, obsessive compulsive).

As shown in Table 23.2, the most prevalent personality disorders found in patients with PNES were those of cluster B followed by those of cluster C and, less frequently, those of cluster A. High percentages of cluster B personality disorders, especially of the borderline type, were found not only in patients with PNES but also in the mixed ES/PNES group. Furthermore, the rates of borderline personality disorder (BPD) in PNES and mixed groups were significantly higher than those found in patients with ES only [4, 28, 29]. One study [4] did not find differences in the prevalence of cluster B diagnoses between the three groups (28% in the PNES group, 34% in the mixed ES/PNES group and 16% in the ES only group), but there were differences when comparing subtypes of personality disorders within the cluster B. For example, patients with PNES and mixed ES/PNES were more likely to exhibit symptoms consistent with BPD and histrionic personality disorder, while patients with ES met criteria of narcissistic personality disorder more frequently.

The reported prevalences of cluster A personality disorders were low in patients with PNES: 0% [4, 5, 28], 3.3% [30], and 4% [27]. Of note, the studies that reported higher frequencies did not use the SCID II but other less specific though highly sensitive questionnaires for DSM personality disorders [10, 12]. Bowman and Markand [10] found that 51% of patients with PNES met criteria of paranoid personality disorder. Yet, they clarified that "despite their endorsement of paranoid personality items, few subjects were clinically paranoid, but many showed avoidant mistrust that they related to traumatic experiences." Patients with mixed ES/PNES exhibited a higher prevalence of cluster A than patients with PNES [12, 27].

The prevalence of cluster C diagnoses were inconsistent among the various studies, with some authors not finding differences between PNES groups and those with ES [28] or mixed ES/PNES [27], while others reported significant differences [4, 12]. Kuyk et al. [12] observed that patients with mixed ES/PNES were more often characterized by cluster C personality disorders than patients with PNES ($p < 0.05$). Also, in one study [4] cluster C personality disorders were not found in the PNES group but they emerged in both control groups – mixed ES/PNES and ES – in the same proportion. That the mixed group displayed the same pattern of cluster C personality pathology as did the ES group cannot be explained at this point and more research is necessary to determine the clinical significance (if any) of these data.

Borderline personality disorder, adaptation to complex trauma and PNES

A recent study [23] evaluated 85 patients with PNES (82.3% female) and 63 patients with ES (38.1% female) using a dimensional assessment of personality patterns. The most typical pattern, found in 50.6% of patients with PNES, resembled the profile seen in patients with BPD. In particular, patients with PNES had significantly higher affect dysregulation – a core feature of BPD – than the healthy and ES control groups ($p = 0.001$).

Affect dysregulation, characterized by rapid shifts from overwhelming emotions (fear, anger, shame, sadness, or dysphoria) to emotional emptiness, together with other clinical features – pervasive instability of interpersonal relationships, self-image, and prominent dissociative symptoms – have adverse implications on the management and prognosis of many patients with PNES. Thus, BPD, more than PNES per se, underlies the main clinical challenges presented by these patients

Table 23.2 Prevalence of personality disorders (clusters A, B, and C) in patients with psychogenic nonepileptic seizures (PNES)

Authors, date	Diagnostic criteria / Assessment instrument	Sample (% women) / N control group (% women)	N (%) PNES patients also with epilepsy	Cluster A % PNES	Cluster A % control group	Cluster B % PNES	Cluster B % control group	Cluster C % PNES	Cluster C % control group
Bowman and Markand, 1996 [10]	DSM-III-R / Personality Diagnostic Questionnaire-Revised	45 PNES (78%)	5 (11)	51 paranoid		49 borderline 40 histrionic		38 avoidant	
Arnold and Privitera, 1996 [28]	DSM-III-R / SCID II	14 PNES (64%) / 27 ES (48%)		0 cluster A		21 borderline	3 borderline	21 avoidant 7 obsessive-compulsive	18 avoidant 3 obsessive-compulsive 3 dependent
Kanner et al., 1999 [5]	DSM-III-R / SCID II	45 PNES (70%)	19 (42)	0 cluster A		11 cluster B		33 cluster C	
Kuyk et al., 2003 [12]	DSM-IV / Questionnaire on Personality Traits	60 PNES (70%) / 25 mixed group (76%)		23 cluster A	40 cluster A	18.3 cluster B	24 cluster B	18 cluster C	40 cluster C*

(cont.)

Table 23.2 (cont.)

Authors, date	Diagnostic criteria / Assessment instrument	Sample (% women) / N control group (% women)	N (%) PNES patients also with epilepsy	Cluster A % PNES	Cluster A % control group	Cluster B % PNES	Cluster B % control group	Cluster C % PNES	Cluster C % control group
Galimberti et al., 2003 [4]	DSM-III-R	31 PNES (77%)		0 cluster A	0 cluster A ES	28 cluster B	16 cluster B ES 3 borderline 0 histrionic 10 narcissistic 3 antisocial	0 cluster C	22 cluster C ES 3 avoidant 6 obsessive-compulsive 13 dependent
	SCID II	31 sex-age matched ES				10 borderline 13 histrionic 3 narcissistic 3 antisocial			
		38 mixed group (89%)			3 paranoid mixed group		34 cluster B mixed group 16 borderline 12 histrionic 5 narcissistic		12 cluster C mixed group 0 avoidant 12 obsessive-compulsive 0 dependent
Baillés et al., 2004 [30]	DSM-IV	30 PNES (90%)		3.3 paranoid		13.3 borderline 26.7 histrionic		6.7 dependent	
	SCID II								
Binzer et al., 2004 [29]	DSM-IV	20 PNES (75%)		65 any personality disorder	25 any personality disorder*	35 borderline	5 borderline*		
	SCID II	20 ES (60%)							
D'Alessio et al., 2006 [27]	DSM-IV	24 PNES (79%)		4 cluster A	31.5 cluster A	33 cluster B	21 cluster B	33 cluster C	16 cluster C
	SCID II	19 mixed group (53%)							

ES, patients with epileptic seizures; Mixed group, patients with PNES and epileptic seizures; Cluster A, paranoid, schizoid, schizotypical; Cluster B, borderline, histrionic, narcissistic, antisocial; Cluster C, avoidant, obsessive-compulsive, dependent; DSM-III-R, Diagnostic and statistical manual of mental disorders – third edition, revised; DSM-IV, Diagnostic and statistical manual of mental disorders – fourth edition; SCID II, Structured Clinical Interview for DSM-III-R/DSM-IV Personality Disorders.
* $p \leq 0.05$.

and is the core of their disability [22]. Furthermore, as stated above, patients with BPD are at increased risk of comorbid psychopathology, explaining the elevated prevalence of depressive and anxiety disorders in many patients with PNES.

The main clinical challenge of BPD arises from the insufficient knowledge of its etiology to guide its treatment [31]. Comparably high frequency of adverse childhood experiences has been reported in patients with BPD (without PNES) and in patients with PNES. For example, one study found higher prevalence of traumatic events, childhood sexual and physical abuse, and PTSD in patients with PNES than in control groups composed of patients with refractory ES [16]. Furthermore, a recent meta-analysis concluded that the probability of having a history of childhood sexual abuse was almost three times greater in patients with PNES than in comparison samples [32]. Moreover, our review of the literature showed significantly higher rates of PTSD in PNES samples than in control groups (see Table 23.1), pointing to a relevant role of traumatic events in the development of PNES. The reason for the development of PNES and BPD in some patients with a history of traumatic experiences and BPD without PNES in others remains unknown. The effect of childhood abuse was predictive of somatic distress in later life and was not specific to PNES [33, 34]. Abuse was also found to be a marker for more significant family dysfunction in patients with PNES [35].

By the same token, in a recent case-control study [29] patients with recent onset PNES were more likely to have BPD ($p < 0.05$) and to recollect less parental emotional warmth and more paternal rejection in childhood ($p = 0.0001$) than patients with recent onset epilepsy. The high rates of early trauma in subjects with BPD and the phenomenological overlap with PTSD have led to the hypothesis that BPD may be a trauma-related disorder or variant of PTSD stemming from early childhood trauma [36–38]. This assumption is supported by the DSM-IV Field Trial for PTSD, which suggested that complex traumas, defined as prolonged traumas of interpersonal nature that first occur at an early age, result in severe personality disturbances, which are not identified by the PTSD diagnostic criteria [39].

A new diagnosis was proposed in 1992 by Herman [40] to describe the psychological reactions to complex traumas: "disorder of extreme stress, not otherwise specified" (DESNOS) or complex PTSD. Complex PTSD comprises the following features overlapping with BPD: affect dysregulation, self-destructive and impulsive behavior, identity disturbance, impaired relationships, and dissociative symptoms. Complex PTSD symptoms are arranged in seven categories, two of them (2 and 6) containing manifestations of PNES: (1) disturbances of affect regulation and impulses (e.g., difficulty modulating anger, persistent sadness, suicidal thoughts), (2) alterations in consciousness (e.g., amnesia for traumatic events, dissociative episodes, including depersonalization), (3) alterations in self-perception (e.g., a sense of being permanently damaged), (4) alterations in perception of the perpetrator (e.g., idealizing a sexually abusive parent or partner), (5) alterations in relationships with others (e.g., inability to trust others, revictimization, a repeated search for a rescuer), (6) somatization (e.g., chronic pain, conversion symptoms), and (7) alterations in systems of meaning (e.g., despair and hopelessness) (for more details, see van der Kolk *et al.* [41, 42]). The construct of complex PTSD may be a useful explanation for the widely reported overlap between BPD and somatoform disorders, among which PNES is one type [43, 44].

Since BPD has been shown to have negative prognostic implications in the course of PNES, the consideration of the diagnosis of complex PTSD in patients with PNES and BPD may have important treatment implications. For example, some patients with PNES presenting symptoms of PTSD could benefit from short-term cognitive-behavioral interventions, in particular trauma exposure [45, 46]. Also, psychotherapeutic techniques especially developed in recent years to manage problems related to complex trauma – dissociation, affect regulation, and altered relationships – might have a positive impact on the outcome [47].

The review of the literature cited so far demonstrates the heterogeneous nature of PNES, as evidenced by the comorbid occurrence of Axis I and Axis II (BPD) disorders. Accordingly, the sole identification of the primary psychiatric disorder operant in PNES is insufficient to achieve a successful treatment; it is critical that the other comorbid psychiatric disorders are recognized and their treatment incorporated into a comprehensive treatment plan.

Impact of psychopathology on the course of PNES after diagnosis

Certain psychiatric disorders may be predictive of the outcome of PNES after diagnosis. Their early identification can be of paramount importance in planning treatment strategies. This is illustrated in a study of 45 consecutive patients with PNES documented with VEEG [5] in which the investigators prospectively evaluated the persistence of PNES at one month and six months after diagnosis. Three outcome patterns of PNES were identified: (1) complete cessation of PNES since diagnosis; (2) transient cessation of PNES for a period of at least three months with subsequent recurrence; and (3) uninterrupted persistence of PNES. The psychiatric profiles associated with these outcome patterns are described below.

Uninterrupted persistence of PNES was found in 20 of the 45 patients. These patients were more likely to have a history of abuse (physical, emotional, sexual, mixed), a history of recurrent major depressive episodes, personality disorders, and a history of dissociative disorder (not presenting as PNES). Given the frequent history of abuse, it is reasonable to expect that PNES may be an expression of a dissociative process. This observation is further supported by the higher frequency of a history of dissociative disorder that preceded and presented in forms other than PNES. Of interest is that despite their severe psychopathology, 17 of these 20 patients readily accepted the psychogenic nature of their events and were able to recognize their PNES as a form of dissociation soon after their diagnosis was discussed with them.

Transient cessation of PNES for a period of at least three months was found in 12 of the 45 patients. Patients with this outcome pattern differed from those with the two other outcomes in two areas: they were more likely to deny the presence of any psychiatric or psychological problems. Eight of the 12 patients with this outcome refused a recommendation to start psychiatric treatment. All patients accepted that their events were not epileptic, however. In addition, patients in this group were more likely to develop new somatic complaints after the diagnosis of PNES was established.

Cessation of PNES since diagnosis occurred in 13 patients, even in the absence of any therapeutic intervention. Most of this group had psychiatric disorders of mild severity, but in 5 of the 13 patients, no current psychopathology was identified during the psychiatric and neuropsychological evaluations. Clearly, the completion of a psychiatric evaluation as soon as the diagnosis of PNES is established can help inform the course of the PNES and help clinicians prepare the patient and family members on how to deal with their recurrence.

Concluding remarks

The present review demonstrates that PNES are the expression of a heterogeneous psychiatric disorder presenting with one or more comorbidity. A careful psychiatric evaluation is in order to identify all present and past psychiatric disorders to plan a comprehensive treatment. It follows from the observations made in this chapter that treatment of PNES may have greater impact if tailored to each patient. Furthermore, the heterogeneity and complexity of the psychopathology operant in PNES may pose challenges for the design and implementation of randomized treatment trials. In most patients with PNES, a combination of pharmacological treatment and psychotherapy (cognitive, insight oriented, supportive, family therapy) may be necessary.

References

1. American Psychiatric Association. *Diagnostic and Statistical Manual of Mental Disorders*, 4th edn. (DSM-IV). Washington, DC: American Psychiatric Association 1994.
2. LaFrance WC, Jr. Psychogenic nonepileptic seizures. *Curr Opin Neurol* 2008;**21**(2):195–201.
3. Reuber M. Psychogenic nonepileptic seizures: answers and questions. Epilepsy Behav 2008;**12**(4): 622–35.
4. Galimberti CA, Ratti MT, Murelli R, *et al*. Patients with psychogenic nonepileptic seizures, alone or epilepsy-associated, share a psychological profile distinct from that of epilepsy patients. *J Neurol* 2003;**250**(3):338–46.
5. Kanner AM, Parra J, Frey M, *et al*. Psychiatric and neurologic predictors of psychogenic pseudoseizure outcome. *Neurology* 1999;**53**(5):933–8.
6. Kanner AM. Is the neurologist's role over once the diagnosis of psychogenic nonepileptic seizures is made? No! *Epilepsy Behav* 2008;**12**(1):1–2.
7. Marchetti RL, Kurcgant D, Neto JG, *et al*. Psychiatric diagnoses of patients with psychogenic non-epileptic seizures. *Seizure* 2008;**17**(3):247–53.
8. World Health Organization. *The ICD-10 Classification of Mental and Behavioural Disorders: Clinical Descriptions and Diagnostic Guidelines*. Geneva, Switzerland: World Health Organization, 1992.
9. Snyder SL, Rosenbaum DH, Rowan AJ, Strain JJ. SCID diagnosis of panic disorder in psychogenic seizure patients. *J Neuropsychiatry Clin Neurosci* 1994;**6**(3):261–6.

10. Bowman ES, Markand ON. Psychodynamics and psychiatric diagnoses of pseudoseizure subjects. *Am J Psychiatry* 1996;**153**(1):57–63.

11. Alper K, Devinsky O, Perrine K, Vazquez B, Luciano D. Psychiatric classification of nonconversion nonepileptic seizures. *Arch Neurol* 1995;**52**(2):199–201.

12. Kuyk J, Swinkels WA, Spinhoven P. Psychopathologies in patients with nonepileptic seizures with and without comorbid epilepsy: how different are they? *Epilepsy Behav* 2003;**4**(1):13–18.

13. Andrade L, Caraveo-Anduaga JJ, Berglund P, et al. The epidemiology of major depressive episodes: results from the International Consortium of Psychiatric Epidemiology (ICPE) Surveys. *Int J Methods Psychiatr Res* 2003;**12**(1):3–21.

14. Ohayon MM. Epidemiology of depression and its treatment in the general population. *J Psychiatr Res* 2007;**41**(3–4):207–13.

15. Ohayon MM. Anxiety disorders: prevalence, comorbidity and outcomes. *J Psychiatr Res* 2006;**40**(6):475–6.

16. Fiszman A, ves-Leon SV, Nunes RG, D'Andrea I, Figueira I. Traumatic events and posttraumatic stress disorder in patients with psychogenic nonepileptic seizures: a critical review. *Epilepsy Behav* 2004;**5**(6):818–25.

17. LaFrance WC, Jr, Kanner AM, Hermann B. Psychiatric comorbidities in epilepsy. *Int Rev Neurobiol* 2008;**83**:347–83.

18. Kanner AM. Epilepsy and mood disorders. *Epilepsia* 2007;**48** Suppl 9:20–2.

19. Kim-Cohen J, Moffitt TE, Taylor A, Pawlby SJ, Caspi A. Maternal depression and children's antisocial behavior: nature and nurture effects. *Arch Gen Psychiatry* 2005;**62**(2):173–81.

20. Fassino S, Amianto F, Gastaldi F, et al. Personality trait interactions in parents of patients with borderline personality disorder: a controlled study using the Temperament and Character Inventory. *Psychiatry Res* 2009;**165**(1–2):128–36.

21. Skodol AE. Longitudinal course and outcome of personality disorders. *Psychiatr Clin North Am* 2008;**31**(3):495–503, viii.

22. Lacey C, Cook M, Salzberg M. The neurologist, psychogenic nonepileptic seizures, and borderline personality disorder. *Epilepsy Behav* 2007;**11**(4):492–8.

23. Reuber M, Pukrop R, Bauer J, Derfuss R, Elger CE. Multidimensional assessment of personality in patients with psychogenic non-epileptic seizures. *J Neurol Neurosurg Psychiatry* 2004;**75**(5):743–8.

24. Dodrill CB, Holmes MD. Part summary: psychological and neuropsychological evaluation of the patient with non-epileptic seizures. In: Gates JR, Rowan AJ, eds. *Non-Epileptic Seizures*. Boston, MA: Butterworth-Heinemann. 2000; 169–81.

25. Owczarek K. Anxiety as a differential factor in epileptic versus psychogenic pseudoepileptic seizures. *Epilepsy Res* 2003;**52**(3):227–32.

26. First MB, Gibbon M, Spitzer RL, Williams JBW, Benjamin LS. *Structured Clinical Interview for DSM-IV Axis II Personality Disorders (SCID-II)*. Washington, DC: American Psychiatric Press, 1997.

27. D'Alessio L, Giagante B, Oddo S, et al. Psychiatric disorders in patients with psychogenic non-epileptic seizures, with and without comorbid epilepsy. *Seizure* 2006;**15**(5):333–9.

28. Arnold LM, Privitera MD. Psychopathology and trauma in epileptic and psychogenic seizure patients. *Psychosomatics* 1996;**37**(5):438–43.

29. Binzer M, Stone J, Sharpe M. Recent onset pseudoseizures–clues to aetiology. *Seizure* 2004;**13**(3):146–55.

30. Baillés E, Pintor L, Fernandez-Egea E, et al. Psychiatric disorders, trauma, and MMPI profile in a Spanish sample of nonepileptic seizure patients. *Gen Hosp Psychiatry* 2004;**26**(4):310–15.

31. Paris J. The treatment of borderline personality disorder: implications of research on diagnosis, etiology, and outcome. *Annu Rev Clin Psychol* 2009;**5**:277–90.

32. Sharpe D, Faye C. Non-epileptic seizures and child sexual abuse: a critical review of the literature. *Clin Psychol Rev* 2006;**26**(8):1020–40.

33. Salmon P, Skaife K, Rhodes J. Abuse, dissociation, and somatization in irritable bowel syndrome: towards an explanatory model. *J Behav Med* 2003;**26**(1):1–18.

34. Slavney PR. Pseudoseizures, sexual abuse, and hermeneutic reasoning. *Compr Psychiatry* 1994;**35**(6):471–7.

35. Salmon P, Al-Marzooqi SM, Baker G, Reilly J. Childhood family dysfunction and associated abuse in patients with nonepileptic seizures: towards a causal model. *Psychosom Med* 2003;**65**(4):695–700.

36. Golier JA, Yehuda R, Bierer LM, et al. The relationship of borderline personality disorder to posttraumatic stress disorder and traumatic events. *Am J Psychiatry* 2003;**160**(11):2018–24.

37. Zanarini MC. Childhood experiences associated with the development of borderline personality disorder. *Psychiatr Clin North Am* 2000;**23**(1):89–101.

38. Thorpe M. Is borderline personality disorder a post-traumatic stress disorder of early childhood? *Can J Psychiatry* 1993;**38**(5):367–8.
39. Whealin JM, Slone L. Complex PTSD: Differences between the effects of short-term trauma and the effects of chronic trauma? http://www.ncptsd.va.gov/ncmain/ncdocs/fact_shts/fs_complex_ptsd.html (accessed January 30th, 2009).
40. Herman JL. *Trauma and Recovery: the Aftermath of Violence from Domestic Abuse to Political Terror.* New York: Basic Books, 1997.
41. van der Kolk BA, Pelcovitz D, Roth S, *et al.* Dissociation, somatization, and affect dysregulation: the complexity of adaptation of trauma. *Am J Psychiatry* 1996;**153**(7 Suppl): 83–93.
42. van der Kolk BA, Roth S, Pelcovitz D, Sunday S, Spinazzola J. Disorders of extreme stress: the empirical foundation of a complex adaptation to trauma. *J Trauma Stress* 2005;**18**(5):389–99.
43. Bass C, Murphy M. Somatoform and personality disorders: syndromal comorbidity and overlapping developmental pathways. *J Psychosom Res* 1995;**39**(4): 403–27.
44. Sar V, Akyuz G, Kundakci T, Kiziltan E, Dogan O. Childhood trauma, dissociation, and psychiatric comorbidity in patients with conversion disorder. *Am J Psychiatry* 2004;**161**(12):2271–6.
45. Bisson JI, Ehlers A, Matthews R, *et al.* Psychological treatments for chronic post-traumatic stress disorder. Systematic review and meta-analysis. *Br J Psychiatry* 2007;**190**:97–104.
46. Mendes DD, Mello MF, Ventura P, Passarela CM, Mari JJ. A systematic review on the effectiveness of cognitive behavioral therapy for posttraumatic stress disorder. *Int J Psychiatry Med* 2008;**38**(3):241–59.
47. Ford JD, Courtois CA, Steele K, Hart O, Nijenhuis ER. Treatment of complex posttraumatic self-dysregulation. *J Trauma Stress* 2005;**18**(5):437–47.
48. Mökleby K, Blomhoff S, Malt UF, *et al.* Psychiatric comorbidity and hostility in patients with psychogenic nonepileptic seizures compared with somatoform disorders and healthy controls. *Epilepsia* 2002;**43**:193–8.

Section 5
Treatment considerations for psychogenic nonepileptic seizures

Section 5 Chapter 24

Treatment considerations for psychogenic nonepileptic seizures

Historical approaches to treatments for psychogenic nonepileptic seizures

W. Curt LaFrance, Jr. and Steven C. Schachter

Hysteria and epilepsy have been recognized and linked by medical practitioners since ancient times [1]. One of the first known descriptions of nonepileptic seizures (NES) is found in the British Museum's "Babylonian Collection" and dates from the first millennium B.C. The tablet describes, "If before he fits he suffers from frontal headaches and is emotionally upset, and afterwards he … [..] his hands and feet, (and) rolls from side to side *(on the ground)* without *deviation (of the eyes)* or foam(ing of the mouth), it is a fall – R: due to emotional shock, or 'hand of Ishtar.' He will recover" [2].

Just as is the case today, treatment of psychogenic NES (PNES) begins with accurate diagnosis, differentiating it from epileptic seizures (ES). Even in the nineteenth century, Reynolds commented about the reliability of certain signs to distinguish ES from hysteria [3]. He wrote, "Nausea, eructations, borborygmi, tympanitis, palpitation of heart, syncopal feelings, and frequent micturation of clear pale urine – sometimes spoken of as diagnostic signs of hysteria – have no value of that kind; for I have witnessed them all, and with as great frequency, after epileptic seizures." This echoes with the recognition of today's medical community that signs that "perfectly distinguish" one condition from the other are hard to come by.

The initial treatments offered for NES were a prayer to exorcise demons that may be causing the fits. From Lennox's published writings of medieval authors on epilepsy we read, "Note that an epileptic, lunatic and demoniac have certain things in common, as Constantine says, *Practica* Book 9, Chapter 5 'On Epilepsy.' Therefore, to discern whether the one who falls to the ground be a lunatic or an epileptic, make this test. Utter these words into the ear of the suspect: 'Depart demon, and go forth, because effimolei (?) command thee.' If he be a lunatic or a demoniac, he immediately becomes (?) dead, for nearly an hour. When he arises, ask him any question whatever, and he will give the answer. If he does not fall when he hears these words, then you know that he is an epileptic." [4]. As we do in modern medicine, the ancient physicians realized the importance of ictal semiology as it influenced diagnosis and prognosis, and they used provocative tests to diagnose and treat PNES (Figure 24.1).

With the incorporation of "Disorders of the Uterus" in the pathology of hysteria, treatment moved from spirit to sexual organs. Aretaeus classified seizures as ordinary and hysterical, the latter of which, he noted, was due to movement of the uterus [5]. His suggested treatment for the disorder was to give fetid-smelling substances or old urine, which would drive the uterus downward, at the same time fragrant oils being "rubbed into the region of the female parts" in order to attract the uterus back to its correct position [6]. Willis proposed the movement of the seat of hysteria from the uterus to the brain, noting, "The distemper named from the womb is chiefly and primarily convulsive, and chiefly depends on the brain and the nervous stock being affected…" [7]. Less than a century later, the first treatments incorporating a behavioral model were implemented, as described below.

Mandeville records the first full description of a hysterical seizure [8]. In 1730, he wrote,

As to Fits, some are seiz'd with violent Coughs; others with Hick-ups; and abundance of Women are taken with Convulsive laughing. There are Fits that have short Remissions, in which you would think the Woman was going to recover, and yet last many Hours. Some are so slight that the Patients only lose the Use of their Legs and Tongue, but remain sensible; others again are so violent that those who are seiz'd with them, foam at the Mouth, rave and beat their

---

Gates and Rowan's Nonepileptic Seizures, 3rd edn. ed. Steven C. Schachter and W. Curt LaFrance, Jr. Published by Cambridge University Press. © S. Schachter and W. C. LaFrance, Jr. 2010.

Section 5: Treatment considerations for PNES

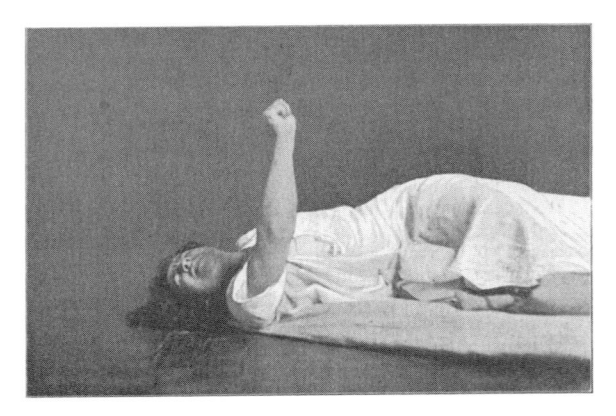

Figure 24.1. First photograph of patient with PNES. From Binswanger [32].

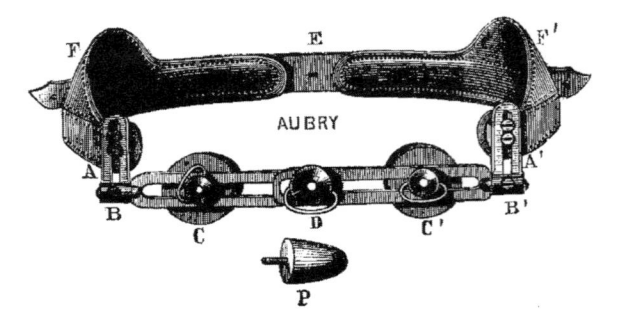

Figure 24.2. Ovarian compression belt, used for treatment of PNES. From Richer [14].

Heads against the Ground; but whether they resemble an Apoplex, or are only fainting, or seem to be Epileptick, they all come under the Denomination of Hysterick…

In a dialogue between a physician and a patient whose daughter also suffers from hysterical convulsions, Mandeville records the first behavioral prescription for PNES:

Philopirio – a physician. "…wherefore if the Lady's Youth and Strength be prudently assisted, I am of the Opinion, Madam, that she'll certainly be cured. In order to it, in the first Place, I would for one Month prescribe a Course of Exercise, and no Medicines at all."

Polytheca – a patient. "A Course of Exercise! and no Medicines at all!"

Interestingly, the patient's dismay at a physician's prescribing behavioral methods and not prescribing a medicine to take away the nonepileptic events is similarly found in patients today, even three centuries later.

Bromides are noted to be the first documented allopathic pharmacological treatment for PNES. Sir Charles Locock mentioned his successful use of potassium bromide in a series of cases that he had "determined to try thin remedy in cases of hysteria in young women, unaccompanied by epilepsy," noting resolution in 14 of 15 cases [9]. Whether the women had "hysterical epilepsy" or bromide was actually treating catamenial epilepsy is unclear [10]. Friedlander notes that "Bromides were tried by Locock for hysterical conditions, because others had considered this drug a genital system sedative" [11].

By the late nineteenth century, the neuropsychiatric syndrome of PNES was established in the Western medical literature (then referred to as hystero-epilepsy). Briquet, Charcot, Richer, and Gowers described PNES, but the French and English differed in treatment approaches [12–15]. Charcot, with his understanding of hypnosis, likely utilized the power of suggestion, and he promoted ovarian compression for treatment of acute attacks (Figure 24.2). Gowers, however, described aversive therapies for PNES such as closing the nose and mouth, faradization (electric shock to the skin), and hydrotherapy. Long-term management for both Charcot and Gowers consisted of environmental changes with removal of the patient from the home, suggesting that family dysfunction can influence PNES recurrence.

Gowers documented his recommendations for treatments of PNES in 1881 [16]. The 1901 second edition of Gowers' monograph on epilepsy updates treatment of hysteroid attacks: "…the most important point is abstinence from that to which there is an invariable tendency – restraint. All restraint intensifies the struggling movements which are the object of restraint." If the attacks do not cease in a few minutes, "it may be desirable to cut them short. This can often be effected by a strong sensory impression of any kind…such as a strong induced current applied to one of the limbs. A magnetoelectric apparatus answers well." He also described the intelligible utility of "a vigorous tug at the pubic hair," as used by "an old country surgeon," in the treatment armamentarium. "Affusion with water is often employed, but more than one jugful is generally needed. A small quantity will suffice, if poured into the mouth of the patient." "Closing the mouth and nose with a towel until the patient is on the point of asphyxia, when all convulsion ceases" was noted as expedient "by the late Dr Hare"; however, he acknowledged that "the chief disadvantage of this method is the impression it conveys to the friends." Finally, "the most effective measure of arresting severe attacks, which would otherwise go on for an hour or two, is the injection of apomorphia." After injection of one-sixth of a grain, he observed, "in two minutes all spasms ceased, and the patient began to look uncomfortable. In three minutes she got up and walked to the nearest sink; and in four minutes vomited copiously" [17].

Charcot's ovarian compression methods were not as readily accepted by Gowers in the UK or in the US as they were in France, as Wood noted in a letter to the *American Journal of Insanity* [18].

> In many of Charcot's cases of grave hysteria, ovarian pain and tenderness have been marked features; and the Professor lays great stress upon the occurrence of such symptoms, and upon the fact that firm ovarian pressure will, in hystero-epilepsy, arrest the paroxysms. Our experience does not coincide with this. In the case of hystero-epilepsy spoken of above, ovarian pressure did not arrest the fits; and this is our common experience. In American women, the ovaries do not seem to be often involved in hysteria, nor are we able to feel them or impress them by the method described by Charcot. Often, too, I have seen very marked ovralgia and ovarian tenderness, without hysterical symptoms.

In the late nineteenth and early twentieth century, students of Charcot, Sigmund Freud and Pierre Janet, developed the historical theories on conversion disorder [19, 20]. With the growth of psychoanalysis in the early twentieth century, dream interpretation and hypnosis were used more frequently to treat PNES. Regarding dream interpretation, Freud wrote [21],

> When one carries out the psycho-analysis of a hysterical woman patient whose complaint is manifested in attacks, one soon becomes convinced that these attacks are nothing else but phantasies translated into the motor sphere, projected on to motility and portrayed in pantomime.... Often a dream takes the place of an attack.... A hysterical attack, therefore, needs to be subjected to the same interpretive revision as we employ for night-dreams.

Moving forward to the twenty-first century, although our treatments now are refined in the sense that we target neurotransmitter abnormalities in patients with drugs or treat them with individualized psychotherapies, after more than 200 years, we have not added one phase III randomized placebo-controlled trial to empirically test the efficacy of treatments for PNES. Despite this, we can learn about PNES treatment from the numerous case reports, case series, and retrospective treatment reports that have been published.

The PNES psychotherapy data include case reports, small uncontrolled trials or medium-size retrospective follow-up studies. In a review of all of the PNES treatment literature, articles were included that gave clear descriptions of their treatment(s) and the individual/population treated (see Table 24.1). (Where repeated treatment descriptions in case reports were found, only the earliest noted article was included.) The majority of treatment trials for PNES to date would be considered class IV data [22]. A handful of class III studies exists, including open-label trials or the retrospective trial that utilized a control group. The chapters following this historical introduction delineate the lessons that can be applied from the treatment literature to PNES treatments. This paucity of controlled treatment data underscores the need to conduct class I level trials to inform effective treatments for patients with PNES.

Learning from past approaches, the current evidence for PNES management is summarized in Table 24.2. Encouragingly, the direct evidence grows annually for treatments for PNES. A current treatment approach involves the patient, family, community, and neurological/psychiatric treatment providers, both in prevention and treatment of PNES (Figure 24.3).

Consolidating literature from past approaches, we see that PNES are likely the result of a complex interaction between psychiatric disorders, psychosocial stressors, dysfunctional coping styles, and CNS vulnerability [23]. Identifying the underlying stressors and providing supportive psychotherapy can help some patients but is often insufficient or ineffective. Studies consistently identify three main comorbid diagnoses in patients with PNES: major depressive disorder, posttraumatic stress disorder, and Cluster B personality traits characterized by impulsivity/hostility [24, 25]. Three additional critical areas of dysfunction in the PNES population are: emotion regulation, family dynamics, and unemployment/disability [26–28]. Poorer outcomes to treatment may be associated with the high number of comorbid psychiatric disorders and psychosocial stressors [29]. Therefore, therapy for patients with PNES may require a clear presentation of the diagnosis by the neurologist, followed by combined psychological education, psychotherapy, and pharmacotherapy, while simultaneously eliminating ineffective antiepileptic drugs. Regarding future directions, a 2005 workshop jointly sponsored by the National Institute of Neurological Disorders and Stroke, the National Institute of Mental Health, and the American Epilepsy Society emphasized that there is a great need

Table 24.1 Classification of PNES treatment reports

Author, Year	N	Treatment	Design	Classification
LaFrance et al., 2009 [33]	38	SSRI vs. placebo	Prospective, randomized, placebo-controlled	I
Ataoglu et al., 2003 [34]	30	Paradoxical intention inpatient therapy vs. outpatient diazepam	Prospective, randomized, open trial	III
Moene et al., 2003 [35]	2 (of 44 w/motor conversion)	Outpatient, H vs. Wait List	Prospective, randomized, controlled clinical trial	III
Moene et al., 2002 [36]	8 (of 45 w/motor conversion)	Inpatient, H vs. No H, with PT, GT, CBT, SST	Prospective, randomized, controlled, open clinical trial	III
Aboukasm et al., 1998 [37]	61 (4 groups – CEP P; CEP N; non-CEP P; No intervention)	"supportive confrontation," P	Observational, retrospective, nonrandomized, with control group, phone follow-up	III
Aldenkamp and Mulder, 1989 [38]	45 adolescents (3 groups)	Inpatient BT, OC, Paradoxical; "wait and see"; Neurological f/u	Prospective, nonequivalent control groups, open clinical trial	III
Hafeiz, 1980 [39]	6 (of 61 w/ various conversion)	Outpatient, Suggestion + Faradization, Sleep machine, IVB, MeAm	Prospective, randomized, uncontrolled, open label	III
Rampello et al., 1996 [40]	4 (of 18 w/ various conversion)	Outpatient, sulpiride or haloperidol (D2 antagonists)	Prospective, randomized, open label	III
Prigatano et al., 2002 [41]	15	Group P	Prospective, open trial	IV
Zaroff et al., 2004 [42]	7	Group PEd	Prospective, open trial	IV
Barry et al., 2008 [43]	7	Group PdP and PEd	Prospective, open trial	IV
LaFrance et al., 2009 [44]	21	CBT	Prospective, open trial	IV
Goldstein et al., 2004 [45]	16	CBT	Prospective, open trial	IV
LaFrance et al., 2007 [46]	8	Sertraline	Prospective, open trial	IV
Lambert and Rees, 1944 [47]	17	IVB; P, OT, E; H	Observational, retrospective, nonrandomized	IV
Ramani and Gumnit, 1982 [48]	9	Inpatient, BT, BM, short-term PdP, FT, OT	Uncontrolled, unblended, phone follow-up	IV
Kuyk et al., 2008 [49]	16	Inpatient CBT, FT, GT	Prospective, uncontrolled, unblinded	IV
McDade and Brown, 1992 [50]	16	ST, OT, OC, AMT, PT, FT	Prospective, uncontrolled, unblinded	IV
Bhattacharyya and Singh, 1971 [51]	8	OC	Prospective, uncontrolled, unblinded	IV
Betts and Boden, 1992 [52]	121	OC; CBT; H; P; FT; MT	Chart review, retrospective	IV
Buchanan and Snars, 1993 [53]	50	"Direct communication," P, PdP, ST	Chart review, retrospective	IV
Kim et al., 1998 [54]	14	Inpatient psychotherapy: H, GT, IT, FT	Chart review, uncontrolled, phone follow-up	IV
Thompson et al., 2005 [55]	48	Shen protocol modified, P	Retrospective, phone followup	IV
Farias et al., 2003 [56]	22 (vs. 10 Ep)	Shen protocol presentation [57]	Retrospective, case-control	IV
Wilder et al., 2004 [58]	52	Shen protocol presentation [57]	Retrospective, phone follow-up	IV
Rusch et al., 2001 [59]	26	CBT; IT; PdP; OC	Series review, retrospective	IV

(cont.)

Table 24.1 (cont.)

Author, Year	N	Treatment	Design	Classification
Hill and Höhn, 1999 [60]	10	P, FT, BT	Case series	IV
Blumer and Adamolekun. 2006 [61]	5	Reduction of AEDs	Case series, mixed PNES/ES	IV
Gardner, 1967 [62]	1	Parental contingency management plan	Case report	IV
Gardner, 1973 [63]	1	H	Case report	IV
Iwata and Lorentzson, 1976 [64]	1	OC with patient	Case report	IV
Parraga and Kashani, 1981 [65]	1	PdP, OC, H, OT	Case report	IV
Miller, 1983 [66]	3	H	Case series	IV
Aylward, 1984 [67]	2	CBT, ST, FT	Case report	IV
Shulman and Silver, 1985 [68]	1	TCA and PdP	Case report	IV
Montgomery and Espie, 1986 [69]	1	BM (differential reinforcement, OC)	Case report	IV
Lachenmeyer and Olson, 1990 [70]	1	BM	Case report	IV
Daie and Witztum, 1994 [71]	1	Abreaction	Case report	IV
Lamiral and Van Rijckevorsel-Harmant, 1994 [72]	2	CD, P	Case report	IV
Mims and Antonello, 1994 [73]	3	IT, FT, E	Case series with comparison group	IV
Baker et al., 1995 [74]	1	FT	Case report	IV
Swingle, 1998 [75]	3	Neurofeedback, P	Case series	IV
Blumer, 2000 [76]	Unspecified	Various medications, P	Chapter report	IV
Chand and al Khalili, 2000 [77]	1	Graded exposure	Case report	IV
McLean and Dyer, 2003 [78]	1	CBT	Case report, mixed PNES/ES	IV
Chemali and Meadows, 2004 [79]	1	EMDR	Case report	IV
Myers and Zaroff, 2004 [80]	1	IT, Group PEd	Case report	IV
Kalogjera-Sackellares, 2004 [81]	Unspecified	PdP	Case reports	IV
Gowers, 1901 [17]	Unspecified	Water, faradization, pulling of hair, apomorphia I.V.	Case reports	IV
Kingdon, 1898 [82]	1	Hyoscine hydrobromate	Case report	IV
Locock (in paper by EH Sieveking, 1857) [9]	14	Bromide of potassium	Case reports of "hysterical epilepsy" (which could be catamenial epilepsy)	IV

AED, antiepileptic drug; AMT, art and music therapy; BM, behavioral modification; BT, behavioral therapy; CBT, cognitive behavioral therapy; CD, communication of diagnosis of PNES; CEP, comprehensive epilepsy program; D, dopamine; E, education; EMDR, eye movement desensitization; Ep, epilepsy patients; ES, epileptic seizures; FT, family therapy; f/u, follow-up; GT, group therapy; H, hypnosis; IT, individual psychotherapy; I.V., intravenous; IVB, intravenous barbiturate; MeAm, methylamphetamine; MT, major tranquilizer (antipsychotic); N, neurologist; PNES, psychogenic nonepileptic seizures; OC, operant conditioning; OT, occupational therapy; P, psychotherapy; PdP, psychodynamic psychotherapy; PEd, psychoeducation; PT, physical therapy; SSRI, selective serotonin receptor inhibitor; SST, social skills training; ST, supportive psychotherapy; TCA, tricyclic antidepressant; w/, with.

Table 24.2 PNES management paradigm and evidence basis

Treatment steps		Direct evidence	Indirect evidence
Diagnosis	Consider early	[26, 83, 84]	
	Investigate (video-EEG, provocation techniques, home video)	[85, 86]	
Assessment	Characterize neurological comorbidity	[85, 87–90]	
	Characterize psychiatric comorbidity	[24, 91]	
	Characterize social/family conflict, trauma history	[28, 92, 93]	
Communication of diagnosis	Explain what PNES are not (epilepsy, syncope)	[94]	[95]
	Explain what PNES are (psychogenic disorder)	[55, 56, 57]	
	Leaflets	[55]	
Psychiatric treatment	Patient engagement/reattribution	[26]	[96]
	Cognitive behavioral therapy	[44, 45]	[97–99]
	Family therapy	[100]	[28, 92, 93, 101]
	Antidepressants	[46]	[102, 103]
	Case management		[104, 105]
	Rehabilitation	[106]	[107, 108]

EEG, electroencephalogram; PNES, psychogenic nonepileptic seizures.
Modified from Reuber and House [109]. With permission, LWW.

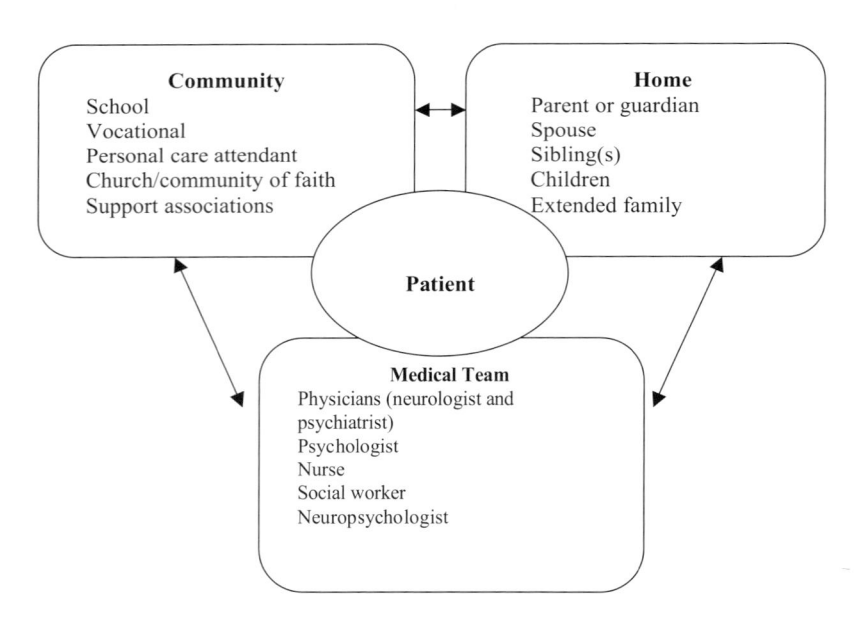

Figure 24.3. Systems model for prevention and treatment of psychogenic nonepileptic seizures. From LaFrance Jr and DeVinsky [110] with permission, *Epilepsia*, and Blackwell Publishing.

for these interventions to be studied in randomized, controlled trials and therefore the workshop established benchmarks for conducting PNES treatment research [30, 31].

Conclusion

Psychogenic nonepileptic seizures commonly occur and patients with PNES are frequently seen by neurologists, psychiatrists, and emergency department physicians. We know much about the phenomenology of the disorder, but we lack controlled data from the literature on specific treatments. While the disorder is treatable, an effective treatment that yields long-term PNES freedom and improved quality of life has yet to be discovered. Prior treatment reports reveal that coordination between neurologists and psychiatrists/psychologists with accurate diagnosis and prompt initiation of psychotherapy and communication between care providers, patient, and family yields higher treatment success.

A review of the historical approaches to PNES reveals that treatments have modified from administering concoctions to medication to behavioral interventions. Pharmacological treatment of the commonly occurring comorbid psychiatric disorders, along with diagnosis-directed psychotherapy, may be the key to improving outcomes in these patients. Therapy will probably need to be individualized based on etiology, level of intelligence, family dynamics, comorbid psychiatric illness, and other factors. Controlled efficacy and effectiveness trials of PNES treatments are greatly needed.

References

1. Temkin O. Epilepsy in ancient medical science. In: *The Falling Sickness: A History of Epilepsy from the Greeks to the Beginnings of Modern Neurology*, 2nd, revised edn. Baltimore: Johns Hopkins Press. 1971; 28–81.
2. Wilson JVK, Reynolds EH. Texts and documents. Translation and analysis of a cuneiform text forming part of a Babylonian treatise on epilepsy. *Med Hist* 1990;**34**(2):185–98.
3. Reynolds JR. *Epilepsy: Its Symptoms, Treatment, and Relation to Other Chronic Convulsive Diseases.* London: Churchill, 1861.
4. Lennox WG. John of Gaddesden on epilepsy. *Ann Med Hist* 1939;**1**:283–307.
5. Aretaeus. On hysterical suffocation. In: *The Extant Works of Aretaeus, the Cappadocian.* London: Sydenham Society. 1856; 285–7.
6. Aretaeus. Cure of the hysterical convulsion. In: *The Extant Works of Aretaeus, the Cappadocian.* London: Sydenham Society. 1856, 449–51.
7. Willis T, Pordage S, tr. *Dr. Willis's practice of physick, being the whole works of that renowned and famous physician: containing these eleven several treatises, viz. I. Of fermentation. II. Of feavers. III. Of urines. IV. Of the accension of the blood. V. Of musculary motion. VI. Of the anatomy of the brain. VII. Of the description and use of the nerves. VIII. Of convulsive diseases. IX. Pharmaceutice rationalis, the first and second part. X. Of the scurvy. XI. Two discourses concerning the soul of brutes. Wherein most of the diseases belonging to the body of man are treated of, with excellent methods and receipts for the cure of the same. Fitted to the meanest capacity by an index for the explaining of all the hard and unusual words and terms of art derived from the Greek, Latine, or other languages for the benefit of the English reader. With forty copper plates.* London: Printed for T. Dring C. Harper and J. Leigh, 1684.
8. Mandeville B. *A Treatise of the Hypochondriack and Hysterick Diseases. In Three Dialogues.* Corrected and enlarged by the author: 2nd edn. London, J. Tonson, 1730.
9. Sieveking EH. Analysis of fifty-two cases of epilepsy observed by the author. *Lancet* 1857;**1**:527–8.
10. Trousseau A. Lecture III. On epilepsy; with a note by the editor on the use of bromide of potassium in epilepsy. In: Bazire PV, ed. *Lectures on Clinical Medicine, Delivered at the Hotel-Dieu, Paris.* London: New Sydenham Society. 1868; 39–104.
11. Friedlander WJ. Treatment. In: *The History of Modern Epilepsy: The Beginning, 1865–1914.* Westport, CT: Greenwood Press. 2001; 151–207.
12. Briquet P. *Traité Clinique et Thérapeutique de l'Hystérie.* Paris: Baillière, 1859.
13. Charcot JM. Lecture XII. Hystero-epilepsy. In: Sigerson G, ed. *Lectures on the Diseases of the Nervous System: Delivered at La Salpêtrière.* London: The New Sydenham Society. 1877; 300–15.
14. Richer PMLP. *Études Cliniques sur l'Hystéro-épilepsie, ou Grande Hystérie.* Paris: Delahaye et Lecrosnier, 1881.
15. Gowers WR. *Epilepsy and Other Chronic Convulsive Diseases: Their Causes, Symptoms, and Treatment.* London: Churchill, 1881.
16. Gates JR. Diagnosis and treatment of nonepileptic seizures. In: McConnell HW, Snyder PJ, eds. *Psychiatric Comorbidity in Epilepsy. Basic Mechanisms, Diagnosis, and Treatment*, 1st edn. Washington, DC: American Psychiatric Press, Inc. 1998; 187–204.
17. Gowers WR. Treatment. Hysteroid Attacks. In: *Epilepsy and Other Chronic Convulsive Diseases: Their Causes, Symptoms, and Treatment*, 2nd edn. London: Churchill. 1901; 299–301.
18. Wood HC. Ovarian compression in hystero-epilepsy. *Am J Insanity* 1881;**37**:444–5.
19. Breuer J, Freud S (Translated by Brill AA). *Studies in Hysteria 1895.* Monograph 61. New York: Nervous and Mental Disease Monographs, 1950.
20. Janet P. *The Major Symptoms of Hysteria; Fifteen Lectures Given in the Medical School of Harvard University.* New York: Macmillan, 1907.
21. Freud S. Some general remarks on hysterical attacks (1909 [1908]) [Allgemeines uber den hysterischen Anfall]. In: Strachey J, Freud A, eds. *The Standard Edition of the Complete Psychological Works of Sigmund Freud*, 1st edn. London: Hogarth Press. 1959; 227–34.

22. Goodin DS, Frohman EM, Garmany GP, Jr, *et al.* Disease modifying therapies in multiple sclerosis: report of the Therapeutics and Technology Assessment Subcommittee of the American Academy of Neurology and the MS Council for Clinical Practice Guidelines. *Neurology* 2002;**58**(2):169–78.

23. Mokleby K, Blomhoff S, Malt UF, *et al.* Psychiatric comorbidity and hostility in patients with psychogenic nonepileptic seizures compared with somatoform disorders and healthy controls. *Epilepsia* 2002;**43**(2):193–8.

24. Bowman ES, Markand ON. Psychodynamics and psychiatric diagnoses of pseudoseizure subjects. *Am J Psychiatry* 1996;**153**(1):57–63.

25. Rechlin T, Loew TH, Joraschky P. Pseudoseizure "status". *J Psychosom Res* 1997;**42**(5):495–8.

26. Walczak TS, Papacostas S, Williams DT, *et al.* Outcome after diagnosis of psychogenic nonepileptic seizures. *Epilepsia* 1995;**36**(11):1131–7.

27. Holmes MD, Dodrill CB, Bachtler S, *et al.* Evidence that emotional maladjustment is worse in men than in women with psychogenic nonepileptic seizures. *Epilepsy Behav* 2001;**2**:568–73.

28. Griffith JL, Polles A, Griffith ME. Pseudoseizures, families, and unspeakable dilemmas. *Psychosomatics* 1998;**39**(2):144–53.

29. Carson AJ, Ringbauer B, MacKenzie L, Warlow C, Sharpe M. Neurological disease, emotional disorder, and disability: they are related: a study of 300 consecutive new referrals to a neurology outpatient department. *J Neurol Neurosurg Psychiatry* 2000;**68**(2):202–6.

30. LaFrance Jr WC, Alper K, Babcock D, *et al.* Nonepileptic seizures treatment workshop summary. *Epilepsy Behav* 2006;**8**(3):451–61.

31. Kelley MS, Jacobs MP, Lowenstein DH; NINDS Epilepsy Benchmark Stewards. The NINDS epilepsy research benchmarks. *Epilepsia* 2009;**50**(2):579–82.

32. Binswanger O. *Die Hysterie*. Wien: Hölder, 1904.

33. LaFrance Jr WC, Blum AS, Ryan CE, Miller I, Keitner GI. Treating comorbidities in patients with psychogenic nonepileptic seizures. *Neurology* 2009;**72**(11(Suppl3)): A328.

34. Ataoglu A, Ozcetin A, Icmeli C, Ozbulut O. Paradoxical therapy in conversion reaction. *J Korean Med Sci* 2003;**18**(4):581–4.

35. Moene FC, Spinhoven P, Hoogduin KA, van Dyck R. A randomized controlled clinical trial of a hypnosis-based treatment for patients with conversion disorder, motor type. *Int J Clin Exp Hypn* 2003;**51**(1): 29–50.

36. Moene FC, Spinhoven P, Hoogduin KA, van Dyck R. A randomised controlled clinical trial on the additional effect of hypnosis in a comprehensive treatment programme for in-patients with conversion disorder of the motor type. *Psychother Psychosom* 2002;**71**(2):66–76.

37. Aboukasm A, Mahr G, Gahry BR, Thomas A, Barkley GL. Retrospective analysis of the effects of psychotherapeutic interventions on outcomes of psychogenic nonepileptic seizures. *Epilepsia* 1998;**39**(5):470–3.

38. Aldenkamp AP, Mulder OG. Pseudoepileptic seizures in adolescents. In: Manelis J, Bental E, Loeber JN, Dreifuss FE, eds. *Advances in Epileptology: XVIIth Epilepsy International Symposium*. New York: Raven Press. 1989; 445–9.

39. Hafeiz HB. Hysterical conversion: a prognostic study. *Br J Psychiatry* 1980;**136**:548–51.

40. Rampello L, Raffaele R, Nicoletti G, *et al.* Hysterical neurosis of the conversion type: therapeutic activity of neuroleptics with different hyperprolactinemic potency. *Neuropsychobiology* 1996;**33**(4):186–8.

41. Prigatano GP, Stonnington CM, Fisher RS. Psychological factors in the genesis and management of nonepileptic seizures: clinical observations. *Epilepsy Behav* 2002;**3**(4):343–9.

42. Zaroff CM, Myers L, Barr WB, Luciano D, Devinsky O. Group psychoeducation as treatment for psychological nonepileptic seizures. *Epilepsy Behav* 2004;**5**(4):587–92.

43. Barry JJ, Wittenberg D, Bullock KD, *et al.* Group therapy for patients with psychogenic nonepileptic seizures: a pilot study. *Epilepsy Behav* 2008;**13**:624–9.

44. LaFrance Jr WC, Miller IW, Ryan CE, *et al.* Cognitive behavioral therapy for psychogenic nonepileptic seizures. *Epilepsy Behav* 2009;**14**(4):591–6.

45. Goldstein LH, Deale AC, Mitchell-O'Malley SJ, Toone BK, Mellers JDC. An evaluation of cognitive behavioral therapy as a treatment for dissociative seizures: a pilot study. *Cogn Behav Neurol* 2004; **17**(1):41–9.

46. LaFrance Jr WC, Blum AS, Miller IW, Ryan CE, Keitner GI. Methodological issues in conducting treatment trials for psychological nonepileptic seizures. *J Neuropsychiatry Clin Neurosci* 2007;**19**(4):391–8.

47. Lambert C, Rees WL. Intravenous barbiturates in the treatment of hysteria. *BMJ* 1944;**2**:70–3.

48. Ramani V, Gumnit RJ. Management of hysterical seizures in epileptic patients. *Arch Neurol* 1982; **39**(2):78–81.

49. Kuyk J, Siffels MC, Bakvis P, Swinkels WA. Psychological treatment of patients with psychogenic non-epileptic seizures: an outcome study. *Seizure* 2008;**17**(7):595–603.

50. McDade G, Brown SW. Non-epileptic seizures: management and predictive factors of outcome. *Seizure* 1992;**1**(1):7–10.

51. Bhattacharyya DD, Singh R. Behavior therapy of hysterical fits. *Am J Psychiatry* 1971;**128**(5):602–6.

52. Betts T, Boden S. Diagnosis, management and prognosis of a group of 128 patients with non-epileptic attack disorder. Part I. *Seizure* 1992;**1**(1):19–26.

53. Buchanan N, Snars J. Pseudoseizures (non epileptic attack disorder) – clinical management and outcome in 50 patients. *Seizure* 1993;**2**(2):141–6.

54. Kim CM, Barry JJ, Zeifert PA. The use of inpatient medical psychiatric treatment for nonepileptic events. *Epilepsia* 1998;**39** Suppl 6:242–3.

55. Thompson NC, Osorio I, Hunter EE. Nonepileptic seizures: reframing the diagnosis. *Perspect Psychiatr Care* 2005;**41**(2):71–8.

56. Farias ST, Thieman C, Alsaadi TM. Psychogenic nonepileptic seizures: acute change in event frequency after presentation of the diagnosis. *Epilepsy Behav* 2003;**4**(4):424–9.

57. Shen W, Bowman ES, Markand ON. Presenting the diagnosis of pseudoseizure. *Neurology* 1990;**40**(5):756–759.

58. Wilder C, Marquez AV, Farias ST, et al. Long-term follow-up study of patients with PNES. *Epilepsia* 2004;**45** Suppl 7:349.

59. Rusch MD, Morris GL, Allen L, Lathrop L. Psychological treatment of nonepileptic events. *Epilepsy Behav* 2001;**2**:277–83.

60. Hill JM, Höhn GE. Psychotherapeutic treatment of patients with nonepileptic seizures (NES). *J Neuropsychiatry Clin Neurosci* 1999;**11**:131.

61. Blumer D, Adamolekun B. Treatment of patients with coexisting epileptic and nonepileptic seizures. *Epilepsy Behav* 2006;**9**(3):498–502.

62. Gardner JE. Behavior therapy treatment approach to a psychogenic seizure case. *J Consult Psychol* 1967;**31**(2):209–12.

63. Gardner GG. Use of hypnosis for psychogenic epilepsy in a child. *Am J Clin Hypn* 1973;**15**(3):166–9.

64. Iwata BA, Lorentzson AM. Operant control of seizure-like behavior in an institutionalized retarded adult. *Behav Ther* 1976;**7**:247–51.

65. Parraga HC, Kashani JH. Treatment approach in a child with hysterical seizures superimposed on partial complex seizures. *Can J Psychiatry* 1981;**26**(2):114–17.

66. Miller HR. Psychogenic seizures treated by hypnosis. *Am J Clin Hypn* 1983;**25**(4):248–52.

67. Aylward GP. Description of a therapeutic approach to pseudoseizures in adolescents. *Community Ment Health J* 1984;**20**(2):155–8.

68. Shulman KI, Silver IL. Hysterical seizures as a manifestation of "depression" in old age. *Can J Psychiatry* 1985;**30**(4):278–80.

69. Montgomery JM, Espie CA. Behavioural management of hysterical pseudoseizures. *Behav Psychother* 1986;**14**:334–40.

70. Lachenmeyer JR, Olson ME. Behaviour modification in the treatment of pseudoseizures: a case report. *Behav Psychother* 1990;**18**:73–8.

71. Daie N, Witztum E. A case of posttraumatic stress disorder masked by pseudoseizures in a Jewish Iranian immigrant in Israel. *J Nerv Ment Dis* 1994;**182**(4):244–5.

72. Lamiral B, Van Rijckevorsel-Harmant K. Crises non epileptiques: quelle strategie therapeutique? [Non-epileptic crisis: which therapeutic strategy to follow?]. *Acta Neurol Belg* 1994;**94**(4):262–5.

73. Mims J, Antonello JL. Treatment of nonepileptic psychogenic events in adolescent patients using the systems model for intervention. *J Neurosci Nurs* 1994;**26**(5):298–305.

74. Baker GA, Moore P, Appleton RE. Non-epileptic attack disorders in children and adolescents: a single case study. *Seizure* 1995;**4**(4):307–9.

75. Swingle PG. Neurofeedback treatment of pseudoseizure disorder. *Biol Psychiatry* 1998;**44**(11):1196–9.

76. Blumer D. On the psychobiology of non-epileptic seizures. In: Gates JR, Rowan AJ, eds. *Non-Epileptic Seizures*, 2nd edn. Boston, MA: Butterworth-Heinemann. 2000;305–10.

77. Chand SP, al Khalili K. Pseudoseizures associated with doll phobia. *Int J Psychiatry Med* 2000;**30**(1):93–6.

78. McLean T, Dyer C. Treatment of psychogenic pseudoseizures in an adolescent with a history of epilepsy. *Clin Psychol* 2003;**7**(2):109–20.

79. Chemali Z, Meadows M-E. The use of eye movement desensitization and reprocessing in the treatment of psychogenic seizures. *Epilepsy Behav* 2004;**5**(5):784–7.

80. Myers L, Zaroff C. The successful treatment of psychogenic nonepileptic seizure using a disorder-specific treatment modality. *Brief Treat Crisis Interv* 2004;**4**:343–52.

81. Kalogjera-Sackellares D. *Psychodynamics and Psychotherapy of Pseudoseizures.* Carmarthen, Wales, UK: Crown House Publishing, Ltd, 2004.

82. Kingdon WR. The diagnosis of hystero-epilepsy from status epilepticus. *Lancet* 1898;**152**(3910):320–1.

83. Wyllie E, Friedman D, Luders H, *et al.* Outcome of psychogenic seizures in children and adolescents compared with adults. *Neurology* 1991;**41**(5):742–4.

84. Lempert T, Dieterich M, Huppert D, Brandt T. Psychogenic disorders in neurology: frequency and clinical spectrum. *Acta Neurol Scand* 1990;**82**(5):335–40.

85. Reuber M, Fernandez G, Bauer J, Helmstaedter C, Elger CE. Diagnostic delay in psychogenic nonepileptic seizures. *Neurology* 2002;**58**(3):493–5.

86. Walczak TS, Williams DT, Berten W. Utility and reliability of placebo infusion in the evaluation of patients with seizures. *Neurology* 1994;**44**(3 Pt 1):394–9.

87. Benbadis SR, Agrawal V, Tatum IV, WO. How many patients with psychogenic nonepileptic seizures also have epilepsy? *Neurology* 2001;**57**(5):915–17.

88. Westbrook LE, Devinsky O, Geocadin R. Nonepileptic seizures after head injury. *Epilepsia* 1998;**39**(9):978–82.

89. Silver LB. Conversion disorder with pseudoseizures in adolescence: a stress reaction to unrecognized and untreated learning disabilities. *J Am Acad Child Psychiatry* 1982;**21**(5):508–12.

90. Kalogjera-Sackellares D, Sackellares JC. Intellectual and neuropsychological features of patients with psychogenic pseudoseizures. *Psychiatry Res* 1999; **86**(1):73–84.

91. Krishnamoorthy ES, Brown RJ, Trimble MR. Personality and psychopathology in nonepileptic attack disorder and epilepsy: a prospective study. *Epilepsy Behav* 2001;**2**:418–22.

92. Krawetz P, Fleisher W, Pillay N, *et al.* Family functioning in subjects with pseudoseizures and epilepsy. *J Nerv Ment Dis* 2001;**189**(1):38–43.

93. Moore PM, Baker GA, McDade G, Chadwick D, Brown S. Epilepsy, pseudoseizures and perceived family characteristics: a controlled study. *Epilepsy Res* 1994;**18**(1):75–83.

94. Ettinger AB, Devinsky O, Weisbrot DM, Ramakrishna RK, Goyal A. A comprehensive profile of clinical, psychiatric, and psychosocial characteristics of patients with psychogenic nonepileptic seizures. *Epilepsia* 1999;**40**(9):1292–8.

95. Coia P, Morley S. Medical reassurance and patients' responses. *J Psychosom Res* 1998;**45**(5):377–86.

96. Fink P, Rosendal M, Toft T. Assessment and treatment of functional disorders in general practice: the extended reattribution and management model–an advanced educational program for nonpsychiatric doctors. *Psychosomatics* 2002;**43**(2):93–131.

97. Kroenke K, Swindle R. Cognitive-behavioral therapy for somatization and symptom syndromes: a critical review of controlled clinical trials. *Psychother Psychosom* 2000;**69**(4):205–15.

98. Ostelo RW, van Tulder MW, Vlaeyen JW, *et al.* Behavioural treatment for chronic low-back pain. *Cochrane Database Syst Rev* 2005(1):CD002014.

99. Barsky AJ, Ahern DK. Cognitive behavior therapy for hypochondriasis: a randomized controlled trial. *JAMA* 2004;**291**(12):1464–70.

100. LaFrance WC, Jr, Blum A, Miller I, Ryan C, Keitner GI. Cognitive behavioral therapy or family therapy for nonepileptic seizures. *Epilepsia* 2008;**49** Suppl 7:273–4.

101. Wood BL, McDaniel S, Burchfiel K, Erba G. Factors distinguishing families of patients with psychogenic seizures from families of patients with epilepsy. *Epilepsia* 1998;**39**(4):432–7.

102. Voon V, Lang AE. Antidepressant treatment outcomes of psychogenic movement disorder. *J Clin Psychiatry* 2005;**66**(12):1529–34.

103. O'Malley PG, Jackson JL, Santoro J, *et al.* Antidepressant therapy for unexplained symptoms and symptom syndromes. *J Fam Pract* 1999;**48**(12):980–90.

104. Smith GR, Jr, Rost K, Kashner TM. A trial of the effect of a standardized psychiatric consultation on health outcomes and costs in somatizing patients. *Arch Gen Psychiatry* 1995;**52**(3):238–43.

105. Smith GR, Jr, Monson RA, Ray DC. Psychiatric consultation in somatization disorder. A randomized controlled study. *N Engl J Med* 1986;**314**(22):1407–13.

106. Clemmons DC, Dodrill CB, Fraser RT. Vocational patterns of patients with nonepileptic seizures. *Epilepsia* 2001;**42** Suppl 7:137.

107. Abbey SE, Lipowski ZJ. Comprehensive management of persistent somatization: an innovative inpatient program. *Psychother Psychosom* 1987;**48**(1–4):110–15.

108. Ness D. Physical therapy management for conversion disorder: case series. *J Neurol Phys Ther* 2007;**31**(1):30–9.

109. Reuber M, House AO. Treating patients with psychogenic non-epileptic seizures. *Curr Opin Neurol* 2002;**15**(2):207–11.

110. LaFrance WC, Jr, Devinsky O. The treatment of nonepileptic seizures: historical perspectives and future directions. *Epilepsia* 2004;**45** Suppl 2:15–21.

Section 5 Chapter 25

Treatment considerations for psychogenic nonepileptic seizures

Managing psychogenic nonepileptic seizures in patients with epilepsy

Roderick Duncan and Meritxell Oto

There is some disagreement in the literature about what proportion of patients with psychogenic nonepileptic seizures (PNES) also have epileptic seizures (ES), with proportions ranging from approximately 5% to 50% in different series [1, 2]. Most series are from tertiary centers, which are likely to have a recruitment bias toward difficult diagnostic cases and patients already known to have epilepsy. More stringent studies estimate a 10% rate of mixed PNES and ES [2]. Patients with PNES and learning disability (LD) appear to have a higher prevalence of epilepsy [3], and are therefore likely to be overrepresented in series of patients with a dual diagnosis. In our series of 288 patients with PNES [3], 9/25 patients with LD (36.0%) had ES, whereas only 23/263 patients without LD (8.7%) had epilepsy.

Patients who have both epilepsy and PNES pose particular management challenges. The patients have two disorders rather than one, each with different underlying causes and treatments. To complicate matters, the manifestations of the two disorders are usually similar in the eyes of the patients and their relatives. The process of getting across the distinction between the two disorders to patients, family, and caregivers can be formidably difficult.

Our main objective in this chapter is to describe the practical management of PNES in patients with epilepsy: this includes the management of the diagnostic process itself, and issues relating to communication with the patient, caregivers, and relatives. We will also discuss the management of epilepsy in patients with PNES.

Overall strategy

One can consider management of PNES in two broad streams: practical management and psychological therapy. The two domains do interconnect, but are usefully considered separately, especially in this patient group, where practical management often assumes great importance. Practical management can be taken to include all aspects relating to explanation and communication of the diagnosis (to patient, relatives, caregivers, family doctors, etc.), advice on management of events, including behavioral management where relevant, and maintaining appropriate diagnostic beliefs, i.e., that all concerned continue to accept the explanation of the events given to them at the time of diagnosis, and have not reverted to believing that all the events are due to epilepsy or some other physical illness.

The last of these is particularly important. We regard establishing and maintaining appropriate diagnostic beliefs as a crucial platform for successful practical management and psychological therapy. Because of this, the term "practical management" may also include some measures normally considered as diagnostic. For example, some experienced clinicians do not require diagnostic video-EEG (VEEG) monitoring in all patients. Nonetheless, the ability to show habitual VEEG-recorded episodes to family or caregivers confers a huge advantage when it comes to convincing patients and those around them of the diagnosis, and "making it stick" in the longer term. Similarly, it is often necessary to re-monitor patients who claim "new" episodes after an initial diagnosis. The episodes may not be clinically new at all, but it is our experience that they have to be recorded in most cases in order to ensure that diagnostic beliefs remain firmly appropriate. In these circumstances, we would regard VEEG recording as being primarily a management step. This of course applies when the diagnosis is one of PNES only, but becomes doubly important when a dual diagnosis of PNES/ES is known or suspected.

Gates and Rowan's Nonepileptic Seizures, 3rd edn. ed. Steven C. Schachter and W. Curt LaFrance, Jr. Published by Cambridge University Press. © S. Schachter and W. C. LaFrance, Jr. 2010.

The question of what constitutes best psychological treatment for PNES remains problematic, as there is only observational evidence and expert opinion at this time. Most authorities agree that psychological therapy is advised [4], and many now use cognitive behavioral approaches [5, 6].

Characteristics of patients with both PNES and ES

Potential differences between patients with PNES who do versus those who do not have epilepsy may impact the diagnosis and management. One important difference is that in patients with mixed PNES/ES there is an excess of patients with learning difficulty (see above): a patient with PNES who also has ES is approximately five times more likely to have LD [7].

Patients with both disorders, particularly those of normal intelligence, tend to present with frequent PNES on a background of well controlled ES [8, 9]. This reflects on the relative difficulty of making the two diagnoses: PNES tend to be relatively easy to record, whereas recording ES may require complete antiepileptic drug (AED) withdrawal [10]. In patients with LD it is our experience that a higher proportion have uncontrolled epilepsy, making it easier to record both types of seizures. However, patients with PNES and ES in general may be less susceptible to induction procedures [11], so inpatient VEEG monitoring may be necessary more often, and diagnostic delay may be longer [11, 12].

In patients with a dual diagnosis, the PNES generally begin at some point after the onset of the ES. The recorded age at onset of PNES is earlier in patients who also have epilepsy [7]. However, the exact point during the course of epilepsy at which PNES supervene may be difficult to determine. It is easy to imagine that difficulty in determining when exactly PNES supervened on top of ES might induce an artificial bias toward recording an earlier age at onset.

Psychogenic nonepileptic seizures in patients who also have epilepsy are not known to be semiologically different from those in patients who do not have epilepsy, but a proportion of patients have PNES that to some degree imitate their ES [8]. This complicates diagnosis and has implications for those management strategies that depend on caregivers and others being able to distinguish PNES from ES.

There is some evidence that PNES patients without epilepsy have a greater tendency to somatization [13, 14]. Attempts to differentiate groups in terms of personality, past personal and family history have failed to show significant differences [8].

Managing the diagnostic process

The diagnoses of ES and PNES need to be considered as separate tasks. The two types of seizures have to be separated in the minds of the patient and his/her relatives if management is to be effective. It is our experience that it is best to separate them at an early stage, indicating clearly to the patient and relatives that two separate diagnoses are being considered, and one or both may finally apply.

The diagnosis of PNES

Where a dual diagnosis is in question, recognition of the PNES is often easier than that of ES. Much has been written on the former subject, and it will not be dealt with in detail here, other than to reiterate its importance as a sound basis for management.

Patients with LD present particular diagnostic difficulties [15]. One problem is worth specific mention, one we term "pseudo PNES." This relates mainly to patients with LD and epilepsy. Such patients may produce PNES-like behaviors in response to epileptic experiences (usually auras, or experiential simple partial seizures) that they find frightening and are poorly equipped to understand or communicate [16]. The EEG during such events may be normal, except when they progress to a complex partial seizure, so it is important to ascertain historically whether the "behavioral" events sometimes lead into complex partial seizures, and to acquire a good sample of events during monitoring. Similarly, when undergoing monitoring, anxious patients with poor coping skills can produce nonhabitual behaviors that may cause diagnostic confusion [17]. Careful comparison of recorded events with descriptions of habitual events is key. Lastly, and uncommonly, auras or seizures may provoke actual PNES. In patients with possible mixed PNES/ES, it is essential to adequately monitor the patient after capturing PNES, which includes tapering AEDs to potentially reveal previously controlled ES.

The diagnosis of epilepsy in patients with PNES

In the past, there has been a tendency to accept some uncertainty regarding whether or not a patient with

PNES also has epilepsy, and to leave the patient on AED therapy. This tendency may be reduced by the increased realization of the potential for serious AED-related side effects, such as teratogenic risk in women of childbearing age (a large part of the PNES population) [18] and increased risk that the patient will have potentially life-threatening treatment at presentation to emergency departments [19], as well as long-term side effects of individual AEDs, such as weight gain or hair loss. In addition to all this, communication of the diagnosis in patients who do not have epilepsy is in a practical sense easier: the diagnostic message is simpler and therefore easier to get across to all concerned, and withdrawing AED treatment can add clarity and conviction. This measure is not available when the patient is thought to have epilepsy as well as PNES. There are therefore highly cogent reasons for making every effort to be clear on whether or not a patient with PNES also has epilepsy.

It is always best to have VEEG evidence for ES. However, in some patients the diagnosis of ES may be made on the basis of clear patient and eyewitness accounts, supported by epileptiform interictal EEG abnormalities. However, in other patients, firm, supporting evidence of ES is lacking, even after a period of EEG monitoring that includes sleep periods. We have shown that if certain simple criteria are adhered to, the risk of AED withdrawal is low, and the patient is unlikely to have epilepsy [20]. In that event, rather than accept uncertainty, we would consider a "diagnostic" withdrawal of AED. This strategy should not be carried out without a formal risk assessment, shared with patients and caregivers.

Diagnostic withdrawal needs to be carried out with appropriate monitoring and safeguards. If carried out with the patient at home, then AEDs should be withdrawn slowly, and sequentially. An assessment of our own simple withdrawal criteria has been published, with the drug withdrawal schedules we used [20]. The criteria used were:

1. All current types of events described by patient and eyewitnesses recorded and identified as PNES.
2. No descriptions of past events raising suspicion of epilepsy.
3. No history of events during childhood.
4. No interictal epileptiform abnormalities on EEG.

If withdrawal is planned, it is crucial that advice to patients and relatives is clear, and that there is rapid access back to the PNES clinic should problematic events occur during withdrawal. Patients who live without a competent relative or caregiver are not usually suitable for withdrawal at home.

If a patient does have a seizure, or seizures, on withdrawal, then a VEEG recording should be obtained if possible but, failing that, the described event should be compared and contrasted with the PNES already recorded, and the information shared with the patient and caregivers, in order to maximize the degree of clarity on the distinction between the patient's ES and PNES.

We do not carry out EEG monitoring during AED withdrawal in all patients. However, some AEDs are known to suppress interictal EEG abnormalities, particularly in primary generalized epilepsies. These include sodium valproate and levetiracetam [21]. If recently introduced, barbiturates and benzodiazepines may do the same [21], and are associated with specific withdrawal problems, including a risk of withdrawal seizures.

For patients presenting increased risk of ES we recommend admission to a short- to medium-term monitoring center (see below) for periods up to 8 weeks in order to establish whether they have ES, and if so, whether it is active or well controlled. The natural untreated seizure frequency may be much lower in some patients, so seizures may occur even after several weeks off medication, and clinical surveillance should continue after discharge from such facilities.

The management of PNES in patients with epilepsy

The population of patients with PNES is heterogeneous, with some evidence suggesting that different mechanisms may apply in different subgroups [7]. It may therefore be inappropriate to apply a single pharmacological or psychotherapeutic intervention across the board.

The use of psychotropic drugs to treat core symptoms, such as anxiety, and depression, has been described by some authors [4, 10]. In patients with the additional diagnosis of ES, greater care is required since many psychotropic drugs may exacerbate seizures. The use of most forms of psychotherapy in the treatment of PNES has been documented, including individual therapy (particularly cognitive behavioral therapy [CBT]), psycho-education, and family therapy [22, 23].

These approaches can be beneficial in patients who also have epilepsy, as long as the patient and therapist are clear about which events are being treated. Cognitive behavioral therapy-based psychotherapy requires however a level of intelligence and understanding of language which may limit its use in some patients with LD. Behavioral modification is, in our experience, more often successful in this group, as patients with PNES and LD have a tendency for their PNES to occur in response to certain situations or stressors [3]. The stressors may be fairly easy to elicit, and in some cases the caregivers may have already correctly identified the PNES through their triggers. Identifying and keeping a record of the context and triggers for the behavior is the first step, followed by the establishment of a consistent approach and response to events, with the overall aim of ensuring minimal reinforcement. While the documentation of event triggers may be relatively easy, establishing a consistent nonreinforcing response is often more challenging.

In cases where seizures are not situational, it may require time and effort to achieve (and maintain) clarity in the minds of the patient and caregivers about the respective nature of the two types of events. At worst, the distinction is not achieved at all. In this circumstance, it is our experience that psychological therapy is usually ineffective, and that the only measures available are those we refer to as "damage limitation." In general, this means working with relatives and caregivers to ensure that the reaction to PNES is appropriate and the possibility of inappropriate treatment and iatrogenic harm is minimized. This would include ensuring that emergency services are not inappropriately called for PNES, as well as informing local emergency services of the diagnosis. Of these two measures, the former is probably the more important: paramedics working in ambulances are likely to administer benzodiazepine drugs on picking up the patient. Benzodiazepines can disinhibit the patient, and, unless given in sufficient dose to render the patient very drowsy or unconscious, may well exacerbate the situation and prolong the PNES. Doctors in emergency rooms may not have the experience necessary to distinguish PNES from ES, assume the patient is presenting with ES and initiate treatment for presumed prolonged seizures or status epilepticus. The most effective way to prevent this sequence of events is to prevent the initial call to the ambulance: the key people in this regard are the relatives and caregivers. The clinician should therefore review the video recordings of the patient's PNES with the caregivers and give them detailed advice about how the PNES should be managed.

Damage limitation measures are easiest to put into practice when PNES are frequent and ES are not. A minority of patients, in whom both types of events are frequent, cause difficulties out of proportion to their numbers. It may not realistically be possible to prevent inappropriate medical management in these cases.

The therapeutic value of AED reduction

In patients without ES, AED withdrawal may be viewed as a step that is congruent with a diagnostic message and therefore a potential therapeutic tool for reinforcing the diagnosis of PNES. This step is not possible in most patients with both disorders since they need to be on AEDs to control the ES. However, in patients with both conditions, the ES are often overtreated [24]. There is some evidence that PNES frequency may go down in patients as AEDs are gradually reduced [10, 25]. Reducing AEDs may also reduce side effects, thereby improving mood and alertness. Occasionally, AED side effects seem to have a direct role in causation of PNES [26].

The management of epilepsy in patients with PNES

In patients with ES only, drug treatment is straightforwardly titrated against seizure frequency. The treatment strategy for patients who also have PNES is no different, in principle. In practice, however, the difficulty is to know the frequency of ES so that sensible decisions on AED treatment can be made. By the time a comprehensive assessment has been made, this difficulty has often resulted in AEDs being titrated against the sum of PNES and ES frequencies, with resulting overtreatment. In this regard, it is worth remembering that in many patients with a dual diagnosis, the ES are controlled, but PNES continue. For example, in our series of 288 patients with PNES, 32 had epilepsy, of whom 15 turned out to be either in complete remission on AEDs (n = 11) or in complete remission off AEDs (n = 4) [3]. In all 17 patients who had active ES, PNES frequency was greater than ES frequency.

Knowing the frequency of ES in a patient with PNES requires that the two types of events be identified, and that their differences are made clear for patients and caregivers. It is well worth going through clinical descriptions and video recordings with caregivers, and this may need to be done on more than one occasion. However, even with good diagnostic information and repeated interactions with caregivers, the frequency of ES may remain uncertain in some patients.

In patients with a dual diagnosis on AED polytherapy, clinicians should reduce AEDs to the minimum number and dosages required to treat the ES. In this circumstance, we use a withdrawal procedure similar to that used for diagnostic purposes; the aim in most patients is the transition to a mid-range dose of a single AED. Antiepileptic drugs are withdrawn sequentially, with appropriate monitoring of frequency of both types of seizures. In high-risk patients (for example, patients who live alone or have incomplete or equivocal spell descriptions), withdrawal takes place partly or wholly in our residential facility.

It is important to note that the coexistence of PNES in patients with refractory ES is not an absolute contraindication for epilepsy surgery [27].

The Quarriers experience

Patients referred to our medium-term inpatient assessment center (The Scottish Epilepsy Centre, Quarriers Village, Bridge of Weir, Renfrewshire, Scotland) are initially assessed as outpatients and at that point a provisional diagnosis is made, and the inpatient admission is planned. The 10-bed unit has a home-like atmosphere. In addition to video and ambulatory EEG, we also have constant CCTV coverage of public areas and selected patient rooms. This allows recordings of events in patients who are unable to tolerate monitoring, and in those for whom ambulatory EEG is the only tolerable option.

During the initial part of the admission, event types are identified, and descriptions and video recordings are reviewed with caregivers to establish whether they represent the patient's typical events. Diagnostic labels are attached to each type of event. Events are managed according to diagnosis.

Factors reinforcing PNES are avoided, and seizure-free periods are rewarded. The opportunity afforded by up to 8 weeks of observed care is used to establish the minimum necessary AED therapy, with particular attention to the use of rescue medication. PNES often last longer than ES, and therefore tend to attract the use of rescue medication. This in itself may have been a reinforcing factor for the PNES, and is addressed with relatives or caregivers.

A behavioral analysis to identify patterns and triggers of the events helps caregivers to be aware of potential causes of PNES, and can allow modification of problematic situations. One simple and common example is provided by the patient with LD who attends a day center. He/she suddenly starts to have new and dramatic events that prevent him/her from attending the day center, which subsequently are found to be PNES. Some inquiries are made, and through straightforward behavioral analysis it becomes evident that this patient is being bullied at the center and that having these events takes him/her away from the distressing situation. Dealing with the situation at the center as well as educating caregivers about the nature of the new types of seizures and how to manage them, in our experience, is usually effective.

The factors leading to PNES may of course be much more complex, requiring an inpatient assessment with a comprehensive care plan on discharge and continuing support thereafter. A multidisciplinary team approach is essential.

Conclusion

The great majority of patients with PNES do not have epilepsy; the coincidence of the two conditions is significantly more common in patients with LD. There is no evidence to suggest that the psychological treatment of PNES should be any different when the patient has epilepsy. However, the presence of ES does make the process of establishing and communicating the diagnosis (or rather, diagnoses) more difficult. Short- to medium-term residential assessment may be necessary to establish the relative frequency of ES and PNES, and to make clear the distinction between the two, allowing appropriate treatment of each type of event.

References

1. Martin R, Burneo JG, Prasad A, *et al.* Frequency of epilepsy in patients with psychogenic seizures monitored by video-EEG. *Neurology* 2003;**61**:1791–2.
2. Benbadis SR, Agrawal V, Tatum IV, WO. How many patients with psychogenic non-epileptic seizures also have epilepsy? *Neurology* 2001;**57**:915–17.
3. Duncan R, Oto M. Psychogenic non-epileptic seizures in patients with learning disability: comparison with patients with no learning disability. *Epilepsy Behav* 2008;**112**:183–6.

4. LaFrance Jr WC, Barry JJ. Update on treatments of psychological nonepileptic seizures. *Epilepsy Behav* 2005;7(3):364–74.
5. Reuber M, House AO. Treating patients with psychogenic non-epileptic seizures. *Curr Opin Neurology* 2002;15(2):207–11.
6. Goldstein LH, Deale AC, Mitchell-O'Malley SJ, Toone BK, Mellers DC. An evaluation of cognitive behavioural therapy as a treatment for dissociative seizures: a pilot study. *Cogn Behav Neurol* 2004;17: 41–9.
7. Duncan R, Oto M. Predictors of antecedent factors in psychogenic non-epileptic attacks: multivariate analysis. *Neurology* 2008;71:1000–6.
8. Owczarek K, Jedrzejczak J. Patients with coexisting psychogenic pseudoepileptic and epileptic seizures: a psychological profile. *Seizure* 2001;10:566–9.
9. Kanner AM, Parra J, Frey M, *et al*. Psychiatric and neurological predictors of psychogenic pseudoseizure outcome. *Neurology* 1999;53:933–8.
10. Blumer D, Adamolekun B. Treatment of patients with coexisting epileptic and nonepileptic seizures. *Epilepsy Behav* 2006;9:498–502.
11. Mari F, Di Bonaventura C, Vanacore N, *et al*. Video-EEG study of psychogenic nonepileptic seizures: differential characteristics in patients with and without epilepsy. *Epilepsia* 2006; 47 Suppl 5;64–7.
12. De Timary P, Fouchet P, Sylin M, *et al*. Non-epileptic seizures: delayed diagnosis in patients presenting with electroencephalographic (EEG) or clinical signs of epileptic seizures. *Seizure* 2002;11:193–7.
13. Kuyk J, Swinkels WAM, Spinhoven P. Psychopathologies in patients with nonepileptic seizures with and without comorbid epilepsy: how different are they? *Epilepsy Behav* 2003;4:13–18.
14. Prueter C, Shultz-Venrath U, Rimpau W. Dissociative and associated psychopathological symptoms in patients with epilepsy, pseudoseizures, and both seizure forms. *Epilepsia* 2002;43(2):188–92.
15. Neil JC, Alvarez N, Differential diagnosis of epileptic versus pseudoepileptic seizures in developmentally disabled persons. *Appl Res Ment Retard* 1986;7: 285–98.
16. Devinsky O, Gordon E. Epileptic seizures progressing into nonepileptic conversion seizures. *Neurology* 1998;51:1293–6.
17. Marchetti RL, Kurcgant D, Neto JG, *et al*. Psychiatric diagnoses of patients with psychogenic non-epileptic seizures. *Seizure* 2008;17:247–53.
18. Szaflarski, JP, Ficker DM, Cahill WT, Privitera MD. Four year incidence of psychogenic seizures in adults in Hamilton County, OH. *Neurology* 2000;55:1561–63.
19. Oto M, Russell AJ, McGonigal A, Duncan R. Misdiagnosis of epilepsy in patients prescribed anticonvulsant drugs for other reasons. *BMJ* 2003;326(7384):326–7.
20. Oto M, Espie C, Pelosi A, Selkirk M, Duncan R. The safety of antiepileptic medication withdrawal in patients with non-epileptic seizures. *J Neurol Neurosurg Psychiatry* 2005;76:1682–5.
21. Duncan R. The withdrawal of antiepileptic drugs in patients with nonepileptic seizures: safety considerations. *Expert Opin Drug Saf* 2006;5:609–13.
22. Baker GA, Brooks JL, Goodfellow L, Bodde N, Aldenkamp A. Treatments for non-epileptic attack disorder. *Cochrane Database Syst Rev* 2007(1): CD006370.
23. Zaroff CM, Myers L, Barr WB, Luciano D, Devinsky O. Group psychoeducation as treatment for psychological nonepileptic seizures. *Epilepsy Behav* 2004;5:587–92.
24. Silva W, Giagante B, Saizar R, *et al*. Clinical features and prognosis of nonepileptic seizures in a developing country. *Epilepsia* 2001;4(3):398–401.
25. Buchanan N, Snars J. Pseudoseizures (non epileptic attack disorder): clinical management and outcome in 50 patients. *Seizure* 1993;2:141–6.
26. Weaver DF. "Organic" pseudoseizures as an unrecognized side-effect of anticonvulsant therapy. *Seizure* 2004;13:467–9.
27. Reuber M, Kurthen M, Fernandez G, Schramm J, Elger CE. Epilepsy surgery in patients with additional psychogenic seizures. *Arch Neurol* 2002;59:82–6.

Section 5 Chapter 26

Treatment considerations for psychogenic nonepileptic seizures

Models of care: the roles of nurses and social workers in the diagnosis and management of patients with psychogenic nonepileptic seizures

Noreen C. Thompson and Patricia A. Gibson

Psychogenic nonepileptic seizures (PNES) are common and very costly to the patient and society. They are a physical manifestation of psychological distress. Lillian Smith (1897–1966), a notable Southern author, once said that "the human heart does not stay away too long from that which hurt it most. There is a return journey to anguish that few of us are released from making" [1]. Sometimes that anguish is more than the heart can bear and the brain has to step in and provide a diversion. For reasons we do not understand, sometimes that diversion takes the form of a seizure-like event.

The purpose of this chapter is to explain the supportive educational role that nurses and social workers can play as part of the multidisciplinary team that provides comprehensive care for patients with PNES. During the first national conference on PNES organized by Dr. John R. Gates in 1990, he made a plea for more than a "diagnose and adios" approach to treatment. It has long been recognized that a comprehensive approach is needed in the care of those with epilepsy, and so it may be that a systems model of care may benefit patients with PNES [2]. This comprehensive approach must include, in addition to medical and psychiatric evaluation and treatment, an assessment of the needs and concerns of the individual patient. Most treatment teams include a social worker and nurse, and for the programs that deal with patients with PNES, preferably staff with experience in conversion disorders and other psychiatric disorders. Whoever on the team has established a closer rapport with the patient is often the best choice to work with the patient and family and to direct the psychological aftercare.

There is a gap between neurology and psychiatry that continues to impair the necessary multidisciplinary approach needed by these most vulnerable patients. There is strong preliminary evidence that mental health professionals may be able to address some of the problems faced by patients with PNES [3–8]. This process begins with psychological support at the time of diagnostic disclosure. Advanced practice psychiatric nurses and social workers can provide that psychological support and education. Studies that have followed patients with PNES referred for psychotherapy found rates of recovery considerably better than those reported from natural history studies [9–11]. Patients with PNES frequently fail to follow through with mental health treatment, and the basis for this observation is the focus of intense interest in the field [3]. Several authors note problems in the manner of presenting the patient with the diagnosis [3, 9, 12]. Most patients with PNES, often naïve to mental health care when given the diagnosis of "pseudoseizures," feel that the diagnosis means that they are "faking" or "crazy," and that the problem is imaginary or "all in their head." Patients also worry that the doctor will abandon them [5, 13, 14]. This may well lead to a lack of follow-up with a mental health professional, and to negative feelings toward the neurologist and hospital.

Several investigators have identified a need to attend to psychosocial factors starting at the time of diagnosis in order to counteract stigmatization, foster realistic hope, and facilitate a mental health referral in a way acceptable to the patient [3, 10, 15–17]. Shen *et al.* provide evidence suggestive of the efficacy through naturalistic follow-up [10]. In one

Gates and Rowan's Nonepileptic Seizures, 3rd edn. ed. Steven C. Schachter and W. Curt LaFrance, Jr. Published by Cambridge University Press. © S. Schachter and W. C. LaFrance, Jr. 2010.

Midwestern university hospital, an educational intervention was created for presenting the diagnosis of PNES to patients. In this approach, an advanced practice psychiatric nurse met with the patient whenever the diagnosis was strongly suspected by the neurologist, and again shortly after the diagnosis was established. The meetings took place while the patient was still in the hospital undergoing the video-EEG diagnostic study. The two meetings took approximately 90 minutes total time. An informational pamphlet that summarized the educational material discussed with the patient was given to the patient at the time of diagnostic disclosure by the neurologist [8].

Thompson *et al.* followed 48 patients for two years in their clinic after the diagnosis of PNES, all of whom had experienced this supportive educational intervention. All 48 patients followed up with a mental health professional as compared to 10% before the procedure was instituted. Furthermore, 50% of the patients reported that their seizures had disappeared altogether, and an additional 40% reported an improvement in frequency and/or intensity. Only five patients reported no improvement in their seizures [8]. The educational intervention delivered by the nurse appears to be a promising intervention for patients with PNES. The study was limited in that it relied on patients' self-report of their involvement in therapy to the individuals who recommended it. A preferable study design would be a randomized, double-blind study with a control and experimental group to compare subjects who receive the psycho-educational intervention with subjects who receive standard care. There is a lack of rigorous validated interventions for PNES, and there is a great need for interdisciplinary collaboration to address the issue of how to best intervene with this vulnerable patient population [6].

The purpose of this chapter is to provide information on how interdisciplinary team collaboration at the time of diagnosis can improve patient outcomes. A multidisciplinary model of care, based on the classic work of Shen *et al.* will be described. The model of care's main purpose is to convey the psychological nature of the events without alienating the patient or harming the patient's self-esteem [10].

Presenting the diagnosis to the patient

Bowman [4] provided a comprehensive review of the studies that examined the characteristics of patients with PNES and the parameters associated with PNES outcomes. The review reveals that the high prevalence of depression in this population is far more than a chance association and suggests that clinicians should always evaluate these patients for depression. Many patients with PNES are unaware of any underlying motivation for the seizures and the nature of conversion disorder is that patients do not consciously cause the seizure.

During the presentation, the term "nonepileptic" is preferable, because it includes both physiological and psychological events and carries less pejorative connotation. Due to the perceived stigma of having a psychiatric diagnosis, the patient may go to yet another physician hoping to hear that they do, in fact, have a physiological rather than a psychiatric problem. Patients may have gone from doctor to doctor looking for a physiological basis for their spells before they actually have a confirmed diagnosis of PNES.

In our opinion, and from our experience, the most hurtful and confusing term for our patients is "pseudoseizures." It is startling how often our patients report the trauma of being told in an emergency department visit that they were having "pseudoseizures." Patients and their family members often leave that encounter feeling angry as they sense they have been told they are faking the seizures. Given the potential negative impact on rapport between the clinician and patient/family, it is vitally important for all clinicians to refrain from using "pseudoseizures" when speaking with patients and their families. Many of our patients need reassurance after hearing that term before they can accept the confirmation of a PNES diagnosis from the physician.

Diagnostic disclosure: an opportunity for psychological support

The Comprehensive Epilepsy Center at the University of Kansas Medical Center employs a psycho-educational intervention when it is determined that the seizure is of the psychogenic, nonepileptic type. One of the authors along with two colleagues used the "Shen Protocol" in a retrospective descriptive study, which reported the positive outcome of an increase in the number of patients willing to seek psychotherapy treatment after disclosure of the diagnosis [8, 10]. The Shen approach was modified in a few ways; for example, the videotape is not always watched with the patients. Patients usually do not request to watch the events, but if they do, we comply. The patient is not specifically asked about past sexual abuse – rather they are questioned about past and current trauma and/or stress in their lives. (Editors' note: An example of the Shen protocol was demonstrated at the 2006 American Epilepsy Society Meeting. The video presentation is used merely as a demonstration of the protocol. Querying a history of trauma is necessary at some point in all patients with conversion disorder, however, as noted above, the manner in which trauma and abuse is explored in the Shen protocol is not necessarily recommended as the most appropriate for all patients with PNES.)

The role of the nurse

In 2008, there were two articles in the nursing literature specific to PNES [8, 18] using Cumulative Index to Nursing and Allied Health Literature (CINAHL) and PubMed. When the search was broadened to include nursing, psychosomatic, and psychogenic as well as PNES, 463 journal articles were revealed. Nurses, especially advanced practice psychiatric nurses, can play an important role in the support, education, and therapeutic interventions of the population with somatoform disorders. Approximately 75% of patients with PNES are women, and many report a history of incest, rape, and physical or emotional abuse [13, 19, 20].

In our protocol, the nurse meets with the patient twice during the epilepsy monitoring unit (EMU) hospital admission. The first meeting involves interviewing the patient about what it has been like for them to live with their seizures. Bowman's paradigm provides a useful set of questions that can be incorporated in the first interview with the patient [8].

During the first assessment, the primary goal is to establish rapport and listen as the patient tells his/her story. After introducing myself as a nurse member of the multidisciplinary team, I suggest to the family member or friend who is staying with the patient to "take a break" and leave us alone for the interview. This request is rarely met with resistance by the patient or the visitor. If it occurs, it often provides more information about how the patient usually copes or the relationship between the pair.

The nurse explains that the purpose of the assessment is to understand the emotional side of living with seizures and to see if there is anything we might suggest or put in place for the patient's support. The next questions asked are: "What has it been like for you to live with your seizures?," "What has been the most difficult part for you?," and "What has helped you to cope?" Additional questions about past or present stressors can be asked towards the end of the interview. It is also important to ask about the past need for psychiatric support or hospitalizations. The nurse can assess through interview if the patient is suffering with untreated psychiatric symptoms. The nurse can then mention that psychiatric consultation is a necessary part of the care plan.

The second meeting occurs at the time of diagnostic disclosure. The epileptologist and the nurse usually give the patient the news together. During this meeting, the nurse utilizes a specific protocol including giving the patient and family an educational pamphlet entitled: "Non-epileptic Seizures: A Guide for Patients and Families" [15]. The pamphlet is subtitled: "Your Passport to Wellness." The patient is also given time to react, ask questions, and is encouraged to frame the diagnosis in a hopeful and nonstigmatizing way. The physician and the nurse impart an optimistic message as to the potential for this type of seizure disorder to lessen or stop with appropriate treatment and most importantly emphasize the unconscious, nondeliberate intent of these seizures with the patient and the family.

The nurse reinforces the positive nature of the diagnosis by stating that with proper treatment, 70% of patients report that the seizures eventually disappear. Emphasis is placed on the "good news" of this diagnosis, including: the potential of being able to drive again with seizure cessation, of coming off the medications for patients with only PNES, and of learning additional ways of coping with life stressors with the help of a therapist. A discussion of the patient's and family member's reactions to the diagnosis and the proposed need for psychiatric services is included. Often it takes much effort to remove the patient's sense of being stigmatized if he/she seeks psychiatric care. At the time of discharge from the EMU, the patient leaves with a neurology appointment in addition to the psychiatry or psychology referral. The patient is given the nurse's contact information in case questions arise after discharge. In this psychiatric nurse author's 30 years of practice experience, the essential elements of compassionate verbal and nonverbal communication, a respectful approach, and nonjudgmental attitude have often led to the formation of a therapeutic relationship with the patient. Hildegard Peplau, nurse scholar and psychoanalyst, emphasizes the importance of interacting with each patient as an individual.

Caring for the individual is intrinsic to nursing practice. It takes focus, time, and creativity. Nursing practice involves helping people to cope with and to learn about their illness [21]. Our experience shows that the PNES population can benefit when the multidisciplinary team includes a psychiatric nurse.

Steps of the diagnostic disclosure protocol

- *Provide good news.* The epileptologist explains that the events that were recorded by video-EEG during the hospital stay were nonepileptic. The terms psychogenic and/or pseudoseizure are never used, unless the patient asks about those terms. We emphasize that the good news is that the events are not the result of brain damage or excessive firing of brain waves. We emphasize that although we do not know the exact cause of the seizure or events, they are more likely the result of excessive psychological stressors. We state that it is good that the patient will be able to stop taking the medications that may produce undesirable side effects (if not needed for concomitant epileptic seizures).
- *Reveal realistic diagnosis.* Then we explain that we cannot tell the patient exactly what is causing these symptoms. However, knowing they are not epileptic is a start in that we know that they will not improve by taking antiepileptic medications. We reassure the patient that though we may not know what is causing the seizures, we want to continue to work with him/her. The patient usually continues to see the epileptologist to be weaned off the antiepileptic medications (when appropriate) but most importantly to maintain the patient–physician relationship. This is done to avoid any feelings of abandonment as the patient begins to form a relationship with the psychotherapist.
- *Suggest psychotherapy.* We tell the patient, "In most patients with this type of seizure we eventually discover that the cause is related to either excessive emotional energy or upsetting emotions. Often the patient is not aware of the cause of these feelings. Our patients report they find help by seeking psychotherapy and we would like to help you discover who you might visit for this support."
- *Reassure patient,* "We do not think you are crazy or faking these spells." This is a very essential part of the discussion. We always address this issue whether the patient mentions this or not. We give the patient two copies of our educational pamphlet (see earlier). Everything we address with the patient is reviewed in more depth in the pamphlet. We encourage the patient to share the pamphlet with their therapist.
- *Use the power of suggestion.* We suggest to the patient that "These events may resolve over time. Many of our patients report that after accepting the diagnosis they notice less frequent spells and/or less intense spells. You may also find that you can have more control over the events. You may say to yourself: 'I am not going to have any events today' or you may concentrate on breathing easily in and out if you feel one coming on."
- *Emphasize hope.* It is important that the patient understands that there is hope the events can improve with psychotherapy support including learning new ways to manage stress.

The role of the social worker

Dr. David Taylor, a neuropsychiatrist in Wales, pointed out some time ago that people suffering from epilepsy are in a particular "predicament" [22]. So, too, is the person with PNES. How any given predicament is being experienced depends on the personal history of that person and his/her environment. The history of a person becomes a crucial aspect of diagnosis that is different from the history of the disorder. It is the role of the social worker to gather that history and understand the patient in full social context.

Patients are often confused when the term "seizure" is used in regard to PNES. This confusion is reflected in the many different terms used by various professionals and in the literature, for instance, "pseudoseizure," "psychogenic seizure," and "nonepileptic seizure." One patient, following the relaying of his diagnosis of PNES, was overheard on the phone telling his family, "I just found out that I have a much worse type of new seizure." He only heard "seizures" in the discussion. The social worker can help clarify the terminology heard by patients with PNES and their families.

Research has suggested that the earlier the diagnosis is made and treatment begun, the better the chances for a good outcome [23, 24]. For this reason, it is important that a social worker be involved early on in the assessment of seizures. A full social history, observation of family dynamics, and, in children, a school assessment is beneficial in early identification of PNES. In terms of prevention, it would be ideal for early referral to a psychiatric social worker for any child or adult whose seizures are not controlled after six months of treatment. The referrals could come from pediatricians, family practitioners, or emergency department staff. It is important that the social worker has expertise in epilepsy and PNES. Research indicates an average of seven years from onset of symptoms of PNES to diagnosis [23]. From a monetary point of view, early social work and nursing intervention could help save healthcare dollars.

The importance of how the diagnosis is relayed was discussed earlier. The impact of how this is given was vividly portrayed by a follow-up note from a patient who called the national Epilepsy Information Service at Wake Forest University. The patient had recently been seen at an EMU and diagnosed with PNES. He wrote:

I wanted to tell you that I followed your suggestion to request further evaluation since my seizures have not been controlled with medication. I went to the hospital and during that time, I had about 25 events. There was no other testing done until the last day when I was referred for psychological testing. In this session, I revealed my history of having been abused as a young boy. Not long after that, the doctor met with me, and in an angry and impatient manner, he informed me that I was not having real seizures, but rather "pseudoseizures." He then informed me that I had to leave, that he had better uses for the room. Only once before in my life have I felt more humiliated. The way he handled this made me feel violated again. Like before, I really had no way to fight back, and I went into a severe depression after this encounter.

Social workers play a variety of roles in the treatment of PNES, even within comprehensive epilepsy programs. Some play a more peripheral role, while others, such as Bruce Molyneaux at Children's Hospital in Pittsburgh, have a more central role in the diagnosis and treatment of children with PNES. Molyneaux works throughout all stages of hospitalization and plays an important role in facilitation of communication between the patient, family, and other members of the team. He is the primary link between the student/patient with school officials in regard to follow-up with treatment recommendations. Using a biopsychosocial approach, he works with families so that they better understand the complexities of the medical diagnosis, participate in the formulation of the PNES response plan, and facilitate the behavioral health consultation and discharge planning. Other psychiatric social workers work in private practice or mental health settings and provide clinical treatment of PNES using a variety of treatment approaches. Some limited work has been done by social workers using a group approach but little has been published in this area. In their pilot studies, Barry *et al.* found group therapy that focused on interpersonal issues to have potential benefit [25].

Sykes *et al.* looked at the role that PNES in adolescents have in reinforcing systemic helplessness: "The issues of psychogenic seizures are filled with helplessness: helplessness of physicians in treatment, leading to their anger and potential rejection of the patient; helplessness of the family in providing for their child, leading to anger at the medical establishment; and helplessness of the patient having a chronic disability, leading to anger at the world and/or depression." [26].

As with epileptic seizures, PNES are quite varied with a multitude of underlying etiologies and often other comorbidities; thus the complexities may defy a simple approach or nonspecific treatment. It is the role of the social worker to gather a comprehensive assessment of the family history, presenting problem, patient's developmental and social history and history of other somatic ailments in the family. Interactional patterns are identified, along with quality of relationships and parenting practices. The family's interpretation of the illness should also be solicited. The social work evaluation, while seeking to assess the root causes of the symptoms and the full social environment of the patient, focuses on identifying the strengths of the patient and family and how best to promote those. As Buckingham and Coffman pointed out:

"People don't change that much.
Don't waste time trying to put in what was left out.
Try to draw out what was left in.
That is hard enough." [27]

Summary

By incorporating a psychiatric social worker or nurse, a multidisciplinary approach to the diagnosis and management of patients with PNES may be cost-effective while still providing the direction of a mental health professional grounded in psychotherapeutic skills. After spending years seeing doctors, especially neurologists, the patient tends to reject the idea of seeing a psychiatrist. The lived experience of the person suffering with PNES must be understood as quickly as possible. In the authors' experience, patients and families are able to accept the diagnosis when time was spent in establishing rapport and when their specific preconceived ideas about psychiatry or psychotherapy were addressed. The approach to each patient and family needs to be individualized while we address their unique understanding of psychiatric services. A psychiatric nurse or social worker is able to answer the questions that arise about psychotherapy and psychiatry as well as address misconceptions. Our efforts using this approach have enlisted acceptance of mental health services in nine out of ten patients. The concept of "body memory" has been found to be particularly helpful in patients' acceptance of the psychological nature of the diagnosis.

It is important that at the point of diagnosis there is a professional who has a working knowledge of psychotherapy to help the patient accept the diagnosis of PNES and the suggested psychiatric treatment. Social workers are essential in the care and support of this patient population as they address the patient's social needs and concerns [28].

Acknowledgments

The authors would like to thank Sue Popkess-Vater RN, PhD, Marguerite F. Hartigan MSN, and Lauren E. Thompson for their encouragement and editorial support.

References

1. Smith LE. *Killers of the Dream*. New York: WW Norton. 1949, 1961; 15.
2. LaFrance WC, Jr, Devinsky O. The treatment of nonepileptic seizures: historical perspectives and future directions. *Epilepsia* 2004;**45** Suppl 2:15–21.
3. Benbadis SR. Psychogenic non-epileptic seizures. In Wyllie E, ed. *The Treatment of Epilepsy: Principles and Practice*. Philadelphia: Lippincott Williams & Wilkins. 2005; 623–30.
4. Bowman ES. Psychopathology and outcome in pseudoseizures. In: Ettinger AB, Kanner AM, eds. *Psychiatric Issues in Epilepsy*. Philadelphia: Lippincott Williams & Wilkins. 2001; 355–79.
5. Martin RC, Lillian FG, Kilgore M, Faught E, Kuzniecky R. Improved health care resource utilization following video-EEG-confirmed diagnosis of nonepileptic psychogenic seizures. *Seizure* 1998;**7**:385–90.
6. LaFrance Jr WC, Alper K, Babcock D, *et al*. Nonepileptic seizures treatment workshop summary. *Epilepsy Behav* 2006;**8**:451–61.
7. Bowman ES. Nonepileptic seizures: psychiatric framework, treatment and outcome. *Neurology* 1999;**53**:S84–8.
8. Thompson NC, Osorio I, Hunter EE. Nonepileptic seizures: reframing the diagnosis. *Perspect Psychiatr Care* 2005;**41**(2):71–8.
9. LaFrance Jr WC, Barry JJ. Update on treatments of psychological nonepileptic seizures. *Epilepsy Behav* 2005;**7**(3):365–74.
10. Shen W, Bowman ES, Markand ON. Presenting the diagnosis of pseudoseizure. *Neurology* 1990;**40**:756–9.
11. Lempert T, Schmidt D. Natural history and outcome of psychogenic seizures: a clinical study of 50 patients. *J Neurol* 1990;**237**:35–8.
12. Roelofs K, Spinhoven P, Sandijck MA, Moene FC, Hoogduin KAL. The impact of early trauma and recent life-events on symptom severity in patients with conversion disorder. *J Nerv Ment Dis* 2005;**193**(8): 508–14.
13. Lancman M, Lambrakis CC, Steinhardt M. Psychogenic pseudoseizures: a general overview. In: Ettinger AB, Kanner AM, eds. *Psychiatric Issues in Epilepsy*. Philadelphia: Lippincott Williams & Wilkins. 2001;341–54.
14. Jedrzejczak J, Owczarek K, Majkowski J. Psychogenic pseudoepileptic seizures treated with psychotherapy: clinical and EEG video-recording. *Eur J Neurol* 1999;**6**:473–9.
15. Benbadis S, Stagno S. Psychogenic seizures: a guide for patients and families. *J Neurosci Nurs* 1994;**26**(5): 306–8.
16. Lesser RP. Psychogenic seizures. *Neurology* 1996;**46**: 1449–52.
17. Clarke MR. Psychogenic disorders: a pragmatic approach for formulation and treatment. *Semin Neurol* 2006;**26**(3):357–65.
18. Mims J, Antonello JL. Treatment of nonepileptic events in adolescent patients using the systems model for intervention. *J Neurosci Nurs* 1994; **26**(5):298.
19. Bowman ES, Markand ON. Psychodynamics and psychiatric disorders of pseudoseizure patients. *Am J Psychiatry* 1996;**153**:57–63.
20. Benbadis SR, Hauser WA. An estimate of the prevalence of psychogenic nonepileptic seizures. *Seizure* 2000;**9**(4):280–1.
21. Peplau HE. *Interpersonal Relations in Nursing: A Conceptual Frame of Reference for Psychodynamic Nursing*. New York: Springer. 1952; 64.

22. Taylor DC. The components of sickness: disease, illness, and predicaments. *Lancet* 1979;**ii**:1008–10.
23. LaFrance Jr WC, Benbadis SR. Avoiding the cost of unrecognized psychological nonepileptic seizures. *Neurology* 2006;**66**(11):1620–1.
24. Shneker BF, Elliot JO. Primary care and emergency physician attitudes and beliefs related to patients with psychogenic nonepileptic spells. *Epilepsy Behav* 2008;**13**(1):243–7.
25. Barry JJ, Wittenberg D, Bullock KD, *et al.* Group therapy for patients with psychogenic nonepileptic seizures: a pilot study. *Epilepsy Behav* 2008;**13**: 624–9.
26. Sykes DK, Kenney MT, Kilpatrick KS. Treatment of psychogenic seizures in adolescents. *Clin Soc Work J* 1991;**19**(2):178.
27. Buckingham M, Coffman C. *First Break all the Rules*. New York: Simon & Shuster. 1999; 7.
28. Gibson P. Social services in epilepsy. In: Ettinger AB, Kanner AM, eds. *Psychiatric Issues in Epilepsy*. Philadelphia: Lippincott Williams & Wilkins. 2001; 297–306.

Section 5 Chapter 27

Treatment considerations for psychogenic nonepileptic seizures

Who should treat psychogenic nonepileptic seizures?

Andres M. Kanner

Psychogenic nonepileptic seizures (PNES) are paroxysmal episodes with pleomorphic presentations that result from underlying psychiatric disorders. Thus, any reader browsing the table of contents of this book would question the purpose of this chapter; after all, if PNES are the expression of psychiatric disorders, shouldn't mental health professionals provide the treatment? While this point is not in question, the role of neurologists in the treatment of patients with PNES has been the source of much controversy. Indeed, while it is not unusual for many neurologists to assume that their involvement ceases once a diagnosis of PNES is established, a recent national survey of neurologists and epileptologists revealed that 69% of neurologists continued to follow the patient after the PNES diagnosis is made [1]. Furthermore, while psychiatrists are expected to play a major role in the treatment of these patients, such is not the case in a significant number of patients and their management is relegated to nonmedical mental health professionals who are not trained in the care of patients with PNES and are unable to plan and/or provide comprehensive treatment. In fact, the treatment of PNES is fraught with multiple obstacles, beginning with the lack of a general consensus on the respective roles of neurologists, psychiatrists, psychologists, and other mental health professionals. The aim of this chapter is to address this problem and suggest some practical solutions to optimize the treatment of patients with PNES.

What is the first goal of treatment?

The management of any pathological condition in medicine calls for the tailoring of the patient's treatment plan to the cause(s) of the disorder and the presence of comorbid conditions and concomitant medications. From a psychiatric standpoint, PNES is a heterogeneous disorder. In addition, comorbid neurological and medical conditions and their pharmacological treatments are not infrequent in these patients.

While the ultimate goal is to achieve complete remission of PNES coupled with a resolution of the underlying psychiatric (and comorbid) disorders, the first goal is to recognize that the patient's most significant morbidity and mortality risks result from the interventions of practitioners who continue treating these episodes as epileptic seizures (ES) [2–4]. Accordingly, the first goal of treatment for the patient with confirmed lone PNES is to ensure that the patient and family members have a clear understanding of the diagnosis, that is, that they understand and *accept* that the patient does not suffer from epilepsy. The achievement of this goal can be expected to avert or at least minimize visits to emergency rooms and, thus, the iatrogenic complications caused by unnecessary pharmacological treatments, which are often associated with high risks. Indeed, PNES may often mimic status epilepticus that is erroneously diagnosed as epileptic status epilepticus, leading to unnecessary admissions to intensive care units, aggressive use of parenteral antiepileptic drugs (AEDs), endo-tracheal intubation, and use of coma protocols with general anesthesia and assisted ventilation [2–4]. The resulting iatrogenic complications (respiratory arrest, toxic effects from AEDs) lead to prolonged and costly hospital stays. For example, in a study by Reuber *et al.*, 51% of patients with PNES presented as "pseudostatus" (lasting more than 30 minutes) and 27.8% were admitted to intensive care units [3]. Howell *et al.* [4] suggested that perhaps 50% of patients admitted to the hospital in the UK with status epilepticus do not actually have epilepsy.

Persistence of PNES can be expected in 50% to 70% of patients after diagnosis [5, 6]. Thus, the prevention

Gates and Rowan's Nonepileptic Seizures, 3rd edn. ed. Steven C. Schachter and W. Curt LaFrance, Jr. Published by Cambridge University Press. © S. Schachter and W. C. LaFrance, Jr. 2010.

of, or at least minimizing exposure to, such iatrogenic risks is one of the fundamental responsibilities of the treating neurologist. Indeed, even when patients accept a diagnosis of PNES, they may be taken to emergency rooms if they have an event in public places or at work. Unnecessary treatment can be avoided if the emergency department physician can contact the treating neurologist to discuss any treatment.

How long should neurologists remain involved?

The first stage in treatment is the presentation of the diagnosis. With confirmatory video-EEG (VEEG) monitoring, neurologists present the diagnosis in the epilepsy monitoring unit (EMU). Research shows that patients who were given no feedback after monitoring actually have no improvement or do worse [7]. Even after the presentation, the involvement of the neurologist *does not end* with the establishment of the diagnosis of PNES. Discontinuation of neurological care and supervision depends on the following factors: (a) an understanding and acceptance of the diagnosis of PNES by patient and family alike; (b) the presence of comorbid ES; (c) the timing of complete discontinuation of AEDs; (d) the existence of other comorbid neurological disorders; and (e) a joint decision by the patient, neurologist, and treating mental health professionals that no further neurological supervision and treatment is necessary. These points warrant a more detailed discussion.

In most epilepsy centers, it falls upon the neurologist/epileptologist to establish a diagnosis of NES with VEEG, to rule out a physiological cause of the NES, and in conjunction with data from the patient's history, the neuropsychological and/or psychiatric evaluations, to identify a psychogenic cause. Paradoxically, despite the "good news" associated with having excluded an epileptic seizure disorder, patients and their families often have difficulties accepting a diagnosis of PNES, which in fact, constitutes one of the most frequent and earliest barriers to treatment of this condition. Some of the reasons for the difficulty accepting the diagnosis of PNES include:

1. The diagnosis of PNES may be often made in patients who had been treated for epilepsy for years. Expecting an automatic "switch" in their conceptualization of their events may be unrealistic in many of these patients. Indeed, patients may be unable to understand why their events were misdiagnosed for such a long time and why they should believe the new diagnosis.
2. Patients are sometimes unable to distinguish the difference between a diagnosis of *psychogenic* NES and *epileptic* seizures. Several case series have identified neuropsychological deficits in patients with PNES. For example, Reuber *et al.* found that 60.5% of 206 patients with PNES (without epilepsy) scored at least 1.5 standard deviations below norm populations in at least one type of testing [8]. For this reason, some epileptologists recommend that the term "seizures" should be avoided and the patients' PNES should be called psychogenic nonepileptic events (PNEE) when the diagnosis is discussed.
3. Patients may interpret the diagnosis of PNES as implying that "they have been faking" these events for years, or "that they are crazy."
4. It is not uncommon for neurologists to "infer" a psychogenic cause of the events without having obtained the actual evidence of a psychogenic cause of the events. Hence, in presenting the diagnosis, the neurologist is unable to provide a reasonable explanation in support of the diagnosis.

It is essential for proper patient care to establish the diagnosis of lone PNES versus mixed ES/PNES. Thus, the clinician should document in the history if the patient has one or more types of seizures. Capturing the typical ictus or multiple ictal events on VEEG, with AED taper in the EMU, provides important data for the clinicians, patient, and family, as to defining the types of seizures the patient is having. A clear understanding of the diagnosis allows a clear presentation of the diagnosis.

After the diagnosis has been presented, it is advisable to keep patients in the VEEG monitoring unit for an additional 24-hour period at the end of which their understanding and reaction to the diagnosis can be reassessed. Furthermore, the family members' reaction to the diagnosis is of utmost importance as well, as any perception that the patient has been "faking" the events for attention or other reasons is likely to result in the patient's rejection of the diagnosis. In my experience, the need for further clarifications about the diagnosis is the rule rather than the exception after a 24-hour observation period. In addition, persistence of PNES during that period should serve as a red flag for the suspicion of (a) severe psychopathology; (b) failure to accept the diagnosis; (c) failure to understand the diagnosis; or (d) all of the above. On the other hand, the absence of recurrent PNES in the 24 hours following the presentation of the diagnosis does not rule out those problems.

Ideally, a psychiatric and neuropsychological evaluation should be carried out while the patient is still in the VEEG monitoring unit. First, the information from these evaluations may provide the neurologists with the necessary evidence to support a psychogenic cause for the PNES. Second, the course of PNES after diagnosis can be predicted on the basis of the patient's psychiatric profile. For example, Kanner *et al.* [6] found that persistent PNES are likely after diagnosis in patients with chronic and untreated mood disorders; patients with dissociative processes associated with a history of physical, sexual, and emotional abuse; and patients with personality disorders. On the other hand, the absence of identifiable psychopathology or mild psychiatric comorbidity (no obvious psychopathology has been identified in up to 20% to 30% of patients in some case series) is predictive of remission of PNES after discharge from the VEEG monitoring unit, even without any further therapeutic intervention [5, 6].

Thus, the availability of a psychiatric profile at the time of diagnosis can assist the neurologist in anticipating persistence of PNES after discharge from the hospital in patients with severe psychiatric comorbidity and to prepare the patient and family members on what to do in case of recurrence. The patient and family members must understand that PNES do not cause brain damage. Family members should be advised to let the event run its natural course without calling an ambulance or bringing the patient to the hospital. By the same token, neurologists will need to reassure (often in a repeated manner) mental health professionals, who frequently question the diagnosis of PNES and keep referring the patient back for further neurological evaluations [9]. The resulting mixed messages to patients and family members only contribute to further delay in their acceptance of the diagnosis and the implementation of the proper treatment.

As stated above, the heterogeneous nature of PNES is also related to the occurrence of comorbid neurological disorders. The most frequent conditions include current or past ES, chronic headaches, and cognitive developmental delay with or without cerebral palsy. In a review of case series in the literature, Reuber *et al.* found a report of abnormal MRI studies in up to 76% of patients with PNES [8]. The prevalence of comorbid ES in patients with PNES has ranged between 5% and 50% [10–12]. The lower rates are derived from studies in fourth-level epilepsy centers [10], while higher rates have been identified in populations from general hospitals [11, 12]. The higher rates approaching 50% have been reported in patients with cognitive developmental delay [13]. These patients will clearly require ongoing treatment by a neurologist.

More often than not, for patients with lone PNES, AEDs are tapered off slowly on an outpatient basis. Discontinuation of AEDs should be supervised by a neurologist and patients should be followed for a minimal period of six months after the tapering process is completed, as recurrence of unsuspected ES that were in remission with the prior AEDs may occur following their discontinuation. In some patients, discontinuation of AEDs can be achieved during the diagnostic VEEG if there is no evidence of electrographic and clinical data suggestive of current and/or past ES, and their AEDs can be discontinued quickly without adverse effects.

Antiepileptic drugs would be continued in lone PNES, however, in a few circumstances, including patients with certain pain syndromes, for migraine prophylaxis, and for treatment of bipolar disorder. Antiepileptic drugs can also be continued at that time if the AEDs have positive psychotropic properties yielding a therapeutic effect on an underlying psychiatric disorder.

Headaches in patients with PNES often present as chronic, daily headaches, which can be the expression of mixed muscle tension or rebound headaches and migraines [Kanner AM, unpublished data]. Clearly, the management of these headaches requires the intervention of the neurologist. Given the frequent association of these headache types with chronic mood disorders, their treatment must be coordinated with the psychopharmacological management of the comorbid psychiatric conditions.

It is not rare for patients to develop *de-novo* "neurological" symptoms after the remission of PNES. Such symptoms may be the expression of a conversion disorder, but require a careful neurological evaluation.

Referral to mental health professionals does not automatically imply acceptance of treatment on the part of the patient and the family and agreement with the diagnosis by the mental health professionals. In fact, a common obstacle to the successful treatment of PNES is a relatively frequent refusal by psychiatrists to accept the diagnosis of PNES, even when established with VEEG. In a survey conducted with neurologists and psychiatrists attending a symposium about PNES, 75% of responding psychiatrists indicated that they "do not trust" the data derived from VEEG sufficiently to reach a diagnosis of PNES [12]. As stated above, the neurologist needs to remain actively involved during the evaluation by the treating mental health team to avoid conflicting messages from neurologists and psychiatrists reaching the patient and their family, with the resulting serious consequences.

In conclusion, the evidence cited above clearly demonstrates that establishing a diagnosis of PNES is only the first step in the involvement of the neurologist in the management of these patients. Following discharge from the inpatient monitoring unit, patients with lone PNES should be followed in the outpatient epilepsy clinic on a regular basis (e.g., every three to four months) until the patient, neurologist, and mental health professional team agree that no further neurological treatment or supervision is necessary.

What type of mental health professionals should be involved?

As stated above, PNES is a psychiatric disorder with a chronic course in many patients, presenting as an expression of both Axis I and Axis II psychiatric diagnoses and developmental/psychosocial stressors [5, 6]. Often, the persistence of the PNES and the severity of the underlying psychiatric disorder have precluded patients from maintaining gainful employment, or in the case of children and adolescents, from attending school. Accordingly, the psychiatric management of many of these patients will require a team approach that includes psychiatrists, psychologists, social workers, and, when the patient is unemployed, vocational therapists. Under ideal circumstances, this multidisciplinary team should be part of the epilepsy center. The specific role of each discipline is discussed below.

Psychiatrists

Given the heterogeneous nature of the psychiatric conditions associated with PNES, a psychiatric evaluation is essential for a comprehensive treatment plan. Unfortunately, such evaluations are not conducted in a significant number of patients. Instead many patients only receive a neuropsychological evaluation as part of a refractory seizure workup, which may augment but does not replace the psychiatric evaluation.

Ideally the psychiatrist evaluating patients with PNES should be part of the epilepsy center's team. Unfortunately, psychiatric involvement at epilepsy centers is uncommon. In a survey of epilepsy centers belonging to the US National Association of Epilepsy Centers, only 10 of the 47 responding centers indicated having a psychiatrist as part of their team. This problem is further compounded by poor communication between neurologists and psychiatrists, which has led to the "discordant" opinions on the diagnosis of PNES alluded to above.

The severity and complexity of the psychiatric disorders of more than 50% of patients with PNES require the use of pharmacotherapy and psychotherapy. Because many of these patients suffer from chronic, pharmacoresistant mood/anxiety and attention deficit disorders with or without concomitant personality disorders, the treating psychiatrist must have significant experience in the pharmacological management of such complex psychiatric conditions. Furthermore, these are patients that may require relatively frequent outpatient visits to stabilize their psychiatric condition, independently of the PNES. In summary, the role of psychiatrists is crucial at the present time in the evaluation and management of PNES. The limited access to psychiatrists and poor communication between neurologists and psychiatrists constitute significant barriers to treatment of patients with PNES.

Neuropsychologists and clinical psychologists

Neuropsychologists play a very important role in the diagnostic evaluation of patients with suspected PNES as well as in their treatment. As stated earlier, a significant number of patients with PNES have been found to have neuropsychological disturbances, and it is therefore important to establish the patient's cognitive level when deciding on the optimal nonpharmacological psychotherapeutic strategy. In addition, several standardized personality tests have been of great assistance in screening for patients in whom the PNES are an expression of a malingering process [14, 15].

It is not unusual for psychologists and neuropsychologists to be responsible for a major part of the treatment of these patients. From the standpoint of nonpharmacological treatments, cognitive behavioral therapy has been reported to be an effective strategy (see Chapter 29) [16]. The efficacy of other forms of psychotherapy in PNES has yet to be tested in a systematic manner, though family therapy can be an option, particularly in adolescents and children with PNES (see Chapter 33).

Social workers and rehabilitation therapists

As stated above, a significant number of patients with PNES are unemployed and in need of a variety of psychosocial services. These services include vocational evaluations with the aim to prepare them for possible work, which can be facilitated by social workers in state and institutional facilities.

Many such patients may have supported themselves and their family with governmental disability assistance. The fear of losing this income without other sources of economic support may pose significant stressors that may further interfere with the psychiatric and psychological treatment of the underlying psychiatric disorders. Thus, attention to these psychosocial problems is critical, particularly in patients with chronic PNES, if psychiatric treatment has any chance of being successful. It should also be noted that in many mental health clinics, social workers are in charge of providing the psychotherapy for patients.

Conclusions

The heterogeneous nature of PNES, the complexity and severity of the underlying psychiatric disorder(s), and the comorbid psychosocial consequences in the lives of patients with PNES require a multidisciplinary approach to the evaluation and management of patients with PNES. Thus, under ideal circumstances, every epilepsy center should have a team of epileptologists, psychiatrists, neuropsychologists, social workers, and vocational therapists. Sadly, this is the exception rather than the rule.

Since the advent of VEEG monitoring, reaching a correct diagnosis of PNES has become relatively straightforward. Nonetheless, treatment of these patients remains rudimentary and, often, nonexistent. The lack of communication among the various disciplines, but particularly between neurologists and psychiatrists, accounts for this problem in large part. It is clear that the role of the neurologist does not cease after the diagnosis is reached and that it continues in order to minimize the risk of unnecessary hospitalizations, which pose the gravest morbidity and mortality risks for these patients. Continuous communication among neurologist, psychiatrist, neuropsychologist, and social worker are absolutely essential to ensure the proper implementation of a comprehensive treatment plan.

References

1. LaFrance Jr WC, Rusch MD, Machan JT. What is "treatment as usual" for nonepileptic seizures? *Epilepsy Behav* 2008;**12**(3):388–94.
2. Rechlin T, Loew TH, Joraschky P. Pseudoseizure "status". *J Psychosom Res* 1997;**42**:495–8.
3. Reuber M, Pukrop R, Bauer J, et al. Outcome in psychogenic nonepileptic seizures: 1 to 10-year follow-up in 164 patients. *Ann Neurol* 2003; **53**(3):305–11.
4. Howell SJL, Owen L, Chadwick DW. Pseudostatus epilepticus. *Q J Med* 1989;**71**:507–19.
5. Bowman ES. Pseudoseizures. *Psychiatr Clin North Am* 1998;**21**:649–57.
6. Kanner AM, Parra J, Frey M, et al. Psychiatric and neurologic predictors of psychogenic pseudoseizure outcome. *Neurology* 1999;**53**:933–8.
7. Aboukasm A, Mahr G, Gahry BR, Thomas A, Barkley GL. Retrospective analysis of the effects of psychotherapeutic interventions on outcomes of psychogenic nonepileptic seizures. *Epilepsia* 1998;**39**(5):470–3.
8. Reuber M, Fernandez G, Helmstaedter C, Qurishi A, Elger CE. Evidence of brain abnormality in patients with psychogenic nonepileptic seizures. *Epilepsy Behav* 2002;**3**:246–8.
9. Harden CL, Tuna Burgut F, Kanner AM. The diagnostic significance of video-EEG monitoring findings on pseudoseizure patients differ between neurologists and psychiatrists. *Epilepsia* 2003;**44**: 453–6.
10. Lesser RP, Lueders H, Dinner DS. Evidence for epilepsy is rare in patients with psychogenic seizures. *Neurology* 1983;**33**:502–4.
11. Holmes MD, Wilkus RJ, Dodrill CB, *et al*. Coexistence of epilepsy in patients with nonpileptic seizures. *Epilepsia* 1993;**34** (Suppl 2):13.
12. Kanner AM, Parra J. Psychogenic pseudoseizures: semiology and pathogenic mechanisms. In: Luders HO, Noachtar S, eds. *The Epileptic Seizures:*

Pathophysiology and Semiology. New York: Churchill Livingstone. 2000; 766–73.

13. Neill J, Alvarez N. Differential diagnosis of epileptic versus pseudoepileptic seizures in developmentally delayed persons. *Appl Res Ment Retard* 1986;7:285–98.

14. Derry PA, McLachlan RS. The MMPI-2 as an adjunct to the diagnosis of pseudoseizures. *Seizure* 1996;5(1):35–40.

15. Storzbach D, Binder LM, Salinsky MC, Campbell BR, Mueller RM. Improved prediction of nonepileptic seizures with combined MMPI and EEG measures. *Epilepsia* 2000;**41**(3):332–7.

16. Goldstein LH, Deale AC, Mitchell-O'Malley SJ, Toone BK, Mellers JD. An evaluation of cognitive behavioral therapy as a treatment for dissociative seizures: a pilot study. *Cogn Behav Neurol* 2004;**17**(1):41–9.

Section 5 Chapter 28

Treatment considerations for psychogenic nonepileptic seizures

Designing treatment plans based on etiology of psychogenic nonepileptic seizures

W. Curt LaFrance, Jr. and Helge Bjørnæs

Patients with psychogenic nonepileptic seizures (PNES) potentially present a formidable challenge to treating clinicians and to researchers designing clinical trials because of the heterogeneity of the population. Comorbid psychiatric disorders, such as depression, anxiety, and posttraumatic stress disorder (PTSD), are the rule in patients with PNES. Up to 80% of patients with PNES have a history of abuse. Psychosocial dysfunction is present in patients with PNES, including disability, loss of job and wages, driving restrictions, social limitations, and family dysfunction. Many patients have neurological disorders such as headaches, cognitive difficulties, or histories of traumatic brain injuries. Approximately 10% of patients with PNES have both epileptic seizures (ES) and PNES. Along with the seizures, these many factors in combination limit the quality of life of patients with PNES, and therefore should be addressed in treatment approaches for PNES. At the same time, the factors can complicate the formulation of treatment approaches and the design of clinical trials.

As discussed in previous chapters, once PNES are definitively diagnosed with video-EEG monitoring, the next step in treatment involves a presentation of the diagnosis of PNES. When done in a clear, nonpejorative, positive manner by the clinician, the presentation can act as a bridge between neurological diagnosis and psychiatric/psychological treatment. The psychiatric treatment that follows the presentation of the diagnosis of PNES begins with an adequate understanding of the individual's developmental history, assessment of comorbid psychiatric diagnoses and treatments, psychosocial environment, and precursors, precipitants, and perpetuating factors in their PNES. Psychogenic nonepileptic seizures are a symptom, not the disease itself. Subgroups of PNES characteristics may respond better to specific interventions directed at the contributing factor to PNES. With an understanding of the etiology of PNES, specific treatments can be directed both at the PNES phenomenon and the underlying contributors to PNES.

In this chapter, we describe etiological models as the bases for the individualized treatment of patients with PNES. We present traditional and newer models associated with the development of disorders where psychological factors or psychiatric mechanisms are involved. The models include: a psychodynamic model, a family systems model, a learning theory model, a stress model, a psychosomatic/psychophysiological model, and the possible role of "organic" brain dysfunction. Within each model section, treatment strategies and methods have been developed. The practical application of this chapter is found in the question "If an etiology for PNES can be found in my patient, can treatment matched to the etiology effectively treat the PNES and the core issue?" This etiological model approach may also inform the design of much needed current and future clinical trials for PNES so that treatment groups are more homogenous from the standpoint of etiological factors.

Psychodynamic model

Seizure disorders without known medical cause have traditionally most frequently been regarded as a special form of symptom neurosis, either hysteria or conversion disorder. The psychodynamic theory for developing symptom neuroses may briefly be described as follows. At the core of the neurosis, an intrapsychic conflict is postulated between the main forces constituting the personality: the id, the ego, and the superego. The id signifies primitive, unconscious psychological drives and desires which are interacting

Gates and Rowan's Nonepileptic Seizures, 3rd edn. ed. Steven C. Schachter and W. Curt LaFrance, Jr. Published by Cambridge University Press. © S. Schachter and W. C. LaFrance, Jr. 2010.

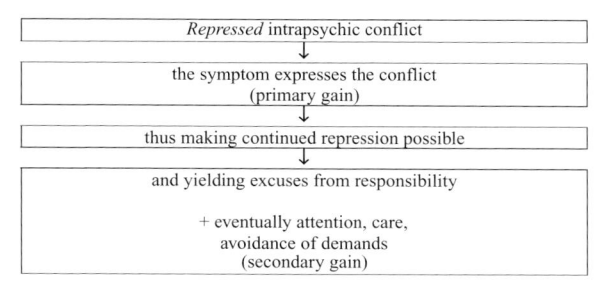

```
Repressed intrapsychic conflict
              ↓
  the symptom expresses the conflict
          (primary gain)
              ↓
  thus making continued repression possible
              ↓
  and yielding excuses from responsibility
              ↓
       + eventually attention, care,
          avoidance of demands
             (secondary gain)
```

Figure 28.1. A psychodynamic model.

with bodily needs and more or less constantly struggle for gratification. The ego is mainly the conscious part of the personality interacting with the outer world and controlling the sense and movement apparatuses, while the superego represents internalized moral norms and values taken over from parents and other persons of authority. In the patient with hysteria, thoughts, affect, and memories that are offensive to the superego cannot be experienced without giving rise to anxiety and are therefore repressed from consciousness.

Repression can be defined as a mental process that enables the individual to forget or not be aware of the forbidden and unpleasant thoughts [1]. But the forbidden mental contents may find some outlet (primary gain) if the balance between the mental forces is interrupted. This "leakage" of forbidden contents, disguised to prevent their recognition by the ego, and unsuccessful attempts by the unconscious part of the ego to prevent the "leakage" constitute the neurotic symptom. The unconscious conflict is thus expressed in a symbolic form through the symptom, which is experienced by the patient as something ego-dystonic or ego-alien. In this way the patient is able to communicate some of the repressed contents without experiencing excessive anxiety or guilt feelings. The draining of id-energies through the expression of the symptom keeps the mental pressure within manageable limits and thus makes it possible for the patient to keep the conflict and the forbidden content further repressed (see Figure 28.1).

In a typical case, for instance an incest victim, the traumatic experiences are too painful to be remembered and are therefore repressed. The symptom, which may be PNES, mimics what happened without the patient being aware of this [2]. The symptom debut is often preceded by some psychological crisis (thought to disturb the dynamic balance between the instances of the personality).

The symptom may also lead to various kinds of secondary gain for the patients, such as obtaining attention and care or avoiding demands and responsibilities. Within this tradition, the differential effect of timing between trauma and developmental stages is also important – emotional traumas in early childhood have more profound pathogenic influence on subsequent development than traumas encountered later on.

In his influential work within this field, Roy [3, 4] considered PNES mainly as hysterical manifestations. Miller [5] likewise maintained that PNES is found most commonly in persons with histrionic personality disorders. Contemporary conceptualizations often use terms like conversion, dissociation, or somatization to describe what is thought to be the core mechanisms of PNES. Studies assessing psychiatric diagnoses in patients with PNES reveal high percentages of conversion disorder, somatization disorder, dissociative disorder, and PTSD [6, 7].

Therapeutic considerations

In accordance with this frequently adopted model (often only implicit in the conception of PNES as conversion neurosis), psychodynamically oriented psychotherapy has been a widely accepted technique in treating PNES [8, 9]. Psychodynamic-oriented therapy would appear to be extremely useful to address the underpinnings of the psychopathology of PNES as discussed earlier. This topic has been reviewed extensively by Kalogjera-Sackellares [10] based on her 15 years of experience with patients with PNES. The monograph provides an excellent overview of psychodynamic conceptualizations of trauma and PNES, along with a review of the psychodynamic concepts used in treatment. Treatment methodology is addressed; however, no quantitative treatment or outcome data are provided. To date, no prospective controlled trials of psychodynamic psychotherapy have been published in the English literature.

Comments on the model

Research on personality characteristics of patients with PNES has not uniformly confirmed the psychodynamic etiology model. Much of the discussion has revolved around whether one can find signs of conversion hysteria (formerly in the *Diagnostic and Statistical Manual of Mental Disorders*, Third Edition (DSM III): hysterical neurosis, conversion type, now conversion disorder with seizures in the DSM-IV) in patients with PNES. Different psychodiagnostic tools such as the Minnesota Multiphasic Personality Inventory (MMPI), the Rorschach inkblot test, or psychiatric interview have been used.

In several studies, the MMPI has been used in attempts to differentiate between groups of patients with PNES or ES. Greater elevation on the scales considered significant for conversion hysteria are reported for patients with PNES compared with patients with ES [11, 12]. Controversy exists on whether the MMPI can be useful in this differentiation, but the MMPI is thought to be helpful especially when using special configural rules developed for classifying the patients [12]. When combined with video-EEG monitoring and characteristics of the events, patients with PNES demonstrated an MMPI pattern like that frequently seen in patients with conversion hysteria, and this can be used to predict development of PNES [13].

Vanderzant et al. [14] could not find significant MMPI profile differences between patients with ES and PNES, even when using Wilkus et al.'s [12] configural rules, nor could they find a typical MMPI profile for the patients with PNES. Only a few of the patients showed a hysterical profile. The authors also draw attention to the fact that many of the MMPI items, especially in the schizophrenia (Sc) scale, describe potentially real experiences of neurologically impaired patients. Schizophrenia-scale elevation would in such instances represent an artifact of disease rather than indicate emotional disturbance.

Henrichs et al. [15], using Wilkus et al.'s [12] configural rules in groups of patients with ES and PNES, found these rules of value in ruling out the probability of PNES, but when inferring PNES on the basis of these rules one was likely to be correct less than 50% of the time. Wilkus and Dodrill [16] again demonstrate the relevance of differentiating between subgroups of patients with PNES and patients with ES by means of the MMPI. Patients with PNES are here divided in groups according to motor and affectual features of their seizures. Patients with PNES with limited motor involvement or with prominently affectual features show a significantly different profile on the MMPI compared with patients with partial ES, while patients with PNES with much motor involvement in their seizures or with few or no affectual features do not differ from patients with generalized tonic-clonic ES.

Stewart et al. [17] studied three groups of patients by means of the MMPI, Rorschach, and the Wechsler Adult Intelligence Scale: one group with ES only, another with PNES only, and a third group with both kinds of seizures. They found more signs of different types of psychopathology in the two latter groups, including suicidal attempts, but signs of hysteria were infrequent. The authors were "surprised by the low percentage of hysterics in any of our study groups."

Findings in children with PNES may differ from those in adults (also see Chapter 17). Goodyer [18] studied five children with PNES and could not find specific personality disorders in any of them, but did find marked emotional problems. Anxiety was the most frequently seen emotional disturbance. Finlayson and Lucas [19] studied 18 patients with PNES ranging in age from 4 to 20 years. They found elevated hysteria scales on the MMPI in 13 of them. In spite of this they believe that conversion mechanisms are not necessarily involved etiologically, as they did not find other signs of conversion disorder such as indifference to the symptom, history of conflictual situation, or dramatic reporting of symptoms. They believe conversion symptoms are an exceptional cause of PNES. These diverse findings concerning the presence of neurotic traits may mean that neurotic mechanisms are not always involved in the etiology of PNES.

In a recent study, personality assessment with the Minnesota Multiphasic Personality Inventory-2 (MMPI-2) and the Revised NEO Personality Inventory (NEO-PI-R) were combined to examine personality characteristics in patients with PNES [20]. Based on NEO-PI-R and MMPI-2 findings, tentative descriptions of personality clusters in PNES were offered. Cluster 1 comprises "depressed neurotics"; cluster 2, "somatic defenders"; and cluster 3, "activated neurotics." The authors suggested the results showed the existence of personality subtypes in patients with PNES that should be considered in the design of interventions for them.

The approach adopted by Wilkus and Dodrill [16], and later extended by Selwa et al. [21], to classify PNES based on seizure semiology was recently chosen by Griffith et al. [22] for their analysis. These authors found patients with no motor involvement in their seizure semiology, described as a "catatonic" type, to respond with normal ranges on the MMPI-2 clinical scales, significantly differing from patients with more motor features in their seizures on the hysteria and hypochondria scales. Significant differences between the groups on several content scales further characterized the groups, supporting the possibility of distinct etiologies of subtypes of PNES. The authors found this important because "it suggests the potential efficacy of targeting treatment to specific aspects of disordered personality or maladaptive coping."

Family systems model

During therapy with families of children with psychosomatic symptoms who did not respond to medical treatment or who showed atypical fluctuations in the symptoms, Minuchin [23] and Minuchin *et al.* [24] realized that certain transactional patterns seemed characteristic of all these families. The characteristics were called *enmeshment*, which refers to an extreme form of proximity and intensity in family interactions; *overprotectiveness, rigidity*, meaning extreme loyalty to family rules; and lack of willingness and ability for *conflict resolution* within the family. The members of such a family are closely attached to each other, show a high degree of mutual concern, share the same opinions, and even speak for each other, but at the expense of individuality. The traditional roles played by different generations may be partly reversed. The family is usually presenting itself as successful and happy, the only sad thing being the presence of a psychosomatic disorder (for instance PNES) in one of the children.

In this model, too, the symptom is assumed to have a communicative function: to express conflicts and personal needs to the environment in such a way that the patient cannot be blamed for it. The symptom is also carrying another function: to draw the attention away from something the family dares not face up to.

Minuchin *et al.* described three necessary (but not independently sufficient) conditions for the development and maintenance of severe psychosomatic problems in children: (1) a certain type of family organization that encourages somatization; (2) involvement of the child in parental conflict; and (3) physiological vulnerability [25]. The pathology of the "symptom carrier" may in some way be an expression of what is wrong within the family, an interpersonal parallel to the intrapersonal conflicts in the psychodynamic model. This could be called a "sociodynamic" model (see Figure 28.2). Within this tradition one is looking more to the special role the symptom plays in the family than to explaining the symptom selection per se.

One of the authors (W. C. L.) has incorporated the McMaster Model of Family Functioning [26] using

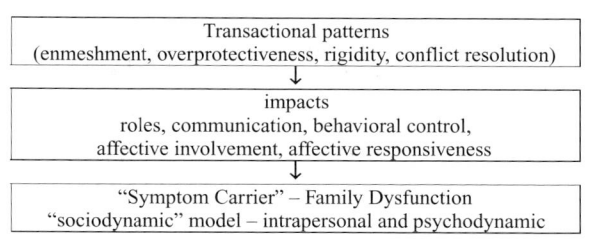

Transactional patterns
(enmeshment, overprotectiveness, rigidity, conflict resolution)
↓
impacts
roles, communication, behavioral control,
affective involvement, affective responsiveness
↓
"Symptom Carrier" – Family Dysfunction
"sociodynamic" model – intrapersonal and psychodynamic

Figure 28.2. A family systems model.

Problems Centered Systems Therapy for Patients for PNES treatment [27] (see also Chapter 33).

Therapeutic considerations

Based on these transactional concepts, powerful therapeutic tools are created to handle the pathogenic interactions. The therapist works towards a change by challenging the family transactions. This must be done "from within" by the therapist joining the family and taking the role as leader in the therapeutic process [24].

Seltzer [28] used a somewhat different approach to families with children showing conversion disorders. She described the family dynamics and structures in cultural or ethnographic terms and found this of value for the therapy because it placed the child's symptom and the family problems in a context of the social reality which these families had to face.

Griffith *et al.* [29] identifies the "unspeakable dilemma" in family interactions as a major contributor to family dynamics in patients with PNES. In the study, an unspeakable dilemma was evident in 13 of 14 families' interviews, with the patient the most silent family member in 13 interviews. In six cases, there was revealed a realistic threat of physical or sexual assault to a person involved in the problem, although not always the patient.

Learning theory models

These models can roughly be divided into classical conditioning and operant conditioning.

Classical conditioning

In a classical conditioning model, a stimulus which is not eliciting a certain response can, because of temporal and situational contiguity to an unconditioned stimulus, which by necessity elicits the response, gradually lead to the release of a similar (but not incidental) response (see Figure 28.3).

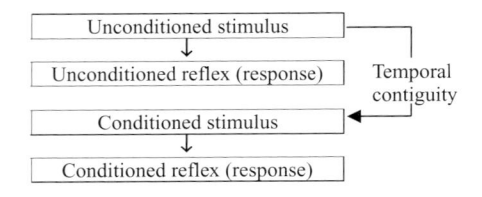

Figure 28.3. A learning theory model 1 for PNES: classical conditioning.

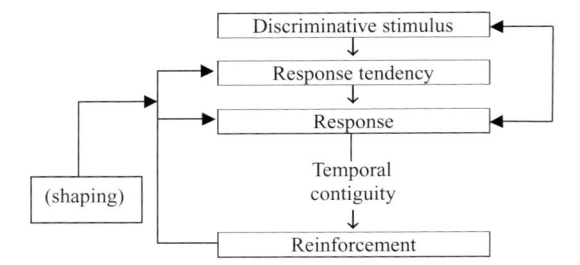

Figure 28.4. A learning theory model 2 for PNES: operant conditioning.

If, for example, a patient has a reflex epilepsy where flickering light, say in the kitchen, repeatedly elicits seizures, initially neutral objects such as the refrigerator might eventually elicit similar but not identical seizures, the difference perhaps being that these seizures do not have epileptiform EEG correlates. Such conditioned responses may generalize so that later on the sight of any refrigerator could elicit a seizure. (We have seen a related case, a patient whose seizures are provoked if she opens the door of any refrigerator, except that these are ES. So far we do not know the mechanisms behind this peculiar "reflex" epilepsy.)

Therapeutic considerations

Gumnit and Gates [30] suggested that PNES may be learned by a classical conditioning paradigm and certain forms of PNES may be classified as "reinforced behaviors" [31]. If certain patients with PNES can be shown to have developed seizures according to this paradigm, it is unknown if one would expect to find the same degree of psychopathology in these patients. Breaking the association may be more readily accomplished with behavioral interventions. Designs aimed at the extinction of the conditioned responses would perhaps be the most plausible in these instances. (One should, however, not overlook possible additional psychological problems even in these "simple" cases.)

Operant conditioning

In an operant paradigm it is assumed that certain subsequent events can reinforce the tendency for a response to be repeated. Such responses need not be correlated with any known stimulus and are designated "operants." A relation to prior stimulation may, however, be acquired, and thus aspects of the situation may influence the operant behavior. Such aspects are designated "discriminative stimuli." Thus any kind of "secondary gain" from a seizure can reinforce the tendency for repeated seizures. The concept of shaping, which means that the forthcoming of the reinforcing event is contingent upon successively greater or more frequent responses (operants), can explain how an initially slight response, say pretending to have a small seizure, can grow into dramatic forms beyond the control of the patient and turn out to be as disabling as comparable ES (see Figure 28.4).

Learning theory models may be applied to symptom formation also at an early age, and may be used to explain the development of severe pathology. Several of the models may be applied in such cases; however, other models may not be as easily applied to symptom formation in otherwise healthy individuals.

Taking classical learning theory and applying it to patients with PNES, we find that fear-avoidance may be relevant to mechanisms and treatments for PNES. Patients with PNES exhibit disproportionately elevated fear sensitivity on self-report measures when compared with patients with epilepsy [32]. Fear of the next seizure and fear of the unknown (future, consequences of seizures, impact on family) are frequently reported by patients with PNES. The fear avoidance model [33] has been used in cognitive behavioral therapy (CBT) for PNES (see Chapter 29) [27, 34, 35] and may impact the dysfunctional learning in PNES (see Figure 28.5).

Stress model

According to Lazarus [36] and Lazarus and Alfert [37], stress can be conceptualized as an unpleasant emotional response to some threatening event. The threat against the person or the person's values initially and most often comes from the outer world, but later on may arise in the inner world of the person as memories, as seen in traumatic neuroses [38]. When exposed to a threatening situation, the person evaluates the possibilities for coping with it. These evaluations are partly objective and realistic, partly

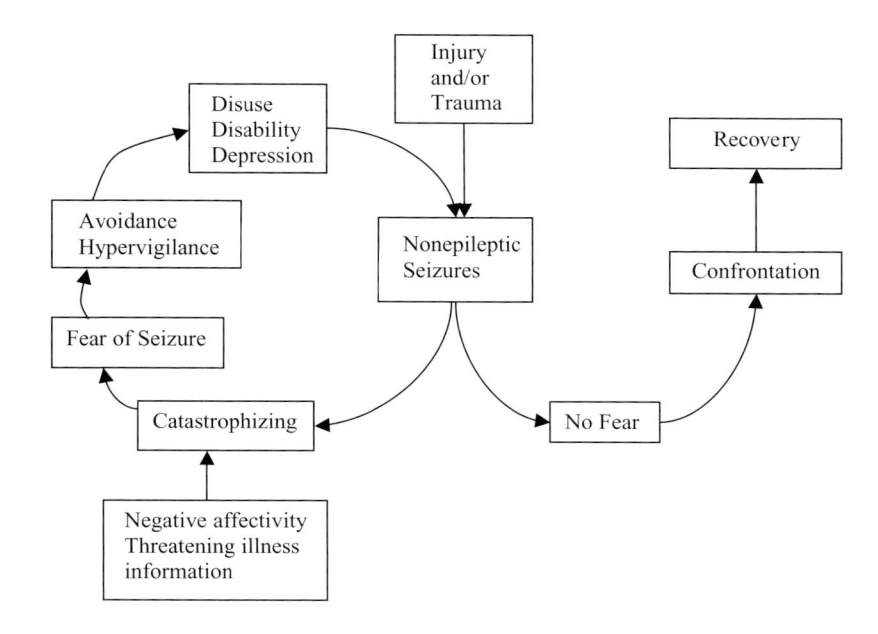

Figure 28.5. A learning theory fear-avoidance model for PNES. Modified from Vlaeyen and Linton [33], used with permission from IASP.

subjective, unrealistic and not necessarily fully conscious mental processes. The person evaluates the relative strength of what is believed to be one's resources on the one hand – knowledge and abilities relevant to the situation – and, on the other hand, aspects of the threatening situation. If the person believes that the situation can in some way be defeated, some assertive, aggressive, or determined kind of emotion emerges together with a response tendency to fight back. If one believes that the threatening situation is too strong to be defeated, fear or anxiety is felt, and one looks for possibilities of escape. If no opportunity for fighting back nor for escaping the threatening situation is seen by the person, the use of intrapsychic defense mechanisms such as denial, repression, or perhaps fainting is near at hand. In accordance with this model, PNES will constitute a maladaptive way to cope with an unbearable stress situation (see Figure 28.6). Several authors recognize this possibility (e.g. [39–41, 42]). The stress condition may be lasting, thus perpetuating the events.

The perception of stress can be influenced by one's experiences, genetics, and behavior. McEwen [43] described the process of allostasis (the ability to achieve stability through change). When the brain perceives a stressful experience, physiological and behavioral responses are initiated, leading to allostasis and adaptation. Over time, the allostatic load (the long-term effect of the body's physiological response to stress) may accumulate, and the overexposure to mediators of neural, endocrine, and immune stress can have adverse effects on various organ systems, leading to disease [43].

Persons under stress can develop individual coping styles which are used in stereotypical ways in situations where they are afraid of being ignored, of getting involved in conflicts, or of demands [39]. Maladaptive coping is found in patients with PNES [44]. Another challenge to healthy coping may be found in people with learning disabilities (LD), who have also been found to develop PNES. While traumatic experiences are not a typical finding in the history of patients with PNES and LD [45], it still seems reasonable to think that this group may be vulnerable to stress because of having fewer coping resources. Case reports have found that stress and distress may trigger PNES in patients with LD [40].

Exposure to an extremely traumatic stressor may result in PTSD. Fiszman et al. conceive of PNES in some patients as a serious form of PTSD combined with dissociative reactions [46].

Comments

The search for special coping styles in patients with PNES was one of the objectives in the study of Brask [41]. Using the MMPI and two health inventories, he assessed whether 12 adult patients with PNES were

Section 5: Treatment considerations for PNES

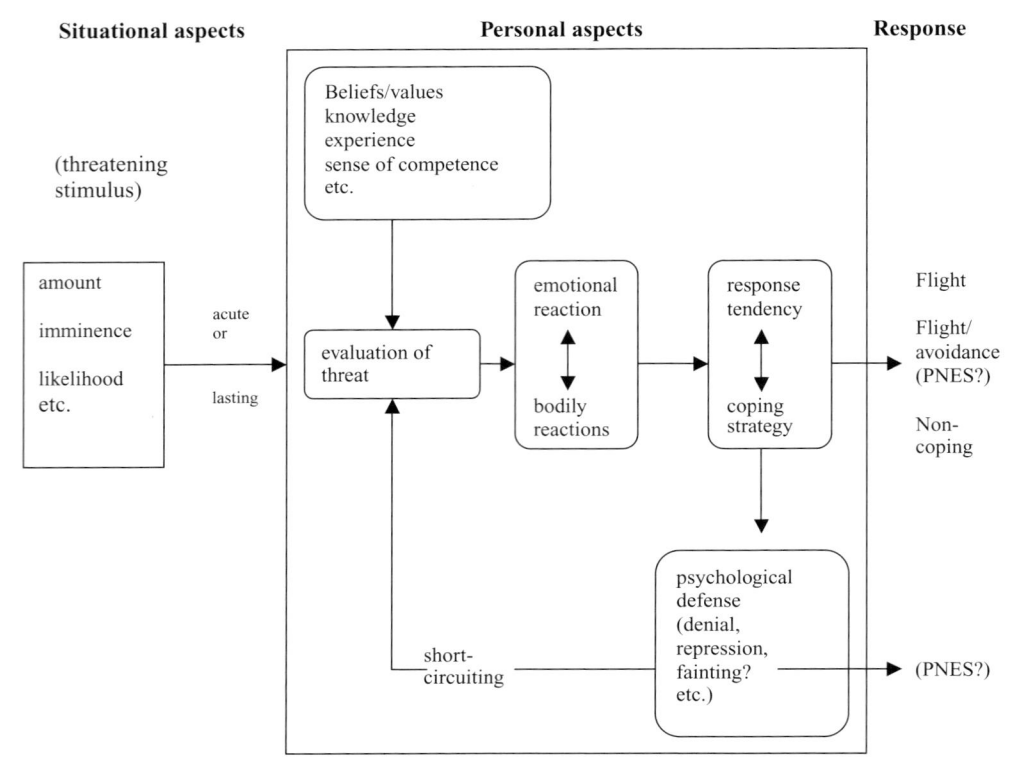

Figure 28.6. A stress model.

characterized in this respect, but he did not find that they differed significantly in coping styles from a group of patients with ES. LaFrance *et al.* [27] found that over the course of time-limited psychotherapy, patients with PNES developed healthier coping styles as assessed by the Ways of Coping instrument.

The age of the patients may play a role in the development of coping styles. Silver [47] studied a group of adolescents with PNES and maintained that the selection of so maladaptive a coping strategy as PNES may be a reflection of the stage of psychological development rather than a generalized personality style that would persist with disabling symptoms throughout their adult lives. Children and adolescents are more helpless and vulnerable than adults, and may therefore more easily use primitive coping strategies like PNES when confronting stress. If so, this may have consequences for the prognosis: seemingly the PNES disappears spontaneously in young people more often than in adults (see [42, 48, 49]). Some of the children with PNES also may change their coping strategies to more adaptive ones.

Therapeutic considerations

This stress model defines the presumed significant forces that interact to make up the stress response in great detail, and may give valuable guidelines in the search for diagnostic clues. Therapy according to this model would consist of diminishing the relative threat by manipulating environmental variables, by strengthening the patients' relevant resources (competence, abilities), or by rendering the patients more objective in the evaluation of the relative strengths and weaknesses perceived in the situation.

Williams *et al.* [50] underline the importance of inducing a feeling of competence and control in patients with PNES. To achieve this they use (among other techniques) hypnotic suggestions of ability to cope successfully with stress in children with PNES and report good results of this treatment.

Interventions to enhance coping strategies as a part of cognitive behavioral treatment programs appear to be effective in the management of stress in adults [51], with promising effects on PNES (see also Chapter 29)

[52]. Similarly, in patients with PTSD, psychotherapeutic techniques, e.g., CBT, have proven to be beneficial [53, 54].

Psychosomatic/psychophysiological models

Traditionally, a psychosomatic disorder can be seen as physical dysfunctions caused by longstanding suppressed emotional responses [55]. The person does not for some reason allow himself to express certain emotional responses, such as depression, anger, sadness, despair, and so on, perhaps because these responses are against the person's standards and if expressed will lead to guilt feelings or shame. The concept of *suppression* means that such withholding of emotional responses is a conscious process, at least in the initial phase. Later on, the suppression may be automatized and not fully conscious, but never unconscious like repression. The patient's life situation may provoke such emotions, and partly because the patient conceals them it may be difficult to clear up the situation, which thus may become lasting, and the un-expressed emotional reactions likewise.

Psychophysiological research has demonstrated that certain situations may give rise to specific physiological responses (situational response specificity), and that persons may tend to respond in more or less stereotyped manners to different kinds of stressors (individual response stereotypy) [56]. These principles might be of value in explaining symptom formation. Consciousness could be conceived of as one possible response system in predisposed individuals, leading to loss of consciousness/PNES under certain conditions (Figure 28.7).

Therapeutic considerations

According to Prick [57] traditional psychotherapeutic treatment of psychosomatic disorders has often met with little success. This may be because the therapeutic tools developed within psychodynamic theory are especially suited to treating the effects of unconscious defense mechanisms, not for the effects of the conscious act of suppression. Interventions in accordance with a stress model or psychophysiological treatment techniques like biofeedback would perhaps be more successful and should be further studied.

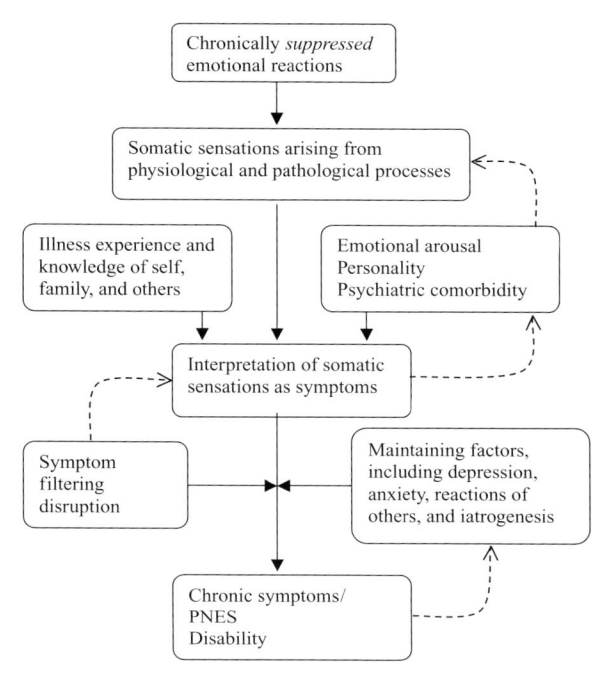

Figure 28.7. A somatic/psychophysiological symptoms model. Modified from Mayou *et al.* [90, 91] with permission from Oxford University Press and the American Journal of Psychiatry (© 2005), American Psychiatric Association.

"Organic" psychosyndrome model

Now an outdated term, "organic" is still used to describe the false dichotomy between mental and physical. Many authors point to the fact that a significant proportion of patients with PNES has different comorbid organic cerebral dysfunction [14, 16, 58–61]. These dysfunctions may turn out to be important etiological factors in PNES, as they may interfere with the patient's attention, executive function, or experience of reality, especially in interpersonal relationships.

On neuropsychological tests, abnormal scores are found as often in patients with PNES as in patients with ES (see Chapter 13). Wilkus and Dodrill [16] maintain that interaction between certain emotional conflicts and organic brain dysfunction may predispose for PNES. Similar views are held by Sackellares *et al.* [58] and Vanderzant *et al.* [14]. Bookheimer and Fedio [59] suspect dysfunction especially of fronto-temporal limbic structures in patients with PNES. Novelly [60] suggested that the different seizure features seen in a group of patients with PNES could be related to specific dysfunctional brain areas. A further subgrouping

Section 5: Treatment considerations for PNES

```
┌─────────────────────────────────────────────────┐
│       Underlying "organic cerebral dysfunction"  │
└─────────────────────────────────────────────────┘
                        ↓
┌─────────────────────────────────────────────────┐
│   Interference of patient's intra- and inter personal │
│                    experiences                   │
└─────────────────────────────────────────────────┘
                        ↓
┌─────────────────────────────────────────────────┐
│       Fronto-temporal limbic circuits dysfunction │
└─────────────────────────────────────────────────┘
                        ↓
┌─────────────────────────────────────────────────┐
│                       PNES                       │
└─────────────────────────────────────────────────┘
```

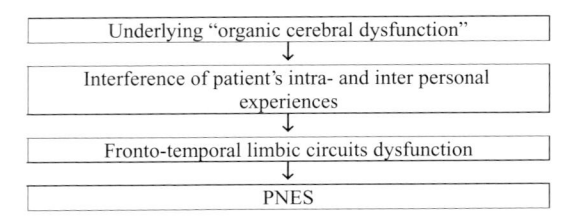

Figure 28.8. An "Organic Psychosyndrome" model of PNES.

of patients with PNES based on seizure features would, however, be difficult since it is reported that 10% to 25% of patients with PNES have more than one type of seizure [42, 62] (see Figure 28.8).

A recent review by Binder and Salinsky [63] points to the possibility that the neuropsychological deficits often found in patients with PNES may be due more to impairment in motivation and the ability to invest effort than to specific brain dysfunction. However, this does not necessarily rule out an "organic" psychosyndrome model, as lack in effort and motivation may be a symptom of apathy, seen in frontal lobe dysfunction, even with little additional cognitive impairment.

Lelliott and Fenwick [61] found that 74% of patients with lone PNES, as contrasted with 24% of psychiatric patients, had abnormal EEGs. They cite Fenton who argues that organic brain disease may facilitate PNES and should be incorporated into models of etiology together with psychosocial stressors, mood state, personality, and secondary gain [64].

Devinsky *et al.* [65] explored the hypothesis that lateralized hemispheric dysfunction may contribute to the development of conversion symptoms. The authors studied frequency of unilateral cerebral physiological or structural abnormalities in 79 consecutive patients with conversion nonepileptic seizures (C-NES), who were also compared with two groups of epilepsy patients without C-NES. Sixty (76%) of the patients with C-NES had unilateral cerebral abnormalities on neuroimaging, of which 85% were structural. Ictal or interictal epileptiform abnormalities on EEG were found in 78% of patients with C-NES and focal slowing in another 10%. Fifty (63%) of the patients with C-NES had both structural and epileptiform abnormalities. Among the 60 with unilateral abnormalities, 43 (72%) had right hemisphere structural lesions or physiological dysfunctions (C-NES > non-C-NES, $p < 0.02$). This study supports prior studies and clinical observations that cerebral dysfunction can contribute to the pathogenesis of conversion disorder, and that nondominant hemisphere dysfunction may play a greater role.

Advances in functional neuroimaging may help to better elucidate the pathophysiology of PNES. At present, however, structural neuroimaging abnormalities neither confirm nor exclude ES or PNES. PNES may occur in the presence of focal lesions, as confirmed by case reports of patients with PNES who have central nervous system lesions [66] and a study showing that 10% of patients with PNES alone have structural abnormalities on MRI scans [67]. A negative ictal SPECT scan does not imply a diagnosis of PNES nor does an abnormal scan mean epilepsy is present. A small series of ictal and interictal SPECT scans of patients with PNES revealed a few scans with lateralized perfusion abnormalities, but the findings did not change when the ictal and interictal images were compared [68]. Patients with ES, in contrast, have dynamic changes when comparing ictal and interictal changes on functional neuroimaging.

In other conversion disorders, advances in assessment of brain physiology may help inform further understanding of PNES. Addressing the psychobiology of somatoform disorders, structural neuroimaging (morphometric MRI) in ten patients with conversion disorder compared to healthy controls revealed smaller mean volumes of the left and right basal ganglia and smaller right thalamus in the patients with conversion disorder [69]. Studies using SPECT and functional MRI have identified the anterior cingulate gyrus and the orbitofrontal cortex as potentially mediating the hypothesized attention and inhibition findings seen in patients with sensory and motor conversion disorders [70, 71]. Bilateral vibrotactile stimulation in three patients with sensory conversion disorders resulted in activation of the contralateral primary somatosensory region (S1), but no contralateral activation was present during unilateral stimulation of the affected limb [72]. Further studies of functional neuroimaging examining striatothalamocortical circuits controlling sensorimotor function and attention may yield insights into the neural and effective connectivity in PNES.

Toward a unified model for PNES

To date, there is no single unifying "lesion" (anatomical or psychological) to explain PNES or any other conversion disorder manifestation. In 2003, prior to the 2005 PNES Treatment workshop [73], the

Chapter 28: Treatment plans based on etiology

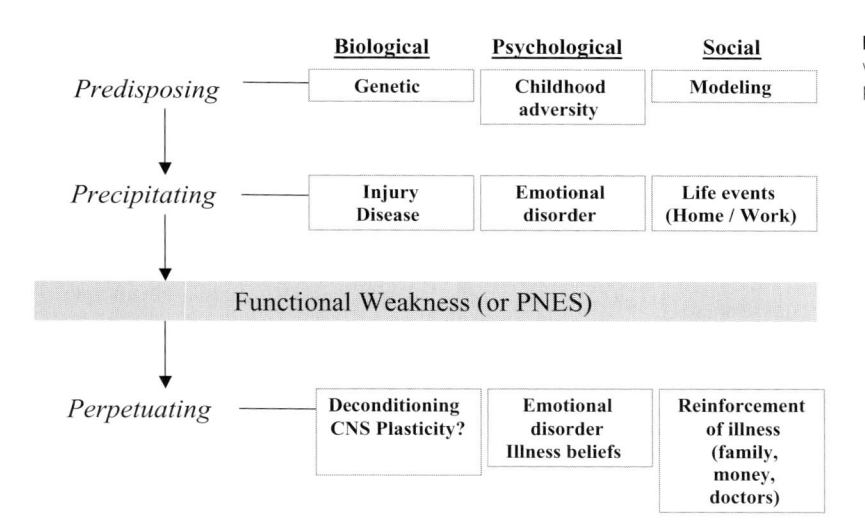

Figure 28.9. What causes "functional weakness"? Modified from Stone [92], with permission.

	Biological	Psychological	Social
Predisposing	Genetic	Childhood adversity	Modeling
Precipitating	Injury Disease	Emotional disorder	Life events (Home / Work)

Functional Weakness (or PNES)

Perpetuating	Deconditioning CNS Plasticity?	Emotional disorder Illness beliefs	Reinforcement of illness (family, money, doctors)

Movement Disorder Society convened a workshop on psychogenic movement disorders [74]. Stone presented an etiological model for functional weakness [75], which is modified here to provide a means of conceptualizing the risks of PNES (predisposing, precipitating, and perpetuating factors) in the context of the biological-psychological-social model (see Figure 28.9).

Along with interpersonal issues and environmental stimuli, as noted in the allostasis discussion, catecholamines and glucocorticoids may play a part in the stress response generated in patients with PNES. Putting all of these developmental, genetic, environmental, and epigenetic mechanisms together can potentially inform clinicians and researchers on mediators of the disorder and may identify treatment targets for patients with PNES. Using the biological-psychological-social model, a working approach to etiological models that lead to PNES is hereby presented (see Figure 28.10).

Combining this information helps develop a biopsychosocial formulation, informing our possible treatments. These pathways take into account the various models and highlight the importance of multifactorial makeup and contributions to pathology.

Arguments for subgroups in PNES (Table 28.1)

Many authors argue from different points of view for the division of patients with PNES into different subgroups. The most obvious division recognized by most authors is of patients with both ES and PNES, and patients with lone PNES. Sackellares *et al.* [58] argue for this differentiation because, in their view, there may well be different etiologies in these groups.

Similarly, in a group of patients with PNES, Vanderzant *et al.* [14] found some with pathological results on the MMPI but normal results on neuropsychological tests, and some patients with the reversed pattern. They believe that these opposite response patterns define two different subtypes of PNES.

Some authors [76] argue for differentiating between three groups of PNES: those with both PNES and ES constitute one subtype; patients with lone PNES can be further divided into those with underlying personality disturbances and those who develop PNES as a conversion reaction to an acute conflict situation. According to some authors, the latter subtype has a very good prognosis, while patients with personality disturbances are in need of long-term treatment and have a poorer prognosis [77].

Brask [41] reports that in one group of patients with partial epilepsy and one group with PNES, the presence of auras are about equally frequent: about 50% in both groups report auras. This is in agreement with Gates *et al.* [78], who found that 39% of patients with PNES report auras of a "simple" type: dizziness, slight sensations, etc. When treating ES with behavior therapy and neuropsychological techniques, the existence of aura is regarded as a possible point of departure for treatment, if the patients are (or can be) motivated to take control of their seizures [79]. Reiter and Andrews found utility of a behaviorally based

275

Section 5: Treatment considerations for PNES

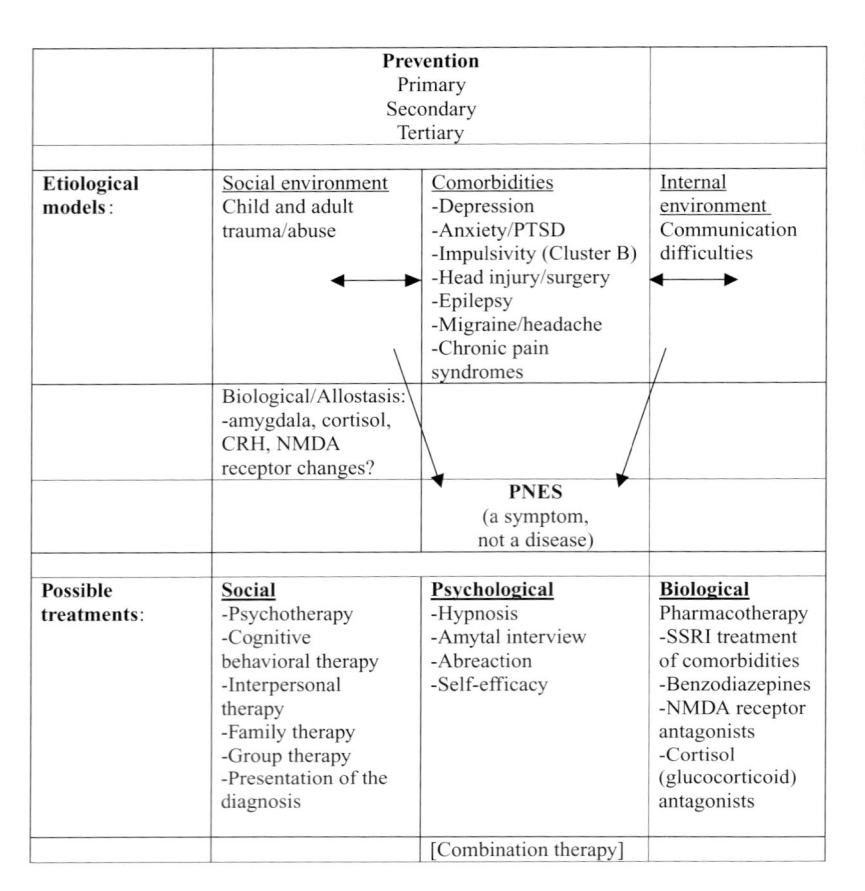

	Prevention Primary Secondary Tertiary		
Etiological models:	Social environment Child and adult trauma/abuse	Comorbidities -Depression -Anxiety/PTSD -Impulsivity (Cluster B) -Head injury/surgery -Epilepsy -Migraine/headache -Chronic pain syndromes	Internal environment Communication difficulties
	Biological/Allostasis: -amygdala, cortisol, CRH, NMDA receptor changes?		
		PNES (a symptom, not a disease)	
Possible treatments:	**Social** -Psychotherapy -Cognitive behavioral therapy -Interpersonal therapy -Family therapy -Group therapy -Presentation of the diagnosis	**Psychological** -Hypnosis -Amytal interview -Abreaction -Self-efficacy	**Biological** Pharmacotherapy -SSRI treatment of comorbidities -Benzodiazepines -NMDA receptor antagonists -Cortisol (glucocorticoid) antagonists
		[Combination therapy]	

Figure 28.10. Pathways in diagnosis and treatment of psychogenic nonepileptic seizures. CRH, corticotropin-releasing hormone; SSRI, selective serotonin reuptake inhibitors. From [87], with permission from Elsevier.

psychotherapy for patients with ES [80, 81]. Realizing that similar psychotherapeutic principles could be applied in patients with PNES, LaFrance et al. demonstrated reduction of PNES in 21 patients with PNES incorporating a functional behavioral analysis to prevent and abort seizures at their subjective onset [27].

Brask [41] also reported that more than half of the patients in both groups describe reduced consciousness during their seizures to a degree where they do not register anything in the environment, while about 40% have no or only slight disturbances of consciousness. Like the existence of auras, this may also indicate differential opportunities for treatment, at least of the symptoms. In patients who are conscious during the initial phase of their seizures, the possibilities for aborting the seizures may be explored.

A naturalistic study examined psychotherapy treatment of patients with PNES based on treatments administered and psychiatric symptomatology [82]. Rusch divided the subgroups of patients with PNES into six categories according to their psychosocial history, PNES etiology, and mechanisms of and response to psychotherapy. These symptom clusters are not mutually exclusive, and many times, overlapping etiologies and comorbidities exist. For a psychological framework to inform treatment, Rusch's six categories could be reframed as: a. Anxious; b. Abused – i. Angry (Borderline personality disorder), ii. Afraid (PTSD); c. Somatic; d. Dysthymic/Depressed; e. Mentally Retarded. Gates described psychiatric approaches to treatment differences based on the chronicity of the PNES, recommending short-term psychotherapy for those with PNES less than six months, and more intensive inpatient therapy for longstanding PNES [83].

Additional arguments for subgroups are found in observations that trauma may not be typical in the history of male patients with PNES, in those with late onset, or in the learning disabled. Likewise, the predominance of females among adult patients with PNES may not be found among younger children [84] and in the elderly [85].

Table 28.1 Summary of factors which may be relevant for subgrouping and prognosis

- Age of patient when the psychological trauma/conflict starts
- Age of onset of PNES
- Duration of PNES
- PNES + ES or PNES alone
- The seizure semiology
- Degree of reduction in consciousness
- Additional psychopathology
- Coping strategies during stressful situations
- Additional cerebral dysfunction
- Presence of aura
- Gender
- Presence of trauma
- Learning disability

Remarks about treatment

Goodyer [18] argued for individually adapted treatment strategies when treating children with PNES. The approach begins with re-educating parents and children about the illness, and then proceeding with selected forms of treatment, ranging from individualized psychotherapy to family therapy and manipulation of the children's environment.

Ramani and Gumnit [39] found that psychiatric intervention usually led to the cessation of the seizures as well as to a better psychosocial functioning of the patients. Preliminary research demonstrates that PNES is a treatable condition [86–88]. Best results are obtained with an individualized, eclectic team approach that employs both psychodynamic and behavioral methods, with attention to reality factors and long-term follow-up care [89]. The involvement of the family in treatment is essential. Longitudinal research is needed to confirm the clinical impression that treatment has an enduring effect.

Gumnit and Gates [30] noted that "the presence of a personality disorder or childhood sexual trauma may greatly complicate diagnostic and treatment efforts." Brief treatment, however, may be very effective in helping patients who simply have a misinterpretation problem or an inappropriate coping mechanism. The converse is that treatment may be quite time consuming and frustrating in patients with deeply buried emotional conflicts.

As stated earlier, the most frequently mentioned emotional problem in children with PNES is anxiety, while depression is the most prominent affective disorder in adult patients [42]. The comorbidities may impact the type of treatment one administers and the patient's prognosis.

Conclusions

From the early literature on the topic, it appears that different authors have had a predetermined concept of the possible etiological factors in PNES and have selected their therapeutic approaches accordingly. But the successive systematization in these patients of demographic information, seizure characteristics and results from different inventories, psychological tests, and therapies has made it increasingly clear that patients with PNES are heterogeneous, with different degrees of disability and different prognoses.

Nonetheless, attempts at establishing subgroups on the basis of such information have proven to be of value both for furthering better understanding of the patients and for selection of the most appropriate treatment strategies. In addition, it is suggested here that patients should also be classified in accordance with possible underlying etiological models, both to learn more about the relative actuality of the different models and to see whether this may be a useful aid in selecting the most appropriate forms of intervention. To enhance the possibilities for individualized and flexible approaches, treatment of patients with PNES should ideally be carried out within a team representing a wide range of treatment strategies.

Portions of Bjørnæs H. Aetiological models as a basis for individualized treatment of pseudo-epileptic seizures. In: Gram L, Johannessen SI, Osterman PE, Sillanpaa M, eds. *Pseudo-Epileptic Seizures*. Petersfield, UK: Wrightson Biomedical Publishing Ltd. 1993; 81–98 were used for this chapter, with permission.

References

1. Fenichel O. *The Psychoanalytic Theory of Neurosis*. London: Routledge, 1999.
2. Goodwin JM. Childhood sexual abuse and non-epileptic seizures. In: Rowan AJ, Gates JR, eds. *Non-Epileptic Seizures*, 1st edn. Stoneham, MA: Butterworth-Heinemann. 1993; 181–91.
3. Roy A, ed. *Hysteria*. Chichester, West Sussex; New York: John Wiley, 1982.
4. Roy A. Pseudoseizures: a psychiatric perspective. *J Neuropsychiatry Clin Neurosci* 1989;**1**(1):69–71.

5. Miller HR. Psychogenic seizures treated by hypnosis. *Am J Clin Hypn* 1983;**25**(4):248–52.

6. D'Alessio L, Giagante B, Oddo S, et al. Psychiatric disorders in patients with psychogenic non-epileptic seizures, with and without comorbid epilepsy. *Seizure* 2006;**15**:333–9.

7. Marchetti RL, Kurcgant D, Neto JG, et al. Psychiatric diagnoses of patients with psychogenic non-epileptic seizures. *Seizure* 2008;**17**(3):247–53.

8. Goodwin J, Simms M, Bergman R. Hysterical seizures: a sequel to incest. *Am J Orthopsychiatry* 1979;**49**(4): 698–703.

9. Brooksbank DJ. Management of conversion reaction in five adolescent girls. *J Adolesc* 1984;**7**(4):359–76.

10. Kalogjera-Sackellares D. *Psychodynamics and Psychotherapy of Pseudoseizures*. Carmarthen, Wales, UK: Crown House Publishing, Ltd, 2004.

11. Matthews CG, Shaw DJ, Klove H. Psychological test performances in neurologic and "pseudo-neurologic" subjects. *Cortex* 1966;**2**:244–53.

12. Wilkus RJ, Dodrill CB, Thompson PM. Intensive EEG monitoring and psychological studies of patients with pseudoepileptic seizures. *Epilepsia* 1984;**25**(1): 100–7.

13. Schramke CJ, Valeri A, Valeriano JP, Kelly KM. Using the Minnesota Multiphasic Inventory 2, EEGs, and clinical data to predict nonepileptic events. *Epilepsy Behav* 2007;**11**(3):343–6.

14. Vanderzant CW, Giordani B, Berent S, Dreifuss FE, Sackellares JC. Personality of patients with pseudoseizures. *Neurology* 1986;**36**(5):664–8.

15. Henrichs TF, Tucker DM, Farha J, Novelly RA. MMPI indices in the identification of patients evidencing pseudoseizures. *Epilepsia* 1988;**29**(2):184–7.

16. Wilkus RJ, Dodrill CB. Factors affecting the outcome of MMPI and neuropsychological assessments of psychogenic and epileptic seizure patients. *Epilepsia* 1989;**30**(3):339–47.

17. Stewart RS, Lovitt R, Stewart RM. Are hysterical seizures more than hysteria? A research diagnostic criteria, DMS-III, and psychometric analysis. *Am J Psychiatry* 1982;**139**(7):926–9.

18. Goodyer IM. Epileptic and pseudoepileptic seizures in childhood and adolescence. *J Am Acad Child Psychiatry* 1985;**24**(1):3–9.

19. Finlayson RE, Lucas AR. Pseudoepileptic seizures in children and adolescents. *Mayo Clin Proc* 1979;**54**(2):83–7.

20. Cragar DE, Berry DT, Schmitt FA, Fakhoury TA. Cluster analysis of normal personality traits in patients with psychogenic nonepileptic seizures. *Epilepsy Behav* 2005;**6**(4):593–600.

21. Selwa LM, Geyer J, Nikakhtar N, et al. Nonepileptic seizure outcome varies by type of spell and duration of illness. *Epilepsia* 2000;**41**(10):1330–4.

22. Griffith NM, Szaflarski JP, Schefft BK, et al. Relationship between semiology of psychogenic nonepileptic seizures and Minnesota Multiphasic Personality Inventory profile. *Epilepsy Behav* 2007;**11**(1):105–11.

23. Minuchin S. *Families & Family Therapy*. Cambridge: Harvard University Press, 1974.

24. Minuchin S, Rosman BL, Baker L, eds. *Psychosomatic Families: Anorexia Nervosa in Context*. Cambridge, MA: Harvard University Press, 1978.

25. Minuchin S, Baker L, Rosman BL, et al. A conceptual model of psychosomatic illness in children. Family organization and family therapy. *Arch Gen Psychiatry* 1975;**32**(8):1031–8.

26. Ryan CE, Epstein NB, Keitner GI, Miller IW, Bishop DS. *Evaluating and Treating Families: The McMaster Approach*. New York: Routledge, 2005.

27. LaFrance WC, Jr, Blum A, Miller I, Ryan C, Keitner GI. Cognitive behavioral therapy or family therapy for nonepileptic seizures. *Epilepsia* 2008;**49** Suppl 7:273–4.

28. Seltzer WJ. Conversion disorder in childhood and adolescence, part II: Therapeutic issues. *Fam Syst Med* 1985;**3**:397–415.

29. Griffith JL, Polles A, Griffith ME. Pseudoseizures, families, and unspeakable dilemmas. *Psychosomatics* 1998;**39**(2):144–53.

30. Gumnit RJ, Gates JR. Psychogenic seizures. *Epilepsia* 1986;**27** Suppl 2:S124–9.

31. Gates JR, Luciano D, Devinsky O. The classification and treatment of nonepileptic events. In: Devinsky O, Theodore WH, eds. *Epilepsy and Behavior*. New York: Wiley-Liss. 1991; 251–63.

32. Hixson JD, Balcer LJ, Glosser G, French JA. Fear sensitivity and the psychological profile of patients with psychogenic nonepileptic seizures. *Epilepsy Behav* 2006;**9**(4):587–92.

33. Vlaeyen JW, Linton SJ. Fear-avoidance and its consequences in chronic musculoskeletal pain: a state of the art. *Pain* 2000;**85**(3):317–32.

34. Chalder T. Cognitive behavioural therapy as a treatment for conversion disorders. In: Halligan PW, Bass CM, Marshall JC, eds. *Contemporary Approaches to the Study of Hysteria: Clinical and Theoretical Perspectives*. Oxford, New York: Oxford University Press. 2001; 298–311.

35. Goldstein LH, Mellers JD. Ictal symptoms of anxiety, avoidance behaviour, and dissociation in patients with dissociative seizures. *J Neurol Neurosurg Psychiatry* 2006;**77**(5):616–21.

36. Lazarus RS. *Psychological Stress and the Coping Process.* New York: McGraw-Hill, 1966.
37. Lazarus RS, Alfert E. Short-circuiting of threat by experimentally altering cognitive appraisal. *J Abnorm Psychol* 1964;**69**:195–205.
38. Grinker RR, Spiegel JP. *Men Under Stress.* New York: McGraw-Hill, 1945.
39. Ramani V, Gumnit RJ. Management of hysterical seizures in epileptic patients. *Arch Neurol* 1982;**39**(2):78–81.
40. Silver LB. Conversion disorder with pseudoseizures in adolescence: a stress reaction to unrecognized and untreated learning disabilities. *J Am Acad Child Psychiatry* 1982;**21**(5):508–12.
41. Brask OD. Funksjonelle anfall. Personlighet og symptomrapportering. *Unpublished dissertation*, University of Oslo, 1988.
42. Lempert T, Schmidt D. Natural history and outcome of psychogenic seizures: a clinical study in 50 patients. *J Neurol* 1990;**237**(1):35–8.
43. McEwen BS. Protective and damaging effects of stress mediators. *N Engl J Med* 1998;**338**(3):171–9.
44. Zaroff CM, Myers L, Barr WB, Luciano D, Devinsky O. Group psychoeducation as treatment for psychological nonepileptic seizures. *Epilepsy Behav* 2004;**5**(4):587–92.
45. Duncan R, Oto M. Psychogenic nonepileptic seizures in patients with learning disability: comparison with patients with no learning disability. *Epilepsy Behav* 2008;**12**(1):183–6.
46. Fiszman A, Alves-Leon SV, Nunes RG, D'Andrea I, Figueira I. Traumatic events and posttraumatic stress disorder in patients with psychogenic nonepileptic seizures: a critical review. *Epilepsy Behav* 2004;**5**(6):818–25.
47. Silver LB. Conversion disorder with pseudoseizures in adolescence: a stress reaction to unrecognized and untreated learning disabilities. In: Gross M, ed. *Pseudoepilepsy: The Clinical Aspects of False Seizures.* Lexington, MA: Lexington Books, D. C. Heath and Company. 1983; 109–18.
48. Wyllie E, Friedman D, Rothner AD, *et al.* Psychogenic seizures in children and adolescents: outcome after diagnosis by ictal video and electroencephalographic recording. *Pediatrics* 1990;**85**(4):480–4.
49. Areng S, Engelskjon T, Lossius R, Skaare H. Follow-up study of adolescent pupils attending Solberg school, the National Center for Epilepsy (Sandvika). *Acta Neurol Scand* 1990;**82** Suppl 133:46.
50. Williams DT, Spiegel H, Mostofsky DI. Neurogenic and hysterical seizures in children and adolescents: differential diagnostic and therapeutic considerations. *Am J Psychiatry* 1978;**135**(1):82–6.
51. Steinhardt M, Dolbier C. Evaluation of a resilience intervention to enhance coping strategies and protective factors and decrease symptomatology. *J Am Coll Health* 2008;**56**(4):445–53.
52. Kuyk J, Siffels MC, Bakvis P, Swinkels WA. Psychological treatment of patients with psychogenic non-epileptic seizures: an outcome study. *Seizure* 2008;**17**(7):595–603.
53. Bisson J, Andrew M. Psychological treatment of post-traumatic stress disorder (PTSD). *Cochrane Database Syst Rev* 2007(3):CD003388.
54. Ehlers A, Clark DM. Post-traumatic stress disorder: the development of effective psychological treatments. *Nord J Psychiatry* 2008;**62** Suppl 47:11–18.
55. Alexander FBT. *Psychosomatic Medicine: Its Principles and Applications.* New York: Norton; 1987.
56. Lang PJ, Rice DG, Sternbach RA. The psychophysiology of emotion. In: Greenfield NS, Sternbach RA, eds. *Handbook of Psychophysiology.* New York: Holt, Rinehart and Winston. 1972; 623–43.
57. Prick JJG. Psychosomatic medicine: its possibilities and limitations. In: Booij J, ed. *Psychosomatics; A Series of Five Lectures.* Amsterdam: Elsevier. 1957; vi, 125 p. ill.
58. Sackellares JC, Giordani B, Berent S, *et al.* Patients with pseudoseizures: intellectual and cognitive performance. *Neurology* 1985;**35**(1):116–19.
59. Bookheimer SY, Fedio P. Ictal psychological changes in non-epileptic seizures and suspected frontotemporal dysfunction. In: Rowan AJ, Gates JR, eds. *Non-Epileptic Seizures*, 1st edn. Stoneham, MA: Butterworth-Heinemann. 1993; 243–55.
60. Novelly RA. Cerebral dysfunction and cognitive impairment in non-epileptic seizure disorders. In: Rowan AJ, Gates JR, eds. *Non-Epileptic Seizures*, 1st edn. Stoneham, MA: Butterworth-Heinemann. 1993; 233–42.
61. Lelliott PT, Fenwick P. Cerebral pathology in pseudoseizures. *Acta Neurol Scand* 1991;**83**(2):129–32.
62. Benbadis SR, Agrawal V, Tatum IV, WO. How many patients with psychogenic nonepileptic seizures also have epilepsy? *Neurology* 2001;**57**(5):915–17.
63. Binder LM, Salinsky MC. Psychogenic nonepileptic seizures. *Neuropsychol Rev* 2007;**17**(4):405–12.
64. Fenton GW. Hysterical alterations of consciousness. In: Roy A, ed. *Hysteria*. Chichester, West Sussex; New York: John Wiley. 1982; 229–46.

65. Devinsky O, Mesad S, Alper K. Nondominant hemisphere lesions and conversion nonepileptic seizures. *J Neuropsychiatry Clin Neurosci* 2001;**13**(3):367–73.

66. Lowe MR, De Toledo JC, Rabinstein AA, Giulla MF. Correspondence: MRI evidence of mesial temporal sclerosis in patients with psychogenic nonepileptic seizures. *Neurology* 2001;**56**(6):821–3.

67. Reuber M, Fernandez G, Helmstaedter C, Qurishi A, Elger CE. Evidence of brain abnormality in patients with psychogenic nonepileptic seizures. *Epilepsy Behav* 2002;**3**(3):249–54.

68. Ettinger AB, Coyle PK, Jandorf L, et al. Postictal SPECT in epileptic versus nonepileptic seizures. *J Epilepsy* 1998;**11**:67–73.

69. Atmaca M, Aydin A, Tezcan E, Poyraz AK, Kara B. Volumetric investigation of brain regions in patients with conversion disorder. *Prog Neuropsychopharmacol Biol Psychiatry* 2006;**30**(4):708–13.

70. Vuilleumier P, Chicherio C, Assal F, et al. Functional neuroanatomical correlates of hysterical sensorimotor loss. *Brain* 2001;**124**(Pt 6):1077–90.

71. Mailis-Gagnon A, Giannoylis I, Downar J, et al. Altered central somatosensory processing in chronic pain patients with "hysterical" anesthesia. *Neurology* 2003;**60**(9):1501–7.

72. Ghaffar O, Staines WR, Feinstein A. Unexplained neurologic symptoms: an fMRI study of sensory conversion disorder. *Neurology* 2006;**67**(11): 2036–8.

73. LaFrance Jr WC, Alper K, Babcock D, et al. Nonepileptic seizures treatment workshop summary. *Epilepsy Behav* 2006;**8**(3):451–61.

74. Hallett M, Fahn S, Jankovic J, et al., eds. *Psychogenic Movement Disorders: Neurology and Neuropsychiatry*. Philadelphia: Lippincott Williams & Wilkins, and American Academy of Neurology Press; 2005.

75. Stone J, Carson A, Sharpe M. Functional symptoms and signs in neurology: assessment and diagnosis. *J Neurol Neurosurg Psychiatry* 2005;**76** Suppl 1:i2–12.

76. Lancman ME, Brotherton TA, Asconape JJ, Penry JK. Psychogenic seizures in adults: a longitudinal analysis. *Seizure* 1993;**2**(4):281–6.

77. Kanner AM, Parra J, Frey M, et al. Psychiatric and neurologic predictors of psychogenic pseudoseizure outcome. *Neurology* 1999;**53**(5):933–8.

78. Gates JR, Ramani V, Whalen S, Loewenson R. Ictal characteristics of pseudoseizures. *Arch Neurol* 1985;**42**(12):1183–7.

79. Dahl JJ. The psychological treatment of epilepsy: a behavioral approach. *Acta Univ Ups* 1987; Dissertation abstract.

80. Reiter JM, Andrews DJ. A neurobehavioral approach for treatment of complex partial epilepsy: efficacy. *Seizure* 2000;**9**(3):198–203.

81. Reiter J, Andrews D, Janis C. *Taking Control of Your Epilepsy. A Workbook for Patients and Professionals*, 1st edn. Santa Rosa, CA: The Basics, 1987.

82. Rusch MD, Morris GL, Allen L, Lathrop L. Psychological treatment of nonepileptic events. *Epilepsy Behav* 2001;**2**:277–83.

83. Gates JR. Diagnosis and treatment of nonepileptic seizures. In: McConnell HW, Snyder PJ, eds. *Psychiatric Comorbidity in Epilepsy. Basic Mechanisms, Diagnosis, and Treatment*, 1st edn. Washington, DC: American Psychiatric Press, Inc. 1998; 187–204.

84. Vincentiis S, Valente KD, Thome-Souza S, et al. Risk factors for psychogenic nonepileptic seizures in children and adolescents with epilepsy. *Epilepsy Behav* 2006;**8**(1):294–8.

85. Duncan R, Oto M, Martin E, Pelosi A. Late onset psychogenic nonepileptic attacks. *Neurology* 2006;**66**(11):1644–7.

86. LaFrance Jr WC, Devinsky O. The treatment of nonepileptic seizures: historical perspectives and future directions. *Epilepsia* 2004;**45** Suppl 2:15–21.

87. LaFrance Jr WC, Barry JJ. Update on treatments of psychological nonepileptic seizures. *Epilepsy Behav* 2005;**7**(3):364–74.

88. Baker GA, Brooks JL, Goodfellow L, Bodde N, Aldenkamp A. Treatments for non-epileptic attack disorder. *Cochrane Database Syst Rev* 2007(1): CD006370.

89. LaFrance Jr WC, Devinsky O. Treatment of nonepileptic seizures. *Epilepsy Behav* 2002;**3**(5 Suppl 1):S19–23.

90. Mayou R, Bass CM, Sharpe M. Overview of epidemiological classification and aetiology. In: Mayou R, Bass CM, Sharpe M, eds. *Treatment of Functional Somatic Symptoms*. Oxford: Oxford University Press. 1995; 42–65.

91. Mayou R, Kirmayer LJ, Simon G, Kroenke K, Sharpe M. Somatoform disorders: time for a new approach in DSM-V. *Am J Psychiatry* 2005;**162**(5):847–55.

92. Stone J. Paralysis and sensory loss. Psychogenic Movements Disorders Workshop. October 11, 2003. Atlanta, GA.

Section 5 Chapter 29

Treatment considerations for psychogenic nonepileptic seizures

Cognitive behavioral treatments

Laura H. Goldstein, W. Curt LaFrance, Jr., Craig Chigwedere, John D. C. Mellers, and Trudie Chalder

Cognitive behavioral therapy (CBT) is one of the most widely offered forms of psychological treatment in current psychiatric practice. Originally developed as a treatment for anxiety disorders and depression, CBT is now applied across the spectrum of psychiatric disorders including an expanding range of somatoform disorders such as chronic fatigue syndrome, chronic pain, and irritable bowel syndrome (e.g., [1–3]). More recently, cognitive behavioral approaches for dissociative seizures [4–7], referred to here as psychogenic nonepileptic seizures (PNES), have been investigated.

Given that ~80% of patients with PNES have a history of medically unexplained presentations [8] and the evidence for CBT in treating somatoform disorders, it seems reasonable to assume that CBT may be helpful for PNES. Patients with PNES share a number of features with patients who have other somatoform disorders. In particular they experience considerable distress, hold strong physical illness attributions [9], avoid engaging in activities [6], and often present clinically with a history of difficult doctor–patient relations. Conventional cognitive behavioral techniques can be used to tackle distress and avoidance, but the symptom complexity of PNES may pose particular challenges for treatment. In particular, the dramatic paroxysmal and often convulsive episodes can include impaired responsiveness and amnesia, and result in injury.

Deary et al. [2] described a cognitive behavioral model of understanding somatoform disorders. General cognitive behavioral approaches, including developing an individualized formulation of the patient's problem, can also be applied to patients with PNES. The approaches include: focusing on disrupting vicious circles of maintaining factors such as avoidance behavior and the cognitive sequelae of childhood traumatic experiences – which are prevalent across the range of somatoform disorders [10] – tackling unhelpful thoughts, and addressing health anxiety and symptom focusing.

In addition to the standard ways in which CBT can be used for somatoform disorders, the special features of PNES suggest that specific cognitive behavioral techniques might be helpful. In particular, the paroxysmal nature of PNES and the associated symptoms of arousal invite comparisons with panic disorder. Although patients with PNES rarely report subjective anxiety during their seizures, somatic symptoms of arousal (e.g., chest tightness, palpitations, hyperventilation) are reported by ~60% of patients and agoraphobic avoidant behavior related to the seizures is three times more common in patients with PNES than in patients with localization-related epilepsy [6]. Based on these findings, Goldstein and Mellers [6] have described a model of PNES in which the seizures are seen as a dissociative response to arousal ("panic without panic") with avoidant behavior acting as an important maintaining factor. This model provides a rationale for applying CBT techniques traditionally associated with the treatment of panic disorder and agoraphobia. Other researchers have found that patients with PNES exhibit disproportionately elevated fear sensitivity on self-report measures when compared with patients with epilepsy [11]. It is of course also relevant that patients with PNES may display significantly distorted beliefs with the development of dysfunctional, often unconscious, repeating behavioral patterns with associated depressive affect. They demonstrate higher levels of general psychopathological symptoms, measured by the Symptom Check List (SCL-90-R), compared to patients with epileptic seizures (ES) [12], including somatization, phobic anxiety, interpersonal sensitivity, anxiety, and depression.

Gates and Rowan's Nonepileptic Seizures, 3rd edn. ed. Steven C. Schachter and W. Curt LaFrance, Jr. Published by Cambridge University Press. © S. Schachter and W. C. LaFrance, Jr. 2010.

To date the literature on psychological treatment of patients with PNES is limited [13], with no adequately designed randomized controlled trials having been reported. Some authors have described how CBT-related interventions may be applied to this patient group [14] and have incorporated elements of CBT into their, as yet uncontrolled, treatment studies [15, 16]. However, two research groups have evaluated CBT more systematically. LaFrance *et al.* conducted an open-label prospective trial of CBT for PNES in 21 patients with video-EEG-confirmed PNES [7, 17] using a protocol modified from a workbook on CBT for epilepsy [18, 19] and from a CBT manual [20]. Additionally, Goldstein *et al.* [5] have examined the outcome from a 12-session CBT intervention in an open trial for patients with PNES. The models underlying these studies and the resulting outcome data will be described in this chapter.

CBT for PNES at Brown Medical School, Rhode Island Hospital

Over the past five years, LaFrance and colleagues have designed, tested, and implemented a Beckian-based CBT structured, time-limited, short-term, present-oriented psychotherapy [21, 22] addressing cognitive distortions and promoting behavioral changes specifically for the PNES population and to address the comorbidities and the PNES directly. As in the epilepsy-based approach [18, 19], the current manualized therapy focused on the patient assuming control over their seizures and incorporated: an introduction contextualizing the individual's environment; a test on identifying moods, situations, and thoughts; training in healthy communication and support seeking; understanding central nervous system medications and seizures; conducting a functional behavioral analysis; learning relaxation techniques; examining external stressors and internal triggers; and preparing for life after completing the time-limited intervention. The therapy addressed mood-cognition-environment connections, automatic thoughts, catastrophic thinking, and somatic misinterpretations.

The CBT was given in 12 individual weekly sessions, each one hour in length, by a therapist trained in CBT for PNES treatment. Cognitive behavioral therapy was administered according to the manualized protocol devised by LaFrance's research group [23], adapted with permission from Reiter *et al.* [18]. The PNES treatment session content was as follows:

- Introduction — Introduction for the Patient: Understanding Seizures
- Week 1 — Making the Decision to Begin the Process of Taking Control
- Week 2 — Getting Support
- Week 3 — Deciding about your Medication Therapy
- Week 4 — Learning to Observe your Triggers
- Week 5 — Channelling Negative Emotions into Productive Outlets
- Week 6 — Relaxation Training
- Week 7 — Identifying your Pre-seizure Aura
- Week 8 — Dealing with External Life Stresses
- Week 9 — Dealing with Internal Issues and Conflicts
- Week 10 — Enhancing Personal Wellness: Learning to Reduce Tensions
- Week 11 — Other Seizure Symptoms
- Week 12 — Taking Control: An Ongoing Process

Missed CBT sessions were made up, if possible, during the same week of the scheduled appointment or by scheduling the session for the following week. Otherwise the next session was scheduled for the following week.

Participants who were unable to attend the CBT office appointments due to transportation limitations had some CBT sessions over the telephone [24–27]. The initial session took place in person to establish patient–therapist rapport, and to provide the patient with the treatment pack (forms, modules, mailing envelopes, etc.) that were to be used in future telephone sessions. Telephone CBT followed the format and duration of face-to-face sessions. All written homework assigned between sessions was reviewed over the phone and the therapist recorded the information for the study chart. Seizure calendars and self-report forms were faxed or mailed in envelopes included in the treatment pack for review every week. With participant consent, office CBT and telephone CBT sessions were audiotaped to ensure adherence and competence of therapy sessions.

Of the 21 patients treated with CBT at Rhode Island Hospital, 17 completed treatment (81% completion rate). Three patients with both ES and PNES who could clearly distinguish between their very different events were included. PNES frequencies decreased from a median of 4 seizures per week at enrollment to 0 per week upon conclusion of the sessions.

Comparing the beginning and end of treatment, a 50% seizure reduction was noted in 16 of the 21 participants, and 11 of the 17 completers reported no seizures by their final CBT session. Secondary outcome variables included depression, anxiety, somatic symptoms, quality-of-life scores, and psychosocial functioning. Mean scores of these scales showed improvement from baseline to final session using paired t-tests (p < 0.05) on intention-to-treat analysis. Depression scores improved, decreasing from an average of 19 to 13 on the Beck Depression Inventory-II [28] over the course of treatment. Davidson Trauma Scale scores [29] improved, decreasing from 58 to 35. Behaviorally, family functioning improved, changing from 2.03 to 1.66 (cutoff < 2.00) on the Family Assessment Device [30]. Coping techniques also improved, changing from self-controlling methods at baseline to positive reappraisal upon completion [31]. Quality-of-life scores improved from 46 to 62 on the Quality of Life in Epilepsy-31 scale [32].

CBT for PNES at the Maudsley Hospital, London

In the context of the general management of patients with PNES at the Maudsley Hospital, London [33] the CBT model, developed by Chalder [34], is based on the two-process, fear escape-avoidance model [35–37]. This proposes that fears are acquired through classical conditioning and maintained by operant conditioning (reinforcement). Within this model, temporally related environmental, cognitive, and sensory events can acquire, through classical conditioning, the qualities of profoundly distressing or life-threatening experiences (e.g., trauma, abuse) to produce intolerable outcomes (e.g., fear and distress). Where the classically conditioned events/triggers are external (e.g., environmental), "active" behavioral avoidance measures are taken by the individual. When triggers are internal/subjective experiences (i.e., cognitive/emotional/physiological cues), inhibitory mechanisms expressed as dissociation may become "best option" ways of *in situ* nonbehavioral escape/avoidance of experiential (cognitive and sensory) distress when the person is confronted with intolerable or fearful circumstances [38]. Such inhibitory experiential avoidance initially allows the person to continue to function, but becomes pathological if used often enough [39], becoming the default coping response in the face of subjective distress. The success of emotional avoidance in preventing the experience of distress reinforces its use. Following a subsequent, critical event (e.g., further trauma, unexpected reminders of the original trauma), more dramatic and intrusive dissociation (i.e., PNES) occurs in response to such cues. Safety behaviors and overt avoidance (e.g., escape and avoidance from feared events/seizure triggers, reassurance seeking) are then employed to avoid or escape from these triggers and thus to prevent PNES from occurring. The success of these strategies in reducing/preventing the experience of distress again reinforces their use. This is counterproductive, since the use of safety behaviors, overt avoidance, and external reinforcements (including responses by relatives), maintain the relationship between seizure cues and PNES, and attention remains focused on the possibility of seizure-related symptoms [5].

Treatment

Goldstein *et al.*'s [5] open study applying this model of CBT to 20 patients with PNES, of whom 16 completed treatment, was developed from Chalder's earlier single case report [34]. Treatment comprised 12 CBT sessions held weekly/fortnightly with a trained CBT therapist. The treatment, which also included seizure diary completion, the use of homework tasks, and a problem-solving approach, was structured as follows.

Stage 1: Engagement and rationale giving

A maintenance and treatment rationale, stressing the non-volitional but "real" nature of PNES, included a discussion of the interaction between cognitions, physiological/emotional responses, and behaviors [40]. As patients may not be able to describe an identifiable trauma, initially focusing on identifying a trauma was felt potentially to be unhelpful. The engagement process outlined the "switching off" nature of PNES in response to cues that represent distressing situations or thoughts. While some consider this as an evolutionary response to threat [41, 42], Goldstein *et al.*'s [5] approach was to explain the nature of dissociation using everyday examples of alterations in selective attention, viewing the manifestation of PNES as an extreme occurrence of this phenomenon and representing a defensive response to anxiety. Finally, the rationale explained that efforts to avoid future risk and the use of safety behaviors maintained PNES occurrence [34], while persisting uncertainty over diagnosis, low mood, over-involvement of family members, and benefits of the sick role maintained fear-related cognitions and the perceived need to use safety behaviors. With their consent, patients' carers/significant others were involved in the process of engagement and later in treatment to facilitate generalization of treatment gains [34].

Stage 2: Seizure control techniques

If an inability to tolerate warning cues, and their interpretation as precursors of severe distress, leads to the occurrence of PNES as a conditioned response, or to the adoption of avoidance or safety behaviors to prevent PNES from occurring, then improved ability to tolerate distress-related cues should result in a reduction of dissociative responses. Initially, exposure to arousal-provoking stimuli leads to the conditioned dissociative response, making the desired outcome (i.e., habituation to such arousal) impossible. To increase opportunities for exposure and habituation, responses that compete with or terminate cues (warning signs) for dissociation were taught, for use at the first sign of seizure-related cues. These were based on approaches used to reduce ES occurrence [43–45] and included attentional distraction and refocusing. Distraction is thought to reduce misinterpretation of sensations and increase acceptance, which might otherwise lead to increased arousal and seizures. Relaxation and controlled breathing were also taught since they may directly reduce physiological sensations (e.g., dizziness, tension, hyperventilation, etc.) and avert the conditioned dissociative response.

Stage 3: Reducing avoidance: exposure techniques

If safety behaviors maintain the fear/arousal inducing effect of triggers, then decreasing their use should reduce fear/arousal and seizure frequency and improve quality of life. Patients were therefore encouraged to face avoided situations using a hierarchy of increasing difficulty, employing competing responses to avert dissociation at the earliest opportunity.

Stage 4: Seizure-related cognitions

Approaching avoided situations may elicit arousal and may lead to the occurrence of negative automatic thoughts (NATs) related to the potential occurrence of seizures and a range of assumptions related to self-esteem and earlier trauma [22, 46]. These may include thoughts such as, "My seizures are dangerous," "If I have a seizure in public, people will shun me," and/or "People are untrustworthy and will not help me if I collapse in public." Treatment involved a range of standard cognitive techniques to challenge NATs, including the identification of thinking errors such as catastrophizing or black-and-white thinking, as well as helpful alternatives. Patients' causal attributions were not challenged directly but were discussed openly, and the therapist attempted to broaden their perspective to encourage the adoption of alternative, healthy coping strategies. Challenging NATs was also undertaken to improve patients' mood more generally and increase positive beliefs about seizure control.

In those individuals for whom trauma had been identified at the start of treatment or had emerged during the process of treatment, a range of strategies was used to encourage appropriate emotional processing using established models (e.g., [47, 48]). Extensive questioning about possible traumatic origins of seizures was not undertaken since this risks eliciting false memories and alienating the patient. In practice, strategies described in stages 3 and 4 were utilized flexibly as appropriate.

Stage 5: Relapse prevention

Therapeutic progress was reviewed towards the end of treatment and goals for any outstanding matters reformulated, with an agreed time scale for their attainment. Issues that might result in relapse and how to tackle them were discussed, along with means of maintaining the achieved goals and the use of problem-solving techniques to deal with setbacks.

Outcome

Following the 12 CBT sessions, a reduction in median frequency of PNES was found not only in the 16 patients completing treatment but also with an intention-to-treat analysis including the 4 patients who did not complete treatment. Mean seizure frequency fell from 18 per month (median 4) to almost 3 per month (median 1.5) at the end of treatment, with a mean of 2.6 seizures (median 1.0) at a 6-month follow up. Of the 16 treatment completers, 13 (81.25%) achieved at least a 50% reduction in seizure frequency at follow-up compared to pretreatment seizure frequency. At 6-month follow-up, 4/16 treatment completers had been seizure-free for the entire follow-up period and another 3 reported no seizures in the month prior to follow-up. A significant improvement was found on the Work and Social Adjustment Scale

[49]. Fear Questionnaire [49] scores indicated a significant reduction in self-reported avoidance of feared situations. Anxiety and depression scores also reduced following treatment and improvement was maintained at follow-up. Following treatment, patients showed a reduction in their beliefs that their seizures had physical causes [50] and in their perceptions of the negative consequences of their seizures. A trend toward improved occupational status was also found.

Therapeutic questions not yet answered by research and therapeutic challenges posed by patients with PNES

LaFrance et al.'s [7, 17] and Goldstein et al.'s [5] studies provided similar feasibility and tolerance data for their respective CBT interventions as well as data to support future multicenter randomized controlled trials for PNES. There are many questions concerning predictors of outcome not yet answered by research as well as therapeutic challenges posed by this patient group.

In terms of predicting outcome, research needs to address the following issues:

1. The CBT approaches described by Goldstein et al. were applied to patients without comorbid ES, but up to 10% of patients with PNES will have a past/current history of actual epilepsy [51]. Rusch et al. [15] suggested that comorbid ES does not reduce the effectiveness of a psychotherapeutic approach in reducing PNES frequency. This idea is supported by a case report in an adolescent boy with mixed ES/PNES and a diagnosis of factitious disorder [52] and by LaFrance et al.'s study, which included patients with mixed ES/PNES, and found reduced frequency of PNES [7]. However, this needs to be determined empirically in controlled trials.
2. It is unclear what impact comorbid psychiatric diagnoses have on outcome and whether differing treatment approaches need to be matched with personality profiles [53, 54] to achieve good outcome. Similarly, the extent to which treatment needs to be highly individualized is unclear, as are the differences between patients who improve very quickly and those who do not [55].
3. No studies have demonstrated whether patients' acceptance/nonacceptance of their diagnosis and acceptance/understanding of a CBT treatment rationale affects treatment outcome. It will also be important to know whether the influence of such factors might be modified by the patient's previous medical and psychosocial history, their cognitive ability, illness attributions, reactions of families/carers to the diagnosis and treatment, and by financial issues such as government or insurance benefits.
4. LaFrance et al. [7, 17] reported an improvement in family functioning, and in quality-of-life measures, and Goldstein et al. [5] reported a trend towards improved work status. It remains unclear just how much CBT can effect broad change in the lives of patients with PNES and over what time course this might occur.
5. Understanding mechanisms of change is helpful in understanding how treatment works. Future studies should assess potential mediating factors such as catastrophizing beliefs or symptom focusing at regular stages throughout treatment and follow-up.
6. In some patients, a history of a specific sexual or physical trauma may simply not exist. Instead, it may be necessary to consider the presence of other less typically reported stressors (e.g., being bullied, developmental neglect) or other psychological difficulties, such as poor coping resources when dealing with stress/illness or low self-esteem. It is not known whether such patients do better following CBT than those with a clear trauma history or whether the type and timing of abuse (childhood vs. adult) determines the severity of the PNES disorder and the response to CBT. No information exists as to whether the different semiologies seen in PNES respond differentially to CBT.

More general therapeutic challenges posed by this patient group include the following:

1. When patients do report an abuse history, the traumatic events' effects upon individuals may be so extensive that they cannot perceive alternatives or that what they experienced may indeed be extraordinary. They may blame themselves or experience significant, unexpressed anger. In such cases, interventions from other CBT-related approaches such as schema therapy [56] may be helpful, but they also require evaluation in this patient group.

2. During therapy it may be difficult for patients to identify warnings/triggers for PNES since they may be "normal" feelings/sensations (e.g., feeling warm). Additionally, triggers may be subtle reminders of past traumas and may be difficult to elicit as may occur more generally in posttraumatic stress disorder [47]. Patients may also have difficulty in expressing their feelings/emotions that may precede seizures, although no conclusive evidence exists for alexithymia in patients with PNES [57, 58].

3. Safety behaviors and fear of stigma can make it difficult for patients to return for treatment in outpatient settings, so that engagement and the smooth flow of therapy become disrupted, leading to high dropout rates. Treatment providers in neurology and mental health contend that there is also a lack of appropriately trained and competent psychological therapists familiar with PNES, which means that patients often have to travel long distances to access specialist care.

4. If patients present to hospital emergency departments, they may receive conflicting messages about the nature of their disorder, which reinforce dysfunctional seizure-related beliefs and behaviors, undermining the CBT intervention. Consistency between all providers involved in the care of patients with PNES is essential [59] although difficult to achieve. In addition, medical and paramedical staff should remember that while patients may not be able to respond to their environment during their seizures, they may recall subsequently hearing ambulance staff making negative comments like "pinch her, she's just pretending."

Conclusions

Given the preliminary positive findings from applications of CBT to patients with PNES, and the rationale derived more broadly from the treatment of medically unexplained symptoms for using this therapeutic approach with PNES, evaluation via randomized controlled trials is now warranted. Reuber *et al.* [16] caution that undertaking controlled studies in this patient group may be difficult and that such studies require well-developed treatment protocols for the assessment of treatment integrity/fidelity, especially where more than one therapist is involved. They also suggest that the uncertainties of randomization may be unattractive to patients if treatment is otherwise available outside the treatment study. While these caveats are important, they should not detract from the development and testing of more specific CBT models to inform treatment. This may require both further open trials as well as more experimentally focused studies that examine psychological and physiological correlates of this disorder [6].

References

1. Kroenke K, Swindle R. Cognitive-behavioral therapy for somatization and symptom syndromes: a critical review of controlled clinical trials. *Psychother Psychosom* 2000;**69**:205–15.
2. Deary V, Chalder T, Sharpe M. The cognitive behavioural model of medically unexplained symptoms: a theoretical and empirical review. *Clin Psychol Rev* 2007;**27**:781–97.
3. Henningsen P. Management of somatoform disorders in neurology. *Neurol Rehabil* 2007;**13**:87–9.
4. Brown RJ, Trimble MR. Dissociative psychopathology, non-epileptic seizures, and neurology. *J Neurol Neurosurg Psychiatry* 2000;**69**:285–9.
5. Goldstein LH, Deale AC, Mitchell-O'Malley SJ, Toone BK, Mellers JD. An evaluation of cognitive behavioral therapy as a treatment for dissociative seizures: a pilot study. *Cogn Behav Neurol* 2004;**17**:41–9.
6. Goldstein LH, Mellers JD. Ictal symptoms of anxiety, avoidance behaviour, and dissociation in patients with dissociative seizures. *J Neurol Neurosurg Psychiatry* 2006;**77**:616–21.
7. LaFrance WC, Jr, Miller IW, Ryan CE, *et al.* Cognitive behavioral therapy for psychogenic nonepileptic seizures. *Epilepsy Behav* 2009;**14**(4):591–6.
8. Bowman ES, Markand ON. Psychodynamics and psychiatric diagnoses of pseudoseizure subjects. *Am J Psychiatry* 1996;**153**:57–63.
9. Stone J, Binzer M, Sharpe M. Illness beliefs and locus of control: a comparison of patients with pseudoseizures and epilepsy. *J Psychsom Res* 2004;**66**:541–7.
10. Roelofs K, Spinhoven P. Trauma and medically unexplained symptoms. Towards an integration of cognitive and neuro-biological accounts. *Clin Psychol Rev* 2007;**27**:798–820.
11. Hixson JD, Balcer LJ, Glosser G, French JA. Fear sensitivity and the psychological profile of patients with psychogenic nonepileptic seizures. *Epilepsy Behav* 2006;**9**:587–92.
12. Prueter C, Schultz-Venrath U, Rimpau W. Dissociative and associated psychopathological symptoms in

patients with epilepsy, pseudoseizures, and both seizure forms. *Epilepsia* 2002;**43**:188–92.

13. Brooks JL, Baker GA, Goodfellow L, Bodde N, Aldenkamp A. Behavioural treatments for non-epileptic attack disorder [Systematic Review]. *Cochrane Database Syst Rev* 2007;(3):CD006370.

14. Reuber M, Howlett S, Kemp S. Psychologic treatment of patients with psychogenic nonepileptic seizures. *Expert Rev Neurother* 2005;**56**:737–52.

15. Rusch MD, Morris GL, Allen L, Lathrop L. Psychological treatment of nonepileptic events. *Epilepsy Behav* 2001;**2**:277–83.

16. Reuber M, Burness C, Howlett S, Brazier J, Grunewald R. Tailored psychotherapy for patients with functional neurological symptoms: a pilot study. *J Psychosom Res* 2007;**63**:625–32.

17. LaFrance WC, Jr, Blum AS, Miller IW, Ryan C, Keitner G. Cognitive behavioral therapy or family therapy for psychogenic nonepileptic seizures (NES). *Epilepsia* 2008;**49** Suppl 7:273–4.

18. Reiter JM, Andrews DJ. *Taking Control of Your Epilepsy. A Workbook for Patients and Professionals.* Santa Rosa, CA: The BASICS Book Company, 1987.

19. Reiter JM, Andrews DJ. A neurobehavioral approach for treatment of complex partial epilepsy: efficacy. *Seizure* 2000;**9**:198–203.

20. Greenberger D, Padesky CA. *Mind Over Mood: Change How You Feel by Changing the Way You Think.* New York: Guilford Press, 1995.

21. Beck JS. *Cognitive Therapy: Basics and Beyond.* New York: Guilford Press, 1995.

22. Beck AT. *Cognitive Therapy and the Emotional Disorders.* New York: International Universities Press, 1976.

23. LaFrance WC, Jr. *CBT NES Treatment Manual.* Providence, RI: Brown Medical School, 2005.

24. Beckner V, Vella L, Howard I, Mohr DC. Alliance in two telephone-administered treatments: relationship with depression and health outcomes. *J Consult Clin Psychol* 2007;**75**:508–12.

25. Mohr DC, Likosky W, Bertagnolli A, et al. Telephone-administered cognitive-behavioral therapy for the treatment of depressive symptoms in multiple sclerosis. *J Consult Clin Psychol* 2000;**68**:356–61.

26. Mohr DC, Hart SL, Julian L, et al. Telephone-administered psychotherapy for depression. *Arch Gen Psychiatry* 2005;**62**:1007–14.

27. Mohr DC, Hart S, Vella L. Reduction in disability in a randomized controlled trial of telephone-administered cognitive-behavioral therapy. *Health Psychol* 2007;**26**:554–63.

28. Beck AT, Steer RA, Brown GK. *Manual for The Beck Depression Inventory – Second Edition (BDI-II).* San Antonio: Psychological Corporation, 1996.

29. Davidson J. *Davidson Trauma Scale.* New York: Multi-Health Systems, Inc, 1996.

30. Miller IW, Epstein NB, Bishop DS, Keitner GI. The McMaster Family Assessment Device: reliability and validity. *J Marital Fam Ther* 1985;**11**:345–56.

31. Vitaliano PP, Russo J, Carr JE, Maiuro RD, Becker J. The ways of coping checklist: revision and psychometric properties. *Multivariate Behav Res* 1985;**20**:3–26.

32. Vickrey BG, Perrine K, Hays RD, et al. *Quality of Life in Epilepsy. QOLIE-31. Scoring Manual.* Version 1.0 edn. Santa Monica, CA: RAND, 1993.

33. Mellers JDC. The approach to patients with 'non-epileptic seizures'. *Postgrad Med J* 2005;**81**: 498–504.

34. Chalder T. Non-epileptic attacks: a cognitive behavioural in a single case approach with a four-year follow-up. *Clin Psychol Psychother* 1996;**3**:291–7.

35. Miller NE. Studies of fear as an acquirable drive. *J Exp Psychol* 1948;**38**:89–101.

36. Mowrer OH. Anxiety reduction and learning. *J Exp Psychol* 1946;**27**:497–516.

37. Mowrer OH. *Learning Theory and Behavior.* New York: Wiley, 1960.

38. Hayes SC, Wilson KG, Gifford EV, Follette VM, Strosahl K. Experiential avoidance and behavioral disorders: a functional dimensional approach to diagnosis and treatment. *J Consult Clin Psychol* 1996;**64**:1152–68.

39. Hilgard ER. *Divided Consciousness: Multiple Controls in Human Thought and Action.* New York: Wiley, 1977.

40. Lang PJ. Fear reduction and fear behavior: problems in treating a construct. In: Shilen JM, ed. *Research in Psychotherapy*, Vol. III. Washington, DC: American Psychological Association. 1968; 90–103.

41. Janet P. L'amnésia et la dissociation des souvenir par l'émotion. *Journal de Psychologie* 1904;**1**:417–53.

42. Nijenhuis ERS, van der Hart O, Kruger K, Steele K. Somatoform dissociation, reported abuse and animal defence-like reactions. *Aust NZJ Psychiatry* 2004;**38**:678–86.

43. Dahl J, Melin L, Lund L. Effects of a contingent relaxation treatment program on adults with refractory epileptic seizures. *Epilepsia* 1987;**28**:125–32.

44. Dahl J, Brorson LO, Melin L. Effects of a broad-spectrum behavioral medicine treatment program on children with refractory epileptic seizures: an 8-year follow-up. *Epilepsia* 1992;**33**:98–102.

45. Dahl JA, Melin L, Leissner P. Effects of a behavioral intervention on epileptic seizure behavior and paroxysmal activity: a systematic replication of three cases of children with intractable epilepsy. *Epilepsia* 1988;**29**:172–83.

46. Beck AT. *Depression: Clinical, Experimental and Theoretical Aspects.* New York: Harper & Row, 1967.

47. Ehlers A, Clark DM. A cognitive model of posttraumatic stress disorder. *Behav Res Ther* 2000;**38**:319–45.

48. Kennerley H. *Overcoming Childhood Trauma.* London: Robinson, 2000.

49. Marks IM. *Behavioural Psychotherapy. Maudsley Pocket Book of Clinical Management.* Bristol, UK: Wright, 1986.

50. Weinman J, Petrie KJ, Moss-Morris R, Horne R. The Illness Perception Questionnaire: a new method for assessing the cognitive representation of illness. *Psychol Health* 1996;**11**:431–45.

51. Benbadis SR, Agrawal V, Tatum IV, WO. How many patients with psychogenic nonepileptic seizures also have epilepsy? *Neurology* 2001;**57**:915–17.

52. McLean T, Dyer C. Treatment of psychogenic pseudoseizures in an adolescent with a history of epilepsy. *Clin Psychol* 2003;**7**(2):109–20.

53. Reuber M, Pukrop R, Bauer J, Derfuss R, Elger CE. Multidimensional assessment of personality in patients with psychogenic non-epileptic seizures. *J Neurol Neurosurg Psychiatry* 2004;**75**:743–8.

54. Goldstein LH. Assessment of patients with psychogenic non-epileptic seizures. *J Neurol Neurosurg Psychiatry* 2004;**75**:667–8.

55. Reuber M. Psychogenic nonepileptic seizures: answers and questions. *Epilepsy Behav* 2008;**12**:622–35.

56. Young JE, Klosko JS, Weishaar ME. *Schema Therapy: A Practitioner's Guide.* New York: Guilford Press, 2004.

57. Bewley J, Murphy PN, Mallows J, Baker GA. Does alexithymia differentiate between patients with nonepileptic seizures, patients with epilepsy, and nonpatient controls? *Epilepsy Behav* 2005;**7**:430–7.

58. Tojek TM, Lumley M, Barkley G, Mahr G, Thomas A. Stress and other psychosocial characteristics of patients with psychogenic nonepileptic seizures. *Psychosomatics* 2000;**41**:221–6.

59. Goldstein LH. Treatment and rehabilitation of neuropsychiatric disorders. In: Halligan PW, Kischka U, Marshall JC, eds. *Handbook of Clinical Neuropsychology.* Oxford: Oxford University Press. 2003; 657–73.

Section 5 Chapter 30

Treatment considerations for psychogenic nonepileptic seizures

Group psychotherapy treatment for psychogenic nonepileptic seizures

Kim D. Bullock

Group psychotherapy was formally developed during World War II in order to care for the large number of psychiatric cases in understaffed military hospitals. It has tended to transcend theoretical orientations and diagnoses, which may make it a highly compatible treatment for the heterogeneous nature of psychogenic nonepileptic seizures (PNES) [1–3]. Corrective emotional experiences, self-awareness, and modeling were originally seen as the mechanisms of change. Psychoanalytic influence encouraged the eliciting of unconscious conflicts in group leaders and members. The 1950s brought about Moreno's [4] development of psychodrama which emphasized spontaneity and action. The early 1960s gave birth to the community mental health movement in the US which led to further growth and application of short-term group therapies to improve ego functioning and social skills. The influential Sullivanian perspective introduced by Irv Yalom [5] focused on here-and-now interpersonal problems. More recent focus has been on integrating cognitive behavioral therapy (CBT) with interpersonal approaches [6]. The above theoretical orientations are just a few of the many that represent contemporary group psychotherapy.

The modern pluralistic approach to group therapy may lend itself well to the treatment of PNES. The efficacy of group therapy is well established across a variety of therapeutic orientations and clinical diagnoses in psychiatry [7]. Individual therapy for PNES involving different theoretical orientations such as cognitive-behavioral and psychodynamic have been reported to be helpful in open trials [8, 9]. Open-label trials of group therapies have also shown utility in PNES, which will be discussed in detail in this chapter. From these studies, it is speculated that group therapies, regardless of orientation, may also be of benefit to patients with PNES.

As research moves forward, it may be possible to tease out which orientations or therapeutic factors may be most helpful in which subpopulations of patients with PNES. An example of this type of progress has been the well documented research on group therapy effectiveness in adults with histories of childhood sexual abuse [10, 11]. Systematic short-term focused treatment has been shown in one study to be significantly superior to prolonged analytic group therapy in patients with a history of intrafamilial childhood abuse [12]. One could foresee the possibility of a PNES subgroup-driven orientation to group therapy based on studies like these.

This chapter will review the current literature and evidence for using group therapy in the treatment of PNES. It will then explore the rationale and motivations for pursuing further research on the effectiveness of this treatment modality. Finally, a summary will be presented of the observational experiences and group format used for the past seven years with patients with PNES at Stanford University's outpatient Behavior Medicine Clinic. This information may help institutions and clinicians who are considering using a group therapy model when treating patients with PNES.

Studies of group therapy for PNES

To date no randomized controlled studies of group therapy have been performed for PNES. The following is a review of the literature involving group therapy specifically for PNES. There are three prospective uncontrolled trials reporting the specific use of group therapy in patients with PNES, all of which show positive findings.

In 2002, Prigatano and coworkers [13] completed the first prospective unblinded study of group

Section 5: Treatment considerations for PNES

therapy for PNES. The therapy was considered psycho-educational in orientation with a focus on the "facts" about PNES. Exploring triggers associated with seizures was encouraged. Two distinctly separate six-month group psychotherapy sessions occurred. The first group had no exclusionary criteria and involved six subjects. The second group involved seven participants with the following exclusionary criteria: ongoing litigation, low intelligence, head trauma, and reluctance to see any connection between seizures and psychological trauma. Subjects in both groups met for 24 weekly 1.5-hour sessions. Participants completed a log of seizures from the past week at the beginning of every session. Following the log, a test of previous session content (typically three to six true-or-false questions) was administered. The previous week's discussion was reviewed. The group was then opened up for discussion of any feelings or topic.

Results of this study combined both groups, consisting of nine patients who attended 50% or more of the sessions. Six out of the nine completers reported a decrease in PNES frequency. Two reported no change. One patient noted an exacerbation of events. Higher self-reported seizure frequency was correlated with paranoid ideation as measured on the Minnesota Multiphasic Personality Inventory-2. Patients in the first group were observed and described as being more hostile and openly angry. The second group was described as internalizing their anger. Both groups were observed to have problems with feelings of being overwhelmed, anger, as well as social isolation and attachment dysfunction. Interestingly, it was noted in both groups that a planned absence of the female psychiatrist coleader negatively affected attendance.

The investigators stressed the need for concomitant individual therapy in order for the group participants to have an additional forum to deal with issues emerging in the group therapy discussions. The authors hypothesized that patients receiving the diagnosis of not "true" epilepsy rekindled earlier life experiences of not being believed when reporting childhood sexual abuse.

In 2004, the second study of PNES group therapy by Zaroff and colleagues [14] was reported and again emphasized psycho-education. At the beginning of each session, subjects were given handouts, read out loud by coleaders, containing information on a single topic. Sequential order of topic presentation included: (1) PNES, (2) anger, (3) trauma and abuse, (4) depression and anxiety, (5) somatization tendencies, (6) quality of life, (7) paths toward health, (8) stress-coping techniques, (9) topic review, and (10) psycho-education termination session. Initial therapy began with a focus on the involuntary nature of motor and psychological symptoms. Subsequent sessions explored the role of anger and trauma. Seeking treatment of comorbid psychiatric problems was highly encouraged. Deep breathing and relaxation techniques were taught. Coping strategies were emphasized.

Ten patients entered this study and seven completed the majority of the ten one-hour weekly sessions. Two patients had a decrease in PNES frequency. One had an increase. Four of the seven completers had no change in seizure frequency, but three of these had already experienced a cessation of events before the group began. The authors reported decreases in posttraumatic and dissociative symptoms. An increase in more direct task-based coping style rather than an emotion-based approach was noted on the Coping Inventory for Stressful Situations (CISS). There was also a trend toward improved quality of life. The recognition and interaction with other people of the same diagnosis was reported as beneficial by PNES subjects. The small sample size and lack of control group limited the power of this study, but the results are promising. The authors suggest more studies of group therapy be designed in the future taking into consideration gender, intellectual level, PNES etiology, and demographics.

The third paper was a pilot study reported in 2008, in which this writer was an author [15]. In contrast to the psycho-educational focus of the studies noted above, this study focused on a psychodynamic group therapy format. The group started with a simple educational format to introduce an understanding of PNES. Psychodynamic therapy encourages the activation of the group in the treatment of the members and minimizes the importance of the therapist. The theory highlights the subjectivity of an individual's experiences based on their internal world. Group process is considered more essential than structural process. The hypothesis supposes that clients improve by relating to each other in an unstructured way. Therapeutic foci are patients' intrapsychic and interpersonal problems. The goal of the therapy is to facilitate the patients' awareness of these problems in order to make changes.

The group in this study focused on the conceptualization of seizures as an expression of hidden or unconscious emotions. Therapy addressed developing conscious and verbal expression of emotional upset instead of somatic displays. Developing direct and assertive communications of aggressive and negative feelings, rather than passive and avoidant ones, was emphasized. The participants were encouraged to investigate the precipitants of their seizures so that they could formulate the connections between the types of situations that appeared to impact the frequency of their events.

During sessions, self-relaxation and hypnosis were used to minimize and contain seizure activity. If a seizure occurred, the session would continue while one of the coleaders would assist the participant using relaxation and self-hypnosis techniques. The group and leaders attempted to send an overall message that PNES should not interrupt normal activity. Outside of the group, the members created a support network. Issues from outside of the group were also revisited during sessions. Of note, five of the patients in this study were seen simultaneously with this author, who was not a group leader, in a cognitive behaviorally oriented individual therapy.

Significant interpersonal changes took place during this group. One subject initiated a divorce with a subsequent remission of all PNES. One subject regained entitled financial independence by assertively confronting family members. Participants better defined interpersonal boundaries and the use of appropriate limit setting. One subject improved once she was able to express negative feelings to her husband and children openly. Several members were able to recognize their behaviors as reenactments of abusive childhood relationships.

Twelve patients entered this study and seven completed at least 75% of the 32 weekly sessions. Two of the noncompleters moved out of the area before being able to complete the study, one noncompleter decided transportation to the group was too difficult, and two subjects did not attend 75% of sessions. In completers, the Beck Depression Inventory and the Global Severity Index of the Symptom Checklist-90 showed statistically significant improvement. There was also a significant overall decrease in PNES frequency. The mean monthly frequency of PNES improved most impressively, declining to less than 10% of baseline level. Seizures remitted completely (except for infrequent mild events due to stress-induced exacerbations) in four of seven patients. Three patients, who upon study entry needed wheelchairs or canes, ended the study fully ambulatory. Long-term follow-up, two years after the trial, revealed that five of the seven completers were seizure free with the exception of occasional but infrequent mild exacerbations of PNES activity during identifiable stress periods. These data suggested that group therapy focusing on interpersonal issues could benefit patients with PNES.

The differing results between the three aforementioned studies of PNES and group therapy most likely represent the differing treatment designs. Comparison of the studies is difficult given these differences. The more robust improvement seen in the last study may be due to differences in duration, treatment modality, and subject variables. The study by Barry et al. [15] involved a relatively long treatment period of 32 weeks compared to 24 and 10 weeks in the previous studies. Perhaps there is a dose-effect response in terms of weeks and hourly session time that mediates a group's effectiveness. The third study was psycho-dynamically oriented rather than psycho-educational. Of note was the weekly CBT that was delivered simultaneous to group therapy in five of the seven completers. It is unclear how many of the subjects in the first two studies had simultaneous individual therapy. If individual therapy was ongoing, the frequency, orientation, and therapist training are unknown and may influence any possible adjunctive or synergistic effects. Perceived experience of group-therapist leaders is also a variable that may influence outcome in group interventions [16, 17]. There may have been differences among study leaders and client's perceptions of their experience. Other unknown variables may be responsible for the differing outcomes between studies of group therapy.

The three studies described show promise regarding possible benefits of group therapy for PNES. Further studies using blinding, randomization, and comparing treatment groups to waitlist/minimal treatment controls are needed to better establish efficacy. If efficacy is documented, further trials to separate treatment-specific effects would also be useful.

Rationale for group therapy

One may wonder why group therapy should be pursued as a treatment option for PNES, especially if individual therapies are found effective. It is often assumed that group therapy is a diluted or less rigorous form of treatment. Meta-analyses reveal there is actually little difference in efficacy between group and individual therapy when directly comparing identical therapy formats within the same study [7]. Efficacy being equal, there are some benefits to group therapy compared to individual therapy that may be particularly meaningful in PNES.

Economy

Although individual treatment can be effective, it can be time consuming and costly. The individual approach may limit the number of patients who could benefit from another model. Group-based interventions can reduce costs and expand the capacity of a treatment program. Perhaps the foremost reason to pursue research and trials of group therapy for PNES comes from this economy-of-scale principle. The cost-effectiveness of group therapy may help patients unable to access mental health treatment through traditional means. In settings where nonsocialized medicine is delivered, this is particularly meaningful. Patients with limited resources or insurance benefits may be able to obtain care that is otherwise unobtainable. Third-party payers may be more willing to pay the cost of weekly group therapy over that of individual psychotherapy, especially if found equally effective and less costly. Managed care patients who have exceeded the number of individual psychotherapy sessions for the year may have group sessions available that can prolong treatment engagement. Reported lifetime cost per patient with PNES in the US has been estimated at $100 000 [18]. Patients with PNES have a high utilization of medical and emergency care as do similar groups with a history of childhood maltreatment [19]. Reducing these costs by using less of limited healthcare resources may have societal benefits as well.

Dose effect

Group therapy may be a way to reach an adequate threshold "dose" of mental health services. Even when individual psychotherapy is available on a once- or even twice-weekly basis, this is often still not the adequate level of care for the severity of some patients' symptoms. Group therapy may be the necessary adjunctive treatment to individual therapy to reach a higher level of care. Many partial psychiatric hospitalization programs are not available to patients with PNES because of programs' safety concerns due to seizure activity. Adjunctive group therapy can act as a bridge between hospitalization and weekly therapy.

Treatment of comorbid conditions

Group therapy can address a patient's comorbid conditions effectively. Proven efficacy in similar and comorbid disorders may be justification for use of group therapy. A small number of patients have both epilepsy and PNES. Interestingly, reduction in epileptic seizure frequency has been found in one case report of short-term group intervention for adults with epilepsy [20]. Group therapy has also been found efficacious in the treatment of depression as evaluated by McDermut et al. [21]. Many patients with PNES are reported to have poorer neuropsychological functioning, which may respond similarly to patients with mild cognitive impairment who received cognitive behavioral group therapy [22]. Finally, group therapy effectiveness is well documented in adults with histories of childhood sexual abuse [10, 11].

Ripple effect

There are therapeutic benefits that a group provides that no other treatment can. A breakthrough in one patient can have a ripple effect within the group as a whole. The change occurring in one patient sometimes elicits changes in another, perhaps via modeling behavior. For example, one patient may have a remission of seizures by including a 20-minute nap in her daily schedule. This witnessed improvement in one member may inspire otherwise ambivalent members to add active relaxation techniques into their day. A quantum group effect thus cascades from a single moment of change in one group member.

Witnessing others in various stages of change may help patients move more quickly from one phase to another. For example, witnessing another member's denial or secondary gain may lead another member to contemplate or to identify his/her own resistance. From motivational interviewing theory, benefits are ensured at whatever stage of change a patient finds him/herself to be: pre-contemplative, contemplative, action, maintenance, or relapse [23].

Social support

Each problem a patient brings up in group is addressed not by a single therapist, but by many others in the room thinking about the problem from different perspectives. Many times fellow patients' experiences have more legitimacy than a therapist's recommendation. Supportive group members can strategize with each other on how to gain appropriate resources to care for themselves. An immediate change in an individual's social support status occurs with the initiation of a group. Formerly isolated patients suddenly have a social network to rely on.

Unique change inducing factors

Irv Yalom [6] suggests there are 11 primary factors unique to a group that induce change: instillation of hope, universality, direct advice, altruism, corrective recapitulation, socializing, imitative behavior, interpersonal learning, cohesiveness, catharsis, and existential factors. The corrective recapitulation of one's family of origin may be particularly important in patients with PNES, who tend to view their families as more dysfunctional in regard to communication compared to patients with epilepsy. Family members of patients with PNES report difficulties defining roles [24], whereas the patients perceive their families as displaying less commitment and support to each other as measured by family cohesion scales. They also report less emphasis on ethical issues and values than both epilepsy and control groups [25].

Suggestions for PNES groups

At present, casting a wide net by using a multidisciplinary approach may be the most prudent when treating PNES using group therapy. This is exemplified by the eclectic group therapy format provided for patients with PNES at Stanford University Medical Center's outpatient Behavior Medicine Clinic. This method draws on strengths from various theoretical orientations for group therapy.

Intake interview

Most patients are referred to this treatment group from the Stanford Comprehensive Epilepsy Center after the diagnosis of PNES has been established through video-EEG monitoring. An individual intake interview by the group leader is then used to assess the appropriateness of a patient's participation. The intake provides an opportunity to introduce the structure of the group to the patient. The group is described as a self-help group designed to develop skills to manage and possibly stop seizures as well as feel better.

The patient is told that each week the leader will introduce a therapeutic technique and its associated paperwork. Homework may be required. A leader may also describe a vignette about how this technique has helped other patients. In this way the leadership is re-established each week and remains directive. Coleaders may be present but usually have less direct and more observational roles. Coleaders or guest presenters may sometimes present a weekly topic and take on a temporary leadership role.

The patient is then told about the ritualized check-in each week that occurs after topic presentations. During this time each person has a chance to voice his or her own concerns. Group members are encouraged and helped to address a life problem using the presented techniques. Group members are encouraged to be co-therapist when a designated member asks for help. The leader determines whose problem and in what order group members will be addressed. The rationale for the highly structured format is to provide some stability for most patients who, at time of entry, are feeling helpless and out of control.

Group member relationships are neither encouraged nor discouraged, but in our experience group members become powerfully bonded. Ground rules such as not discussing issues or information disclosed in group outside of group are required of members. Safety issues around seizures are also discussed at this time. Privacy and preserving the autonomy of all members is emphasized especially in regard to health information.

It is at this intake interview the inevitable question arises; what to do if someone has a seizure in the group? To manage behavioral events during meetings, our groups have had tremendous success implementing operant conditioning techniques to minimize seizure frequency, duration, and severity. When seizures occur, a patient's safety is quickly assessed and ensured by the group leader. Minimal attention is paid to the seizure and a business-like attitude is assumed. The group is instructed to do the same and ignore the seizure as much as possible. If the event is too disruptive (i.e., verbal outbursts), patients are moved to another room until seizures stop. This process allows the group to keep running without disruption by behavioral events. This approach also avoids the seizures becoming the focus of the group. Honesty and consensus about this method is maintained with all group members. Empirical validation with the technique comes from operant conditioning reports from inpatient settings [26, 27]. Information about the conduct of the group is shared in a transparent way with the patient during the intake interview and can model how they decide to behave outside the group.

Psycho-education

The first week of group is purely psycho-educational. A formal presentation on the current state of knowledge about PNES is presented to patients with a question-and-answer period. The presentation establishes the leader as having expertise and experience with PNES [16, 17]. The group is presented to patients as being cognitively and behaviorally oriented with a solution-focused format. Ground rules are reviewed.

Active-relaxation/behavioral activation

Early sessions focus on physical symptoms. Emphasis is placed on teaching skills patients can use during and between events. Active relaxation techniques are encouraged and demonstrated such as: self-hypnosis [28], mindfulness meditation [29], and scheduling 20-minute daily naps into daily activity charts.

Cognitive restructuring

Cognitive restructuring techniques are gently introduced with attention paid to changing locus-of-control beliefs from external factors to internal [26]. Thought records and mood logs are introduced so patients can see how changing their beliefs can change their emotions.

Exposure techniques

If patients have issues with anxiety such as panic, phobias, or posttraumatic stress, exposure and response prevention training are introduced. Sometimes revisiting past traumas in order to solve current problems becomes necessary. Imaginal exposure with rescripting, as described by Edna Foa [30], is taught when appropriate.

Interpersonal skills training

Interpersonal communication techniques are taught using role play and written materials. Education is provided regarding active listening using empathy. Emphasis on decreasing blaming and criticizing statements in order to improve relationships is presented. Particular care is taken to insure patients understand the importance of communicating negative feelings constructively and assertively and its effect on their health [31]. Boundary setting in relationships is also discussed and modeled.

Over time, group members begin to form relationships with one another. Inevitably conflicts arise between members and leaders. The conflicts also give opportunity to practice assertiveness training and interpersonal skills. Processing of aggressive and negative feelings in a constructive way is encouraged and continually modeled.

Motivational techniques and awareness of secondary gain

Using a simple cost–benefit analysis, patients are encouraged in a nonthreatening way to look at the unconscious benefits or reinforcers of their seizures. Shame and defensiveness are reduced because other group members share similar unconscious patterns, hidden emotions, and secondary gain. The concept of seeing problems as poor solutions is introduced. Modifying solutions to be more adaptable is encouraged.

Relapse prevention/radical acceptance

Relapse prevention training is taught soon after patients experience improvement. The idea is that return of symptoms should not devastate a patient or their family. Being vulnerable to seizures for a lifetime is possible. Radical acceptance of symptoms as being chronic can paradoxically help improve symptoms. Getting "back on track" quickly by using what worked in the past is emphasized. Seizure logs are kept to document these improvements and avoid discounting progress. Paying attention to decreases in frequency and severity of episodes, instead of unrealistic goals of complete remission, avoids depressive cognitions sometimes experienced with relapse. Patients are encouraged to use symptom relapses as a compass to guide them back to implementing those techniques that were effective in the past.

Adjunctive treatment

Another helpful strategy is having group members involved in simultaneous individual and/or family therapy. The experience of the group can be overwhelming and intense. Having an individual therapist for support and processing of group material can help a patient make substantial gains more quickly and comfortably. Coping with the myriad of emotions that may arise is facilitated by individual therapy. It also helps the group leader not to be overburdened by sole responsibility for a patient's well-being. It is difficult to accurately access and provide all of a patient's needs within the constraints of the relatively short group meeting time. Caseworkers and social workers are invaluable resources for those patients with access to them. Collaboration and creativity are necessary ingredients in working successfully with a patient.

Summary

The empirical data presented thus far, both observational and experimental, create hope for establishing an accessible and evidence-based group therapy for PNES. Each patient with PNES represents a fascinatingly complicated human being and to assume one cookie cutter treatment approach could be universally helpful is naïve. A flexible and compassionate approach based on experimental evidence is potentially of benefit. Continued research and funding provided to rigorously designed studies of group therapy for PNES are needed. In the meantime, given the state of knowledge on this subject, group therapy appears to be a rational treatment choice for those with PNES who have access to it.

References

1. D'Alessio L, Giagante B, Oddo S, *et al.* Psychiatric disorders in patients with psychogenic non-epileptic seizures, with and without comorbid epilepsy. *Seizure* 2006;**15**(5):333–9.
2. Bowman ES, Markand ON. Psychodynamics and psychiatric diagnoses of pseudoseizure subjects. *Am J Psychiatry* 1996;**153**(1):57–63.
3. Rusch MD, Morris GL, Allen L, Lathrop L. Psychological treatment of nonepileptic events. *Epilepsy Behav* 2001;**2**(3):277–83.
4. Moreno JL. *Who Shall Survive*. New York: Beacon House, 1953.
5. Yalom I. *The Theory and Practice of Group Psychotherapy*. New York: Basic Books, 1975.
6. Yalom I. *The Theory and Practice of Group Psychotherapy*, 5th edn. New York: Basic Books, member of Perseus Books Group. 2005; 668.
7. McRoberts C, Burlingame GM, Hoag MJ. Comparative efficacy of individual and group psychotherapy: a meta-analytic perspective. *Group Dyn* 1998;**2**(2):101–17.
8. LaFrance WC, Jr, Barry JJ. Update on treatments of psychological nonepileptic seizures. *Epilepsy Behav* 2005;**7**(3):364–74.
9. Brooks JL, Baker GA, Goodfellow L, Bodde N, Aldenkamp A. Behavioural treatments for non-epileptic attack disorder. *Cochrane Database Syst Rev* 2007(1):CD006370.
10. De Jong T, Gorey K. Short-term versus long-term group work with female survivors of childhood sexual abuse: A brief meta-analytic review. *Soc Work Groups* 1996;**19**:19–27.
11. Kessler MR, White MB, Nelson BS. Group treatments for women sexually abused as children: a review of the literature and recommendations for future outcome research. *Child Abuse Negl* 2003;**27**(9):1045–61.
12. Lau M, and Kristensen E. Outcome of systemic and analytic group psychotherapy for adult women with history of intrafamilial childhood sexual abuse: a randomized controlled study. *Acta Psychiatr Scand* 2007;**116**(2):96–104.
13. Prigatano GP, Stonnington CM, Fisher RS. Psychological factors in the genesis and management of nonepileptic seizures: clinical observations. *Epilepsy Behav* 2002;**3**(4):343–9.
14. Zaroff CM, Myers L, Barr WB, Luciano D, Devinsky O. Group psychoeducation as treatment for psychological nonepileptic seizures. *Epilepsy Behav* 2004;**5**(4):587–92.
15. Barry JJ, Wittenberg D, Bullock KD, *et al.* Group therapy for patients with psychogenic nonepileptic seizures: a pilot study. *Epilepsy Behav* 2008;**13**(4):624–9.
16. Bright JI, Baker KD, Neimeyer RA. Professional and paraprofessional group treatments for depression: a comparison of cognitive-behavioral and mutual support interventions. *J Consult Clin Psychol* 1999;**67**(4):491–501.
17. Fals-Stewart W, Birchler GR. Behavioral couples therapy with alcoholic men and their intimate partners: the comparative effectiveness of bachelor's and master's level counselors. *Behav Ther* 2002;**33**:123–47.
18. Martin RC, Gilliam FG, Kilgore M, Faught E, Kuzniecky R. Improved health care resource utilization following video-EEG-confirmed diagnosis of nonepileptic psychogenic seizures. *Seizure* 1998;**7**(5):385–90.
19. Arnow BA, Relationships between childhood maltreatment, adult health and psychiatric outcomes, and medical utilization. *J Clin Psychiatry* 2004;**65** Suppl 12:10–15.
20. Spector S, Tranah A, Cull C, Goldstein LH. Reduction in seizure frequency following a short-term group intervention for adults with epilepsy. *Seizure* 1999;**8**(5):297–303.

21. McDermut W, Miller IW, Brown RA. The efficacy of group psychotherapy for depression: a meta-analysis and review of the empirical research. *Clin Psychol (New York)* 2001;**8**:98–116.

22. Joosten-Weyn Banningh LW, Kessels RP, Olde Rikkert MG, Geleijns-Lanting CE, Kraaimaat FW. A cognitive behavioural group therapy for patients diagnosed with mild cognitive impairment and their significant others: feasibility and preliminary results. *Clin Rehabil* 2008;**22**(8):731–40.

23. Walters ST, Ogle R, Martin JE. Perils and possibilities of a group-based motivational interviewing. In: Miller WM, Rollnick S, eds. *Motivational Interviewing: Preparing People for Change*, 2nd edn. Guilford Press: New York. 2002; 377–90.

24. Krawetz P, Fleisher W, Pillay N, *et al.*, Family functioning in subjects with pseudoseizures and epilepsy. *J Nerv Ment Dis* 2001;**189**(1):38–43.

25. Moore PM, Baker GA, McDade G, Chadwick D, Brown S. Epilepsy, pseudoseizures and perceived family characteristics: a controlled study. *Epilepsy Res* 1994;**18**(1):75–83.

26. Stone J, Binzer M, Sharpe M. Illness beliefs and locus of control: a comparison of patients with pseudoseizures and epilepsy. *J Psychosom Res* 2004;**57**(6):541–7.

27. McDade G, Brown SW. Non-epileptic seizures: management and predictive factors of outcome. *Seizure* 1992;**1**(1):7–10.

28. Brooks JL, Goodfellow L, Bodde NM, Aldenkamp A, Baker GA. Nondrug treatments for psychogenic nonepileptic seizures: what's the evidence? *Epilepsy Behav* 2007;**11**(3):367–77.

29. Jain S, Shapiro SL, Swanick S, *et al.* A randomized controlled trial of mindfulness meditation versus relaxation training: effects on distress, positive states of mind, rumination, and distraction. *Ann Behav Med* 2007;**33**(1):11–21.

30. Foa E, Olasov Rothbaum B. *Treating the Trauma of Rape*. New York: Guilford Press, 1998.

31. Kiecolt-Glaser JK, Loving TJ, Stowell JR, *et al.* Hostile marital interactions, proinflammatory cytokine production, and wound healing. *Arch Gen Psychiatry* 2005;**62**(12):1377–84.

Section 5 Chapter 31

Treatment considerations for psychogenic nonepileptic seizures

Hypnosis in the treatment of psychogenic nonepileptic seizures

Franny C. Moene and Jarl Kuyk

Hypnotic phenomena have been used and described since ancient times under numerous terms such as "trance states" and "possession". The history of hypnosis (in Greek: ypnos = sleep) has been reviewed by many and it is said that scientific research on hypnosis began in the eighteenth century with Mesmer, who believed that hypnotic phenomena were induced by "animal magnetism", a force originating from his own hands [1]. Nowadays, hypnosis is considered as an altered state of consciousness in which people can enter if they have the skill and in which absorption (the ability to focus attention excluding other stimuli), dissociation (the ability to fragment perception from the external world), and suggestibility (the ability to suspend critical evaluation of incoming stimuli) are underlying factors [1, 2].

Hypnosis occurs within the context of a special hypnotist–subject relationship, during which suggestions are given pertaining to cognition, perception, memory, and affect [3]. The susceptibility for hypnosis [4] is measured with standardized tests by asking people to experience phenomena that seem similar to dissociative symptoms (e.g., amnesia, paralysis, anesthesia, involuntary movements). The susceptibility for hypnosis is a more or less normally distributed stable trait [5] that may be partly genetically based [6].

Psychogenic nonepileptic seizures (PNES) have been accurately described since the time of Charcot and Gowers in the second half of the nineteenth century. Charcot, when he was chief of the Salpêtrière Hospital in Paris, had to reorganize the hospital because of the defective state of several buildings and therefore separated patients diagnosed with hysteria and others with epilepsy but without psychosis from other patients. The patients with hysteria soon began to display epileptic-like seizures, which he called hystero-epilepsy or hysteria major [7].

The close association between hysteria and hypnosis was demonstrated by Charcot in his famous lectures in which he showed that PNES could be easily induced by hypnosis [8]. Charcot's pupil, Sigmund Freud, used hypnosis prior to developing psychoanalysis to explore and treat hysteria [9]. Pierre Janet [10] suggested that dissociation was the crucial mechanism in both hysteria and hypnosis, and he considered hypnosis as an artificially induced hysterical condition. Janet was the first to describe the hysterical seizure as an attack of dissociation. He argued that there is a relationship between childhood traumatization and dissociative symptoms that is mediated by a process in which the traumatized individual uses his/her hypnotic capacities to induce self-hypnosis as a defense response to overwhelming traumatic events. Modern authors have also argued that conversion symptoms, including PNES, may result from spontaneous self-hypnosis involving a dissociation of sensory and/or motor functions as a reaction to overwhelming traumatic events [11–14]. Indeed, many studies find childhood sexual, physical, and emotional abuse, as well as recent traumatic life events, in the histories of patients with PNES [15]. Bowman and Markand [16] suggested four pathways to the development of PNES, including a history of childhood sexual or physical abuse, recent sexual assault, multiple life stresses that overwhelmed the patient's coping abilities, and panic attacks that were mistaken for PNES.

Not surprisingly, there are striking similarities in the phenomenology of conversion (previously known as hysterical) symptoms and hypnotic phenomena. They are experienced as involuntary, seem feigned as objective tests are applied, and in both cases there is an implicit knowledge that should be not present if the symptoms or hypnotic acts were physiologically real [14]. Moreover, recent neuroimaging

Gates and Rowan's Nonepileptic Seizures, 3rd edn. ed. Steven C. Schachter and W. Curt LaFrance, Jr. Published by Cambridge University Press. © S. Schachter and W. C. LaFrance, Jr. 2010.

studies (PET) provide support for the suggested overlap between hypnotically suggested phenomena and conversion symptoms. A neurophysiological overlap is suggested by the finding of increased regional blood flow in both conditions, particularly in the orbitofrontal and anterior cingulate regions [17]. Hypnotically induced paralysis shows involvement of the same frontal inhibitory structures as those identified in patients with conversion paralysis [18–21].

Several studies show heightened levels of hypnotic susceptibility in patients with dissociative disorders and conversion disorders [22–26] both in comparison with healthy people and other patient groups [24]. Likewise, a high level of hypnotic susceptibility is found in patients with PNES [12, 22, 27–31]. Kuyk and coworkers found that patients with PNES scored higher on a hypnotic susceptibility scale than patients with epileptic seizures (ES), while patients with ES scored in the same range as healthy subjects [29–30].

Hypnosis is also used in the differential diagnosis between PNES and ES. During hypnosis it is possible to recover amnesia for the seizure in PNES but not in ES with loss of consciousness. With this technique, the recall technique, a positive criterion can be obtained for the diagnosis of PNES, while other diagnostic methods, such as ictal EEG and neurohormonal indices, are directed to prove that seizure manifestations are not epileptic. With this technique, a specificity of 100% and a sensitivity of 80% was found [30].

Also, seizure provocation by hypnosis may provide diagnostic indications. If it can be demonstrated that a hypnotically provoked seizure is a typical one for the patient (e.g., recognized by relatives) and the event is not accompanied by epileptiform activity on EEG, then the seizure is not epileptic [32–34]. Barry and coworkers showed that measuring hypnotizability is a useful technique to aid in the diagnosis of PNES, because of the aforementioned fact that patients with PNES are more susceptible than patients with ES [31].

All these phenomena seem to justify the supposition that the mechanisms underlying PNES and hypnosis have at least some isomorphic characteristics, and it is not surprising that therapeutic techniques involving hypnosis can often be used successfully in patients with PNES. The use of hypnosis in patients with conversion disorders is extensively described in numerous studies [14]. Evidence of the benefits of hypnosis in the treatment for PNES has been described in various, often somewhat dated, case studies [27–28, 35–38]. Controlled trials, however, are scarce. There are only two randomized controlled trials with hypnosis for conversion disorder, motor type [39, 40]. In one study, 15 of the 45 patients, beside motor symptoms, also suffered from PNES as did 8 of the 44 participants in the second study. In these trials, hypnosis was significantly more effective in an outpatient trial compared to a waiting list condition, but hypnosis appeared not to add significantly to treatment results in a comprehensive, inpatient treatment program.

In general, hypnosis is considered as an adjunctive technique to be used in support of a broad-based treatment approach, such as cognitive-behavioral, psychodynamic, and rehabilitation therapies [41, 42]. In a review of research on hypnosis as an adjunct to cognitive-behavioral psychotherapy, Schoenberger [43] concludes that hypnosis and cognitive behavioral therapy (CBT) is more successful than CBT alone in the treatment of patients with anxiety, depression, and dissociative identity disorders.

Clinical applications

Hypnotic techniques in the treatment of PNES

In this section several symptom-oriented and expressive/explorative approaches will be described and illustrated. In order to make successful use of hypnosis, the patient must be hypnotizable and have the ability to concentrate on their sensory as well as motor experiences. A hypnotizability test can be applied to assess the hypnotic capacities of the patient as well as to accustom the patient to the hypnotic experience [4]. Carrying out such a test can also be used as a "motivation technique," to underline the strength of the hypnotic capacities the patient possesses and the possibilities it gives them to enhance treatment results. It is important to discuss the existing prejudices and provide the patient with information about PNES and its relation to hypnosis.

Preparing the patient
Information about PNES and hypnosis
Most important is that the patient is convinced of the nonepileptic origin of the seizures. Many patients are

treated for years as having ES [44] and the transition from a somatic to a psychological interpretation of the seizures is often difficult for patients and their families. Explanation of the negative EEG results and extensive psychological assessment including exploration of life events can help to make a psychological explanation plausible.

The patient is told that PNES are generally the result of a recent or past long-term mental overload, and further, in one way or another, the body reacts with seizures in which the release of tension takes place in the muscles without there being an electrical release in the brain. That is why people with PNES tremble or shake or sometimes drop to the floor, when the muscles give way all together. Most patients with PNES experience amnesia for the ictus, while brain functions are not disturbed. So, it can be assumed that patients shift into another state of consciousness during the seizure. The patient is told that one of the reasons for the occurrence of PNES is that the handling of certain emotions, experiences, or memories cannot take place in a "normal" way. Talking about these experiences and expressing the accompanying emotions seems to be mentally blocked, which is why these experiences stay out of the daily, normal consciousness, and instead they are registered in another, a so-called "dissociated," state of consciousness [9, 45]. It is then explained that hypnosis, of which dissociation is a core phenomenon, is a state of mind in which one can enter into this dissociated state of consciousness, and can explore what happened before as well as during a seizure [14, 30, 42]. This explanation makes it clear to the patient that by learning this method it will be possible for him/her to come into contact with dissociated experiences and to learn to be more in control of them.

It is also made clear to the patient what influence (long-term) stress has on physical and mental functioning. In trauma-related PNES, such as sexual abuse, the explanation is put into a wider context and illustrated by examples of animal and human reactions to life-threatening situations. In these situations, the body can react with defensive reactions like "fight" and "flight" responses, but also with a "freezing" response, meaning not being able to move, "sham death," or "falling down" [46]. This explanation may lead to a better understanding of their symptoms and they learn that their bodies can react actively and forcefully to find "a way out." Patients often blame themselves for not having done something to fight off or escape the traumatic event or the stressor. The information about stress and defensive reactions enhances their empowerment and reduces a feeling of guilt and shame about their experiences [47].

It is also important for the patient to learn that what spontaneously happens if they have a seizure is in essence, the same as what happens when someone goes into a hypnotic trance state. This is called "self-hypnosis" and it can help the patient to create a mental distance from stressful or traumatic situations. The deliberate and purposeful use of this capacity in treatment is called hypnotherapy. The patients are told that their trance capacities will be used therapeutically to help them, within the broader context of their overall treatment, to master and understand their seizures. This is motivating for the patient because they often feel powerless about the occurrence of seizures. Moreover, because of their amnesia, there is often a feeling of uncertainty and shame about what has occurred or concern about the patient's behavior during a seizure.

Utilization of trance capacities

To become aware of the patient's spontaneously used induction technique

First, the therapist explores in detail the kind of induction technique the patient spontaneously uses or what family and friends have observed. Patients are often not aware of what happens during their induction process. The first step to get more control is that they learn what they do when they do their induction automatically. In many cases patients use "staring" as a spontaneous induction technique. In the hypnotic literature this is called "eye-fixation" and it is widely used as a formal induction technique [48].

Working with trance, hypnosis, and self-hypnosis

The patient is made familiar with trance and hypnosis by learning a fractioned, step-by-step induction, deepening, and deduction technique. Mostly, patients are surprised (and sometimes a bit disappointed) that what they experience very much resembles their spontaneous use of trance. Many formal induction and deepening techniques are described, as well as therapeutic techniques, which can be used in the clinical application of hypnosis [49]. Nonformal induction procedures include techniques tailored to the characteristics of the individual patient [50]. After the therapeutic work, hypnosis is brought to an end by a deduction technique.

The above-mentioned "eye fixation induction technique" is often a suitable method to enter into a trance. It is important that the patients familiarize themselves with what happens as the trance deepens and that they learn to master induction, deepening, deduction, and relaxation, preferably by fixed and structured procedures, which are helpful by learning self-hypnosis.

In many cases the therapist gives direct or indirect suggestions for mastery and control (e.g., "the more experienced you become, the faster you can go into a calm and relaxing trance; the more you are familiar with hypnosis, the more you understand how it can work for your benefit").

Home practice of self-hypnosis can be a therapeutically significant aspect of symptom reduction strategies. In the sessions the patient also learns what to do if possible complications arise when doing home practice, such as difficulty with trance deduction, or the intrusion of past traumatic memories [51]. Generally, these reactions are described to the patient as idiosyncratic responses to hypnotic suggestions, which are really an opportunity for them to enhance control over the presentation of symptoms and improve their understanding of them [52].

Becoming aware of body signals

Preparatory to working with hypnosis and PNES also requires a basic awareness of body sensations and body signals. Often body sensations are dissociated or patients have no "contact" with what their body feels [53]. The therapist can help them to become more aware of these somatic processes by letting them focus on and register their body sensations like muscle tension or small muscle contractions, heaviness, lightness, temperature differences, tingling sensations, or a feeling of relaxation, several times during the day.

The use of hypnotic symptom-oriented self-control procedures

When patients understand the information about hypnosis and have learned the above described techniques, they are ready to learn self-control procedures. These symptom-focused strategies predominantly involve cognitive-behavioral approaches, as well as the direct and indirect influencing of symptoms by operant conditioning techniques and cue conditioning. In these strategies hypnosis is used formally [42].

Interfering in the sequence of stimuli that lead to a seizure

Registration of antecedent stimuli The more aware that patients become of their (body) signals or stimuli that precede the seizures, the more they are able to control these stimuli by self-hypnotic techniques.

Using the information obtained from the registration tasks and observations about the seizures, the emotional or body signals that precede the seizures are mapped in a specific, hierarchical way: the "green-orange-red" model. Green means that the situation is fairly safe, there are no specific body signals or tension-evoking stimuli. Orange means that there is some danger, a sense of distress or anxiety, or certain body signals such as tension in the shoulders or a cold feeling in the legs that is unpleasant. Red means danger, a seizure is underway: tension is rising fast, body signals intensify, there is an overload of stimuli, or there are new signals such as dizziness, sounds coming from afar, or fast breathing. An illustration of the model and how it is used is described in Figure 31.1.

Counterconditioning antecedent stimuli The therapist teaches the patient to intervene as soon as possible in the sequence of the perceived physical sensations or emotions, preferably while the patient is in the green/orange region. The interventions are aimed to transform, reduce, or stop the increasing tension by practicing antagonistic reactions during hypnosis and in a waking state. An example of such a method is called cue-conditioning. This can be done by a variety of techniques, such as cue-conditioned learning of deep relaxation; breathing management; ego-strengthening techniques, or relaxing visualizations. A short "time-out," such as withdrawing to a situation with reduced stimuli or bed rest, may also be helpful. First, the antagonistic reactions are practiced with the therapist. Then the patient has to utilize them during hypnosis. After that, the patient goes into a trance and is asked to go back to the beginning of the last seizure. Evocation of this experience is done as vividly as possible by asking about the sensory, as well as the emotional, signals and experiences. The therapist asks which signals the patient perceives and then the patient applies the already learned antagonistic reaction(s) [54].

After the patient has mastered these techniques in the therapy room, self-practice begins. Possible pitfalls or complications are talked through in the sessions.

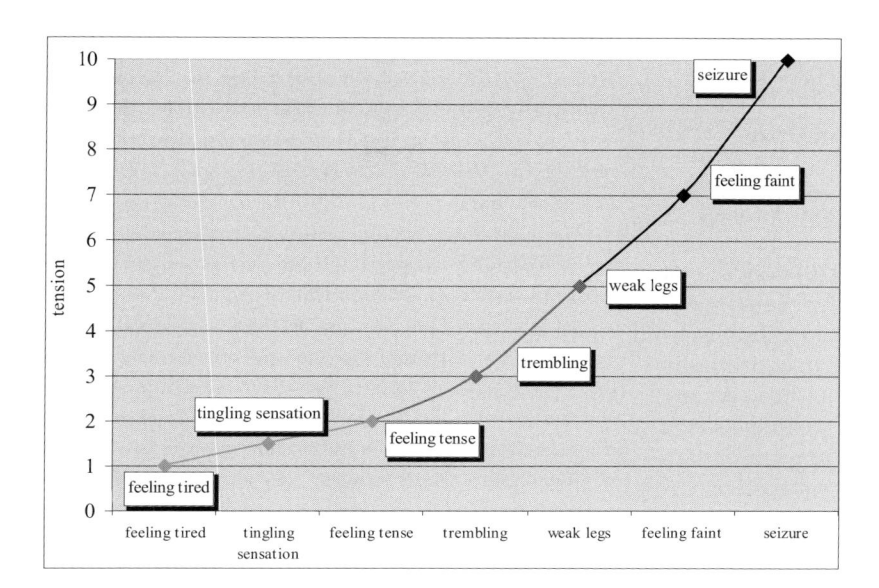

Figure 31.1. Registration of antecedent stimuli.

When the patient is ready, the practicing in "real-life" situations begins.

Illustration: *"Cue-conditioning"*

For Mrs. H, a trembling sensation in the legs is the first warning that a seizure is underway. In hypnosis, Mrs. H learns to relax quickly. When she feels the trembling sensation, she stops doing whatever she is doing and goes into a quick trance by thinking of her boat trips during the weekend, which are for her a symbol of deep relaxation and rest. Then she takes a deep breath, holds it for a few seconds, breathes out, and lets all tension leave her body.

Provoking seizures: prescribing the symptom Hoogduin et al. [55] described this hypnotic approach, which is indicated when the occurrence of the seizures is strongly determined by anticipatory anxiety or when the patient, just by thinking of the situation and emotions that preceded a former seizure, generates a new one. First, the relationship between this kind of anxiety and the seizure is explained and the rationale behind the approach is described in detail. During hypnosis the patient is given suggestions to vividly relive one of the more recently occurring seizures and to describe the antecedent situation and antecedent (physical) sensations or emotions. Then, still during hypnosis, a seizure is induced by deliberately using these situational triggers with attendant emotions. As the symptoms recede, the therapist emphasizes that if the patient can "turn on" the seizures by becoming anxious, then the patient can learn to control them by becoming relaxed in the face of the situational triggers. As this process of elicitation and recovery is repeated, the patient learns to provoke the seizure and how to return to reality more independently. The final goal is that the patient learns to avoid seizures by becoming more conscious of the antecedent events and by interrupting the anxiety before it escalates.

Illustration: Joanna, a 22-year-old woman, goes back in time to the moments before her last seizure, while under hypnosis. The therapist asks her to concentrate on the first signals, and lets her intensify them. Then, the first signs of the seizure appear. The therapist compliments her on being able to activate the seizure herself, and suggests that she also will be able to learn to reduce it. Then he describes what happens: "I see your arms tremble, you now begin to shake your right leg, too, and your breathing speeds up. It's going well, and now we're going to help you get out of the seizure by counterconditioning the symptoms. You will first notice that your breathing will calm down, and your arms will feel heavier and stop trembling. This is the first sign that your body will feel more relaxed, calmer, and heavier. Then the shaking of your right leg will become less and less and eventually your legs will feel heavy and relaxed, too." Every change in the appearance of Joanna's situation is therapeutically utilized and is coupled to the suggestions that the relaxation shall increase and that this is a sign that she is returning to normal consciousness.

Subsequently, an exercise program is discussed and practiced with Joanna. The core of this program is that she learns to go increasingly deeper into hypnosis and arouses the signals prior to a seizure herself in order to countercondition them by self-suggestions of deeply relaxing, calmly breathing, and feeling heavier.

Exploratory and expressive hypnotic approaches
The use of hypnotherapy based on etiologies

There are several techniques which can be used to explore the emotions, experiences, and memories that may trigger a patient's seizures. Kuyk [30] showed that it was possible to hypnotically recover the memory of the events occurring during a seizure. This technique, *hypnotic recall*, can also be used therapeutically to explore the mental state of the patient when a seizure began as well as during it. Exploratory techniques such as revivification or age-regression [51] or working with ego-states [56] can be used when symptom onset is associated with specific distressing situations or experiences that trigger the seizure. In this case, patients can learn to handle this kind of behavior or experience in a more satisfying way by behavior rehearsal, cognitive techniques, or other psychological interventions. When indicated, it can be suggested to the patient that going back to the distressing experience, giving expression to the pent-up or dissociated emotions, and dealing with them both during hypnosis and in the waking state may positively influence the symptoms [42].

Illustration: *Revivification*

Mrs. V, a 42-year-old married woman has a history of several sexual assaults and an extensive history of being bullied at school. She has problems in expressing her anger. During her seizures, she kicks with her legs and cries "no, no." The therapist discusses the possible function of the kicking with her and tells her that it seems like she finds it difficult to express her anger, anger that might be related to traumatic episodes in the past in which she was humiliated, felt helpless, and could not do anything to stop it. It is decided to explore this hypothesis in hypnosis. During the session hypnotic recall is used to go back in time to the situation before her most recent seizure onset, and Mrs. V explains what happened. A man in the supermarket asked her why she wore a helmet (a device to prevent self-harm during her seizures). Mrs. V says that the manner and the tone in which the man asked the question infuriated her. However, she clammed up completely and could not reply. Soon after this encounter a serious seizure occurs.

The therapist explores her feelings with her and relates the experience with this man to her traumatic experiences with men in her past. The therapist explains that the anger is "put away," dissociated, and now, it may find a way out through these seizures. She is told that she can still express her feelings about the actual experience but in another way, using the technique of "changing history" [57]. In hypnosis she goes back to where the interaction with the man began. The therapist encourages her to say to the man what's on her mind. While she verbally expresses her anger, her legs start making small, kicking movements. She is asked to make the movements bigger and to focus on what happens and what she feels. She says that she feels very angry and wants to kick the man. Her legs are making vigorous kicking movements.

She is surprised when she experiences the relationship between her feelings and her symptoms. Thereafter, the hypnotic procedure is repeated several times, focused on similar social situations. The session is tape-recorded. She has to practice this technique of expressing her anger first in a hypnotic state, "in vitro." The therapist explains that she will gradually be more able to succeed in expressing this emotion in a more normal, nonsymptomatic way. To generalize the effects, she learned expression and handling of her feelings of anger in group therapy. Outcome: a year after termination of inpatient treatment she is still seizure-free.

Seizures can be provoked by means of exposure to parts of dissociated (traumatic) material from recent or past experiences. Moene [58] describes two patients with PNES wherein the use of age-regression played an important role in the treatment. As an example, the first illustration will be described here.

Illustration: *Age regression*

William, 22 years old, has seizures during which he seems agitated and confused. He is heard saying things like, "Where is the murderer of my father?" and "Where is the surgical knife?" Afterwards, there is a dissociative period of several hours, in which he behaves as if he were younger. There is complete amnesia for his behavior. It is hypothesized that William, who was very close to his father, could not accept his death, which occurred during a complicated surgical operation when William was 19 years old. The seizures can be seen as a sign of the stagnation of his mourning process. William is told that hypnosis can help him to explore what happens during his seizures, so he can understand what causes them. In the first session, after induction and deepening by visualization of an elevator that descends, the therapist suggests that when the elevator door opens, something will happen that is related to his seizures. He is in a hospital corridor and in one of the rooms he sees his father being operated on. When asked his age, he says that he is 19. The therapist encourages William to relive his emotions and to express his feelings to his father and the doctors. Then he also relives the deathbed of his father. In subsequent sessions, William, in hypnosis, goes back in time to the beginning of his first seizure and tells the therapist what happens. He says that his father is gone and that he must go and find him and that he is calling him, but he does not answer. The therapist acknowledges this and tells William that she knows how difficult it is for him that his father has died, that he must miss him terribly, but that he has to accept that he is dead. William is getting sad, says that his father will never come back.

Other seizures are explored in the same way and they all have the same dynamic content. Finally, the therapist asks if William would like to remember what happened during the seizures, also in the waking state. William agrees and says that it is also a relief that he can see his father during hypnosis. The therapist then gives the post-hypnotic suggestion that he will also be able to see him in the waking state by remembering him vividly. After hypnosis is brought to an end, William is stimulated to talk a lot about his father in a "normal" way, to express his grief and frustration caused by his death, and accept what has happened. Outcome: two years after termination of outpatient treatment, William is still symptom-free.

The dissociated (traumatic) material by which seizures can be provoked can also present itself in the form of so-called ego-states. An ego-state is a dissociated or split-off part of the personality. The observation that dissociated ego-states cause conversion seizures is evident in published cases and is noted in 27% to 49% of cohorts of patients who have PNES [59]. When working with patients with PNES whose seizures are provoked by ego-states, it is important that a positive, trustful working relationship is built up with the patient because of their traumatic background. It should then be explored under whatever conditions possible to work in this way with the patient (necessary ego-strength, stability, and supporting network). Next, it has to be determined by therapist and patient how and in what place the emotional burden of these experiences will be integrated into normal consciousness. In the literature several hypnotic techniques are described that are especially suited for treatment of trauma-related disorders that can be used in the treatment of PNES like: "going to a safe place"; the "vault or library technique" to store away emotionally difficult memories; the "double-screen technique" to teach patients to distance themselves from their memories; and enhancing ego-strength by "empowering" techniques [51, 60–62].

Illustration: *Ego-states*

Seizures in which the patient feels like a six-year-old

Charlotte, 23 years old, has had seizures two to three times a week since she was 17. She could not complete her education and has had to live on welfare. Apart from being unable to work, she cannot lead a normal social life because of her symptoms. After her seizures she has difficulty speaking, standing, and walking and feels like a six-year-old. This can last as long as two days. She has a history of emotional neglect and has lived in foster homes, some of them unsafe and sexually intimidating. Her mother had unpredictable outbursts of anger in which she physically abused Charlotte. She obeyed her mother to prevent the worst abuse. When she was six years old, a plane crashed into the block of flats in which she lived, and many people were killed. She knows that this happened, but she is emotionally blank when she relates it.

It is remarkable that Charlotte feels like a six-year-old during the seizures. It is obvious that somewhere around this age, a traumatic experience took place that was too difficult to handle and was (partly) dissociated, like the plane crash.

The therapist explains what dissociation is and the function it can have in coping with traumatic experiences. She tells Charlotte that from the age of six, the association and integration of various states of consciousness has faltered, probably because of something that happened to her during this period. That is why she feels and expresses herself like a six-year-old. As a result of the many difficulties that have taken place in her life, integrative processes have hampered her until now, despite the fact that her life is more stable and happy. Therefore, the aim of the treatment can be to help associate the experiences of her dissociated part, the "child state of feeling," into consciousness in a way that she can handle. In hypnosis she learns to apply the technique of finding a "safe place," where she can stay during trance and safely meet, in a sort of "meeting" room, her younger ego-state, which is called "small Charlotte." This is always a very emotional experience, because in many cases it is the first time that the patient experiences feelings and sensations that are dissociated, thus new and often upsetting for them. The aim of the treatment is explained to her and "small Charlotte" is asked for her cooperation. After the trance work is done, "small Charlotte" is asked to go back to where she came from with the promise that the patient will return in the next session. During the following sessions, the plane crash and the other events in the life of Charlotte which were too difficult emotionally to integrate are reported by the "small Charlotte." The patient is asked to help and comfort her ego-state and be trustful to her. This process can be described as a form of "limited parenting" [47]. The adult patient gives to her ego-state those things that were missed in the past like support, care, and trust.

In the next phase of the treatment Charlotte is able, by means of psychotherapy and other therapeutic interventions, to integrate her experiences and to learn to cope with the effects of her traumatic experiences. She chooses to integrate "small Charlotte" with the help of a hypnotic ritual. In this ritual she leaves the meeting room, hand in hand with "small Charlotte," and fuses with her in a white light.

Outcome: after inpatient treatment Charlotte is assigned to outpatient aftercare for fifteen months. During this period she has ten seizures of very short duration, which are a reaction to difficult decisions she has to make.

Conclusions

The purpose of this chapter was to discuss the parallel between hypnosis and PNES phenomena, including the rationale for the use of hypnotic techniques. Although hypnosis is not a necessary factor in the treatment of PNES, and randomized controlled studies with hypnosis are up until now nonexistent, it can be a valuable tool. Because patients with PNES constitute a heterogeneous group with differing etiological backgrounds, a comprehensive treatment program focused on the etiologies and on the consequences of the symptoms is advisable and is probably effective [44].

Expressive hypnotic techniques, focused on the emotional experiencing of trauma or conflict, although being helpful in achieving clinical improvement, should be applied with care and should not be focused on the literal recovery of lost memories given the danger for iatrogenic suggestion during therapy [63]. If expressive techniques are applied in trauma patients, this has to be integrated in a therapeutic context in which trauma-related problems are carefully treated. This may be particularly important for patients with PNES, because several authors emphasize the role of sexual abuse in the etiology of PNES [45, 64, 65].

Janet [10] was the first to describe several unexpected responses in the hypnotherapy of patients with PNES. Recent authors [52] describe them for conversion disorders, including PNES. They occurred during the hypnotherapeutic part of the treatment, but their occurrence is a function of the overall therapy and of the higher scores on hypnotic susceptibility of the described patients. Several authors describe the relationship between sexual abuse in the etiology of PNES, hypnotizability, and dissociation [25, 26, 44, 59, 65, 66, 67, 68]. Particularly when the seizures are trauma related, it is expected that these responses in this subgroup of patients with PNES are more prone to occur. They may vary from having seizures during or after hypnotic trance, to having more or different types of seizures outside of sessions. Janet [10] and Moene and Hoogduin [52] use the trance state itself to utilize and change these kinds of responses by giving a rationale for their occurrence and (post-hypnotic) suggestions for transforming or reducing them.

As far as we know there is no literature on the occurrence of ES in hypnotized patients with epilepsy or patients with mixed PNES/ES. Kuyk et al. [29, 30] describe two patients with epilepsy who have ES during hypnosis [28]. The authors suggested that these cases may be an illustration of emotionally induced ES. In their other group of 17 patients with ES [30], however, no seizures occurred at all during hypnosis. So, it seems that the use of hypnosis is not contraindicated in patients with ES.

References

1. Kihlstrom JF. The domain of hypnosis, revisited. In: Nash MR, Barnier AJ, eds. *The Oxford Handbook of Hypnosis. Theory, Research and Practice*. Oxford: Oxford University Press. 2008; 21–52.

2. Roche SM, McConkey KM. Absorption: nature, assessment, and correlates. *J Pers Soc Psychol* 1990;**59**:91–101.

3. Lazarus AA. A multimodal framework for clinical hypnosis. In: Kirsch I, Capafons A, Cardeña-Buelna E, Amigó S, eds. *Clinical Hypnosis and Self-Regulation*. Washington, DC: American Psychological Association. 1998; 181–210.

4. Woody EZ, Barnier AJ. Hypnosis scales for the twenty-first century: what do we need and how should we use them? In: Nash MR, Barnier AJ, eds. *The Oxford Handbook of Hypnosis. Theory, Research and Practice*. Oxford: Oxford University Press. 2008; 255–83.

5. Piccione C, Hilgard ER, Zimbardo PG. On the degree of stability of measured hypnotizability over a 25-year period. *J Pers Soc Psychol* 1989;**56**:289–95.

6. Morgan AH. The heritability of hypnotic susceptibility in twins. *J Abnorm Psychol* 1973;**82**:55–61.

7. Veith I. *Hysteria: The History of a Disease*. Chicago: University of Chicago Press, 1965.

8. Charcot JM. *Leçons du Mardi à la salpêtrière: policliniques, 1887–1888*. Paris: Bureaux du Progrès Médical, 1887.

9. Breuer J, Freud S (translated by Brill AA). *Studies in Hysteria 1895*. Monograph 61. New York: Nervous and Mental Disease Monographs, 1950.

10. Janet P. *The Major Symptoms of Hysteria*. London/New York: Macmillan, 1907. Reprint of second edition: New York: Hafner, 1965.

11. Kuyk J, Van Dyck R, Spinhoven P. The case for a dissociative interpretation of pseudo-epileptic seizures. *J Nerv Ment Dis* 1996;**184**:468–74.

12. Bliss EL. Hysteria and hypnosis. *J Nerv Ment Dis* 1984;**172**:203–6.

13. Oakley DA. Hypnosis and conversion hysteria: a unifying model. *Cogn Neuropsychiatry* 1999;**4**:243–64.

14. Oakley DA. Hypnosis and suggestion in the treatment of hysteria. In: Halligan PW, Bass C, Marshall JC, eds. *Contemporary Approaches to the Study of Hysteria*. New York: Oxford University Press. 2001; 312–29.

15. Sharpe D, Faye C. Non-epileptic seizures and child sexual abuse: a critical review of the literature. *Clin Psychol Rev* 2006;**26**:1020–40.
16. Bowman ES, Markand OM. The contribution of life events to pseudoseizures occurrence in adults. *Bull Menninger Clin* 1999;**1**:70–88.
17. Barry JJ. Hypnosis and psychogenic movements disorders. In: Hallett M, Cloninger CR, Fahn S, *et al.* eds. *Psychogenic Movement Disorders*. Philadelphia: Lippincott Williams & Wilkins/American Academy of Neurology. 2005; 241–8.
18. Halligan PW, Athwal BS, Oakley DA, Frackowiak RS. Imaging hypnotic paralysis: implications for conversion hysteria. *Lancet* 2000;**355**:986–7.
19. Marshall JC, Halligan PW, Fink GR, Wade DT, Frackowiak RS. The functional anatomy of hysterical paralysis. *Cognition* 1997;**64**(1): B1–B8.
20. Roelofs K, Näring GWB, Keijsers GPJ, *et al.* Motor imagery in conversion paralysis. *Cogn Neuropsychiatry* 2001;**6**:21–40.
21. Roelofs K, Hoogduin CAL, Keijsers GPJ. Motor imagery in hypnotic paralysis. *Int J Clin Exp Hypn* 2002;**50**;51–66.
22. Bliss EL. *Multiple Personality, Allied Disorders and Hypnosis*. New York: Oxford Press, 1986.
23. Frischholz EJ, Lipman LS, Braun BG, Sachs RG. Psychopathology, hypnotizability and dissociation. *Am J Psychiatry* 1992;**149**:1521–5.
24. Frischholz EJ, Lipman LS, Braun BG, Sachs R. Suggested posthypnotic amnesia in psychiatric patients and normals. *Am J Clin Hypn* 1992;**35**: 29–39.
25. Roelofs K, Hoogduin CAL, Keijsers GPJ, *et al.* Hypnotic susceptibility in patients with conversion disorder. *J Abnorm Psychol* 2002;**111**:390–5.
26. Moene FC, Spinhoven P, Hoogduin CAL, Sandyck P, Roelofs K. Hypnotizability, dissociation and trauma in patients with a conversion disorder: an explorative study. *Clin Psychol Psychother* 2001;**8**:400–10.
27. Caldwell TA, Stewart RS. Hysterical seizures and hypnotherapy. *Am J Clin Hypn* 1981;**23**:294–8.
28. Glenn TJ, Simonds JF. Hypnotherapy of a psychogenic seizure disorder in an adolescent. *Am J Clin Hypn* 1977;**19**:245–9.
29. Kuyk J, Jacobs LD, Aldenkamp AP, *et al.* Pseudo-epileptic seizures: hypnosis as a diagnostic tool. *Seizure* 1995;**4**:123–8.
30. Kuyk J, Spinhoven P, Van Dyck R. Hypnotic recall: a positive criterion in the differential diagnosis between epileptic and pseudo-epileptic seizures. *Epilepsia* 1999;**40**:485–91.
31. Barry JJ, Atzman O, Morell MJ. Discriminating between epileptic and nonepileptic events: the utility of hypnotic seizure induction. *Epilepsia* 2000;**41**: 81–4.
32. Zalsman G, Dror S, Gadoth N. Hypnosis provoked pseudoseizures: a case report and literature review. *Am J Clin Hypn* 2002;**1**:47–53.
33. Martinez-Taboas A. The role of hypnosis in the detection of psychogenic seizures. *Am J Clin Hypn* 2002;**1**:11–20.
34. Olsen DMO, Howard N, Shaw RJ. Hypnosis-provoked nonepileptic events in children. *Epilepsy Behav* 2008;**12**:456–9.
35. Gardner CG. Use of hypnosis for psychogenic epilepsy in a child. *Am J Clin Hypn* 1973;**15**: 166–9.
36. Miller HR. Psychogenic seizures treated by hypnosis. *Am J Clin Hypn* 1983;**25**:228–52.
37. Spiegel D. Hypnosis with medical/ surgical patients. *Gen Hosp Psychiatry* 1983;**5**:265–77.
38. Montgomery JM, Espie CA. Behavioral management of hysterical pseudoseizures. *Behav Psychother* 1986;**14**:334–40.
39. Moene FC, Spinhoven P, Hoogduin CAL, Van Dyck R. A randomized controlled clinical trial on the additional effect of hypnosis in a comprehensive treatment programme in patients with conversion disorder of the motor type. *Psychother Psychosom* 2002;**71**:66–76.
40. Moene FC, Spinhoven P, Hoogduin CAL, Van Dyck R. A randomized controlled clinical trial of a hypnosis-based treatment for patients with conversion. *Int J Clin Exp Hypn* 2003;**51**:29–51.
41. Wade DT. Rehabilitation for hysterical conversion states. A critical review and conceptual reconstruction. In: Halligan PW, Bass C, Marshall J, eds. *Contemporary Approaches to the Study of Hysteria: Clinical and Theoretical Perspectives*. Oxford: Oxford University Press. 2001; 330–46.
42. Moene FC, Roelofs K. Hypnosis in the treatment of conversion and somatization disorders. In: Nash MR, Barnier AJ, eds. *The Oxford Handbook of Hypnosis. Theory, Research and Practice*. Oxford: Oxford University Press. 2008; 625–47.
43. Schoenberger NE. Research on hypnosis as an adjunct to cognitive-behavioral psychotherapy. *Int J Clin Exp Hypn* 2000;**48**:154–69.
44. Kuyk J, Siffels M, Bakvis P, Swinkels WAM. Psychological treatment of patients with psychogenic seizures: an outcome study. *Seizure* 2008;**17**: 595–603.

45. Bowman ES. Etiology and clinical course of pseudoseizures: relationship to trauma, depression and dissociation. *Psychosomatics* 1993;**34**:333–42.
46. Ogden P, Minton K, Pain C. Defensive subsystems: mobilizing and immobilizing responses. In: *Trauma and the Body. A Sensorimotor Approach to Psychotherapy*. New York: Norton. 2006;85–107.
47. Herman JL. Een helende relatie. In: *Trauma en herstel*. Amsterdam, Wereldbibliotheek, 1994, 3rd edn. Dutch translation from Herman JL. *Trauma and Recovery*. New York: Basic Books. 1992; 175–200.
48. Brown DP, Fromm E. The most widely used induction and deepening techniques. In: *Hypnotherapy and Hypnoanalysis*. New Jersey, Lawrence Erlbaum Associates. 1986; 77–110.
49. Kirsch I. Clinical hypnosis as a nondeceptive placebo. In: Kirsch I, Capafons A, Cardeña-Buelna E, Amigó S, eds. *Clinical Hypnosis and Self-Regulation*. Washington, DC: American Psychological Association. 1998; 211–25.
50. Erickson MH, Rossi EL, Rossi I. *Hypnotic Realities: The Induction of Clinical Hypnosis and Forms of Indirect Suggestion*. New York: Irvington, 1976.
51. Brown DP, Fromm E. Techniques of hypnotherapy. In: *Hypnotherapy and Hypnoanalysis*. New Jersey, Lawrence Erlbaum Associates. 1986; 149–95.
52. Moene FC, Hoogduin CAL. The creative use of unexpected responses in the hypnotherapy of patients with conversion disorders. *Int J Clin Exp Hypn* 1999;**47**:209–27.
53. Ogden P, Minton K, Pain C. Principles of treatment: putting theory into practice. In: *Trauma and the Body. A Sensorimotor Approach to Psychotherapy*. New York: Norton. 2006; 165–87.
54. Moene FC, Rümke M. *Behandeling van de conversiestoornis*. Praktijkreeks Gedragstherapie, deel 20. Houten: Bohn Stafleu Van Loghum, 2004.
55. Hoogduin CAL, Moene FC, Näring G, Sonneveld J, Brans H. Insultprovocatie bij de diagnostiek van de conversiestoornis met toevallen. *Tijdschrift voor Directieve therapie*, 1996;**4**:371–85.
56. Edelstien MG. *Trauma, Trance and Transformation*. New York: Brunner Mazel, 1981.
57. Erickson MH. *De februari man*. Rossi EL, eds. Amsterdam, Karnak, 1991. Dutch translation from MH Erickson & E Rossi. *The February Man*. New York: Brunner/Mazel, 1989.
58. Moene FC. Aanvalsgewijs optredende dissociatieve klachten. In: Van der Hart O, ed. *Trauma, dissociatie en hypnose*, 3rd edn. Amsterdam: Swets & Zeitlinger. 2003; 329–51.
59. Bowman ES. Why conversion seizures should be classified as a dissociative disorder. *Psychiatr Clin North Am* 2006;**29**:185–211.
60. Spiegel D. Hypnosis in the treatment of posttraumatic stress disorders. In: Rue IJW, Lynn SJ, Kirsch I, eds. *Handbook of Clinical Hypnosis*. Washington, DC: American Psychiatric Association. 1993; 493–508.
61. Kingsbury SJ. Hypnosis in the treatment of post-traumatic stress disorder: an isomorphic intervention. *Am J Clin Hypn* 1988;**31**:81–90.
62. Watkins JG. Hypnoanalytic techniques. *The Practice of Clinical Hypnosis*, Vol. 2. New York: Irving, 1992.
63. McNally RJ. *Remembering Trauma*. Cambridge: The Belknap Press of Harvard University Press, 2003.
64. Betts T, Boden S. Diagnosis, management and prognosis of a group of 128 patients with non epileptic attack disorder. Part II. Previous childhood sexual abuse in the aetiology of these disorders. *Seizure* 1992;**1**:27–32.
65. Bowman ES, Markand OM. Psychiatric diagnoses and psychodynamics of pseudoseizure subjects. *Am J Psychiatry* 1995;**153**:57–63.
66. Salmon P, Suad M, Al-Marzooqi SM, Baker G, Reilly J. Childhood family dysfunction and associated abuse in patients with nonepileptic seizures: towards a causal model. *Psychosom Med* 2003;**65**:695–700.
67. Roelofs K, Keijsers GPJ, Hoogduin CAL, Näring GWB, Moene FC. Childhood abuse in patients with conversion disorder. *Am J Psychiatry* 2002;**159**:1908–13.
68. Roelofs K, Spinhoven P, Sandijck P, Moene FC, Hoogduin CAL. The impact of early trauma and later life-events on symptom severity in conversion disorder. *J Nerv Ment Dis* 2005;**193**:508–14.

Section 5 Chapter 32

Treatment considerations for psychogenic nonepileptic seizures

Pharmacological treatments for psychogenic nonepileptic seizures

W. Curt LaFrance, Jr. and Dietrich Blumer

As demonstrated in the extensive literature on psychogenic nonepileptic seizures (PNES), much is known about the phenomenology of PNES, including an understanding of risk factors and prognostic features. A number of studies exist on the diagnosis of PNES, ictal semiology, comorbid psychiatric diagnoses, and neurological and neuropsychological characteristics of patients with PNES. We lack, however, controlled data on specific treatments for PNES. Treatment of PNES has been reviewed many times [1–7]. Although we can learn much from prior retrospective reports on treatments, it is essential that controlled prospective trials of pharmacological, psychotherapeutic, and combined treatment trials for PNES be conducted.

A recent overview on PNES by Reuber and Elger describes the striking extent of the difficulty this condition still presents to the medical profession [8]. Up to 50% of patients with refractory seizures may have PNES, and the mean latency between their manifestation and their correct diagnosis has remained as long as 7 to 16 years. Three-quarters of patients with PNES (and no additional epilepsy) are treated with antiepileptic drugs (AEDs) initially. Sixty-nine percent of patients with PNES were shown to be working at the time of manifestation of seizures, but only 20% were still working at the time the diagnosis was made. After an average of 11 years from onset and 4 years after diagnosis, two-thirds continue to have seizures, and over one-half are on social security. No method of treatment has so far been accepted to improve the natural history in patients diagnosed with PNES.

In contrast to the overall dismal outcome among patients with PNES documented above, Bowman and Markand report a much better outcome by the collaboration of a neurologist and a psychiatrist, combining early diagnosis with skillful psychiatric treatment for the painful and traumatic past events of their patients with PNES [9]. Therapy begins by reducing shame and providing patients with an understanding of their symptoms, then exploring the early traumata and identifying the emotions that past events raised; antidepressants and, if necessary, anxiolytics are prescribed. Based on outcome studies, the authors state that, with motivation of the patients and their understanding the causes of PNES, most of their patients with PNES of less than two years duration do well and attain remission [10–12].

The significance of the nearly ubiquitous early history of emotional traumata among patients with PNES must be recognized. Based on the pertinent literature and our experience at an epilepsy center over the period of ten years, we had previously discussed the psychobiology of PNES and proposed the term "startle seizures," noting that the posttraumatic startle response is involved in PNES [13]. Our PNES treatment experience over the past 20 years has been similar to the one outlined by Bowman and Markand and has been at least partially helpful to patients. The lesser success may be due to the fact that the majority of our patients had suffered from PNES for a period of many years and had already lost their ability to maintain work. We prescribed antidepressant medication combined, if needed, with an anxiolytic drug and with analgesic medication, together with psychotherapy, whenever possible; psychotherapy was readily combined with hypnotherapy. We also used propranolol, often at a high dose, as used for individuals who had been exposed to severe abuse in early childhood and had developed a dissociative identity disorder [14].

The significant early history of painful traumatic events in the life of patients with PNES explains their common suffering from headaches and more generalized pains: as they suppress the unbearable mental agony of the past, their pain persists as physical suffering. Indeed, a prodrome of pain, often in crescendo pattern, tends to be pathognomonic for PNES [15]. The vast prevalence of females among patients with PNES had led to the early term hysteria for the disorder, when it was assumed that wandering of the uterus caused the mental disturbances. Females, unfortunately, tend to be all too often victimized by the more aggression-prone male sex.

While the disorder is treatable, an effective treatment that yields long-term PNES freedom and improved quality of life has yet to be discovered. Prior treatment reports reveal that coordination between neurologists and psychiatrists/psychologists with early accurate diagnosis and prompt initiation of psychotherapy and communication between care providers, patient, and family yields higher treatment success. Psychogenic nonepileptic seizures are likely the result of a complex interaction between psychiatric disorders, psychosocial stressors, dysfunctional coping styles, and CNS vulnerability [16]. Pharmacological treatment of the commonly occurring comorbid psychiatric disorders, along with diagnosis-directed psychotherapy, may be the key to improving outcomes in these patients. Therapy will probably need to be individualized based on etiology, level of intelligence, family dynamics, comorbid psychiatric illness, cultural background, and other factors. Psychotherapy for PNES is addressed elsewhere in the book. In this chapter, we discuss potential psychopharmacological agents for PNES.

Treatment strategies

We learn in medical school the physician's dictum, "*Primum no nocere.*" But in fact, in the PNES population, harm is done, many times, with inappropriate treatments and aggressive therapy to stop seizures. Although PNES are not responsive to treatment by AEDs, most patients with PNES receive unnecessary AEDs [17]. One series found that 24 of 31 (77.4%) consecutive patients with PNES were on at least one AED at the time of diagnosis [18]. In some cases, potentially dangerous invasive diagnostic studies [19], toxic parenteral medications [20], port lines [21], venous cutdowns [22], emergent intubation [23], intensive care unit admission [24], vagus nerve stimulator placement [25], and evaluations for temporal lobectomy [26] are administered. When recommendations for mental health treatment are made, only half of patients with PNES pursue recommended psychiatric follow-up [27]. The patients, their families, and society bear an enormous cost if psychiatric care is not provided or if inappropriate neurological therapy is instituted for PNES.

Antiepileptic drugs: data on AED use in PNES

Extensive observational data suggest that AEDs are ineffective or may worsen PNES. Niedermeyer *et al.* first described the effects of AEDs in PNES, showing that toxicity could exacerbate PNES [28]. Krumholz and Niedermeyer found AED toxicity on admission to Johns Hopkins Hospital in 22% of patients with PNES, and this "often coincided with increasing seizure frequency or dramatic changes in seizure pattern" [29]. With the potential toxic effect of AEDs on PNES, one pharmacological question that has been addressed more recently has been the impact of withdrawing AEDs from patients with lone PNES. Given that the majority of patients with PNES are prescribed AEDs, Oto *et al.* [30] studied whether withdrawal of AEDs can be carried out safely in patients with PNES in a prospective evaluation of safety and outcome. Seventy-eight patients with PNES who satisfied a standardized set of criteria for excluding the diagnosis of coexisting or underlying epilepsy had their AEDs withdrawn (64 as outpatients, 14 as inpatients). PNES frequency declined in the group as a whole over the period of the study (follow-up 6 to 12 months) in all individuals except for eight patients in whom there was a transient increase. Fourteen patients reported new physical symptoms after withdrawal; however, no serious adverse events were reported. The authors concluded that with appropriate diagnostic investigation and surveillance during follow-up, withdrawal of AEDs can be achieved safely in patients with PNES. A review of the literature on AED withdrawal in PNES concluded that patients with PNES and no evidence of epilepsy should be referred to an epilepsy center so that AEDs can be withdrawn under safe conditions [31].

With the potential positive and negative psychotropic effects of AEDs on mood, clarifying the role of AEDs in patients with PNES is a major pharmacotherapy issue to be addressed by the treating neurologist and psychiatrist. During the process of withdrawing anticonvulsant medication, psychological symptoms may emerge (e.g., a previously undiagnosed mood disorder with carbamazepine withdrawal or significant anxiety symptoms with benzodiazepine withdrawal). Some have argued for the mood stabilizing benefits of AEDs as a reason to continue the AEDs. While depression is common in PNES, bipolar disorder is not [32, 33]. Given that AEDs do not treat PNES, that AED toxicity may exacerbate PNES, and only a minority of patients with PNES have bipolar disorder, limited numbers of patients with PNES will require "mood stabilization" with an AED. This underscores the need for good communication between neurology and psychiatry providers during the medication tapering process.

AED use in patients with mixed ES/PNES

Historical estimates of comorbid epileptic seizures (ES) and PNES have been overinflated. To more stringently investigate the actual mixed ES/PNES numbers, Benbadis *et al.* reported the results of a review of 32 patients diagnosed with PNES in their video-EEG monitoring unit over a one-year period [34]. With the criteria of "unequivocal epileptiform discharges, focal or generalized, including sharp waves or spikes, spike-wave complexes, polyspikes or any ictal pattern," but not "transients that met criteria for benign variants," the study found only 10% of patients had PNES *and* epileptiform activity. Prior reports estimated comorbid ES/PNES rates of up to 50% [29, 35, 36]. The authors account for prior overreporting of mixed PNES and ES by the lack of tightly defined criteria for establishing the diagnosis of epilepsy.

Acknowledging that both ES and PNES occur in a minority of patients with PNES, we recommend pharmacotherapy with AEDs targeting only recognized ES. Asking patients and their family members to give a detailed description of their events is essential in obtaining the history. Many times, the PNES and ES have markedly different phenomenology in the same patient [37]. Once documented historically, we give the patient a seizure calendar and ask patients and family members to chart their events prospectively, noting the characteristics of the seizures, and any particular triggers or precipitants. The frequencies of ES and PNES are established and at the following visit, the results are discussed. This process clarifies treatment targets not only for the patient, but also for the physician. We explain that for one seizure type, we will use AEDs (e.g., "the seizure that occurs nocturnally, with lateral tongue biting, incontinence, and sore muscles upon regaining consciousness"). For the other type of seizure (e.g., "the one that occurs when watching a show on TV that reminds you of the past trauma of the assault, with "zoning out" for a brief period of time and coming to just afterwards"), we will use a combination of medications for anxiety and psychotherapy. This method is a problem-oriented, practical approach that patients and their families understand and with which they can comply.

Blumer and Adamolekun explored the relationship between ES and PNES in a series of five patients with both paroxysmal disorders [38]. The authors based the treatment approach on the hypothesis that PNES have a psychobiological basis and the proposal that PNES be recognized as posttraumatic startle seizures [39]. The authors posited that excessive suppression of epileptic paroxysmal activity appears to favor the expression of posttraumatic paroxysmal activity in patients with both paroxysmal disorders, and the manifestation of ES and PNES tends to alternate [40]. The authors reported a treatment approach for these patients that proved effective: reduction of the AED dose(s) to the minimum required to achieve optimal freedom from seizures. The same findings have led to the successful use of electroconvulsive treatment for patients with severe and intractable PNES [41].

Psychiatric treatment (pharmacotherapy and psychotherapeutic interventions) for lone PNES

Inpatient treatment

Intensive treatment using behavioral therapy, psychodynamic psychotherapy, occupational therapy, and education on an inpatient unit was the norm in earlier references to PNES treatment [42, 43]. Success levels were higher than in the current outcomes reports. With the current restrictions imposed by health insurance policies, inpatient care for PNES is now less common, and current treatments incorporate a less intensive, outpatient treatment model, with up to 70% of patients with PNES continuing to have events after treatment [44]. It may behoove insurance providers to realize that with the challenges of treating PNES and other somatoform disorders, with their chronic nature, implementing a "cost saving" approach to avoid an intensive hospitalization may ultimately cost the patient and the company more in the long run.

Psychiatric assessment

Ideally, a psychiatrist asked to manage a patient with PNES should have had some experience in this area, should be part of the team that has been assessing the patient, should have confidence in the diagnosis of PNES, and, in particular, should not feel (as sometimes happens) that a difficult patient has been dumped in their lap by a neurological service eager to be rid of the patient. Patients who are dismissed sometimes "bounce back," resulting in their rapid return to the neurological facility or, worse, the patient being abandoned by everybody and the whole diagnostic process having to be re-undertaken.

Psychiatric assessment of the patient should start long before the diagnosis of PNES is finally given so that the patient's upbringing, social background, personality development, present living circumstances, and relationships with other family members (plus the presence or absence of contributing traumas such as abuse) are already established.

Pharmacological interventions

Medication treatment approaches historically have been prophylactic or symptomatic. As of yet, no acute pharmacological treatment for PNES has been developed, except for stopping convulsions with excessive sedation and paralytic agents, used in "pseudostatus" [45]. Open-label trials of antidepressants in patients with conversion disorders have shown some response [46, 47]. Phase III controlled studies of the benefit of psychotropics in patients with PNES, however, have not been conducted, and apart from anecdotal reports, their effect is unknown [6, 43]. The pharmacological references for PNES treatment using intravenous barbiturates, tricyclic antidepressants, selective serotonin reuptake inhibitors (SSRIs), dopamine receptor antagonists, β-blockers, analgesics, or benzodiazepines are largely anecdotal references in case reports, journal review articles, or book chapters, with only two prospective open-label trials [13, 48–54].

The first report of a medication used for NES was by Locock, who used bromides for "hystero-epilepsy" [55]. Dr. Locock determined to try bromide of potassium in cases of hysteria in young women, unaccompanied by epilepsy. Out of 14 or 15 cases treated by this medicine, only one had remained uncured. Injection of one-sixth of a grain of apomorphia was used by Gowers [56]. He described it as "Unquestionably the most effective measure of arresting severe attacks, which would otherwise go on for an hour or two." He described a case where, "In two minutes all spasm ceased, and the patient began to look uncomfortable. In three minutes she got up and walked to the nearest sink; and in four minutes vomited copiously." Barbiturates, including sodium amytal, have been used in diagnosing and treating patients with conversion disorder effectively for over a half a century [48].

Benzodiazepines

Benzodiazepines have been shown to reduce PNES in open-label studies [54, 57]. In a randomized trial of patients with PNES, Ataoglu et al. tested inpatient paradoxical intention therapy (PI) versus oral outpatient diazepam [54, 57]. Paradoxical intention therapy consisted of encouraging patients to intentionally engage in their unwanted conversionary symptoms. Thirty patients diagnosed with PNES of a conversion type (diagnosed by Diagnostic and Statistical Manual of Mental Disorders, Fourth Edition [DSM-IV] criteria) were evaluated by an emergency unit psychiatrist. Patients with another Axis I or II disorder were excluded from the study. Although patients with an abnormal EEG were excluded, it is unclear how the diagnosis of PNES was made. Patients were randomly assigned to an oral benzodiazepine (diazepam 5 to 15 mg/day) outpatient group or an inpatient PI-treated group. The latter cohort was encouraged to self-provoke their events with the therapist giving suggestions of anxiety-provoking situations in twice-a-day treatment. The inpatient therapy lasted three weeks and patients were reassessed three weeks later. Anxiety scores for each group (measured with the Hamilton Rating Scale for Anxiety) were compared. The therapy group showed a significant decrease in symptoms compared to the diazepam treated group. Of those patients in the PI group, 14/15 had no conversion symptoms for two weeks, prior to the six-week assessment point. In contrast, 9/15 in the diazepam group were considered responders (t = 2.27, p = 0.03). The weaknesses of the study were that there was no placebo control group, and the interventions were conducted in two different settings (outpatient and inpatient). The study was also not blinded.

Serotonin hypothesis

Research reveals that patients with PNES often have comorbid psychiatric conditions such as major depressive disorder, anxiety disorders including posttraumatic stress disorder (PTSD), or symptoms of depression, anxiety, and impulsivity, in addition to their PNES [33]. Mood, anxiety, and impulsivity disorders are characterized by serotonin system dysregulation, and have been shown to be responsive to serotonergic medications [58]. It is known that reducing other medical illnesses or risk factors associated with stroke, such as diabetes, hypertension, and hypercholesterolemia, reduces the frequency of stroke. A study assessing risk factors for persistent PNES revealed that patients with unremitting PNES had a markedly higher frequency of recurrent major depression and personality disorders, and a history of chronic abuse [12]. Therefore, by analogy, we hypothesized that treating the most frequently occurring comorbid conditions associated with PNES will reduce PNES. Serotonin modulating drugs, specifically SSRIs, are a reasonable pharmacological choice to safely treat these comorbid conditions. We proposed designing a treatment strategy that targets depression, anxiety, and impulsivity, the comorbid diagnoses that frequently accompany PNES (and are risk factors for PNES persistence [12]), for which the pathophysiology may be more responsive to pharmacological intervention.

Independent of the anxiety and depression, the serotonin system may respond directly to SSRIs in patients with conversion symptoms. Trauma, especially in childhood, appears to be important in the etiology of conversion disorders in general and PNES in particular [33, 59, 60]. Serotonin may modulate behavioral inhibition in the brain and is useful in the treatment of PTSD [61–63]. Serotonin deficiency may also be associated with impulsivity, aggression, and the compulsive behavioral reenactments seen in victims of trauma [64]. It is well known that symptoms of depression and anxiety respond to pharmacological treatment. Preliminary evidence suggests that some somatoform disorders, such as noncardiac chest pain (NCCP) and psychogenic movement disorder, may respond to antidepressant medications as well [46, 65, 66]. Varia et al. performed a double-blind, placebo-controlled study of sertraline in 30 patients with NCCP. Pain scores in the placebo group decreased from 3.50 to 2.96, versus 3.94 to 1.47 in the sertraline group. The −1.92 pain difference between drug and placebo was statistically significant ($p = 0.02$). The importance of the Varia study has relevance on a few different levels [65]. The study showed that the hypothesis of using SSRIs for other somatoform disorders is reasonable and that SSRIs are effective in treating another form of a somatoform disorder, NCCP. Even more interestingly, the authors hypothesized that the SSRI would *directly* treat the somatoform symptom. The authors found that the reduction in Beck Depression Inventory (BDI) scores within groups and between the placebo and treatment group was insignificant. The bivariate tests of baseline to end-of-study differences in the two groups' BDIs were all nonsignificant. The SSRI may have had a treatment effect on somatoform symptoms *independent of the comorbid depression*.

Treatment trials

Whether treating the comorbid depression seen in many patients with PNES, or treating the actual conversion events themselves, antidepressants and anxiolytics may be able to reduce the frequency of PNES. An open-label trial of sertraline for PNES supported our hypothesis that pharmacotherapy for psychiatric comorbidities of PNES with an SSRI or related compounds may be useful in the treatment of patients with PNES [53]. Pharmacological treatment of PNES has not been studied extensively in a controlled fashion. It is unknown whether medications will effectively treat PNES through direct mechanisms, indirect mechanisms, or not at all. A pilot randomized controlled trial using an SSRI, with flexible dose sertraline versus placebo, to treat the comorbid depression and anxiety in 38 patients with PNES was recently concluded [67]. The authors found a reduction in mean PNES in the sertraline group, but not in the placebo group. Examining the baseline values for the patients reveals that they were symptomatic across psychological and social measures. (For a reference point, the cutoff scores found in healthy control populations or in asymptomatic populations for each of the scales are listed in brackets.) On average, these patients with PNES had moderate to severe depression scores (Hamilton [< 7] and Beck Depression scales [< 14]), symptoms related to trauma (Davidson Trauma Scale [< 17]), moderate to severe impulsivity (Barrett Impulsivity Scale [< 70]), dissociative experiences (Dissociative Experiences Scale [< 5]), elevated somatic scores (Symptom Checklist 90 [< 85]), impaired social functioning (Global Assessment of Functioning [> 81] and LIFE-RIFT [< 9 (in recovery)]), family dysfunction (Family Assessment Device [FAD General Functioning subscale < 2.0]), and maladaptive coping patterns (Ways of Coping [seek social support, planful problem solving]).

Medication plus psychotherapy has demonstrated a synergistic effect in controlled trials for depression and anxiety [68–73] and may have a synergistic effect in PNES. A pilot combined treatment trial for PNES is now being conducted at Brown Medical School/Rhode Island Hospital.

Dopamine hypothesis

Rampello *et al.* explored an alternative possibility, namely a dopaminergic (D2) hypothesis in conversion disorders [52]. The authors followed 18 patients with conversion disorders, 4 of whom had PNES, as they were treated with D2 receptor antagonists. After a washout period of at least one week, two groups matched for sex and age were randomly treated with oral haloperidol (n = 6) or sulpiride (n = 12), over four months. Symptom scales and serum prolactin (PRL) levels were followed. The sulpiride treatment led to greater improvement in symptoms, compared to haloperidol, with decrease or disappearance of PNES. Mean PRL levels were higher in the sulpiride treated group. The authors concluded that the therapeutic efficacy of sulpiride suggested that hyperactivity of dopaminergic transmission is involved in the pathophysiology of conversion symptoms. The prolactinemia reflected the effectiveness of the sulpiride, with greater potency and clinical effect than haloperidol.

Other potential agents

Other potential pharmacological treatments for PNES may include NMDA antagonists, potentially addressing the learning and stress response that occurs in traumatic experiences [74]. McEwen notes that circulating stress hormones play a key role, and, in the hippocampus, excitatory amino acids and NMDA receptors are important mediators of neuronal atrophy [75]. At the same time, excitatory amino acids and NMDA receptors mediate important types of plasticity in the hippocampus. Glucocorticoid antagonists may be of benefit with the potential for cortisol dysfunction in patients with PNES [6, 76]. (See Table 32.1)

Treatment for PNES at the University of Memphis consists of prescribing an antidepressant combined with an antianxiety drug or the β-adrenergic

Table 32.1 Possible medication treatments for psychogenic nonepileptic seizures (PNES)

Hypothesis considerations for PNES medication studies:
Treating the PNES (somatoform disorder) versus treating the comorbidities of PNES
Potential agents for PNES treatment:
SSRIs – serotonergic associated comorbidities
Mixed mechanism antidepressants
Barbiturates
Benzodiazepines
AEDs used in PTSD (e.g., topiramate)
NMDA receptor antagonists
Glucocorticoid antagonists
Beta-adrenergic antagonists in combination with an antidepressant
Analgesics
Combination therapy (medications and psychotherapies)

blocker propranolol (often at high dose), or both, and if possible with psychotherapy [13]. Antidepressants alone have been effective for PNES in a small number of patients. Propranolol has been useful for PTSD and, at high doses, for patients with dissociative identity disorder who were exposed to extremes of early abuse [14].

Pain frequently occurs in patients with PNES [77]. In a study comparing medication usage in patients with PNES to those with ES, the authors found that 20 of 178 (11.2%) patients with ES used analgesics compared to 79 of 170 (46.5%) patients with PNES ($\chi^2 = 51.3$, $p < 0.001$) [78]. Blumer described the use of analgesics in PNES, noting being "able to terminate PNES status by the intramuscular injection of a strong analgesic." He observed that prolonged experience of severe pain appeared to have prolonged the individual's attack [13].

Summary and recommendations

Given the frequency of depression and anxiety in patients with PNES, coupled with theoretical conceptualizations of the disorder that focus on depression as a significant etiological factor, pharmacotherapy is postulated to be a potentially useful intervention in combination with the interventions described in this and other treatment chapters in this book.

Based on the clinical and research reports to date, we suggest the following assessment and treatment

Table 32.2 Neuropsychiatric treatment of psychogenic nonepileptic seizures (PNES)

1. Proper diagnosis: Inpatient video-EEG
2. Presentation: PNES to patient and family
3. Psychiatric treatment:
   a. *Problem* list identifying: → b. Informs *prescription of*:
   Predisposing factors   Psychotherapy(ies) and/or
   Precipitants to seizures   Pharmacotherapy:
   Perpetuating factors
          i. Tapering of AEDs
          ii. Titration of psychotropics

From LaFrance Jr. and Devinsky [1], with permission from Elsevier.

approach by a multispecialty neuropsychiatric team [1] (see Table 32.2):

1. Proper diagnosis: video-EEG for each patient with suspected PNES, refractory, or pharmacoresistant seizures. During or before the monitoring, as part of the video-EEG workup, conduct a thorough psychiatric assessment to identify predisposing factors (including comorbid psychiatric disorders), seizure precipitants, and perpetuating factors.
2. Presentation of the diagnosis: explain the PNES diagnosis in a clear, positive, nonpejorative manner. The patient may make the diagnosis presentation to the family members if cognitively and emotionally capable. This process helps reveal the level of understanding and initial acceptance of the diagnosis by the patient. Clarifications can be made by the physician who is present. Communicate the diagnosis unambiguously to the referring physician and explain the need to eliminate unnecessary medications.
3. Psychiatric treatment: as diagnosis informs treatment, a dual armed approach ensues with pharmacotherapy and/or psychotherapy, as indicated by the individual needs of the patient with PNES.

Pharmacological management begins with tapering and discontinuing ineffective AEDs for patients with lone PNES, unless a specific AED has a documented beneficial psychopharmacological effect in the patient. In patients with mixed ES/PNES, reduce high-dose or multiple AED therapy if possible. Use psychopharmacological agents to treat mood, anxiety, or psychotic disorders. No research exists on specific dosing recommendations of psychotropic medications in patients with PNES. Monitor for side effects of psychotropics and AEDs, which could exacerbate PNES. Enroll the patient in individual therapy with a psychiatrist or psychologist familiar with PNES and somatoform disorders, if a history of trauma, illness behavior, or specific interpersonal issues is identified in the assessment. Consider family therapy (Chapter 33) if the family functioning is found to be unhealthy, noting it to be a potential contributor to the symptoms [6]. Medication may be an adjunct to the whole patient treatment approach, which appears to be beneficial in treating patients with PNES.

References

1. LaFrance WC, Jr, Devinsky O. Treatment of nonepileptic seizures. *Epilepsy Behav* 2002;**3**(5 Suppl 1):S19–23.
2. Gates JR, Luciano D, Devinsky O. The classification and treatment of nonepileptic events. In: Devinsky O, Theodore WH, eds. *Epilepsy and Behavior*. New York: Wiley-Liss. 1991; 251–63.
3. Devinsky O. Nonepileptic psychogenic seizures: quagmires of pathophysiology, diagnosis, and treatment. *Epilepsia* 1998;**39**(5):458–62.
4. Kanner AM, Palac SM, Lancman ME, Lambrakis CC, Steinhardt MI. Treatment of psychogenic pseudoseizures: what to do after we have reached the diagnosis? In: Ettinger AB, Kanner AM, eds. *Psychiatric Issues in Epilepsy: A Practical Guide to Diagnosis and Treatment*. Philadelphia, PA: Lippincott Williams & Wilkins. 2001; 379–90.
5. Iriarte J, Parra J, Urrestarazu E, Kuyk J. Controversies in the diagnosis and management of psychogenic pseudoseizures. *Epilepsy Behav* 2003;**4**(3):354–9.
6. LaFrance WC, Jr, Barry JJ. Update on treatments of psychological nonepileptic seizures. *Epilepsy Behav* 2005;**7**(3):364–74.
7. Baker GA, Brooks JL, Goodfellow L, Bodde N, Aldenkamp A. Treatments for non-epileptic attack disorder. *Cochrane Database Syst Rev* 2007(1): CD006370.
8. Reuber M, Elger CE. Psychogenic nonepileptic seizures: an overview. In: Schachter SC, Holmes GL, Kasteleijn-Nolst Trenité D, eds. *Behavioral Aspects of Epilepsy: Principles and Practice*. New York: Demos. 2008; 411–19.
9. Bowman ES, Markand ON. Diagnosis and treatment of pseudoseizures. *Psychiatr Ann* 2005;**35**(4):306–16.
10. Lempert T, Schmidt D. Natural history and outcome of psychogenic seizures: a clinical study in 50 patients. *J Neurol* 1990;**237**(1):35–8.

11. Betts T, Boden S. Diagnosis, management and prognosis of a group of 128 patients with non-epileptic attack disorder. Part I. *Seizure* 1992;**1**(1): 19–26.

12. Kanner AM, Parra J, Frey M, et al. Psychiatric and neurologic predictors of psychogenic pseudoseizure outcome. *Neurology* 1999;**53**(5):933–8.

13. Blumer D. On the psychobiology of non-epileptic seizures. In: Gates JR, Rowan AJ, eds. *Non-Epileptic Seizures*, 2nd edn. Boston, MA: Butterworth-Heinemann. 2000; 305–10.

14. Braun B. Unusual medication regimens in the treatment of dissociative disorder patients. Part 1: Noradrenergic agents. *Dissociation* 1990;**3**: 144–50.

15. Blumer D, Phillips B, Montouris G, Silverman S, Hermann B. Pain associated with epileptic and non-epileptic seizures. *Epilepsia* 1995;**36** Suppl 4:158.

16. Mökleby K, Blomhoff S, Malt UF, et al. Psychiatric comorbidity and hostility in patients with psychogenic nonepileptic seizures compared with somatoform disorders and healthy controls. *Epilepsia* 2002; **43**(2):193–8.

17. Reuber M, Fernandez G, Bauer J, Helmstaedter C, Elger CE. Diagnostic delay in psychogenic nonepileptic seizures. *Neurology* 2002;**58**(3):493–5.

18. Benbadis SR. How many patients with pseudoseizures receive antiepileptic drugs prior to diagnosis? *Eur Neurol* 1999;**41**(2):114–15.

19. Wyler AR, Hermann BP, Blumer D, Richey ET. Pseudo-pseudoepileptic seizures. In: Rowan AJ, Gates JR, eds. *Non-Epileptic Seizures*, 1st edn. Stoneham, MA: Butterworth-Heinemann. 1993; 73–84.

20. Pakalnis A, Paolicchi J, Gilles E. Psychogenic status epilepticus in children: psychiatric and other risk factors. *Neurology* 2000;**54**(4):969–70.

21. Holtkamp M, Othman J, Buchheim K, Meierkord H. Diagnosis of psychogenic nonepileptic status epilepticus in the emergency setting. *Neurology* 2006;**66**(11):1727–9.

22. Gunatilake SB, De Silva HJ, Ranasinghe G. Twenty-seven venous cutdowns to treat pseudostatus epilepticus. *Seizure* 1997;**6**(1):71–2.

23. Pakalnis A, Drake ME, Jr, Phillips B. Neuropsychiatric aspects of psychogenic status epilepticus. *Neurology* 1991;**41**(7):1104–6.

24. Rechlin T, Loew TH, Joraschky P. Pseudoseizure "status". *J Psychosom Res* 1997;**42**(5):495–8.

25. Britton J, Rathke K, Cascino G, Cicora KM, Schauble B. Vagus nerve stimulator implantation in patients with nonepileptic events: a costly result of misdiagnosis. *Epilepsia* 2002;**43** Suppl 7:161.

26. Henry TR, Drury I. Non-epileptic seizures in temporal lobectomy candidates with medically refractory seizures. *Neurology* 1997;**48**(5):1374–82.

27. Krahn LE, Reese MM, Rummans TA, et al. Health care utilization of patients with psychogenic nonepileptic seizures. *Psychosomatics* 1997;**38**(6):535–42.

28. Niedermeyer E, Blumer D, Holscher E, Walker BA. Classical hysterical seizures facilitated by anticonvulsant toxicity. *Psychiatr Clin (Basel)* 1970;**3**(2):71–84.

29. Krumholz A, Niedermeyer E. Psychogenic seizures: a clinical study with follow-up data. *Neurology* 1983; **33**(4):498–502.

30. Oto M, Espie C, Pelosi A, Selkirk M, Duncan R. The safety of antiepileptic drug withdrawal in patients with non-epileptic seizures. *J Neurol Neurosurg Psychiatry* 2005;**76**(12):1682–5.

31. Duncan R. The withdrawal of antiepileptic drugs in patients with non-epileptic seizures: safety considerations. *Expert Opin Drug Saf* 2006;**5**(5): 609–13.

32. Mondon K, de Toffol B, Praline J, et al. Comorbidité psychiatrique au cours des événements non épileptiques: étude rétrospective dans un centre de vidéo-EEG [Psychiatric comorbidity in patients with pseudoseizures: retrospective study conducted in a video-EEG center]. *Rev Neurol (Paris)* 2005;**161**(11): 1061–9.

33. Bowman ES, Markand ON. Psychodynamics and psychiatric diagnoses of pseudoseizure subjects. *Am J Psychiatry* 1996;**153**(1):57–63.

34. Benbadis SR, Agrawal V, Tatum IV, WO. How many patients with psychogenic nonepileptic seizures also have epilepsy? *Neurology* 2001;**57**(5): 915–17.

35. Ozkara C, Dreifuss FE. Differential diagnosis in pseudoepileptic seizures. *Epilepsia* 1993;**34**(2): 294–8.

36. Walczak TS, Williams DT, Berten W. Utility and reliability of placebo infusion in the evaluation of patients with seizures. *Neurology* 1994;**44**(3 Pt 1): 394–9.

37. Devinsky O, Gordon E. Epileptic seizures progressing into nonepileptic conversion seizures. *Neurology* 1998;**51**(5):1293–6.

38. Blumer D, Adamolekun B. Treatment of patients with coexisting epileptic and nonepileptic seizures. *Epilepsy Behav* 2006;**9**(3):498–502.

39. Matsumoto J, Hallett M. Startle syndromes. In: Marsden CD, Fahn S, eds. *Movement Disorders 3*. Oxford, Boston: Butterworth-Heinemann. 1994; 418–33.

40. Blumer D. The biologic basis of hysteria and its polarity to epilepsy. *Szondiana* 2005;**5**:16–19.
41. Blumer D, Rice S, Adamolekun B. Electroconvulsive treatment for nonepileptic seizure disorders. *Epilepsy Behav* 2009;**15**(3):382–7.
42. Ramani V, Gumnit RJ. Management of hysterical seizures in epileptic patients. *Arch Neurol* 1982;**39**(2): 78–81.
43. LaFrance WC, Jr, Devinsky O. The treatment of nonepileptic seizures: historical perspectives and future directions. *Epilepsia* 2004;**45** Suppl 2:15–21.
44. Reuber M, Pukrop R, Bauer J, et al. Outcome in psychogenic nonepileptic seizures: 1 to 10-year follow-up in 164 patients. *Ann Neurol* 2003;**53**(3): 305–11.
45. Walker MC, Howard RS, Smith SJ, et al. Diagnosis and treatment of status epilepticus on a neurological intensive care unit. *QJM* 1996;**89**(12):913–20.
46. O'Malley PG, Jackson JL, Santoro J, et al. Antidepressant therapy for unexplained symptoms and symptom syndromes. *J Fam Pract* 1999;**48**(12): 980–90.
47. Voon V. Treatment of psychogenic movement disorder: psychotropic medications. In: Hallett M, Fahn S, Jankovic J, et al., eds. *Psychogenic Movement Disorders: Neurology and Neuropsychiatry*. Philadelphia: Lippincott Williams & Wilkins, and American Academy of Neurology Press. 2005; 302–10.
48. Lambert C, Rees WL. Intravenous barbiturates in the treatment of hysteria. *BMJ* 1944;**2**:70–3.
49. Shulman KI, Silver IL. Hysterical seizures as a manifestation of "depression" in old age. *Can J Psychiatry* 1985;**30**(4):278–80.
50. Ramani V. Review of psychiatric treatment strategies in non-epileptic seizures. In: Rowan AJ, Gates JR, eds. *Non-Epileptic Seizures*, 1st edn. Stoneham, MA: Butterworth-Heinemann. 1993; 259–67.
51. Bowman ES. Nonpileptic seizures. *Curr Treat Options Neurol* 2000;**2**(6):559–70.
52. Rampello L, Raffaele R, Nicoletti G, et al. Hysterical neurosis of the conversion type: therapeutic activity of neuroleptics with different hyperprolactinemic potency. *Neuropsychobiology* 1996;**33**(4):186–8.
53. LaFrance WC, Jr, Blum AS, Miller IW, Ryan CE, Keitner GI. Methodological issues in conducting treatment trials for psychological nonepileptic seizures. *J Neuropsychiatry Clin Neurosci* 2007;**19**(4): 391–8.
54. Ataoglu A, Sir A, Ozkan M. Paradoxical therapy in conversion disorder. *Turk J Med Sci* 1998;**28**: 419–21.
55. Sieveking EH. Analysis of fifty-two cases of epilepsy observed by the author. *Lancet* 1857;**1**:527–8.
56. Gowers WR. Treatment. Hysteroid attacks. In: *Epilepsy and Other Chronic Convulsive Diseases: Their Causes, Symptoms, and Treatment*, 2nd edn. London: Churchill. 1901; 299–301.
57. Ataoglu A, Ozcetin A, Icmeli C, Ozbulut O. Paradoxical therapy in conversion reaction. *J Korean Med Sci* 2003;**18**(4):581–4.
58. Vaswani M, Linda FK, Ramesh S. Role of selective serotonin reuptake inhibitors in psychiatric disorders: a comprehensive review. *Prog Neuro Psychopharmacol Biol Psychiatry* 2003;**27**(1):85–102.
59. Brown RJ, Schrag A, Trimble MR. Dissociation, childhood interpersonal trauma, and family functioning in patients with somatization disorder. *Am J Psychiatry* 2005;**162**(5):899–905.
60. Roelofs K, Keijsers GP, Hoogduin KA, Naring GW, Moene FC. Childhood abuse in patients with conversion disorder. *Am J Psychiatry* 2002;**159**(11): 1908–13.
61. Southwick SM, Paige S, Morgan III, CA, et al. Neurotransmitter alterations in PTSD: catecholamines and serotonin. *Semin Clin Neuropsychiatry* 1999;**4**(4):242–8.
62. Nutt DJ. The psychobiology of posttraumatic stress disorder. *J Clin Psychiatry* 2000;**61** Suppl 5:24–9; discussion 30–2.
63. Pearlstein T. Antidepressant treatment of posttraumatic stress disorder. *J Clin Psychiatry* 2000; **61** Suppl 7:40–3.
64. Van der Kolk BA. The body keeps the score: approaches to the psychobiology of posttraumatic stress disorder. In: Van der Kolk BA, McFarlane AC, Weisaeth L, eds. *Traumatic Stress: The Effects of Overwhelming Experience on Mind, Body, and Society*. New York: Guilford Press. 1996; 214–41.
65. Varia I, Logue E, O'Connor C, et al. Randomized trial of sertraline in patients with unexplained chest pain of noncardiac origin. *Am Heart J* 2000;**140**(3):367–72.
66. Menza M, Lauritano M, Allen L, et al. Treatment of somatization disorder with nefazodone: a prospective, open-label study. *Ann Clin Psychiatry* 2001;**13**(3): 153–8.
67. LaFrance WC, Jr, Blum AS, Ryan CE, Miller I. Comorbidities in patients with psychogenic nonepileptic seizures. *Neurology* 2009;**72**(11(Suppl 3)):A328.
68. March JS, Silva S, Petrycki S, et al. The Treatment for Adolescents With Depression Study (TADS): long-term effectiveness and safety outcomes. *Arch Gen Psychiatry* 2007;**64**(10):1132–43.

Section 5: Treatment considerations for PNES

69. Glass RM. Fluoxetine, cognitive-behavioral therapy, and their combination for adolescents with depression: Treatment for Adolescents with Depression Study (TADS) randomized controlled trial. *J Pediatr* 2005;**146**(1):145.

70. Lenze EJ, Dew MA, Mazumdar S, *et al.* Combined pharmacotherapy and psychotherapy as maintenance treatment for late-life depression: effects on social adjustment. *Am J Psychiatry* 2002;**159**(3): 466–8.

71. Sammons MT, Schmidt NB. *Combined Treatments for Mental Disorders. A Guide to Psychological and Pharmacological Interventions*, 1st edn. Washington, DC: American Psychological Association, 2001.

72. Pettit JW, Voelz ZR, Joiner TE, Jr. Combined treatments for depression. In: Sammons MT, Schmidt NB, eds. *Combined Treatments for Mental Disorders. A Guide to Psychological and Pharmacological Interventions*, 1st edn. Washington, DC: American Psychological Association. 2001;131–59.

73. Barlow DH, Gorman JM, Shear MK, Woods SW. Cognitive-behavioral therapy, imipramine, or their combination for panic disorder: a randomized controlled trial. *JAMA* 2000;**283**(19):2529–36.

74. Berlin HA. Antiepileptic drugs for the treatment of post-traumatic stress disorder. *Curr Psychiatry Rep* 2007;**9**(4):291–300.

75. McEwen BS. Allostasis, allostatic load, and the aging nervous system: role of excitatory amino acids and excitotoxicity. *Neurochem Res* 2000;**25**(9–10):1219–31.

76. McEwen BS. Allostasis and allostatic load: implications for neuropsychopharmacology. *Neuropsychopharmacology* 2000;**22**(2):108–24.

77. Benbadis SR. A spell in the epilepsy clinic and a history of "chronic pain" or "fibromyalgia" independently predict a diagnosis of psychogenic seizures. *Epilepsy Behav* 2005;**6**(2):264–5.

78. Hantke NC, Doherty MJ, Haltiner AM. Medication use profiles in patients with psychogenic nonepileptic seizures. *Epilepsy Behav* 2007;**10**:333–5.

Section 5 Chapter 33

Treatment considerations for psychogenic nonepileptic seizures

Family therapy for patients diagnosed with psychogenic nonepileptic seizures

Richard C. Archambault and Christine E. Ryan

A central principle in family therapy is that the pattern of the whole is reflected in the behavior of the parts and that the parts (individual family members) can affect the whole (family system). The major focus of most family therapy models is to assist families in identifying and resolving those issues and concerns that are impacting the physical and emotional wellbeing of its members. Unresolved issues, whether originating from childhood or emerging over the course of the family's life cycle, become the focus of family treatment. The residue impact of such issues can be expressed in a variety of maladaptive behaviors in family members, ranging from anxiety to more serious psychiatric conditions such as depression.

One paradigm to study the etiological factors of psychogenic nonepileptic seizures (PNES) is as a manifestation of family system dysfunction (disturbed family system relationships). What is known about the relationship between family functioning and PNES, however, is based primarily upon studies comparing the perceptions of patients with PNES to those with epileptic seizures (ES). Although research has not been able to provide a definitive answer to the causes of PNES, the limited research that has been reported has pointed to a reciprocal relationship between family functioning and PNES. Current research on PNES and family functioning has revealed that patients with PNES perceive conflicts in how family members show interest and concern for each other and how they verbally express feelings [1]. Patients with PNES have been found to view their families as more controlling and having more difficulty expressing emotions [2] and not being supportive [3]. They have also been found to have more marital and family problems [4, 5], and more often report a history of psychological stress [6–9]. The limited research on the relatives of patients with PNES has found that family members are more critical and hostile [10]; report more anxiety, depression, somatization symptoms, and health problems [11]; and report more difficulties with defining their roles [1] than families of patients with epilepsy. Griffith et al. [12] studied 14 adult patients with PNES and their families and found that there was a relationship between the family's suppression of emotional distress, or what the authors termed "unspeakable dilemmas," and PNES. Although limited, the research to date provides some credence to the hypothesis that PNES is a somatoform symptom disorder that helps the patient cope with unspeakable family distress [9, 10, 12].

In addition to the lack of research, the scope of the research is also limited as it focuses mostly on either the patient with PNES or a family member's perceptions of family functioning and in the methodology (data primarily collected through questionnaires). Research is needed that integrates objective with subjective self-report perspectives and which includes the entire family unit.

This chapter will describe a method of family assessment and therapy that has been used over the past 40 years with a variety of psychiatric and medical illnesses and which is currently being used in research conducted at Brown University. The McMaster Model of Family Functioning (MMFF) [13, 14] provides the conceptual model for a series of assessments and procedures that encompass the "McMaster Approach" for evaluating and treating families. The McMaster approach grew out of research and clinical work in the Departments of Psychiatry at McGill and McMaster Universities in Canada and Brown University in the US. The overall model encompasses a view of healthy and unhealthy family functioning, techniques for assessing the family's functioning, and an approach to treating families. A comprehensive account of the McMaster Model and related instruments and clinical procedures is contained in Ryan *et al.* [14]. The description of the McMaster Approach presented in this chapter is taken from this text and from the article of Keitner *et al.* [15].

McMaster Model of Family Functioning

An important feature of the McMaster Model is that it conceptualizes and assesses family functioning along six dimensions of family life as well as an overall rating of the family. It assesses the entire family system rather than a collection of dyads. This broad perspective encourages a comprehensive and systematic assessment of families leading to a more thorough understanding of the strengths and weaknesses of the family including interactions among members (e.g., parent–child, spousal partners) which are then integrated into a treatment program. The six dimensions and the overall General Functioning dimension are as follows:

1. Problem Solving: examines how instrumental problems (e.g., making household repairs, planning family events) and affective problems (e.g., helping family members resolve emotional upsets) are resolved.
2. Communication: focuses on how family members listen to, talk with, and make observations about one another's behavior and understanding of one another.
3. Roles: assesses how family members allocate and complete instrumental (e.g., household chores, finances) and affective tasks (e.g., giving and receiving affection) and how extended family relationships are managed. The Roles dimension also assesses the personal development of family members (e.g., how children are performing in school, health concerns) and adult sexual intimacy.
4. Affective Responsiveness: assesses how family members experience welfare emotions (pleasure, joy, and happiness, love, caring, and tenderness) and emergency emotions (sadness, anger, and fear).
5. Affective Involvement: evaluates how family members show interest in and value the interests and activities of one another.
6. Behavior Control: focuses on the expectations and rules that family members have for dangerous situations (e.g., child playing with matches, adults drinking too much), meeting psychobiological drives (e.g., eating, hygiene, aggression) and interpersonal relations (e.g., how family members treat one another).
7. General Functioning: overall understanding of how the family generally manages the instrumental and affective functions common to daily family life.

Assessment instruments

The Brown University Family Therapy and Research Group has developed a number of instruments to assess these family dimensions both from an objective and subjective perspective, including the Family Assessment Device (FAD), the McMaster Clinical Rating Scale (MCRS) and the McMaster Structured Interview of Family Functioning (McSIFF).

The Family Assessment Device (FAD)

The FAD [14, 16] is a 60-item self-report instrument that was designed to be filled out by all family members who have at least an eighth-grade reading level. The FAD evaluates the family's perception of their functioning on the six dimensions of the McMaster Model as well as on the general functioning scale. Family members respond using a 4-point scale (strongly agree, agree, disagree, and strongly disagree). Cutoff scores for healthy and unhealthy functioning have been established for each of the family dimensions. The higher score denotes *worse* family functioning. The instrument has been validated and translated into 23 languages [14].

The McMaster Clinical Rating Scale (MCRS)

The MCRS [14, 17] is an objective rating scale that uses data collected in a family interview to provide a rating on each of the family dimensions as well as on the overall family functioning. Ratings are assessed on a 7-point Likert Scale using anchor points for ratings of 1–2 (severe dysfunction), 3–4 (moderate dysfunction), 5 (borderline-nonclinical), and 6–7 (superior functioning).

The McMaster Structured Interview of Family Functioning (McSiff)

The McSiff [14, 18] is a semi-structured interview schedule that gathers standardized clinical data on how the family structures and organizes itself within and across the family dimensions. The McSiff also identifies specific problems in each dimension (e.g., communication) and the salient transactional pattern that characterizes the family's presentation across dimensions. The McSiff was developed as a result of methods used for training and supervising psychiatry residents and psychology interns at the Brown University School of Medicine and later became a valued research tool. The McSiff is typically used by less experienced clinicians or those new to the model to ensure that sufficient clinical information is obtained from the family and to derive a clinical score on all McMaster family dimensions.

The Problem Centered Systems Therapy of the Family (PCSTF)

The PCSTF [14, 19] is the treatment component of the MMFF. The PCSTF operates on the assumption that changing the systemic process within the family can change individual behavior. The PCSTF draws from system theory to explain the processes by which families function. The major assumptions of the PCSTF are [14]:

1. The parts of the family are interrelated. One part of the family cannot be understood in isolation from the rest of the family system.
2. Family functioning cannot be understood fully by understanding each of the parts (e.g., discrete individuals or dyads).
3. A family's structure and organization are important factors in determining the behavior of family members.
4. Transactional patterns of the family system are among the most important variables that shape the behavior of family members. A transactional pattern is a set of beliefs, feelings, and behaviors that structure, organize, and give meaning to family interactions.

The PCSTF is composed of four major stages: (1) assessment; (2) contracting; (3) treatment; and (4) closure. A distinction of the PCSTF is its emphasis on the therapist moving systematically through these four stages of treatment, each of which contains a set of specific goals and a sequence of substages. In addition, the model recognizes the importance and usefulness of a therapist's individual style, the importance of identifying transactional styles within the family, and dealing with process issues within the family.

Assessment stage

In many ways the assessment stage is the most important stage. It is the stage in which the therapist orients the family to the treatment process and establishes an open collaborative relationship with the family. The therapist and the family identify all current problems in the family including the presenting problem, as well as those delineated during a comprehensive assessment of the family along the six dimensions of the MMFF. It is important not to get bogged down. If the family comes up with several examples of their problems, the therapist can condense these examples into one or two problems (e.g., "It looks like there is a communication problem that affects the way that Dan and Rose get along"). At the end of the assessment the therapist formulates hypotheses regarding the factors and/or processes that appear to be causally associated with the family's identified problems. The therapist and the family together clarify and agree on a problem list that then becomes the foundation for the next stage of treatment.

Contracting stage

In the contracting stage the goal is for the therapist and family to prepare a contract that delineates mutual expectations, goals, and commitments regarding therapy. Problems are prioritized according to their importance to the family. The therapist may have to preempt this priority list if issues of safety are involved, and the family does not identify risk situations as problematic.

Treatment stage

In the treatment stage the therapist and family members implement strategies and negotiate ways to change the identified behaviors that contribute to the problems. The goal is to produce behavioral change in the family by the family identifying and setting tasks that the family will work on between sessions. Subsequently, the therapist and family members evaluate the success or failure of the tasks.

Closure stage

In the closure stage the course of treatment is reviewed with the family and long-term goals as well as optional follow-up visits are discussed.

Limited research is available on treatment of PNES incorporating family therapy. One recent study enrolled patients with PNES into family therapy using

Table 33.1 The family's rating of their family functioning. Prior to the initial assessment, Dan and Rose completed the Family Assessment Device (FAD)

FAD ratings of the family		
	The A family FAD score	Healthy/unhealthy cutoff score
Problem Solving	2.75	2.20
Communication	2.89	2.20
Roles	2.90	2.30
Affective Responsiveness	2.75	2.10
Affective Involvement	2.50	2.20
Behavior Control	2.11	1.90
General Functioning	2.92	2.00

(higher scores denote *worse* family functioning, range = 1 – 4) Their individual scores were averaged for the family rating. The mean family FAD scores were all in the unhealthy range for all dimensions. All family FAD scores indicated that family functioning was rated as problematic across dimensions. Individual FAD scores, often used by the clinician to compare individual perceptions of family functioning, are listed in Table 33.2.

Table 33.2 Individual FAD ratings of the A family

	Mr. A	Mrs. A
Problem Solving	2.67	2.83
Communication	2.89	2.89
Roles	2.82	3.00
Affective Responsiveness	3.00	2.50
Affective Involvement	2.57	2.43
Behavior Control	2.44	1.78
General Functioning	3.17	2.67

FAD scores indicated that except for Rose's rating of Behavior Control, Dan and Rose perceived all family functioning dimensions as problematic. They rated Problem Solving, Communication, Roles, Affective Responsiveness, Affective Involvement, and General Functioning as very difficult areas in their family's functioning.

PCSTF [20]. Five patients were enrolled in PCSTF for PNES, and three discontinued, one transferred and one did not require further family sessions. The pilot study was not powered to evaluate efficacy; however, individual patients improved with the treatment. The remainder of this chapter describes the application of the McMaster Approach in assessing and treating a couple with one member diagnosed with PNES who enrolled in the family therapy for PNES pilot study.

The case reported in this chapter participated in the full McMaster Assessment, the contracting stage, and the treatment stage. Usually the entire family is involved but the couple requested that their three children not participate in the therapy. The couple completed the FAD (subjective rating) before the McSiff (objective rating) was administered to them. (Refer to Tables 33.1 and 33.2.) The therapist provided a McSiff rating and then scored the FAD.

Mr. and Mrs. A

Mr. and Mrs. A (Dan and Rose) had been married for 16 years. Dan was 46 and had been unemployed as a computer technician for two years due to seizures and depression. Rose was 44 and worked full time in a public utilities company. Prior to Dan's unemployment Rose worked part time while she cared for their children. The couple had three children, two sons ages 14 and 12 and a daughter age 10. Dan was diagnosed with PNES two years prior to seeking treatment. He reported that his illness and job loss has made him feel depressed and hopeless. In addition to the couple's therapy, Dan was receiving individual therapy from a psychotherapist in the community. Rose had never received any type of psychotherapy.

Assessment stage

Orientation to family treatment

The therapist oriented Dan and Rose to the assessment by providing the following introduction: "It has been our experience when treating families that what happens to one person in the family affects everyone in the family. In order to better understand your particular situation I'm going to be asking questions that will help me better understand your relationship. I'll be jumping around from topic to topic and asking a number of questions about how you work as a couple. If there are any questions that you cannot or do not feel comfortable answering, please let me know. From time to time I may share my observations as to what I think is going on. Please let me know if my observations are correct and feel free to correct me. The important thing is to relax and be as honest and direct as you can with your responses." After this brief introduction the therapist asked and gained permission to begin the interview.

Presenting problems

The next step was to elicit the presenting problems. Dan and Rose stated that their relationship had progressively deteriorated over the past two years. They argued over everything and their arguments had become more frequent and intense. Minor disagreements often escalated into full-blown heated arguments until Dan gave up and withdrew. A central theme in these arguments was Rose's belief that Dan was not motivated to secure employment. Rose stated that for the past two years she felt overwhelmed that the burden of providing for the family fell on her shoulders. Dan stated that he would like nothing more than for their lives to return to the way things used to be when he was employed, and he and Rose spent enjoyable time together raising their children. He expressed a desire for Rose to better understand his illness and to be more affectionate. She expressed a desire for her husband to become more motivated to "pick up the slack" of managing the house and to actively seek employment. And, finally, Dan and Rose commented that they have different parenting styles that were sometimes a source of disagreements.

Dan and Rose identified the following concerns:
1. Couple arguments.
2. Dan not receiving enough affection from Rose.
3. Rose's belief that Dan was using his seizures as an excuse not to help out more around the house and to not find employment.
4. Dan's belief that Rose does not believe that he has a legitimate medical problem.
5. The couple's different parenting styles.
6. Financial stresses due to Dan's unemployment.
7. Rose feeling overwhelmed with working full time, caring for the children, and performing household tasks.

Dan and Rose commented that talking about these issues usually turned into an argument and that they have learned that it was best to avoid differences of opinion whenever possible. "Leave things the way they are" had become their rule for living. Following the McMaster protocol the therapist then asked if it was OK to proceed with the assessment. After obtaining permission, he proceeded to assess the six areas of family life according to the guidelines set forth in the MMFF. The following summarizes the data gathered on each dimension.

Problem solving

Dan and Rose stated that they were unable to sit down and address daily issues, whether it be instrumental (e.g., finances, replacing their stove) or affective (e.g., Dan's sadness over his unemployment). When instrumental issues arose, it often reminded them of their limited financial situation, which, in turn, elicited strong feelings. The couple's style for addressing strong feelings was to initially avoid the issue so as not to disagree. The couple reported a pattern of circumventing or ignoring the issue in hopes that it would take care of itself. Attempts to resolve emotional upsets often resulted in disagreements over how best to handle the situation, leaving Dan feeling sad and Rose angry. These unresolved emotional upsets created "bad feelings" in the relationship.

Communication

The couple reported that a pattern of communication had emerged characterized by not listening, making critical remarks, and misinterpreting what the other was feeling or trying to say. Dan and Rose stated that they did not share feelings with one another. Rose turned to friends when she had a bad day or needed to vent her feelings citing that she didn't want to overburden Dan. Dan reported that he felt that Rose did not understand him, especially his depression and his seizures, and rather than risk what he felt was criticism from Rose he kept feelings to himself. The couple stated that the conversation they were having in the session was avoided at home for fear of arguing, especially in front of their children.

Roles

Although a struggle, and with some financial support from their families, Dan and Rose were able to provide adequate food, clothing, and shelter to their children and to pay their mortgage and monthly bills. In the area of completing routine household tasks, Rose commented that she felt overworked and that Dan could help out more around the house. The couple was satisfied with their children's personal development, but Dan reported a variety of health concerns in addition to depression and seizures (e.g., high blood pressure). Rose's work schedule, coupled with Dan's lack of interests, prevented them from pursuing individual and couple interests. They reported stress in their relationships with their respective extended families. Adult sexual intimacy and affection were also reported to be problematic.

Affective Responsiveness

Dan and Rose agreed that the stress they experienced over the past two years had diminished their capacity for appropriately experiencing joy, happiness, love, and concern, especially for one another. Dan stated that he experienced too much anger, becoming angry too quickly and having a difficult time getting past his anger. His anger often turned to sadness, and he reported that he was sad most of the time. Rose stated that she was uncomfortable with how Dan was managing his job loss and depression and at times she became too angry with Dan and with her children. She also reported that she often experienced too much sadness over all that has happened to the family and was afraid for the future.

Affective Involvement

Dan and Rose both stated that while they still cared about one another's welfare they have grown apart. Dan stated that Rose was not affectionate, and he felt that she no longer found him attractive. Rose acknowledged her husband's feelings and added that over the years Dan stopped taking an interest in her and showed her little affection. Marital discomfort was most intense for Rose when she felt Dan was feeling sorry for himself. The issue of separation recently came up but was not acted upon; neither felt divorce would be in their best interest at this time, especially for their children. Dan and Rose expressed deep concern for their children. Both acknowledged that they felt the other was active in their children's lives. However, Rose observed that Dan was "too lenient," while Dan stated that Rose was "too strict." Rose acknowledged that at times she yelled too much at her children, attributing this to the stress that she was experiencing in her marriage.

Behavior Control

Rose and Dan disagreed on how to discipline their children. A significant issue was that the couple's differing parenting styles could result in arguments over how to best discipline their children. There were no reports of substance abuse, engaging in dangerous behavior (driving excessively fast, smoking, etc.), experiencing legal problems, physically aggressive behavior, or domestic violence. Dan and Rose were generally comfortable with how they treated one another in public. They stated that their arguments never become verbally or physically abusive. Dan reported that he would never hurt himself because he was aware of how this would impact his children.

Table 33.3 The clinician's rating of the family's functioning. After the initial assessment, the therapist rated the family's functioning following the guidelines outlined in the McMaster Clinical Rating Scale (MCRS)

MCRS ratings of the A family	
Problem Solving	3 moderately problematic
Communication	2 severely problematic
Roles	2 severely problematic
Affective Responsiveness	2 severely problematic
Affective Involvement	3 moderately problematic
Behavior Control	4 mildly problematic
General Functioning	2 severely problematic

(higher scores denote *better* family functioning, range = 1 − 7) The clinician's ratings of family functioning were in the moderate to severely problematic range on all dimensions.

Clinical Formulation

Dan and Rose felt they were locked in an impasse over how they viewed each other's beliefs, feelings, and behavior, primarily around Dan's seizures and depression. Dan believed that Rose was disappointed in the way he was managing his depression and seizures. Rose expressed a belief that her husband was not working hard enough to overcome his depression. She stated that she wasn't sure whether his seizures were "real" and insinuated that he could exercise more control over them. The more Rose verbalized her displeasure with what she considered Dan's lack of effort to overcome his problems, the more Dan felt unsupported and that his efforts would never satisfy Rose's expectations. Dan felt hopeless to change the situation, which negatively impacted his motivation to work on his depression and return to work. Rose also felt powerless to change the situation and expressed great displeasure that she has had to become the primary economic provider. "Bad" feelings had developed and a collective feeling of sadness and hopelessness characterized their family life. (Refer to Table 33.3.)

Sharing clinical impressions

In the McMaster Approach, the therapist reserves time to share with the family what he/she learned about the family's functioning. The therapist ended the session by summarizing his impressions and then asking the couple if they felt that he obtained an accurate picture of how they function as a couple and if there were any other areas that needed clarification. Dan and Rose stated that they felt understood and that the therapist appeared to have a good understanding of their relationship. The therapist then asked the couple to think about whether they wanted to use family therapy to work on their relationship and to give the therapist a call regarding their decision. Dan and Rose immediately stated that they would like to come back for another session. They agreed to think about what was discussed so that they could decide with the therapist what issues they felt they could work on in family therapy. The therapist explained that in the next session they would be asked to identify issues that they thought they could work on to improve their relationship.

Contracting stage

The contracting stage began with the therapist asking the couple if they had any thoughts about the first session. Dan and Rose stated that after the initial assessment they both discussed issues that were identified but they were unable to agree on what issues they could work on in therapy. The therapist shared with the couple their FAD scores and then the discussion moved to the couple agreeing on issues to work on in therapy.

Dan and Rose negotiated the following behavioral changes with each other:

1. Develop a more consistent weekend schedule that would allow Rose to rest when she comes home from work. Dan agreed to take care of the children while his wife slept and not to allow the children to disturb her while she was sleeping.
2. Work together to develop some house rules for the children.
3. Refrain from blaming one another for their current situation. Focus on how each is working to make things better. Dan agreed to let Rose know the behaviors he is working on in individual therapy and once he receives medical clearance to drive he will return to work.
4. Rose agreed to offer her husband positive comments when she sees him making an effort to help out more around the house and to refrain from making comments that can be taken as not making an effort to change.

The initial contracting expectations served as a frame of reference for treatment. As treatment progressed, these expectations were adjusted to the couple's ability to move forward and identify new issues. The therapist also noted his expectations.

Therapist's expectations
1. Keep all scheduled appointments (or call in advance to reschedule if needed).
2. Work hard on using what they have learned about one another to improve their relationship.
3. Telephone the therapist if any family member experienced a serious setback or crisis.

Treatment stage: overview

Dan and Rose participated in three additional treatment sessions over a period of two and a half months. The dominant themes that were revealed in the assessment and that organized their treatment was Dan's belief that his wife didn't believe that his problems were truly medical, that he was responsible for his family's struggles over the past two years, and Rose's contention that Dan was not working hard enough to "fix" his problems. Treatment sessions followed a pattern. Each session began with the couple's reflections of the previous meeting. This was followed by a discussion of what had worked and what hadn't worked since the previous session and why. When tasks were successfully completed, the therapist reinforced their efforts. If tasks were not followed, the reason preventing task completion was reviewed.

In each session, Dan and Rose discussed and worked on applying their "new" expectations for one another so they could address their respective problems. The therapist had the couple engage in face-to-face conversations and then he would reframe the content and themes of these conversations into formulations intended to help the couple more clearly understand one another's perspectives. The therapist pointed out perspectives and behaviors that were working and not working and then helped the couple reshape identified behaviors that they felt would improve their relationship. Sessions ended with Dan and Rose agreeing to work on these "new" behaviors and expectations between sessions.

The sessions were often emotionally intense. A major obstacle preventing the couple from resolving their differences was Rose's struggle with providing Dan with positive support when he did make efforts to change and Dan's adherence to the belief that nothing he could do would win his wife's approval. Initially these beliefs hindered the couple's ability to refine and transform their contracting expectations into concrete behaviors that they agreed to practice between sessions. However, as Dan and Rose experimented with and became more comfortable with new relationship behaviors and were better able to understand each other's perspective, they reported some improvement in their relationship.

Treatment session 1

The session took place two weeks after the contracting session and consisted of a series of interrelated revelations about their relationship. Dan and Rose began the session by stating that they experienced some success with following the new schedule and that this had motivated them to attend a barbecue at a neighbor's home. Rose commented that her husband's mood at the barbecue was more upbeat. She stated that "he participated, went in the pool, and smiled." Dan acknowledged Rose's observation and stated, "I haven't done anything in two years." The couple acknowledged that working together on implementing the new schedule agreed to in the contracting session motivated them to talk more without arguing. As Dan stated, "I made sure she slept."

The conversation then turned to the couple's dilemma. Dan began the conversation with the comment: "I went from being an active, productive husband and father to having to have my wife care for me." He went on to state how Rose compared him to her older brother who Rose believed was able to successfully work himself out of his depression. The couple agreed with the therapist's formulation that "The more Dan feels that Rose doesn't think that he is taking enough initiative to change, the less motivated he becomes, which only serves to confirm Rose's belief." They agreed that these behaviors were a "vicious circle" that left them feeling hopeless. The children worried about their father, especially when Rose took them out and Dan stayed home, too tired to participate. This only served to make Rose angrier with Dan.

The conversation ultimately worked its way into an issue that Dan had never discussed with Rose. The conversation began when Dan contrasted their style at the neighbor's barbecue to other couples. He observed: "We're not a traditional couple ... she won't sit next to me and rub the back of my head." He stated that what made them "nontraditional" was the lack of expressed affection between them. He repeated this observation when describing what he would like to happen when Rose comes home from work, saying that he wanted "a hug and a smile." This opened up a discussion of Rose's upbringing and how affection was not expressed in her house. A discussion ensued over the contrast in how each experiences and expresses emotions and affection. The couple agreed with the therapist's observation that when Dan sought support and affection, Rose withdrew and withheld affection, expecting Dan to overcome his depression "on his own," the way her older brother did.

The discussion of expressing emotions and affection opened up a space where Dan confessed that he has felt that he was "unlovable" since he and Rose married.

Dan: "I didn't think you loved me ... I never thought that I would measure up."

Rose (softly crying): "I never knew you thought that." Rose went on to state that in the early years of their relationship Dan was "fun, great ... everyone loved being around him ... he stopped being fun ... he's a different person. People are afraid of him not knowing what his mood will be."

Rose (continuing the discussion): "I'm still in love with him."

Dan and Rose then engaged in a conversation that revealed how their conflict was amplified by misinterpretations about one another's intentions and behaviors. Dan responded to Rose's comment that she still loves him by commenting that he interpreted her lack of demonstrative affection and what he termed her unpredictable mood as signs that she did not love him and did not find him attractive.

Dan: "I don't know which Rose is going to show up."

Rose: "You do know ... you know how it makes me feel when I come home to a mess. Sometimes you just don't care ... no one respects me."

Dan: "I do care."

Rose: "Then what is it?"

Dan: "The motivation ...." (referring to his lack of energy to clean the house).

Rose: "You don't even have the kids do anything."

Dan: "I want them to have fun ... I love them. I don't want to be mean. I don't want them to have to go through what I did when I was a kid. My parents were always yelling and screaming at us."

The session then turned to how the couple referred to each other as being "bitchy." The therapist then asked, "What would it look like for Rose to come home at night and not to get the 'bitchy Dan' and for Dan not to get the 'bitchy Rose'?"

Rose: "Not to trip over shoes and toys when I come through the door ... cups on the floor, food stains.... I would like to be able bring a friend home with me. I can't do that."

   Dan: "Smile, say hello. Give me a hug...ask me how was my day."

   Therapist: "Why can't you get there?"

   Rose: "Motivation."

   Dan: "Blame me to let the kids mess up the house."

The session ended with the couple agreeing to the following:

1. To discuss rules for the children to be more responsible for keeping the house clean.
2. Continue to follow the schedule agreed to in the contracting session.
3. Dan to take Rose out on a "date."
4. Rose to provide positive feedback whenever Dan shows that he is working on his emotional issues.

Treatment session 2

The second treatment session took place two weeks later. The session began with Dan reporting that he took Rose out to dinner over the weekend. The couple reported that at first they felt a little awkward but that the evening went well. Dan stated that he was making more of an effort to help out around the house and Rose stated how she was trying to be more supportive to Dan. The couple then requested that the rest of the session be devoted to developing a plan to use with their children.

The couple developed the following list of rules for their children:

1. Put toys and/or materials away when they finished an activity.
2. Clean up their bedrooms before going to bed.
3. Restrict play to their bedrooms and computer room. Clean up TV room after watching TV.
4. Eating restricted to the kitchen.

The session ended with the couple agreeing to the following:

1. Follow through with the plan for the children.
2. Continue with the plan developed in the contracting session.
3. Dan to continue following through with tasks developed in individual therapy.
4. Rose to continue to provide positive feedback to her husband's efforts to "get back on track."
5. The couple will go out on another "date."

Treatment session 3

Vacation schedules along with the couple canceling a session delayed the third and final treatment session for one month. (Parenthetically, cancellations after progress are not uncommon in therapy, with the challenge of a new pattern of functioning.) The couple began the session by reporting that there had been some regression over the past month. Dan, however, reported that there had been a significant decrease in his seizures and that he has scheduled an appointment with his neurologist to be medically re-evaluated to drive. Dan and Rose then proceeded to use the session to discuss the following: (1) Implementation of the rules for their children; (2) Dan's health issues; (3) Rose's feeling that Dan still needed to be motivated to regain his health; (4) Rose providing positive feedback to Dan's efforts to regain his health. The couple agreed to work on the above issues. Rose also stated that she felt that Dan and she should be able to work on these issues by themselves and, although therapy had been helpful to "put their issues on the table," she believed that one more session should be sufficient.

Closure

Unfortunately, a closure session did not take place. Dan called two days before the scheduled session to cancel, stating that Rose did not feel the need for therapy. Dan stated that things had been going better and that he found the therapy helpful but that Rose was a private person who felt that they should be able to resolve their issues without the assistance of therapy. A follow-up conversation with Dan's community therapist who was following his care reported that Dan had returned to work, his mood improved, he was seizure free, and he and Rose were still together.

Summary of the case and conclusion

The treatment of PNES may benefit from involving the patient's family. However, there is virtually no research documenting the effectiveness of family therapy as an intervention in the treatment of PNES [21]. Over the course of brief family therapy, Dan and Rose (1) learned how to discuss their disagreements, (2) modified their behaviors in small ways which helped them understand each other's perspectives, (3) addressed their family roles and responsibilities, and (4) cleared up some misconceptions each had of the other's feelings.

As alluded to above, the new transactional pattern sometimes presents a relational challenge. Many times families stop therapy only to return at a later date. If so, a new assessment should be completed to evaluate current functioning and to identify behaviors impacting family relationships. Rose and Dan did not feel the need for a final closure session, a decision that the therapist respected. He expressed encouragement that they continue to practice what they learned in family therapy and that he would be available should they need to discuss any other family issues. The therapist and family parted on a cordial note.

In sum, the treatment of PNES may benefit from an integrated treatment approach combining pharmacotherapy, individual and family therapy. As illustrated in this case, the reciprocal relationship between the patient's PNES symptoms and family functioning may be treated with family therapy.

References

1. Krawetz P, Fleisher W, Pillay MB, et al. Family functioning in subjects with pseudoseizures and epilepsy. *J Nerv Ment Dis* 2001;**189**(1):38–43.
2. Salmon P, Al-Marzooqi SM, Baker GA, Reilly J. Childhood family dysfunction and associated abuse in patients with nonepileptic seizures: towards a casual model. *Psychosom Med* 2003;**65**:695–700.
3. Moore PM, Baker GA, McDade G, Chadwick D, Brown S. Epilepsy, pseudoseizures, and perceived family characteristics: a controlled study. *Epilepsy Res* 1994;**18**(1):75–83.
4. Roy A. Hysteria. *J Psychosom Res* 1980;**24**:53–6.
5. Lempert T, Schmidt D. Natural history and outcome of psychogenic seizures: a clinical study of 50 patients. *J Neurol* 1990;**237**:35–8.
6. Blumer D, Adamolekun B. Treatment of patients with coexisting epileptic and nonepileptic seizures. *Epilepsy Behav* 2006;**9**:498–502.
7. Bowman ES, Markand ON. The contribution of life events to pseudoseizure occurrences in adults. *Bull Menninger Clin* 1999;**63**(1):70–88.
8. Fleisher W, Staley D, Krawetz P, et al. Comparative study of trauma-related phenomena in subjects with pseudoseizures and subjects with epilepsy. *Am J Psychiatry* 2002;**159**:660–3.
9. Moore PM, Baker GA. Non-epileptic attack disorder: a psychological perspective. *Seizure* 1997;**6**:429–34.
10. Stanhope N, Goldstein LH, Kuipers E. Expressed emotion in the relatives of people with epileptic or nonepileptic seizures. *Epilepsia* 2003;**44**(8):1094–102.
11. Wood BL, McDaniel S, Burchfiel K, Erba G. Factors distinguishing families of patients with psychogenic seizures from families of patients with epilepsy. *Epilepsia* 1998;**39**(4):432–7.
12. Griffith JL, Polles A, Griffith ME. Pseudoseizures, families and unspeakable dilemmas. *Psychosomatics* 1998;**39**:144–53.
13. Epstein NB, Bishop DS, Levin S. The McMaster Model of Family Functioning. *J Marriage Fam Couns* 1978;**4**:19–31.
14. Ryan CE, Epstein N, Keitner GI, Miller I, Bishop D. *Evaluating and Treating Families: The McMaster Approach*. New York: Routledge Taylor & Francis Group, 2005.
15. Keitner GI, Archambault R, Ryan CE, Miller IW. Family therapy and chronic depression, *J Clin Psychol* 2003;**59**(8):873–84.
16. Epstein NB, Baldwin LM, Bishop DS. The McMaster Family Assessment Device. *J Marital Fam Ther* 1983;**9**(2):171–80.
17. Epstein NB, Baldwin LM, Bishop DS. *The McMaster Clinical Rating Scale*. Providence, RI: Brown University Family Research Program, 1982.
18. Bishop DS, Epstein NB, Keitner GI, et al. *McMaster Structured Interview of Family Functioning (MCSIFF)*. Providence, RI: Brown University Family Research Program, 2000.
19. Epstein NB, Bishop DS. Problem centered systems therapy of the family. *J Marital Fam Ther* 1981;**7**(1):23–31.
20. LaFrance Jr WC, Blum A, Miller IW, Ryan CE, Keitner GI. Cognitive behavioral therapy or family therapy for nonepileptic seizures. *Epilepsia* 2008;**49** (Suppl 7):273–4.
21. Kanner AM, LaFrance Jr WC, Betts T. Psychogenic non-epileptic seizures. In: Engel Jr J, Pedley TA, eds. *Epilepsy: A Comprehensive Textbook*, 2nd edn. Philadelphia: Wolters Kluwer Health/Lippincott Williams & Wilkins. 2008; 2795–2810.

Appendix: Care coordination letters

School/individualized educational plan (IEP) template letter for student with psychogenic nonepileptic seizures

Department of Health and Human Services or to whomever it may concern:

I am writing to provide a brief overview of the clinical condition and educational needs of NAME. NAME has been continuing in treatment here at our office for nonepileptic seizures. He has multiple learning disabilities as well. He receives some family based treatment as well as medications. He has shown that he becomes easily overwhelmed in situations with excessive stimuli, and may respond with nonepileptic seizure episodes. These episodes may seem like seizures but are actually related to a stress condition. They are not medically dangerous.

If these episodes occur, I recommend that a calm and reassuring stance be taken. It is extremely unlikely that emergency medical attention will be required, but a visit to the school nurse and watchful waiting for the episode to end would be an adequate response. It may be counterproductive to call emergency medical services as we are trying to teach NAME to manage these events with coping strategies and stress management.

I would strongly recommend that an individualized educational plan be formulated based on an "other health impaired" distinction. Emphasis should be placed on reducing environmental stimulation, structuring transitions, and fostering social development with a facilitated social skills group or similar intervention. Please contact me for any questions. Thank you.

NAME OF PROVIDER, DEGREE
Letter format developed by Jay Salpekar, M.D.

Appendix: Care coordination letters

Mixed epilepsy-PNES generic response plan brief

NAME shows two types of seizures: (A) Epileptic Complex Partial Seizures and (B) Nonepileptic Seizures (NES)

Epileptic Complex Partial Seizures for NAME typically look like: [ENTER DESCRIPTION] EXAMPLE: twitching of her left upper extremity or twitching of both her upper and lower left extremities – twitching of muscles would be rhythmic; lying in bed appearing to be fidgeting but in a purposeless manner with purposeless movements, followed by stiffening of her extremities. *Eyes are open, pupils dilated.*

Nonepileptic Seizures, which are *NOT* medically dangerous for NAME typically look like: [ENTER DESCRIPTION] EXAMPLE: unresponsive, sitting with *eyes closed*, no associated movements; *eyes closed* with flailing of extremities in a random, nonrhythmic manner with changes from flailing extremities to stiffening extremities and then back to flailing; flailing or stiffening may worsen when other people approach her; sitting in chair, head slumped forward, *eyes closed* and then slumped slightly to right side; may have some stiffening and flailing of extremities in nonrhythmic manner with crying/tears towards the end of the episode; NES episodes may be precipitated by hyperventilation, feelings of panic, tightening of chest, and increase in heart rate.
[IF PANIC IS TRIGGER TO NES]

If you see NAME is hyperventilating with increased heart rate, feelings of panic, and feeling a tight chest, she may be having a panic attack. With these symptoms or developing a headache, you should:

- Stay calm.
- Minimize stimulation – dim lights, lower volume of sounds from TV or radio, decrease number of people interacting with NAME to one person.
- Tell her she is safe in calm, soothing voice.
- Let her know she is having a panic attack and that it will pass within a few minutes.
- Give gentle reassurance she is in a safe place and that she will be okay.
- Coach her to concentrate on taking slow, deep breaths up to minimum of ten breaths.
- Help her think about calm thoughts such as a favorite place to be – help her imagine what the place looks like, smells like, sounds like, feels like... Use whatever you can to distract her from focusing on her feelings of panic or worries about having NES.

If you see NAME is having a seizure: Talk to her briefly to see if she is responsive. Will she nod her head in response to a question? Will she speak? Look to see which type of seizure she may be having. Notice what time it is so you can time how long the event lasts.

If she is having an Epileptic Partial Seizure:

1. Provide her calm reassurance that she is okay and is safe.
2. Note the time the seizure began. Her partial seizures typically last 30 seconds or less.
   a. If she is having these types of seizures repeatedly, then call 911.
   b. If this type of seizure lasts longer than 10 minutes, call 911.
3. Monitor her for any changes.
   a. Note whether both sides of her body begin jerking in a rhythmic manner (Rhythmic = pace of jerks of all muscles are in sync and at the same pace, not flailing of extremities), with drooling or foaming of mouth, it may be generalizing to a Tonic-Clonic seizure. If you notice changes in any of these ways, call 911 or take her to the nearest Emergency Room for evaluation.
4. If no changes occur and the seizure is brief, note the date and duration of seizure and then return back to normal activities as soon as possible.

If she is having a Nonepileptic Seizure (NES):

1. Give her brief reassurance such as: "You are having a nonepileptic seizure. It's OK. You will be fine. Your body is asking for some time to calm. I am going to leave you to rest. I will stay close and check in on you."
2. Give her a safe and comfortable place to finish having the NES. She should not be near any potentially sharp or dangerous surfaces where she could bump herself during the NES. Televisions, video-games, and radios should be turned off. Lights should be dimmed. All people should be removed from the room. Check on her periodically to make sure nothing has changed.
   a. Check her eyes – are her pupils dilated? If so, she may be having a partial seizure, see above directions.

    b. Check the jerking/flailing of extremities – is it rhythmic? If so, she may be having an epileptic seizure and then see above directions.

    c. If no changes, then leave her alone with continued checking and nearby supervision to ensure safety.

3. Note the date and duration of the NES. Note what was happening just before it started happening. Can you connect any stress or strong emotion to the event?

4. Once the NES is done, return to normal activities as soon as is possible to reinstate normalcy and minimize disruption to her daily life. If she still you stressed, seems may want to allow her some time to rest until she is ready to resume activities.

Appendix: Care coordination letters

Response plan for child with both epileptic seizures and nonepileptic seizures

CHILD shows two types of events: (A) Epileptic Seizures, most often Complex Partial Seizures and (B) Psychogenic Nonepileptic Seizures (NES)

Epileptic Seizures for CHILD typically look like: [describe in detail most typical event, include eyes open, pupils dilated, rhythmic movements, etc…as applicable]

Non-epileptic events, which are *NOT* medically caused for CHILD typically look like: [describe in detail most typical NES, include eyes closed, non-rhythmic movements, etc.…as applicable] [Also include any known triggers or warning signs that often precipitate NES]

If you see CHILD is [insert known warning signs of NES]:

- Stay calm.
- Minimize stimulation – dim lights, lower volume of sounds from TV or radio, decrease number of people interacting with CHILD to one person.
- Tell her she is safe in calm, soothing voice.
- Give gentle reassurance she is safe and that she will be okay.
- Coach her to concentrate on taking slow, deep breaths up to minimum of ten breaths.
- Help her think about calm thoughts such as a favorite place to be – help her imagine what the place looks like, smells like, sounds like, feels like… With goal of trying to distract her from focusing upon worry about an impending NES.

If you see CHILD is having an event:

Talk to her briefly to see if she is responsive. Will she nod her head in response to a question? Will she speak? Look to see which type of seizure she may be having. Notice what time it is so you can time how long the event lasts.

If she is having an Epileptic Seizure:

1. Provide her calm reassurance that she is okay and is safe.
2. Note the time the seizure began. Her complex partial seizures typically last XX seconds or less.
3. Follow instructions given to you by her neurologist. This may include:
   a. If she is having these types of seizures repeatedly, then call 911.
   b. If this type of seizure lasts longer than XX minutes, call 911.
4. Monitor her for any changes.
   a. Note whether both sides of her body begin jerking in a rhythmic manner (Rhythmic = pace of jerks of all muscles are in sync and at the same pace, not flailing of extremities), with drooling or foaming of mouth, it may be generalizing to a Tonic-Clonic seizure. If you notice changes in any of these ways, call 911 or take her to the nearest Emergency Room for evaluation.
5. If no changes occur and the seizure is brief, note the date and duration of seizure and then return back to normal activities as soon as possible.

If she is having a Nonepileptic Seizure (NES):

1. Give her brief reassurance such as: "You are having a nonepileptic seizure. It's OK. You will be fine. Your body is asking for some time to calm. I am going to leave you to rest. I will stay close and check in on you."
2. Give her a safe and comfortable place to finish having the NES. She should not be near any potentially sharp or dangerous surfaces where she could bump herself during the NES. Televisions, video-games, and radios should be turned off. Lights should be dimmed. All people should be removed from the room.
3. Check on her periodically to make sure nothing has changed.
   a. Check her eyes – are her pupils dilated? If so, she may be having a partial seizure, see above directions.
   b. Check the jerking/flailing of extremities – is it rhythmic? If so, she may be having an epileptic seizure and then see above directions.
   c. If no changes, then continue to monitor her without interacting with her.
4. Note the date and duration of the NES. Note what was happening just before it started happening. Can you connect any stress to the event?
5. Once the NES is done, return to normal activities as soon as is possible to minimize disruption to her daily life. If she seems still stressed, you may want to allow her some time to rest until she is ready to resume activities.

NAME OF PROVIDER, PhD, LP   Date
Licensed Psychologist
LOCATION

XXXXXX XXXXX, MD   Date
Pediatric Epileptologist/Neurologist
LOCATION

PNES generic response plan (brief)

The attending epileptologist/neurologist working with your child has determined that your child has episodes of psychogenic nonepileptic seizures (NES) that may look very similar to epileptic seizures but are not actually caused by abnormal brain activity. Nonepileptic seizures are not medical in nature and therefore do not warrant medical intervention. The NES will not stop in response to antiepileptic medications. In most cases, these episodes are not purposeful and are not intentional. The NES are resulting from an inability to recognize and properly cope with stress, anxiety, frustration, or other strong negative emotions. Nonepileptic seizures may also result from unrecognized or unaddressed underlying mental health issues or traumas. Nonepileptic seizures are real. The mind is causing the body to respond physically to negative emotions, similar to when some people get stomach aches or hives when nervous or headaches when stressed.

The first line of defense against NES is to obtain individual psychotherapy with the goal of decreasing the frequency or eliminating altogether the NES. We specifically recommend a mental health professional (e.g., a licensed psychologist) with specialized training in working with children and adolescents. Goals for psychotherapy to address NES typically include, but may not be limited to, (1) reducing physiological arousal through relaxation techniques, (2) enhancing activity regulation through increasing exercise and pleasurable, meaningful activities and pacing those activities, (3) increasing awareness of emotions including physical, behavioral, and cognitive signals of various feelings, (4) modifying dysfunctional beliefs, (5) enhancing communication of thoughts and emotions, (6) reducing reinforcement of illness behaviors by others (family, peers, teachers, etc...), and (7) increasing social support network. Sometimes individuals with NES also benefit from seeing a psychiatrist who can prescribe psychotropic medications to decrease anxiety, depression, or to address other mental health issues. As needed and with appropriate permission from you, our team can work collaboratively with these professionals to maximize benefit of services.

In addition to these services, it is essential that family members and school staff members respond consistently to NES in order to minimize the impact of the NES on daily functioning. Regular visits with the school counselor often serve as a source of additional support during school for both academic- and social-related stress. The school counselor should work on a regular basis with your child's psychologist/therapist to ensure consistency. The counselor can reinforce new skills the child learns in psychotherapy by prompting them to use the skills while in the school setting (e.g., relaxation exercises). We also recommend the following plan be implemented at both home and school for the NES.

<u>You should obtain a description of the specific ways you can tell that an event is an NES from the physician or nurse treating the child with the NES. The description of the NES should be put in writing and given to school staff and other caretakers involved with the child, and ideally would be attached to this response plan for reference as needed.</u>

Response Plan for NES:

1. If you see that the child may be having a NES or if she states that she is worried that she may have a NES, talk to the child briefly. Will they nod their head in response to a question? Will they speak? Look at their symptoms and make note of the time and date.

2. It is okay to give the child brief reassurance and tell them what you are going to do in response to the NES, such as:

   a. "You are having one of your nonepileptic seizures. It's OK. You will be fine. Your body is asking for some time to calm down. I am going to stay close but step away to give you that time to calm down." <u>Or</u>

   b. "You're having a nonepileptic seizure, but you are okay and you are safe. I am going to turn off the TV and step away to give you time to rest."

   c. **After this brief reassurance, it is best to stop interacting with the person until the NES has stopped.**

3. Ensure the child is in a physical position where they cannot get hurt but where they can finish having the NES. We do not recommend they be moved to another location such as the nurses' office, as this will not help them learn how to manage their stress on their own. Removing to another location can sometimes actually backfire

because the child is able to avoid the very thing that triggered the strong emotion to begin with, which does not give them a chance to learn how to cope with those stress-related feelings in a healthy way.
4. Keep them away from potentially sharp or dangerous surfaces where they could bump something during the NES.
5. Televisions, radios, and video-games should be immediately turned off. Lights should be dimmed.
6. It is best to avoid holding or restraining the child having the NES.
7. **Do not** attempt to put anything in the child's mouth.
8. If others are present in the room, if possible, they should be instructed to return to their normal activities without interacting with the person until the NES is finished.
    a. We encourage you to use language such as: "NAME is having a nonepileptic seizure, but she's okay. Let's let her be so she can get better."
    b. If the child is at home during the NES, all others should leave the room except for one person who can stay near to monitor their safety.
9. Monitor the child to make sure nothing has changed.
10. It is not appropriate to give the child medications, to send them home from school, to send them away from class, to call the paramedics, to give them prizes, or to allow them to avoid any particular tasks in response to NES.
    a. However, if there are new or unusual physical symptoms such as loss of consciousness we do recommend that 911 be called and that the child be evaluated by a physician to rule out other seizure activity.

After the NES:
11. Note the duration of the NES. Note what was happening just before it started happening. Can you connect any stress or strong emotion to the event?
12. It is essential that "normal" activities typical for the child be resumed as soon as is possible to reinstate normalcy and minimize disruption to their daily life. Neutral, calm responses by others to these events will help to make them feel safe and calm.
13. If the child still appears stressed, worried, or fearful, you may want to allow them a very brief period of time to rest before resuming activities. However, this rest time should take place in the same location where the NES occurred. The child should not be removed to an alternate location as this will only increase disruption to their activities and may send them the signal that something *is* wrong.
14. Please keep others informed of occurrences of NES, including parents, school staff, and therapists.

Appendix: Care coordination letters

Response plan for Child with lone nonepileptic seizures

Student/Patient: NAME
Date of Birth:
Date Plan Developed:
Providers:

Presenting Issue: The attending neurologist working with NAME has determined that she has episodes of psychogenic nonepileptic seizures (NES) that may look very similar to epileptic seizures but are not actually caused by abnormal brain activity. Nonepileptic seizures are not medical in nature and therefore do not warrant medical intervention. In most cases, these episodes are not purposeful and are not intentional. The NES are resulting from an inability to recognize and properly cope with stress, anxiety, frustration, or other strong negative emotions. Nonepileptic seizures may also result from unrecognized or unaddressed underlying mental health issues or trauma. Nonepileptic seizures are real. The mind is causing the body to respond physically to negative emotions, similar to when some people get stomach aches or hives when nervous or headaches when stressed.

The first line of defense against NES is to obtain individual psychotherapy with the goal of decreasing the frequency or eliminating altogether the NES. **Note here if patient is already seeing a psychologist or psychiatrist** We specifically recommend a mental health professional with specialized training in working with children and adolescents. Goals for psychotherapy to address NES typically include, but may not be limited to, (1) reducing physiological arousal through relaxation techniques, (2) enhancing activity regulation through increasing exercise and pleasurable, meaningful activities and pacing those activities, (3) increasing awareness of emotions including physical, behavioral, and cognitive signals of various feelings, (4) modifying dysfunctional beliefs, (5) enhancing communication of thoughts and emotions, (6) reducing reinforcement of illness behaviors by others (family, peers, teachers, etc...), and (7) increasing social support network. Sometimes individuals with NES also benefit from seeing a psychiatrist who can prescribe psychotropic medications to decrease anxiety, depression, or to address other mental health issues. As needed and with your permission, our team can work collaboratively with these professionals to maximize benefit of services.

In addition to these services, it is essential that family members and school staff members respond consistently to NES in order to minimize the impact of the NES on daily functioning. Regular visits with the school counselor often serve as a source of additional support during school for both academic- and social-related stress. The school counselor should work closely with the person's psychologist/therapist to ensure consistency. The counselor can reinforce new skills the person learns in psychotherapy by prompting them to use the skills while in the school setting (e.g., relaxation exercises). We also recommend the following plan be implemented at both home and school for the NES.

<u>Description of NAME's nonepileptic seizures (e.g., psychologically based or psychogenic nonepileptic seizures that are not medical in nature):</u>

*NAME typically refers to her NES as "(insert term used by family)"
*NAME'S NES are often precipitated by (stressing events?)
*NAME'S NES often begin with (symptoms)
*DESCRIBE NES in detail.
*Sometimes, NAME's NES can be interrupted or stopped quicker by
*NAME's NES often last approximately (duration)
*After the NES, NAME usually (behaviors, responsiveness, state of mind)

<u>Response Plan for NES:</u>

1. If you see that the child may be having NES or if she states that she is worried that she may have a NES, talk to the child briefly. Will they nod their head in response to a question? Will they speak? Look at their symptoms and make note of the time and date.
2. It is okay to give the child brief reassurance and tell them what you are going to do in response to the NES, such as:

   a. "You are having one of your nonepileptic seizures. It's OK. You will be fine. Your body is asking for some time to calm down. I am going to stay close but step away to give you that time to calm down." <u>Or</u>

   b. "You're having a nonepileptic seizure, but you are okay and you are safe. I am going to turn off the TV and step away to give you time to rest."

c. **After this brief reassurance, it is best to stop interacting with the person until the NES has stopped.**

3. Ensure the person is in a physical position where they cannot get hurt but where they can finish having the NES. We do not recommend they be moved to another location such as the nurses' office, as this will not help them learn how to manage their stress on their own. Removing to another location can sometimes actually backfire because the person is able to avoid the very thing that stressed them out to begin with, which does not give them a chance to learn how to cope with those stress-related feelings in a healthy way.
4. Keep them away from potentially sharp or dangerous surfaces where they could bump something during the NES.
5. Televisions, radios, and video-games should be immediately turned off. Dim lights.
6. It is best to avoid holding or restraining the person having the NES.
7. **Do not** attempt to put anything in the person's mouth.
8. If others are present in the room, if possible, they should be instructed to return to their normal activities without interacting with the person until the NES is finished.
    a. We encourage you to use language such as: "NAME is having a nonepileptic seizure, but she's okay. Let's let her be so she can get better."
    b. If the person is at home during the NES, all others should leave the room except for one person who can stay near to monitor their safety.
9. Monitor the person to make sure nothing has changed.
10. It is not appropriate to give the person medications, to send them home from school, to send them away from class, to call the paramedics, to give them prizes, or to allow them to avoid any particular tasks in response to NES.
    a. However, if there are new or unusual physical symptoms such as loss of consciousness we do recommend that 911 be called and that the person be evaluated by a physician to rule out other seizure activity.

After the NES:

11. Note the duration of the NES. Note what was happening just before it started happening. Can you connect any stress to the event?
12. It is essential that "normal" activities typical for the person be resumed as soon as is possible to reinstate normalcy and minimize disruption to their daily life. Neutral, calm responses by others to these events will help to make them feel safe and calm.
13. If the person still appears stressed, worried, or fearful, you may want to allow them a very brief period of time to rest before resuming activities. However, this rest time should take place in the same location where the NES occurred. The person should not be removed to an alternate location as this will only increase disruption to their activities and may send them the signal that something *is* wrong.
14. Please keep others informed of occurrences of NES, including parents, school staff, and therapists.

This plan was developed collaboratively by NAME's medical/psychosocial team at LOCATION.

PROVIDER, PhD	XXXXX, MD
Licensed Psychologist	Attending Epileptologist/ Neurologist
Pediatric Psychology Services	SERVICE LOCATION
SERVICE LOCATION	

Format developed by Anastasia Sullwold Ristan, Ph.D.

Index

abridged somatization disorder, 27
abuse/trauma
　association with PNES, 213–15
activation procedures. *See* diagnosis of PNES
acute life-threatening event (ALTE) neonates and infants, 94–7
adolescents with PNES, 104
　perceptions about PNES, 187–9
　perceptions of family members, 187–9
　See also diagnostic approach for children; paroxysmal events in children.
advanced practice psychiatric nurse role in care of patients with PNES, 255–6
afebrile infantile convulsions, 69
affective disorders
　comorbidity with PNES, 11
affective functioning in PNES patients
　objective neuropsychological findings, 144–5
　subjective appraisal, 144–5
age-related macular degeneration, 71
aggressive outbursts, 71
alternating hemiplegia of childhood, 101
Alzheimer's disease, 116
amobarbital
　use in PNES diagnosis, 42
antiepileptic drugs (AEDs)
　resistance in PNES, 38
　See also pharmacological treatments for PNES.
antihistamines, 65
anxiety disorders
　comorbidity with PNES, 11, 226–7
anxiety in PNES patients, 145–6
aortic stenosis, 64, 65

apnea (neonatal and infantile), 94–7
Arnold-Chiari malformation, 67
ataque de nervios (attack of nerves). *See* Puerto Rican culture and PNES
athetosis, 102, 115
atrial myxoma, 65
atrioventricular block, 64
attention deficit disorder, 101, 102
autistic spectrum disorder, 100
autosomal dominant nocturnal frontal lobe epilepsy (ADNFLE), 69

ballism, 102, 115
benign myoclonus of infancy, 99–100
benign neonatal sleep myoclonus, 97
benign nonepileptic infantile spasms, 99–100
benign paroxysmal positional vertigo, 68, 70
benign paroxysmal torticollis of infancy, 99
benign paroxysmal vertigo, 98
BNI Screen for Higher Cerebral Functions (BNIS), 144
body rocking in children, 100
borderline personality disorder, 142, 228–31
Boston Naming Test, 144
bradyarrhythmias, 65
brain injury
　and PNES, 43
breath-holding spells in children, 46, 98
Breuer, Joseph, 22, 82
Brief Visuospatial Memory Test-Revised, 143
Briquet, Pierre, 19–20
Briquet's hysteria, 19–20, 24

bromides
　early use in PNES treatment 238, 310
Brugada syndrome, 64, 65, 67
bruxism (sleep-related), 79
burden of PNES. *See* costs of PNES

California Verbal Learning Test, 137
carcinoid syndrome, 72
cardiac events, 3
cardiogenic syncope, 64, 65–6
cardiomyopathy, 65
cardiomyopathy, inherited, 65
care of patients with PNES
　benefits of psychological support and education, 253–4
　comprehensive care, 253–4
　diagnostic disclosure protocol, 256
　multidisciplinary approach, 253–4
　multidisciplinary model of care, 254–8
　presenting the diagnosis to the patient, 254–5
　psychological support, 254–5
　role of the advanced practice psychiatric nurse, 255–6
　role of the nurse, 255–6
　role of the social worker, 256–7
carotid sinus hypersensitivity, 65
Carter, Robert Brudenell, 19
cataplexy, 67–8
　in children and adolescents, 105
catatonia, 203
causation of PNES
　legal implications, 159–60
cerebrogenic cardiac dysfunction, 66
Charcot, Jean-Martin, 20–1, 82, 83, 132, 297
Charles Bonnet syndrome, 71
childhood neglect
　association with PNES, 214

Index

children with PNES
  adolescents' perceptions about PNES, 187–9
  approaches to diagnosis and treatment, 183–5
  clinical vignettes, 171–4
  cognitive evaluation, 179
  comorbid psychiatric diagnoses, 165–6
  diagnostic challenges, 166–7
  diagnostic feedback to parents and child, 169–71
  diagnostic process, 167–9
  etiological theories, 187
  familiy conflict and psychopathology, 179–80
  history of multiple stressors, 179–80
  history of sexual abuse, 179
  individual child's experience of stress, 185
  learning difficulties, 179–80
  models of pediatric PNES, 163–5
  parents' perceptions about PNES, 187–9
  peer relationship problems, 180
  perceptions of PNES in India, 189
  prevalence related to age, 187
  primary diagnosis, 165
  psychological assessment, 179
  risk factors for pediatric PPNES, 163
  study of stressor types and responses, 180–3
  timing of diagnosis, 167
  treatment goals, 174–6
  See also diagnostic approach for children; paroxysmal events in children.

chorea, 69, 101, 115

chronic fatigue syndrome, 27–8, 39

chronic pain, 39

chronic pelvic pain, 216

Chvostek's sign, 101

circadian rhythm sleep disorders, 77

Clarke, Pierce, 22

classical conditioning model for treatment, 269–70

classification of nonepileptic seizures
  catatonia, 203
  conversion disorders, 203
  dissociative states, 202–3
  DSM, 199, 202
  episodic dyscontrol, 204
  etiologic approach, 201–2
  issues concerning consciousness, 204–5
  malingering, 203–4
  nosological approach, 202–4
  panic attacks, 203
  PNES, 204
  purpose, 201
  semiological approach, 202
  semi-structured clinical interview for diagnosis (SCID), 209
  tool to classify PNES, 209

classifications of PNES
  as symptom or disease, 12
  based on etiology, 8, 11
  based on personality testing, 7
  based on semiology, 5–7
  based on semiology and personality testing, 8
  based on suspected psychological mechanism, 8
  clinical relevance of subtypes of PNES, 5
  comorbidities of PNES, 11–12
  descriptive vs. etiological approach, 11
  differential diagnosis, 8–9
  DSM, 11, 12–13
  ICD, 11
  proposed dissociative subtype, 12
  somatoform vs. dissociative nature, 10–11
  sources of confusion, 10–13
  suggested changes to DSM, 12–13
  within existing psychiatric taxonomies, 9–13

clinical features of PNES. *See* diagnosis of PNES

clinical psychologist
  role in treatment of PNES, 263–4

clinical types of PNES, 79

cognitive behavioral therapy (CBT) for PNES, 281–2
  Brown Medical School, Rhode Island Hospital, 282–3
  Maudsley Hospital, London, 283–5
  questions not yet answered by research, 285
  therapeutic challenges posed by this patient group, 285–6

cognitive complaints of PNES patients, 144
  and level of self-perceived anxiety, 145–6
  implications for clinical practice and research, 146–7
  memory dysfunction, 145–6

cognitive functioning in PNES patients
  objective neuropsychological findings, 144–5
  subjective appraisal, 144–5

colloid cysts, 67

comorbid ES and PNES, 5, 43
  and developmental delay, 58
  case examples, 51–2
  characteristics of NES versus ES, 55–6
  definition of ES, 51
  definition of PNES, 51
  delay in diagnosis, 52–3
  diagnosis, 53–4
  EEG, 57
  epilepsy surgery and PNES, 58
  healthcare costs, 53
  historical reports, 51
  ictal semiology, 55
  incidence and prevalence, 52–3
  indications for suspicion, 51
  medical treatment, 53
  negative VEEG using scalp recordings, 56
  neuropsychological evaluations, 56–7
  prolactin measurement, 58
  pseudostatus and status epilepticus, 56
  quality of life (QOL) effects, 53
  risk factors, 53–4
  social impacts, 53
  temporal relationship of seizures, 54–5
  VEEG, 57–8
  See also epilepsy with PNES.

comorbidities with PNES, 11–12
  anxiety disorders, 226–7
  associations with trauma, 215–17
  mood disorders, 226–7
  personality disorders, 227–31

complaisant overadjustment, 122

confidentiality
  legal implications of PNES, 158–9

confusional arousals, 45, 72, 78

confusional states (prolonged), 72–3

congenital heart disease, 64

Conversation Analysis, 85–6

conversion, 22
  symptoms in PNES patients, 29

conversion disorder, 203
  DSM criteria, 11
  in children and adolescents, 105
  in patients with PNES, 27

337

Index

convulsionnaires, 17

convulsive movement episodes, 68–70

costs of PNES
- antiepileptic drug use, 31
- changes in employment status, 32
- comorbid medical and psychiatric conditions, 31–2
- comparison with intractable epilepsy, 29–30
- comparison with well-defined disorders, 28–9
- estimating costs, 29–32
- extent of MUS in neurology practice, 28–9
- financial assistance, 32
- pre-diagnosis costs, 30
- prognosis, 32
- tertiary care, 30–1

cough syncope, 65

creatine kinase
- postictal testing, 44

culture and PNES
- culturally embodied metaphors, 121
- development of culturally appropriate treatments, 128
- India, 126–8
- Puerto Rico, 124–6
- socio-cultural factors in psychopathology, 121–2
- theoretical background, 121–2
- Turkey, 122–4

culture-specific startle syndromes, 70

DAPP-BQ (Dimensional Assessment of Personality Pathology-Basic Questionnaire), 7

daydreaming in children, 101

decision tree to diagnose seizure-like events, 205–9

dementia, 111, 115, 116

denial in PNES patients
- brain structures involved, 145–6

depression
- in the elderly, 111

DES (Dissociative Experiences Scale), 11

descriptive approach to classification of PNES, 11

developmental delay
- and comorbid ES and PNES, 58

diabetes
- in the elderly, 115

diagnosis of comorbid ES and PNES, 53–4

diagnosis of PNES, 3–4
- abnormal movements in the ICU, 46
- ambulatory EEG, 39
- analysis of ictal semiology, 40–2
- circumstances in which attacks occur, 38
- coexisting epilepsy, 43
- coexisting neurological disease, 43
- differential diagnosis, 8–9, 45–6
- differentiation from epilepsy, 8–9, 83–4
- differentiation from parasomnias, 45–6
- differentiation from paroxysmal movement disorders, 46
- differentiation from syncope, 45
- difficult and special issues, 43
- difficulties in accepting the diagnosis, 261–2
- errors in EEG interpretation, 43
- ES and PNES, 77
- events which occur during sleep, 77
- examination, 39
- frequency of events, 38
- home video recordings, 39
- in the elderly, 43
- induction of seizures, 42
- lack of ictal EEG changes, 43–4
- late-onset PNES, 43
- limitations of VEEG monitoring, 43–4
- linguistic analysis, 85–8
- misdiagnosis as epilepsy, 38
- multiple seizure types, 43
- neuropsychological evaluation, 45
- nocturnal seizures, 79–80
- physiological nonepileptic events, 45–6
- PNES after epilepsy surgery, 43
- postictal laboratory tests, 44–5
- presenting the diagnosis to the patient, 254–6
- previous abnormal EEG, 43
- provocative techniques, 42
- psychological profiling, 45
- resistance to AEDs, 38
- role of VEEG, 8–9, 38
- routine EEG, 39
- short-term outpatient VEEG with activation, 42
- sources of confusion, 10–13
- specific triggers, 38
- suspicion by patient history, 38–9
- transient loss of awareness, 62–3
- use of hypnosis, 83–4
- use of hypnosis to induce PNES, 83–4
- VEEG monitoring, 39–42, 43–4

diagnosis of seizure-like events decision tree, 205–9

Diagnostic and Statistical Manual of Mental Disorders. *See* DSM

diagnostic approach for children
- clinical clues from the history, 91–2
- clinical event description, 91
- confirmatory tests for nonepileptic events, 92–3
- differential diagnosis. *See* paroxysmal events in children
- ES differential diagnosis, 92
- nonepileptic differential diagnosis, 92
- particular challenges in children, 105
- patient history, 91–2
- risk factors from the history, 91–2
- routine EEG, 92
- simultaneous VEEG and polysomnography, 92–3

diagnostic disclosure protocol
- patients with PNES, 256

diagnostic issues in the elderly. *See* elderly people

Digit Memory Test, 137

digoxin, 65

disability
- legal implications of PNES, 159

discrimination against patients with PNES, 159

dissociation
- and trauma, 82–3

dissociation in PNES, 10–11
- proposed dissociative subtype, 12

dissociative disorder
- comorbidity with PNES, 11

dissociative identity disorder (DID), 83

dissociative states, 202–3

driving
- legal implications of PNES, 157–8

drop attacks, 67–8

DSM (Diagnostic and Statistical Manual of Mental Disorders)
- approach to psychiatric classification, 11
- classification of nonepileptic seizures, 199, 202
- classification of PNES, 11

Index

personality disorder classifications, 7
suggested changes to PNES classification, 12–13
dysautonomia, 9
dyskinesias
  in children, 101–2
dystonia, 69, 102, 115

echolalia, 70
echopraxia, 70
elderly people
  age-related diagnostic issues, 111
  diabetes, 115
  diagnostic issues, 110
  diagnostic steps and problems, 111–12
  diagnostic VEEG monitoring, 110, 112, 116
  encephalopathy, 111, 115–16
  epidemiology of NES, 110–11
  hyperkinetic symptoms, 115
  hypoglycemia, 115
  ischemic events, 114
  late-onset PNES, 43
  movement disorders, 115
  NES treatment and outcome, 116
  physiological NES, 114
  PNES treatment and outcome, 116
  psychogenic NES (PNES), 114
  REM sleep behavior disorder, 115
  routine EEG monitoring, 111–12
  sleep disorders, 115
  syncope, 114
  TIAs (transient ischemic attacks), 114
electroencephalogram (EEG)
  markers for the hypnotic state, 83
emotional abuse
  association with PNES, 213–14
emotional adjustment evaluation and PNES, 138–40
encephalopathy
  in the elderly, 111, 115–16
epidemiology of NES in the elderly, 110–11
epidemiology of PNES, 3–5
  diagnosis of PNES, 3–4
  ES comorbidity, 5
  incidence, 4
  prevalence, 4–5
epilepsy
  association with hysteria, 22–3
  association with sleep, 71–2

historical association with hysteria, 19
misdiagnosis of PNES, 38
PNES after epilepsy surgery, 43
epilepsy diagnosis
  analysis of ictal semiology, 40–2
  differentiation from migraine, 70
  ES and PNES, 77
  nocturnal seizures, 79–80
  rates of misdiagnosis, 62
  transient loss of awareness, 62–3
  use of hypnosis, 83–4
  See also diagnosis of PNES.
epilepsy surgery and PNES, 58
epilepsy with PNES, 43
  diagnosis of epilepsy, 248–9
  diagnosis of PNES, 248
  incidence, 247
  management challenges, 247
  management of epilepsy, 250–1
  management of PNES, 249–50
  managing the diagnostic process, 248
  overall management strategy for PNES, 247–8
  patient characteristics, 248
  Quarriers inpatient assessment process, 251
  therapeutic value of AED reduction, 250
  See also comorbid ES and PNES.
epileptic myoclonus, 68
epileptic personality concept, 23
epileptic seizures (ES)
  comorbidity with PNES, 5
  differentiation from PNES, 3, 8–9
episodic ataxia
  in children, 102
episodic ataxia (EA1 and EA2), 69
episodic dyscontrol, 204
  in children, 102
episodic dyscontrol syndrome, 71
episodic phenomena in sleep, 71–2
essential tremor, 98
etiological classification of nonepileptic seizures, 201–2
etiological approach to classification of PNES, 8, 11, 266–74
etiological models for treatment
  classical conditioning model, 269–70
  family systems model, 269
  individualized treatment plans, 277

learning theory models, 269–70
operant conditioning model, 270
"organic" psychosyndrome model, 273–4
psychodynamic approach, 266–9
psychosomatic/psychophysiological models, 273
stress model, 270–3
subgroups in PNES, 275–6
towards a unified model for PNES, 274–5
etiology of PNES
  attachment trauma theories, 218
  complexity and variability, 219
  dissociation theories, 217–18
  dissociation vs. somatization, 10–11
  family dysfunction theories, 218
  historical theories, 213
  information from comorbidities, 12
  PNES as brain trauma, 219
  PNES as panic attacks, 218–19
  PTSD theories, 218
  somatization vs. dissociation, 10–11
  theories linking trauma or PTSD, 217–19
  use in classification schemes, 8
excessive fragmentary hypnic myoclonus, 77, 79

faciomandibular myoclonus, 79
factitious disorder, 28
  See also Munchausen syndrome.
familial dilated cardiomyopathy, 65
Family Assessment Device (FAD), 318
family conflict and psychopathology
  children with PNES, 179–80
family dysfunction
  association with PNES, 214–15
family members
  perceptions about children with PNES, 187–9
family system dysfunction in PNES, 317
family systems model of treatment, 269
family therapy
  assessment instruments, 318–19
  case study (McMaster Assessment), 320–6
  McMaster Model of Family Functioning (MMFF), 317–18
  principles and focus, 317

339

family therapy (*cont.*)
  Problem Centered Systems Therapy of the Family (PCSTF), 319–20
  role of family dysfunction in PNES, 317
fibromyalgia, 27–8, 39, 217
"forced obedience" response, 70
frequency of PNES, 82
Freud, Sigmund, 21–3, 82, 85, 131, 132, 297
fugue states (prolonged), 72–3
functional somatic syndromes, 27–8
furor uterinus, 18

generalized epilepsy with febrile seizures (GEFS+), 69
geste antagoniste, 69, 102
glaucoma, 71
globus hystericus, 17
grand chorea epidemics, 17
group psychotherapy
  history of development, 289
  theoretical orientations, 289
group therapy for PNES
  active relaxation/behavioral activation teaching, 294
  adjunctive treatment, 294–5
  as adjunctive treatment, 292
  awareness of secondary gain, 294
  cognitive restructuring techniques, 294
  contribution to threshold dose of care, 292
  cost-effectiveness, 292
  exposure techniques, 294
  format at Stanford University outpatients Behavior Medicine Clinic, 293–5
  intake interview, 293–4
  interpersonal skills training, 293–4
  motivational techniques, 294
  potential benefits for patients, 289
  psycho-educational presentation, 294
  radical acceptance of symptoms, 294
  rationale, 291–3
  relapse prevention training, 294
  ripple effect within the group, 292
  social support, 292–3
  studies, 289–91
  treatment of comorbid conditions, 292

unique change-inducing factors, 293
Gulf War syndrome, 27

hallucinations, 9, 71, 77, 105
  in children, 104
haloperidol, 312
head banging, 46, 71, 100
head injury
  and PNES, 43
headrolling in children, 100
Health Related Quality of Life, 139
  concept, 149
  limitations of measures for PNES patients, 154–5
  measures, 149–50
  PNES, 150–1
  PNES compared with anxiety and depression, 153
  PNES compared with ES, 151
  self-report questionnaires, 149–50
hereditary hyperekplexia, 97
historical approaches to PNES treatment, 237–43
history of hysteria
  ancient Egyptians, 17
  ancient Greeks, 17
  association with epilepsy, 18–19, 22–3
  association with trauma, 22
  association with witchcraft, 17
  beginnings of neurology, 18
  Briquet's hysteria, 19–20, 24
  eighteenth and nineteenth centuries, 18–19
  epileptic personality concept, 23
  implication of sexual causes, 18, 19
  link between body and mind, 18–19
  link with emotions, 18
  Middle Ages, 17
  new hysteria studies, 24
  outbreaks of mass hysteria, 17
  posttraumatic hysteria, 19
  role of subconscious ideas, 21
  role of unconscious conflicts, 22
  socio-historical studies, 24
  stress as trigger for seizures, 23–4
  supernatural explanations, 17
  the French school, 19–21
  twentieth century, 23–4
  wandering womb concept, 17
  war-related neuroses, 23–4
  work of Briquet, 19–20, 238
  work of Charcot, 20–1, 238–9
  work of Freud, 21–3

work of Janet, 21, 239
work of Laycock, 18–19
work of Sydenham, 18
work of Whytt, 18
work of Willis, 18
hyperekplexia, 69–70
  in neonates and infants, 97
hyperkalemic periodic paralyses, 68
hyperkinetic movement disorders
  in children, 101–2
hyperkinetic symptoms
  elderly people, 115
hypersomnias of central origin, 77
hypertrophic cardiomyopathy, 64, 65
hypertrophic obstructive cardiomyopathy, 65
hyperventilation in children, 101
hypnic jerks (sleep starts), 71, 77
hypnosis
  and hysteria, 22
  clinical applications, 298–304
  comparison with other induction procedures, 84–5
  differentiation between ES and PNES, 83–4
  exploratory and expressive approaches, 302–4
  history of uses, 82–3
  induction procedure in PNES diagnosis, 83–4
  parallels with PNES phenomena, 297–8
  pathophysiology of the hypnotic state, 83
  physiological basis, 83
  preparing the patient, 298–300
  susceptibility for hypnosis, 297
  therapeutic aspects in PNES, 85
  use in PNES diagnosis, 42
  use in posttraumatic hysteria, 20
  use of self-control procedures, 300–2
Hypnotic Induction Profile (HIP), 83
hypnotizability
  and psychopathology, 83
  trait hypothesis, 83
hypocalcemia, 72
hypochondriasis, 27
hypoglycemia, 72
  in elderly people, 115
hypokalemic periodic paralyses, 68

Index

hysteria. *See* history of hysteria
hysteria libidinosa, 18
hysteria major, 20
hysterical neurosis, 11
hysterical pseudoseizures, 3
hystero-epilepsy, 3, 19

ICD (International Classification of Diseases)
 classification of PNES, 11
illusions or hallucinations, 71
incidence of PNES, 4
India
 perceptions about PNES in children, 189
Indian culture and PNES, 126–8
 clinical phenomenology, 126
 comorbidity, 127–8
 epidemiology, 126
 precipitating factors, 127
 psychopathogenesis, 126–7
 variability of clinical course, 127–8
induction of PNES
 comparison of techniques, 84–5
 use of hypnosis, 83–4
induction of seizures
 diagnosis of PNES, 42
infantile masturbation, 100
inpatient treatment for PNES, 309–10
insomnias, 77
intermittent explosive disorder, 71, 204
 in children, 102
intracranial monitoring, 44
ion channel disorders, 69
irritable bowel syndrome, 27, 28, 217
ischemic cardiomyopathy, 64
ischemic events
 in elderly people, 114
ischemic heart disease, 65

Jackson, Hughlings, 18, 19
jactatio capitis, 46
jactatio capitis nocturna, 71, 100
Janet, Pierre, 21, 82, 83, 297
Jorden, Edward, 17
Jumping Frenchmen of Maine, 70
juvenile myoclonic epilepsy, 102

Lange-Neilson syndrome, 65
Latah from Indonesia, 70
Laycock, Thomas, 18–19
learning difficulties
 children with PNES, 179–80
learning theory models for PNES treatment, 269–70
left atrial myxoma, 64
legal implications of PNES
 causation of PNES, 159–60
 comparison with epilepsy, 157, 160
 confidentiality, 158–9
 disability, 159
 discrimination, 159
 driving, 157–8
 privacy, 158–9
Letter Memory Test, 137
linguistic analysis
 Conversation Analysis, 85–6
 metaphoric conceptualizations of seizures, 87
 seizure labels, 87–8
 therapeutic potential, 88
 use in diagnosis of PNES, 85–8
long QT syndromes, 64, 65
Lyme disease, 39

malingering, 28, 203–4
 definition, 190
mass hysteria outbreaks, 17
McMaster Clinical Rating Scale (MCRS), 318
McMaster Model of Family Functioning (MMFF), 317–18
McMaster Structured Interview of Family Functioning (McSiff), 318–19
medically unexplained symptoms (MUS)
 burden of healthcare costs, 28
 connection with PNES, 27–8
 conversion symptoms in PNES patients, 29
 costs associated with, 28
 in patients with PNES, 29
 level of occurrence in neurology practice, 28–9
 pain disorders in PNES patients, 29
 prevalence, 27–8
 research implications for PNES, 32–4

memory dysfunction in PNES patients
 brain structures involved, 145–6
Ménière's disease, 70
Mesmer, Franz Anton, 82
metaphoric conceptualizations of seizures, 87
migraine, 3, 46
 differentiation from epilepsy, 70
 in children and adolescents, 103–4
 in the elderly, 111
migrainous phenomena
 differentiation from PNES, 9
mitral stenosis, 65
MMPI (Minnesota Multiphasic Personality Inventory), 7, 57
MMPI/MMPI-2 (Minnesota Multiphasic Personality Inventory-2), 138–9
models for treatment. *See* etiological models for treatment
mood disorders
 comorbidity in PNES, 226–7
motor neuron disorders, 69
movement disorders
 in elderly people, 115
multidisciplinary approach to PNES patient care, 253–4
multidisciplinary approach to treatment of PNES, 264
multidisciplinary model of PNS care, 254–8
multiple chemical sensitivities, 27
multiple sclerosis, 43, 69
multisomatoform disorder, 27
Munchausen by proxy syndrome, 102–3
Munchausen syndrome
 consequences and costs, 191
 definition of factitious disorder, 28, 190
 impacts on the patient–doctor relationship, 190–1
 issues of special concern, 192–3
 literature review, 191
 neurological history and examination, 191–2
 origin of the term, 190
 professional vignette, 193–4
 prognosis, 190–1
 psychiatric consultation, 192
 psychiatric treatment, 193

Index

Munchausen syndrome (cont.)
  suicide risk, 192
  suspicion of deceit, 191–2
  variant of factitious disorder, 190
myalgic encephalomyelitis, 27
Myers, Frederick, 82
myoclonic jerks
  during a syncopal episode, 66
myoclonus, 68
Myriachit from Siberia, 70

narcolepsy, 46, 67–8, 77
  in children and adolescents, 105
NEO-PI-R personality measure, 7
neurally mediated hypotension, 64
neurocardiogenic syncope, 64
neurological disease
  comorbidity with PNES, 43
neurologist
  role in treatment of PNES, 260, 261–3
neuropsychological testing, 136
  cognitive and affective aspects in PNES, 144–5
  effort testing, 137–8
  inability to differentiate ES and PNES, 138
  similarity of results in ES and PNES patients, 136–8
  test-taking motivation in PNES, 137–8
neurosis
  early use of the term, 20
night terrors, 45, 72, 103
nightmares, 72
  in children, 103
nocturnal epileptic seizures
  differential diagnosis, 79–80
nocturnal hypnogenic paroxysmal dyskinesia, 69
nocturnal panic attacks, 78
nocturnal paroxysmal dystonia, 46
nocturnal sleep-related eating disorder, 78
nonepileptic attack disorder, 3
nonepileptic myoclonus, 9, 46
nonepileptic nonpsychogenic episodes.
  See physiological nonepileptic events

nonepileptic physiologic events, 45–6
non-REM parasomnias, 72, 77–8
nonstate dependent parasomnias, 78
nurse
  role in care of patients with PNES, 255–6

obsessive compulsive disorder, 102
obstructive sleep apnea, 72
  in the elderly, 111
Oedipus complex, 22, 23
operant conditioning model for treatment, 270
opsoclonus in children, 100
"organic" psychosyndrome model, 273–4
orthostatic syncope, 64–5

pain disorders, 27
  in PNES patients, 29
panic attacks, 46, 71, 203
  in children, 104
  nocturnal, 78
parasomnias, 9, 38, 44, 45–6, 71, 77–8
  non-REM parasomnias, 72, 77–8
  REM parasomnias, 72, 78
parents
  perceptions about PNES in children, 187–9
Parkinson's disease, 111, 114, 115
paroxysmal dyskinesias, 69
  in children, 98–9
paroxysmal dystonias, 46
paroxysmal dystonic choreoathetosis, 69
paroxysmal events in children, 93–105
  acute life-threatening event (ALTE), 94–7
  adolescents, 103–5
  alternating hemiplegia of childhood, 101
  apnea (neonatal and infantile), 94–7
  approaches to classification, 93–4
  benign myoclonus of infancy, 99–100
  benign neonatal sleep myoclonus, 97
  benign nonepileptic infantile spasms, 99–100
  benign paroxysmal torticollis of infancy, 99

benign paroxysmal vertigo, 98
breath-holding spells, 98
cataplexy, 105
conversion disorder, 105
daydreaming, 101
dyskinesias, 101–2
episodic ataxia, 102
episodic dyscontrol, 102
hereditary hyperekplexia, 97
hyperekplexia, 97
hyperkinetic movement disorders, 101–2
hyperventilation, 101
hypnagogic hallucinations, 105
infancy (2 months to 2 years), 98–101
infantile masturbation, 100
intermittent explosive disorder, 102
jitteriness (infants), 97
migraine, 103–4
Munchausen by proxy syndrome, 102–3
narcolepsy, 105
neonatal period (birth to 8 weeks), 94–7
nightmares, 103
opsoclonus, 100
paroxysmal dyskinesia, 98–9
paroxysmal tonic upward gaze, 97
pavor nocturnus (night terrors), 103
PNES in children and adolescents, 104
psychiatric disorders, 104–5
rage attacks, 102
rhythmic movement disorder of sleep, 100–1
rumination, 99
Sandifer syndrome, 99
shuddering attacks in infants, 98
sleep attacks, 105
sleep paralysis, 105
somnambulism (sleepwalking), 103
spasmus nutans, 100
staring spells, 101
startle response (neonates), 97
stereotypies, 100
stool withholding activity, 101
syncope in children and adolescents, 104
tics, 102
paroxysmal hypnogenic dyskinesias
  in children, 102
paroxysmal kinesiogenic dyskinesia, 69
paroxysmal kinesiogenic dyskinesia
  in children, 102
paroxysmal limb movements of sleep, 46

Index

paroxysmal movement disorders
  differential diagnosis, 46
paroxysmal nonkinesiogenic dyskinesia
  in children, 102
paroxysmal tonic upward gaze (infants), 97
pavor nocturnus, 103
pediatric PNES (PPNES). *See* children with PNES
peer relationship problems
  children with PNES, 180
perceptions about PNES in children and adolescents, 187–9
periodic limb movement disorder, 78
periodic limb movements in sleep, 72
Personality Assessment Inventory (PAI), 139
personality disorders
  comorbidity with PNES, 12, 227–31
personality profiles of PNES patients, 7
personality testing and PNES, 138–40
phantom limb pain, 71
pharmacological treatments for PNES
  AED use in patients with mixed ES/PNES, 309
  AED use in PNES, 308–9
  analgesics, 307, 312
  antidepressants, 307
  anxiolytics, 307
  assessment and treatment recommendations, 312–13
  barbiturates, 310
  benzodiazepines, 310
  bromides, 310
  dopamine hypothesis, 312
  historical approaches, 310
  NMDA antagonists, 312
  propranolol, 307, 312
  role in combination with other therapies, 307–8
  serotonin hypothesis, 311
  sodium amytal, 310
  SSRIs, 311–12
  treatment strategies, 308
  University of Memphis approach, 312
pheochromocytoma, 72

physical abuse
  association with PNES, 213–14
physiological nonepileptic seizures
  definition, 3
physiological nonepileptic events, 45–6
PNES. *See* psychogenic nonepileptic seizures
Portland Digit Recognition Test, 137
positron emission tomography (PET)
  physiology of hypnosis and hysteria, 83
posttraumatic hysteria, 19
  use of hypnotism, 20
posttraumatic stress disorder (PTSD), 82, 111, 134
  association with PNES, 215
  comorbidity with PNES, 11
  indirect association with PNES, 215–17
  link with PNES, 12
  role in PNES etiology, 217–19
postural orthostatic tachycardia syndrome (POTS), 64–5
postural syncope, 64
presyncope, 64
prevalence of PNES, 4–5
privacy
  legal implications of PNES, 158–9
Problem Centered Systems Therapy of the Family (PCSTF), 319–20
progressive encephalomyelitis with rigidity and tetanus, 70
prolactin levels
  patients with comorbid ES and PNES, 58
  postictal testing, 44–5
prolonged confusional or fugue states, 72–3
propranolol, 307, 312
propriospinal myoclonus, 77
provocative techniques
  diagnosis of PNES, 42
pseudoepileptic seizures, 3
pseudoparasomnias, 79
pseudoseizures, 3
"pseudosleep"
  clinical features of PNES during, 79
pseudostatus and status epilepticus, 56

psychiatric assessment of PNES patients, 310
psychiatric disorders
  in children and adolescents, 104–5
psychiatric disorders in PNES
  borderline personality disorder, 228–31
  comorbid anxiety disorders, 226–7
  comorbid mood disorders, 226–7
  comorbid personality disorders, 227–31
  heterogeneity and complexity, 232
  impact on outcome after PNES diagnosis, 231–2
  primary psychiatric disorders, 225
psychiatric features of pediatric PNES
  clinical vignettes, 171–4
  comorbid psychiatric diagnoses, 165–6
  diagnosis, 166–9
  diagnostic feedback to parents and child, 169–71
  models of pediatric PNES, 163–5
  primary diagnosis of pediatric PNES, 165
  risk factors, 163
  treatment goals, 174–6
psychiatric taxonomies
  classification of PNES, 9–13
psychiatrist
  role in treatment of PNES, 260, 263
psychic experiences
  causes, 71
psychoanalysis, 21, 22
psychodynamic approach to PNES treatment, 266–9
psychogenic movement disorders, 44
psychogenic nonepileptic seizures (PNES)
  alternative terminology, 3
  definitions, 3
  differentiation from ES, 3
psychogenic seizures, 3
psychological mechanism of PNES, 8
psychological support. *See* care of patients with PNES
psychoneurosis, 22
psychosomatic/psychophysiological models for PNES treatment, 273
PTSD. *See* posttraumatic stress disorder

343

Index

Puerto Rican culture and PNES, 124–6
  childhood trauma, 124–5
  clinical phenomenology of *ataque de nervios*, 124
  comorbidity, 125–6
  cultural predisposition to dissociation, 125
  epidemiology of *ataque de nervios*, 124
  gender roles, 125
  precipitating factors for *ataque de nervios*, 125
  psychopathogenesis, 124–5
  relationship between *ataque* and dissociation, 125
  variability of clinical course, 125–6

quality of life. *See* Health Related Quality of Life
Quality of Life in Epilepsy Inventory-89 (QOLIE-89), 143, 150

rage attacks, 204
  in children, 102
reflex epilepsies, 71
reflex hypotension, 64
reflex startle epilepsy, 70
reflex syncope, 64
rehabilitation therapist
  role in treatment of PNES, 264
REM parasomnias, 72, 78
REM sleep behavior disorder, 45, 46, 72, 78, 115
REM sleep-associated parasomnias
  in the elderly, 111
repression, 267
repression in PNES patients
  brain structures involved, 145–6
research on PNES
  funding support, 32–4
restless legs syndrome, 46, 71
  in the elderly, 115
Rett's syndrome, 100
Rey Auditory Verbal Learning Test, 145
rhythmic movement disorder of sleep
  in children, 100–1
rhythmic movement disorders, 46, 71, 79

rhythmie du sommeil, 100
right ventricular dysplasia, 64, 65
Riley Day syndrome, 98
Romano-Ward syndrome, 65
rumination in children, 99

saline injection (IV)
  use in PNES diagnosis, 42
Sandifer syndrome, 99
scalp EEG, 44
seizure labels, 87–8
semiological classification of nonepileptic seizures, 202
semiology of PNES
  clinical types, 79
sensory starts, 77
sertraline, 311
sexual abuse
  association with PNES, 213–14
  children with PNES, 179
shell shock, 23
Shorter, Edward, 24
Showalter, Elaine, 24
shuddering attacks
  in infants, 98
  in young children, 46
situational syncope, 64
sleep
  occurrence of PNES events, 77
sleep apnea, 72
  in the elderly, 115
sleep arousal disorders, 72
sleep attacks, 105
sleep disorders, 3, 45–6
  episodic phenomena in sleep, 71–2
  in elderly people, 115
  major categories, 77
  See also narcolepsy; parasomnias.
sleep events
  differential diagnosis, 80
  nocturnal epileptic seizures, 79–80
sleep paralysis, 72, 77, 105
sleep-related breathing disorders, 77

sleep-related movement disorders, 77, 78–9
sleep terrors, 78
sleep transition parasomnias, 77
sleepwalking, 45, 72, 78
  in children, 103
social worker
  role in care of patients with PNES, 256–7
  role in treatment of PNES, 264
socio-historical studies of hysteria, 24
somatization
  role in PNES, 10–11
somatization disorder, 24, 27
somatoform disorders
  comorbidity with PNES, 11
  presence of medically unexplained symptoms, 27
somatoform pain disorder, 216
somnambulism, 45, 72, 78
  in children, 103
somniloquy, 45
spasmus nutans in children, 100
St Vitus' dance, 17
Stanford Hypnotic Susceptibility Scale Form C, 83
staring spells in children, 101
startle epilepsy, 69, 70
startle syndromes, 69–70
stereotypies in children, 100
stiff-person syndrome, 70
stool withholding activity in children, 101
stress
  as trigger for seizures, 23–4
stress model for PNES treatment, 270–3
stress seizures, 3
stressors
  link with PNES in children, 179–80
stroke, 43, 111
  in children, 105
subconscious ideas
  role in hysteria, 21
subgroups in PNES, 275–6

Index

sudden unexpected death in epilepsy (SUDEP), 66
suggestibility and hysteria, 21
sulpiride, 312
supraventricular tachycardia, 64, 65
swallowing syncope, 65
Sydenham, Thomas, 18
syncope, 38, 44, 45, 62–7
   cardiogenic, 64, 65–6
   causes, 64–6
   definition, 63–4
   diagnosis, 66–7
   differential diagnosis, 45
   differentiation from PNES, 9
   in children and adolescents, 104
   in the elderly, 111, 114
   incidence, 64
   presence of myoclonic jerks, 66
   prevalence, 64
   prognosis and treatment, 67
   recurrence, 64
   structural heart disease, 65–6
   transient loss of awareness, 62–3
   vascular causes, 64–5
   vasovagal syncope, 64

tachyarrhythmias, 65
Tarantism, 17
terminology relating to nonepileptic seizures, 199–200
Test of Memory Malingering, 137
tetralogy of Fallot, 104
TIAs. See transient ischemic attacks
tics, 69
   in children, 102
"torsade de pointes", 65
torticollis in children, 99
Tourette, Gilles de la, 82
Tourette's syndrome, 102
transient epileptic amnesia, 73
transient focal hypermotor episodes, 68–70
transient focal sensory attacks, 70–1
transient global amnesia, 46, 72–3
   in adolescents, 105
transient global cerebral hypoperfusion. See syncope

transient ischemic attacks (TIAs), 46, 70
   differentiation from PNES, 9
   in children, 105
   in the elderly, 111, 114
transient ischemic events, 73
   differentiation from PNES, 9
transient loss of awareness, 62–3
   See also syncope.
transient retrograde amnesia, 62
trans-theoretical model of intentional human behavior change, 193
trauma
   and dissociation, 82–3
   causal role in hysteria, 22
   effects on the central nervous system, 82
   indirect association with PNES, 215–17
   role in PNES etiology, 217–19
trauma/abuse
   association with PNES, 213–15
treatment of PNES
   clinical psychologist's role, 263–4
   first goal of treatment, 260–1
   historical approaches, 237–43
   issues relating to who should treat, 260
   need for a multidisciplinary approach, 264
   neurologist's role, 260, 261–3
   neuropsychologist's role, 263–4
   psychiatrist's role, 260
   psychiatrist's role, 263
   rehabilitation therapist's role, 264
   role of mental health professionals, 260, 263–4
   social worker's role, 264
   See also specific therapies
treatment plans
   classical conditioning model, 269–70
   family systems model, 269
   individually adapted strategies, 277
   learning theory models, 269–70
   operant conditioning model, 270
   "organic" psychosyndrome model, 273–4
   psychodynamic approach, 266–9
   psychosomatic/psychophysiological models, 273
   stress model, 270–3
   subgroups in PNES, 275–6
   towards a unified model for PNES, 274–5

tremor, 68
   See also shuddering attacks in young children.
tremors
   in children, 102
Trousseau's sign, 101
Turkish culture and PNES, 122–4
   alexithymia, 123
   childhood trauma and dissociation, 122–3
   clinical phenomenology, 122
   comorbidity, 123–4
   complaisant overadjustment, 122
   difficulty in self-perception and self-expression, 123
   disadvantageous effects of exaggerated gender roles, 123
   epidemiology, 122
   family dynamics, 122
   insecure attachment, 122–3
   precipitating factors, 123
   psychopathogenesis, 122–3
   psychosocial stress factors, 123
   special role in the family, 122
   variability in clinical course, 123–4

unconscious conflicts
   role in hysteria, 22
undifferentiated somatoform disorder, 27

vascular causes of syncope, 64–5
vasodepressor hypotension, 64
vasovagal hypotension, 64
ventricular fibrillation, 64
ventricular tachycardia, 64, 65
vertebrobasilar ischemia, 68
vertigo, 70–1
video-EEG (VEEG) monitoring
   analysis of ictal semiology, 40–2
   comorbid ES and PNES, 57–8
   diagnosis of epilepsy, 23
   diagnosis of PNES, 3–4
   diagnostic use in the elderly, 110, 112, 116
   limitations and pitfalls, 43–4
   role in diagnosis of PNES, 38, 39–42
   role in PNES diagnosis, 8–9
   short-term outpatient VEEG with activation, 42
   use of hypnosis to induce PNES, 83–4
   use of provocative techniques, 42
vocal outbursts, 71

Index

wandering womb concept of hysteria, 17, 190
war-related neuroses, 23–4
war-related trauma, 83
Whytt, Robert, 18
Willis, Thomas, 18
Wolff-Parkinson-White syndrome, 65

women and PNES
  epidemiology, 132–3
  gender difference in medical disorders, 131
  gender differences in PNES, 131
  gender-related difference in symptomatology, 134
  gender-related differences in prognosis, 134
  historical views of women and hysteria, 131–2
  nature of the relationship, 134
  role of age, 132–3
  sexual trauma and PNES, 133–4
  subtypes of PNES and gender, 133

Word Memory Test (WMT), 137